CANCER STEM CELLS THEORIES AND PRACTICE

Edited by **Stanley Shostak**

Cancer Stem Cells Theories and Practice
Edited by Stanley Shostak

Published by InTech
Janeza Trdine 9, 51000 Rijeka, Croatia

Publishing Process Manager Ana Nikolic

Technical Editor Teodora Smiljanic

Cover Designer InTech Design Team

Additional hard copies can be obtained from orders@intechopen.com

Cancer Stem Cells Theories and Practice, Edited by Stanley Shostak
p. cm.
ISBN 978-953-307-225-8

For EU product safety concerns:
IN TECH d.o.o., Prolaz Marije Krucifikse Kozulić 3, 51000 Rijeka, Croatia,
info@intechopen.com or visit our website at intechopen.com.

Meet the editor

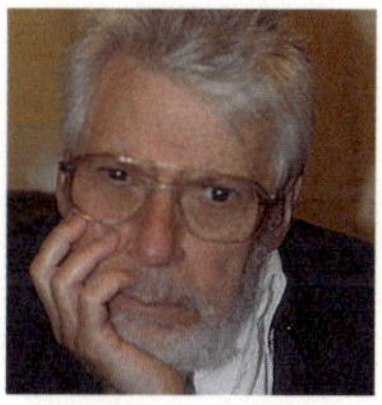

For fifty years, I have studied the evolution of growth's integration with form. Hydras' ability to move excess cells into buds was my model for cancer's ability to support metastasis (e.g., Vegetative reproduction by budding in Hydra: A perspective on tumors. Perspectives in Biology and Medicine, 20:545–68; 1977; "Hydra and cancer: Immortality and budding," pp. 275-86 in C.J. Dawe, J.C. Harshbarger, S. Kondo, T. Sugimura, and S. Takayama, eds., Phyletic Approaches to Cancer. Tokyo: Sci. Soc. 1981). I have concentrated on the origins of stem cells (Symbiogenetic origins of cnidarian cnidocysts. Symbiosis, 19:1–29; 1995 [with V. Kolluri]; "Speculation on the Evolution of Stem Cells," Breast Disease, 29:3–13; 2007–8) and have developed my ideas further in books (Evolution of Death: Why We Are Living Longer. Albany: SUNY Press; 2006; Becoming Immortal: Combining Cloning and Stem-Cell Therapy. Albany: SUNY Press; 2002; Evolution of Sameness and Difference: Perspectives on the Human Genome Project. Amsterdam: Harwood Academic Publishers, 1999; Death of Life: The Legacy of Molecular Biology. London: Macmillan, 1998).

Contents

Preface

Cancer Stem Cells Theories and Practice does *not* "boldly go where no one has gone before!" Rather, *Cancer Stem Cells Theories and Practice* boldly goes where the cutting edge of research theory meets the concrete challenges of clinical practice. *Cancer Stem Cells Theories and Practice* is firmly grounded in the latest results on cancer stem cells (CSCs) from world-class cancer research laboratories, but its twenty-two chapters also tease apart cancer's vulnerabilities and identify opportunities for early detection, targeted therapy, and reducing remission and resistance.

The chapters reflect the current diversity of research on CSCs and are distributed among six parts that inevitably overlap rather than isolate cubbyholes of research. Part I examines CSC models, from questions about what stem cells are and where they come from to issues of plasticity and reprogramming. Part II takes a close look at the CSCs in particular cancers. Part III examines issues surrounding CSC niches and their neovascularization. Part IV concentrates on signaling pathways, cross talk, and regulatory mechanisms in CSCs. Part V looks at possibilities offered by CSCs for improving diagnosis, therapeutics, and prognosis. And Part VI confronts CSCs' role in resistance.

Part I: Cancer Stem Cell Models

Chapter 1

"The Dark Side of Cellular Plasticity: Stem Cells in Development and Cancer," by Fernando Abollo-Jimenez et al., makes a subtle and often overlooked observation: "it is the case in tumors … [that] cellular identity is reprogrammed by oncogenic alterations to give rise to a new pathological lineage. This aberrant deviation of the normal developmental program is only possible if the initial cell suffering the oncogenic insults posses[s] enough plasticity so as to be reprogrammed by them."

The authors provide a brief lexicon of developmental terms before coming to the crucial contrast: "the genetic potential of cells did not diminish during differentiation, and … there were no genetic changes occurring during development," while "for many types of tumors, specific mutations have been described to be tightly associated to the tumor phenotype, especially in the case of mesenchymal tumors caused by chromosomal aberrations."

The authors use B-cell differentiation as an example of plasticity from committed undifferentiated stem cells. Until relieved, Pax-mediated repression keeps cells from downstream terminal differentiation. Reprogramming in tumorigenesis is "wrong" reprogramming.

The "cancer cell-of-origin would therefore be a normal cell that has undergone reprogramming by the oncogenic events to give rise to a CSC, a new pathological cell with stem cell properties." The cancer cell-of-origin's "loss of the [initial] identity ... is an essential step in tumorigenesis." The loss lowers the stem cell's resistance to change, which would be higher in a differentiated cell than in an undifferentiated cell, and increases plasticity resulting in the cell's acquiring the tumor phenotype. Were the cell not a stem-cell to begin with, it would have to acquire stem-cell properties such as self-renewal, but if it were already a stem cell, it would bring its qualities along with it to the cancer state.

Hence, "the initiating lesion would have an active function in the reprogramming process, but afterwards it would become just a passenger mutation." Thus, "cancer does not only depend on genetic mutations, but also on epigenetic changes that establish a new pattern of heritability, providing a cellular memory by which the new tumoral cellular identity can be maintained."

The hope is that "differentiation therapies" will force the terminal loss of cancer cells. In the meantime, "epigenetic therapies are already in use or in very advanced clinical trials against cancer ... restor[ing] the normal levels of expression of genes that are required for the normal control of cellular proliferation and/or differentiation."

Chapter 2

Stéphane Ansieau, Anne-Pierre Morel, and Alain Puisieux's chapter, "From where do Cancer Initiating Cells Originate?" takes a close look at "several of the experimental assays commonly used to evaluate stem-like properties" and finds them wanting. In particular, the authors conclude that the "potential filiation between normal stem-cells and CSCs ... remains a matter of discussion."

"A significant example [of inconsistency] is provided by the contradictory results generated by using the transmembrane protein CD133 as a stem-cell marker." Cells with high expression levels of stem cell transporters and cells carrying the marker for "CSC populations do not always match." Indeed, hardly "any of these markers are strictly allotted to stem-cells." The same criticism also applies to methods of xenografting, "challenging the concept that tumours arise from rare CSCs." Finally, the authors conclude that, "the stem-like properties harboured by numerous cancer cells do not rely on any particular relationship to normal stem-cells but rather reflect the Darwinian selection that operate[s] within a tumor." But all is not lost. Alternatively, novel transgenic mouse models on the horizon may obviate these problems.

Chapter 3

Linda Li, Laura Borodyansky, and Youxin Yang look for "Connections between Genomic Instability and Cancer Stem Cells." The text is sharply focused as they ponder, "What causes the transformation from normal stem cells to cancer stem cells?" The authors suggest that "cancer stemloid (or stem cell-like cancer cells)" might be more precise than CSCs when referring to cells "exist[ing] only as a minority within the cancer cell population ... [and] contribut[ing] to tumor growth, metastasis, and resistance to therapy."

Genomic instability (GIN) "could be a potential driving force in the transformation of normal stem cells into cancer stem cells," but it might also be a consequence of long-term culture in vitro and not an intrinsic characteristic of stem cells. On the other hand, "After a long term culture of human adult non-tumorigenic neural stem cells, ... [cells with] a high level of genomic instability [emerged] and a spontaneously immortalized clone ... developed into a cell line with features of cancer stem cells."

All told, data suggest that, CSCs "may present a relatively less heterogeneous cell population for targeting than their progeny." On the other hand, CSCs "may be derived from clonal selection for resistance to growth limiting conditions imposed by mutagens or carcinogens"?

Chapter 4

The chapter, "Cancer Stem Cells as a Result of a Reprogramming-Like Mechanism," by Carolina Vicent-Dueñas et al. asks more questions than it answers, but its questions are crucial: "[W]hat are the mechanisms of tumor relapse by which tumors evolve to escape oncogene dependence?" Is "the maintenance of oncogene expression ... critical for the generation of differentiated tumor cells"? Are "the oncogenes that initiate tumor formation ... dispensable for tumor progression and/or maintenance"?

The authors seek answers mainly by tracing CSCs in chronic myeloid leukemia (CML). CML is a CSC disease typically traced to rare, malignant hematopoietic stem cells (HSCs). But could "the combination of the reprogramming capabilities of the oncogenic alteration and the [cell's] intrinsic plasticity [i.e., susceptibility to reprogramming] determine the final outcome of a CSC"?

Answers rely on "[r]ecent breakthroughs [that] have shown that reprogramming of differentiated cells can be achieved by the transient expression of a limited number of transcription factors that can 'reset' the epigenetic status of the cells and allow them to adopt a new plethora of possible [cancerous] fates." Since "the absence of the tumor suppressor does not have an instructive role in tumorigenesis but just a permissive one ... the driving force[s] of the reprogramming process are the reprogramming factors themselves." Is it possible that "the oncogenes that initiate tumor formation might be dispensable for tumor progression"? Are these "hands-off regulation mechanisms ... found in other cancer types"? Is cancer "a reprogramming-like disease"?

Part II: Stem Cells in Specific tumors

Chapter 5

"Breast Cancer Stem Cells" by Marco Velasco-Velázquez, Xuanmao Jiao, and Richard Pestell takes a sober and sobering look at "the potential role of cancer stem cells (CSCs) in the initiation, maintenance, and clinical outcome of breast cancers." The loss of tumorigenicity following serial propagation of cells of mammospheres shows that "only a subgroup within the CD44+/CD24$^{-/low}$ cells are self-renewing." Subsequently, increased tumorigenicity was found among cells with "the CD44+/CD24-/ALDH+ phenotype ...

in comparision with CD44+/CD24- or ALDH+ cells." Likewise, PKH26 proved a reliable marker for rare CSCs. But did "these cells with different immunophenotypes represent different breast CSCs?

The authors suggest that the "CD44+/CD24- population most likely represent basal breast CSCs and cells with the $CD24^{hi}CD29^{low}$ signature most likely originate from the mammary luminal progenitor cells." In addition, "CSCs isolated from cancer cell lines exhibited increased invasiveness and elevated expression of genes involved in invasion (IL-1α, IL-6, IL-8, CXCR4, MMP-1, and UPA), … [while] ALDH+ cells isolated from breast cancer cell lines were more migratory and invasive than the ALDH- cells."

The role of CSC in resistance to chemotherapy was dramatically demonstrated when mammosphere formation was found to be enriched 14-fold and the proportion of $CD44+/CD24^{-}/^{low}$ cells increased approximately 10-fold in tumor cells from patients after neoadjuvant chemotherapy. Mouse models followed the same pattern.

In general, "molecular signals that promote 'stemness' in cancer cells also promote the acquisition of metastatic ability." Indeed, "a single cellular proto-oncogene is necessary to both activate signaling pathways that promote features of CSC and maintain the invasive phenotype of mammary tumors." Overall, a variety of strategies are now on the table for eradicating breast CSCs from antagonists and inhibitors, blocking antibodies, radioligands, and siRNAs. In addition, specific promoters of oncolytic virus are targeted on ABC transporters, membrane markers, intracellular signaling molecules, onco-specific metabolites, and the micro- and global environments.

Chapter 6

Candace Gilbert and Alonzo Ross tell another "dismal" tale of low expected survival in their chapter, "Glioma Stem Cells: Cell Culture, Markers and Targets for New Combination Therapies." Hope for finding the glioma stem cell rose in the mid-20th century when the discovery of neural stem cells in the subventricular zone and dentate gyrus shattered the dogma that the adult brain contained no mitotic figures. But it "is currently unknown what is the cell of origin for glioma stem cells," and raising glioma cells in vitro is problematic.

"Gene expression in serum cultures can be drastically different from the original tumor … [while] glioma neurosphere cultures [in serum-free media supplemented with growth factors] maintain genetic profiles similar to the original patients' tumors and form invasive tumors in intracranial xenografts." When cultured on laminin-coated plates in serum-free, defined medium glioma cells "grow as an adherent culture … [in which] almost all of the cells express glioma stem cell genes, such as Sox2, Nestin, CD133 and CD44 … [but all the cells] are capable of tumor formation … [when] intracranially injected into immunocompromised mice." Inasmuch as the "gold standard to classify a cell as a glioma stem cell is that it can form a xenograft tumor capable of serial transplantations in immunodeficient mice," these results demonstrate a high percentage of tumor-initiating glioma stem cells, and suggest "that CD133 is not a universal stem cell marker for all gliomas."

Glioma is notoriously resistant to treatment. "Glioma stem cells disrupt tumor immunosurveillance and result in both ineffective adaptive and innate immune responses."

Furthermore, "[g]lioma stem cells express a variety of proteins that promote survival following cancer treatment, ... and anti-apoptotic genes ... [are] upgraded ... [indicating] that CD133+ glioma stem cells['] resistance to radiotherapy is partially due to enhanced DNA repair."

Chapter 7

Koji Okudela et al. devote their chapter, "Cancer Stem Cells in Lung Cancer: Distinct Differences between Small Cell and Non-Small Cell Lung Carcinomas," to demonstrating differences in biological properties and in abundance of CSC in small cell lung carcinoma (SCLC) and non-small cell lung carcinoma (NSCLC). The authors review recent results with a variety of markers, transcription factors, and intermediates in signaling pathways (e.g., Sonic hedgehog, Wnt/β-catenin) before concentrating on aldehyde dehydrogenase (ALDH), "a marker for stem cells in a variety of cancers."

Initially, "overall findings revealed low levels of ALDH activity in SCLC cell lines, while higher levels were detected in some, but not all, NSCLC cell lines." But results of screening several SCLC and NSCLC cell lines with quantitative reverse transcription polymerase chain reaction (RT-PCR) for the mRNAs of three ALDH and Western blotting for ALDH protein yielded contradictory results. But the results of immunohistochemistry with non-selective antibody showed "significantly higher levels [of ALDH] in NSCLC than in SCLC."

Ultimately, the issue seems to be settled by the high concentration of CSC in a samples demonstrated by levels of CD133 mRNA which "could be one [of the] causes of [the] highly malignant activity of SCLC." At the same time, "there is considerable heterogeneity in the mechanism maintaining the stemness of CSCs of SCLCs and NSCLCs."

Chapter 8

Galina Botchkina and Iwao Ojima's chapter, "Prostate and Colon Cancer Stem Cells as a Target for Anti-Cancer Drug Development" removes most doubts that prostate and colon cancer are stem-cell cancers, possessing "a minor subpopulation of stem cells and a major (or bulk) mass of progenitors at different stages of their maturation." This functionally, genomically and morphologically distinct subpopulation "possess[es] exclusive tumor-initiating capacity in vivo ... [and is, therefore] likely to be the most crucial target in the treatment of cancer." Of potential clinical importance, a new generation of taxoid, SB-T-1214, is effective against advanced colon cancer and prostate cancer spheroids in vitro by inhibiting the expression of stem cell-related genes.

Part III: Niches and Vascularization

Chapter 9

Farrokh Asadi, Gwendal Lazennec, and Christian Jorgensen ask why prostate cancer is recalcitrant to treatment in the "Importance of Stromal Stem Cells in Prostate Carcinogenesis Process." The chapter begins with a tour of prostate anatomy and an account of the ambiguity surrounding the sources of prostate stem cells. Evidence suggests, "that prostate cancer may arise from ... immature cell types located within the basal or luminal cell layer ... [i.e.,] from stem or progenitor cells rather than from a terminally differentiated cell type." Moreover, "basal cells from primary benign human prostate tissue can initiate prostate cancer in immunodeficient mice." Consequently, "histological characterization of cancers does not necessarily correlate with the cellular origins of the disease." Moreover, the "prostate tumors may contain a small population of androgen-insensitive cells that survive [androgen ablation therapy] and can expand in the absent of androgen … Since normal adult prostate stem cells (PSCs) are androgen-insensitive, it is reasonable to suspect they may be the source of these cells." What is more, "[c]ommon anticancer treatments such as radiation and chemotherapy do not eradicate the majority of cancer stem cells." And making matters worse, "the tumor suppressor gene PTEN, polycomb gene *Bmi1* and the signal transduction pathways such as the Sonic Hedgehog (Shh), Notch and Wnt that are crucial for normal stem cell regulation, have been shown to be deregulated in the process of carcinogenesis."

Chapter 10

In "Cancer Stem Cells and Their Niche," Guadalupe Aparicia Gallego et al. scrutinize CSCs' "metastatic cascade" between "tumor cell intravasation, transport and immune evasion within the circulatory systems, arrest [at] a secondary site, extravasations and finally colonization and growth" in their new home. The chapter begins by classifying and surveying niches before going on to discuss what can go wrong in niches apropos of CSCs: "disruption of cell cycle inhibition may contribute to the formation of the so-called cancer stem cells (CSCs) that are currently hypothesized to be partially responsible for tumorigenesis and recurrence of cancer."

Niches for CSCs in solid tumors involve "intratumoral areas" more like zones than specific sites in an organ: "The inner, highly hypoxic/anoxic core, characterized by stem cells with low proliferation index, and intermediate, mildly hypoxic layer, lining the anoxic core, with immature and proliferating tumor precursor cells, and the peripheral, more predominantly committed/differentiated cells." In contrast to core cells, cells from the intermediate area form the largest spheroids in vitro and display a higher proliferation rate, while cells from peripheral areas are more differentiated and do not form spheroids. Niche-bound carcinoma-associated fibroblasts (CAFs), endothelial progenitor cells (EPCs), cytokines, and growth factors all play roles in preparing and maintaining metastatic sites.

Chapter 11

Maguer-Satta Véronique's chapter, "The Stem Cell Niche: The Black Master of Cancer" lives up to its title. As mythology portends, niches harboring CSCs have only evil consequences. Véronique begins with a model for the hematopoietic niche that "regulates the dormancy, survival and non-differentiation of hematopoietic stem cells [HSCs] … but also receives feedback from stem cells which actively contribute to the organization of their own niche." The adhesion of HSCs "to both matrix proteins and stromal cells and exposure to their soluble factors (cytokines, morphogens) controls the[ir] self-renewal and differentiation." In effect, the niche is "the guardian of key features of stem cells" such as asymmetric cell division, quiescence, plasticity or potency and fate, and niches also drive stem-cell transformations "inducing cancer stem cell escape, resistance, and persistence."

Crucial evidence for the role of the tumor microenvironment in tumor initiation and progression is the occurrence of leukemia "in normal donor hematopoietic cells transplanted to leukemia patients." The list of circulatory and solid cancers affected by their microenvironment includes myeloid or lymphoid leukemias, myeloma, chronic myelogenous leukemia, acute myeloid leukemia, and solid tumors, including breast cancer. "Altogether, these data indicate that most cancers are likely associated with modifications of the stem cell environment."

"Of particular interest in the context of cancer, niches have been demonstrated to be capable of reprogramming cells." It "is intriguing that factors deregulated in the cancer niche, such as hypoxia, have recently been reported to significantly improve the iPS [induced pluripotent stem cell] process." Véronique is "tempted" to suggest that, "one of the first steps in tumor initiation is the generation of cancer 'iPS' induced by alterations occurring in the niche, such as a change in rigidity, extracellular matrix remodeling or oxygen concentration." The author also makes a case for niches as "an important target in anti-cancer therapy," first by awakening quiescent cancer stem cells from dormancy and second by making them leave their protective niche! Certainly the time has come to stand up "against the strong wave of genetic promoters as the only explanation for the etiology of cancer, and … [proclaim] that 'mutations [a]re not all' in oncogenesis."

Chapter 12

Yi-fang Ping et al. "provide the evidence for the role of CSCs in tumor vascularization and discuss the potential therapeutic significance based on the interaction between CSCs and their vascular niches" in their chapter, "Cancer Stem Cells Promote Tumor Neovascularization." First of all, CSCs produce "high levels of proangiogenic factors … for instance VEGF [vascular endothelial growth factor] and interleukin 8." In addition, "[c]hemokines and their receptors are believed to be involved in CSCs-mediated production of angiogenic factors." Second, the authors find genetic abnormalities shared by endothelial cells (ECs) and cancer cells, suggesting "a link in their common origin." Do CSCs "generate or transdifferentiate into ECs"? Do "Tumor cells with high degree[s] of differentiation plasticity … contribute to the de novo formation of tumor cell-lined blood channels"? Conspicuously favoring positive answers, "angiogenesis inhibitors abrogate new vessels formed by human vascular endothelial cells in vitro, while under the same conditions did not affect tumor cell tuber network formation, and even induced the formation of VM [vascular mimicry] as an escape route by tumor tissue for progressive growth." But the most novel suggestion the authors bring to the field is that the "CSC compartment of a tumor may be involved in VM formation, by differentiating/transdifferentiating into endothelial-like cells. Such a potential function of CSCs might represent one of the mechanisms by which CSCs initiate neoplastic formation and promote tumor progression."

Part IV: Signaling Pathways and Regulatory Controls

Chapter 13

Noriko Gotoh makes an astonishing claim in "Possible Signaling Pathways Activated in Cancer Stem Cells in Breast Cancer," namely, that "inflammatory cytokines and chemokines are critical components for the maintenance of breast cancer stem cells." Specifically, cancer-associated fibroblasts (CAFs) secreting growth factors, cytokines, and chemokines "can induce inflammatory responses and angiogenesis by paracrine mechanisms ... [and t]umor cells appear to use these activities for tumor progression ... In this sense, TICs [tumor initiating cells; aka CSCs] may actively generate and maintain a microenvironment conducive to the progression of tumorigenesis, or in other words, a cancer stem cell niche."

The evidence is copious. "Activation of several pathways involved in inflammatory responses has recently been detected in breast cancer stem cells." Moreover, the nuclear factor NF-κB, activated in breast cancer stem-like cells "has roles in inflammation, angiogenesis, inhibition of apoptosis, and tumorigenesis." What is more, several "target genes of the NF-κB pathway, such as those encoding for proinflammatory cytokines and chemokines, have been identified as regulators of the breast cancer stem cell phenotype."

Most importantly, in "clinical trials, it was found that several anti-inflammatory drugs reduce tumor incidence when used as prophylactics and slow down tumor progression and reduce mortality when used as therapeutics." Is it possible that "the critical molecules involved in inflammatory pathways in cancer stem cells are appropriate targets for breast cancer treatment"?

Chapter 14

"Signalling Pathways Driving Cancer Stem Cells: Hedgehog Pathway" by Vanessa Medina Medina Villaamil et al. reveal that "altered Hh [Hedgehog] signaling contributes to the development of up to one third of all human malignancies." Mutations in the genes encoding Hh components are associated with medulloblastoma, basal cell carcinoma, and rhabdomyosarcoma, while aberrant activation of Hh signally without any known mutational basis is associated with glioma, breast, esophageal, gastric, pancreatic, prostate, chrondrosarcoma, and small-cell lung carcinoma. The authors analyze the role of mutations and gene over-expression on components of the signaling pathway leading up to its role "as a pathological player in the growth of a group of human cancers." Happily, Hh pathway antagonists are widely sought, and "[t]herapeutic approaches are in development to block embryonic pathways that play a role in cancer stem cells, including Notch, sonic hedgehog and Wnt."

Chapter 15

Jeffrey DeSano, Theodore Lawrence, and Liang Xu's chapter, "MicroRNAs: Small but Critical Regulators of Cancer Stem Cells" heralds in the new age of nanoparticle therapy: "effective and efficient packaging, targeting, and delivery of these miRNA-based therapeutics." The authors develop their message methodically and convincingly, beginning with the ability of small interfering RNA (siRNA) and microRNA (miRNA) to "negatively regulate gene and protein expression via the RNA interference (RNAi) pathway." Moreover, "specific cross talk [takes place] between epigenetic regulation and the miRNA pathway." There are, in addition, "widespread changes in miRNA expression profiles during tumorigenesis."

The oncogenic miRNAs (aka oncomiRs) are "dominant, gain-of-function mutation[s] ... up-regulated in cancer cells ... [whereas the] expression of other miRNAs ... is depressed in tumors suggesting that these "miRNAs are tumor suppressor miRNAs

[TSmiRs] ... usually a loss-of-function, recessive mutation [which,] when normally expressed, prevent tumor formation and development ... [but] in cancer their expressionis down-regulated, allowing increased disease progression."

The "latest research ... proposes that the dysregulation in cancer stem cells is a result of an antagonism network between different miRNAs that stabilizes the switch between self-renewal and differentiation." Hence, "confronting abnormal miRNA expression levels with molecular miRNA therapy can be a promising and powerful tool to tackle oncogenesis"

Clearly, one can imagine many "molecular therapeutic possibilities ... [with] the distinct purpose of regulating aberrant miRNA levels," but, "in order to be clinically ready, the miRNA-based therapeutics must be effectively, efficiently, and functionally delivered to the cancerous tumor [and t]his has been a great challenge." The approach favored by the authors focuses "on nanotechnology for systemic delivery of therapeutics *in vivo*." So far, the approach has worked with "a [targeted] synthetic nanoparticle delivery system ... and siRNA designed to reduced the expression of ... [a specific] mRNA."

Chapter 16

Massimo Zollo, Immacolata Andolfo, and Pasqualino De Antonellis' chapter, "MicroRNAs and Cancer Stem Cells in Medulloblastoma," examines "the potential use of miRNAs as 'shuttle' [molecules] to impair Cancer Stem Cells in medulloblastoma." Human medulloblastoma (MB) is frequently studied in a well-established murine model: CD133 positive cells are transplanted into the brains of immunodeficient (NOD/SCID) six-week old mice and tumors are harvested in 12 to 24 weeks. Remarkably, "cells derived from classic medulloblastomas showed small round blue cell morphology characteristic [of] histologic structures ... while CD133+ cells derived from a different MB variant, desmoplastic medulloblastoma, recapitulate the cytoarchitecture associated with this subtype."

Not surprisingly, "[p]athways, such as Shh [Sonic Hedgehog], Wnt, Notch and AKT/PI3K, regulating the normal cerebellum development, play a crucial role in the MB tumorigenesis." For example, "Notch pathways are upregulated in MB and increased expression of [the gene] HES1 [hairy and enhancer of split 1], a target of both the canonical notch pathway and the non-canonical shh pathway, is associated with poor prognosis in MB patients." What is more, "cross talk among these pathways provides an interpretation for the synergy in the regulation of MB progression and in CSCs maintenance."

Small noncoding RNAs (i.e., microRNAs) "are often expressed aberrantly in tumors as compared to normal tissues and are likely to contribute to tumorigenesis by dysregulating critical target genes." But microRNAs are also useful for silencing cancers. The latter RNAs bind to cis-regulatory elements mainly present in the 3′ UTR of mRNAs, resulting in the inhibition of mRNA translation or its degradation. "Typically, miRNAs that serve as oncogenes are present at high levels, which inhibit the transcription of genes encoding tumor suppressors. Conversely, tumor suppressor miRNAs are present at low levels, resulting in the overexpression of transcripts encoded by oncogenes."

Happily, the authors report success with an in vivo "microRNA that regulate[s] the Notch pathway and depletes the tumor stem cells [sic] compartment" delivered by an adenovirus type 5 as carrier. Specifically, an miRNA (miR199b-5p) which targets HES1, the principal Notch effector, reduced the proliferation rates of "clones overexpressing the miRNA 199b-5p … when compared to the control clone," enhanced markers of differentiation, decreased the size of the CSC population with transporter activity, and reduced significantly the cells' colony formation potential in NOD-SCID. "Overall, these data indicate a beneficial effect of over-expression of miR199b-5p, as a negative regulator of tumor growth of MB cells." What is more, results with human patients suggest that "the expression levels of miR-199b-5p … might be due to genetic and epigenetic regulation during carcinogenesis."

"It is becoming clear that miRNAs are essential regulators of many of the key pathways implicated in tumor pathogenesis. While adding another layer of complexity, the discovery of the role miRNAs in brain tumors has also revealed a new category of therapeutic targets. As miRNA research continues to evolve, novel therapeutic targets for the treatment of brain tumors will continue to emerge in the near future."

Part V: Diagnosis, Therapeutics, and Prognosis

Chapter 17

Paola Marcato and Patrick Lee's chapter, "The Rocky Road from Cancer Stem Cell Discovery to Diagnostic Applicability" travels over a vast terrain encompassing outcome and survival, risk factors and tumor regrowth, differentiation, metastasis, Gleason score, tumor grade, and size. Marcato and Lee come to the discouraging but not unrealistic conclusion that "patients with elevated levels of CSCs would more likely suffer from an aggressive form of disease that is comparatively resistant to currently employed therapeutics." In the case of acute myeloid leukemia (AML), patients with CD34+CD38- cancer cells at time of diagnosis have the worse outcomes. Breast cancer patients with CD44+ tumor cells have the worse outcome, and for glioblastoma (brain cancer) and colon cancer patients, CD133+ cells are the culprit, although not all CD133+ cells are tumor cells and some colorectal cancer cells are CD133-. Indeed, the "analysis of the literature reveals a large disparity in the prognostic potential of the identified cell surface colon CSC markers" which, the authors add, "highlight[s] the importance of employing multiple markers in the accurate identification of a CSC population in illustrating its potential prognostic applicability." The prognostic value of the current array of prostate CSC markers is "ambiguous at best," although "CD133 in combination … with the ABC transporter, ABCG2, was a much more powerful prognostic tool than either marker alone."

Chapter 18

The chapter by Renata Zobalova, et al., "Drugs that Kill Cancer Stem-Like Cells" begins with a critique of stem cell definitions. The authors draw attention to ambiguity surrounding the use of "prominin-1 [the mouse homologue of human CD133] … as a marker for the increase in the 'stemness' of the cell subpopulation, in particular in combination with other markers, such as CD44 and CD24." A review follows of mechanisms by which a host of agents kill (or fail to kill) CSCs.

The authors characterize three types of CSCs, namely, breast and prostate cancer and mesothelioma cultured as cancer cell spheres *in vitro*. The analysis of their "stemness" is then taken to a new plane by using microarray analysis and the tools of bioinformatics to search for shared characteristics among spheres and other types of CSC cultures. The study of CSCs of solid tumors in vitro in spheres in minimum medium demonstrates "an overall increase in the 'stemness signature' of such cultures, i.e., enrichment in markers of several types of stem cells." Surprisingly, "the tryptophan pathway was the most activated of all pathways whose activation was common to the cancer cells studied suggesting that inhibitors of indoleamine-2,3-dioxygenase (IDO), an enzyme in the tryptophan to N-formyl kynurenin pathway, would be useful for killing CSCs."

The authors develop their "principle of mitochondrial targeting" by synthesizing a "mitochondrially targeted vitamin E succinate [MitoVES] that crosses the mitochondrial inner membrane and "acts by targeting the mitochondrial complex II (CII), whereby causing generation of high levels of ROS [reactive oxygen species], which then induces apoptosis by destabilizing the mitochondrial outer membrane." Indeed, "MitoVES ... [is] probably thus far the best characterized agent toxic to CSCs."

According to the authors, cancer attacks in two waves. First, at the time of their "malignant conversion," mutant pre-CSCs escape the wrath of natural killer (NK) cells, natural killer T-cells (NKTs), and cytotoxic T cells or macrophages. Second, "the 'second-line' tumors, derived from the CSCs that survived the therapeutic intervention, is resistant to the 'first-line' treatment, which considerably jeopardizes any therapeutic modalities applicable to such patients." Taking a two-pronged approach to therapy, therefore, might be desirable: a "combination of agents like MitoVES that would kill the bulk of the tumor cells, while the IDO inhibitor would allow for the cells of the immune system to attack the remaining tumor cells, likely those with higher level of 'stemness'."

Chapter 19

In their chapter, "Cancer Stem Cells as a New Opportunity for Therapeutic Intervention," Victor Bolós, Ángeles López, and Luis Anton Aparicio suggest that "new anti-target agents designed to block the signaling pathways that rule the activity of stem cells may be considered a new promising therapeutic strategy to avoid relapses to conventional treatments." Their target pathways are Notch, Wingless (Wnt)-β-catenin, and Hedgehog (Hh).

According to the authors, the defining characteristics of CSC is uncontrolled "alterations in genes that encode for key signaling proteins or in the niche control ... [that] give[s] rise to aberrant tumorigenic tissues." The Hh gene family encodes several secreted glycoproteins that trigger pathways leading to the release and translocation to the nucleus of transcription factors for "target genes involved in proliferation and differentiation such as cyclin D and c-myc." Therefore, "[t]herapeutic inhibition of the Hh signaling destroys CSC, improves outcome, and even may effect a cure when ... combined with gemcitabine."

The Wnt family of genes also transcribe secreted glycoproteins that operate the "master switch" for controls of proliferation versus differentiation. In the differentiated cells, the canonical Wnt pathway is in the "off state." In the absence of Wnt, β-catenin fails to translocate to the nucleus thereby repressing Wnt target genes. In the "on state," Wnt binds to its receptor and co-receptor setting in motion events leading to the accumulation of β-catenin that enters the nucleus, binds T cell factor (TCF), and activates transcription of target genes thereby inducing cell division. The non-canonical Wnt pathway has much the same effect independently of β-catenin. Hope and expectations surround the use of fungal derivatives "which specifically disrupt nuclear β-catenin/TCF interaction."

The Notch signaling pathway regulates stem cell self-renewal, cell fate, and differentiation. Notch genes encode transmembrane receptors that, in the presence of their ligand, cleave their Notch intracellular domain (NICD) that, in turn, is translocated to the nucleus where it binds transcription factor CBF1 releasing a co-repressor (CoR) protein and binding co-activator protein (CoA). "Deregulated expression of this pathway is observed in a growing number of hematological and solid tumors." Thus, "with the possible exception of keratinocyte derived tumors … Notch signaling may be oncogenic … and its inhibition may be an effective strategy to combine with current therapeutic agents." Happily, "monoclonal antibodies that target Notch receptors … also lead to an antitumoral effect."

Part VI: Targeting Resistance

Chapter 20

Miaorong She and Xilin Chen's chapter, "Targeting Signal Pathways Active in Leukemic Stem Cells to Overcome Drug Resistance," aims at a small sub-population of leukemia stem cells (LSCs) among hematopoietic stem cells (HSCs) in bone marrow and peripheral blood. The authors' "studies focus on a number of signaling pathways that regulate chemoresistance of LSCs through survival pathway[s]."

Beginning with hedgehog (HH), "one of the main pathways that control stem cell fate, self-renewal and maintenance" may also play a role in drug resistance by ... control[ling] the cell cycle fate during cell proliferation." Selectively targeting "HH pathway may lead to more effective cancer therapies."

The use "of farnesyltransferase blockade [has evolved] as a targeted therapy against oncogenic Ras." Moreover, since upregulating the PI3Ks/AKT cell survival pathway plays a critical role in the chemotherapy resistance of AML cells and hence poor prognosis and chemoresistance, it is gratifying that "[i]nhibition of the PI3K/AKT pathway by the specific pathway inhibitors [sic] LY294002 leads to a dose-dependent decrease in survival of LSCs." The drug's efficacy may result from an increase in apoptosis and potentiating the response to cytotoxic chemotherapy.

Finally, the nuclear factor NF-κB is constitutively activated in poorly differentiated LSCs but not in their normal counterpart, suggesting a possible specific target for therapy while sparing normal HSCs. Happily, "the single plant-derived compound parthenolide (PTL) effectively eradicates AML LSCs by inducing robust apoptosis via induce[d] oxidative stress" while sparing normal HSCs.

Chapter 21

Suebwong Chuthapisith's chapter, "Cancer Stem Cells and Chemoresistance" begins by acknowledging that "resistance to chemotherapy is a major cause of failure in the treatment of solid organ malignancies." The chapter takes aim, therefore, at mechanisms alleged to be involved in chemotherapy resistance, namely CSCs' high expression of transporter proteins, their active DNA repair capacity, and their resistance to apoptosis.

The main types of transporters known to be present at high levels in CSCs are adenosine triphosphate-binding cassettes (ABC). Their function would seem to be to excrete toxins and filter toxins that have entered cells. Hence, they are only doing their job when over-expressed and effluxing drugs out of tumors, but it's a job that promotes resistance to chemotherapeutic agents.

More than 40 ABC transporter genes are classified into 8 subfamilies (ABCA through ABCG plus ANSA) each with several genes whose products play various roles in the cell membrane. Subfamily B (aka MDR), for example, has 11 member proteins including P-gp (aka MDR1/ABCB1) that confers resistance to anthracyclines, vinca, alkaloids, colchicines, epipodophyllotoxins and taxanes.

The second model of impairment linked to chemoresistance is "malfunction of the apoptotic process ... mediated by the tumour-suppressor protein p53." Thus, "a disabled/ deregulated apoptotic pathway [due to a] (p53 mutation or over-expression of BCL-2 protein) ... will prevent death of the cancer cell through drug-induced apoptosis."

Regrettably, Chuthapisith ends on a somber note. "[A]ll the strategies proposed above are speculative. Published data, so far, has not yet confirmed the benefit of these approaches in chemoresistant patients where CSCs are believed to be the predominant factor."

Chapter 22

The title of Michal Sabisz and Andrzej Skladanowski's chapter, "Cancer Stem Cells in Drug Resistance and Drug Screening: Can We Exploit the Cancer Stem Cell Paradigm in Search for New Antitumor Agents?" asks the crucial question. Unfortunately, the answer is that "more detailed fundamental knowledge is still required about molecular mechanisms responsible for CSC formation ...[before it will be possible] to kill or arrest CSC growth by inhibiting critical intracellular pathways associated with stemness or CSC differentiation or both."

The path that leads to their conclusion is brilliantly laid out and illustrated. It begins with an historic review of the "new paradigm of cancer origin ... in which malignant stem cells with de-regulated self-renewal and differentiation mechanisms are responsible for tumor initiation and growth." But how good is the evidence? The authors look for data in the case of human colon carcinoma HCT-116 and glioblastoma C6. Contrary to expectations, "the majority of cell[s] ... formed tumors *in vivo* ... Does it mean that in these tumor cell populations all cells have features of CSC?" It "has never been firmly established" after all that the CSC fraction can be clearly distinguished from non-CSC cells. Nor is it "clear whether longer doubling times are characteristic for CSCs in all types of tumors and if they result from fundamental differences in cell cycle regulation between CSCs and differentiated tumor cells."

Possible solutions to these conundrums are examined throughout the chapter, and promising developments are noted. For example, "new compounds which are able to kill CSCs" have been discovered through drug screening using tumor cells cultivated *in vitro*. Hence, many tumor types are shown to differentiate reversibly or irreversibly into different cell types, and the role of the tumor microenvironment for the maintenance of tumor cell phenotype would seem to offer a point of tumor vulnerability.

The discovery of senescent cell progenitor (SCP) and immortal cell progenitor (ICP) cell types may also provide a new model for drug resistant CSCs versus non-drug resistant non-CSCs. Indeed, the authors summarize several mechanisms responsible for CSC therapeutic resistance shared by different tumors and results of efforts to combat damage done to different intracellular pathways in tumors.

In sum, *Cancer Stem Cells Theories and Practice* examines CSCs' contribution to tumorigenesis and metastasis, recurrence and resistance in a host of malignancies, but it also touches on features of cancer beyond CSCs as such. Assuming that CSCs are real and not artifacts of experimentation, tumors take on a new look when seen as organs built by the progeny of CSCs; reprogramming pre-CSCs and CSC plasticity enter the calculus of cancer initiation; CSC dynamics become an issue in tumorigenesis and cancer promotion; vascularization, tissue interactions, inflammatory responses and immune-responsiveness become challenging features of CSCs' niches; mutations in CSCs are complicated by genomic rearrangements, transcriptional and chromatin aberrations, and epigenetic modification; dormancy and gaps in CSCs' mitotic cycle fall out on both therapeutic and pathologic sides of DNA repair; and marker maturation, signaling pathways, differentiation, apoptosis, and cell disposal figure in cancers' progress.

The results of many experiments are suggestive of clinical applications. From the molecular to the organismal, CSCs figure in prospects for improved diagnosis, treatment, and extending remission: devices are or will soon target transporters, membrane markers, elements of intracellular signaling cascades, promoters of oncolytic viruses; a variety of anti-inflammatory drugs, antagonists and inhibitors, blocking antibodies, and radioligands will be deployed; mitochondrial, epigenetic, and differentiation therapies, viral and nanoparticle delivery systems, and small interfering RNAs for reprogramming and inducing apoptosis will become generally available.

Not unexpectedly, the work reported in *Cancer Stem Cells Theories and Practice* contained many surprises and posed many questions. Of course, many technical problems remain, notably for identifying, isolating, raising, and destroying CSC, and a great deal more work remains to be done. But, without doubt, *Cancer Stem Cells Theories and Practice* will give this work direction and impetus.

Stanley Shostak
Associate Professor Emeritus
Department of Biological Sciences,
University of Pittsburgh,
USA

Part 1

Cancer Stem Cell Models

1

The Dark Side of Cellular Plasticity: Stem Cells in Development and Cancer

Fernando Abollo-Jimenez[1,*], Elena Campos-Sanchez[2,*], Ana Sagrera[3,*], Maria Eugenia Muñoz[4], Ana Isabel Galan[4], Rafael Jimenez[4] and Cesar Cobaleda[2,4]

[1]*Experimental Therapeutics and Translational Oncology Program; Instituto de Biología Molecular y Celular del Cáncer; CSIC/Universidad de Salamanca; Campus M. Unamuno s/n; Salamanca*

[2]*Centro de Biología Molecular "Severo Ochoa, "Consejo Superior de Investigaciones Científicas-Universidad Autónoma de Madrid, C/Nicolás Cabrera 1, Universidad Autónoma, Cantoblanco, 28049 Madrid*

[3]*Estacion de Atocha, 1, 28740 Colmenar Viejo, Madrid*

[4]*Departamento de Fisiología y Farmacología, Universidad de Salamanca, Edificio Departamental, Campus Unamuno s/n, 37007-SALAMANCA, Spain*

1. Introduction

All multicellular organisms require a continuous homeostatic control of cellular proliferation and differentiation in order to maintain the numbers of the different types of cells and the global size of the organism, while at the same time compensating for all the permanent loss of cells due to aging and to the attacks from the environment. In general, this control is achieved by the use of a hierarchical system where a small number of multipotential, slow-dividing, stem cells give rise to more differentiated, actively proliferating intermediate progenitors, which in turn will originate large numbers of cells committed to a specific cellular fate. These cells will then terminally differentiate and integrate functionally into the mature organs or tissues. Along this process there is a gradient of developmental potential, in such a way that, as they mature into a certain fate, the cells lose the capacity of giving rise to other cell types.

This process is tightly controlled by extrinsic environmental signals (either permissive or inductive) and, more importantly, by the intrinsic transcriptional and epigenetic profiles of the developing cells. These profiles change and evolve along with development and are the responsibles for establishing both the cellular identity and the susceptibility of the cell to

---

* These authors contributed equally to this work.

alterations that might alter the outcome of cellular differentiation. The nature of these alterations can be environmental (new signals) or, more frequently, internal to the cells (genetic or epigenetic alterations). In this context, it is therefore easy to understand that any deregulation of the transcriptional or epigenetic equilibrium will lead to an unwanted final outcome, like it is the case in tumors, were the cellular identity is reprogrammed by oncogenic alterations to give rise to a new pathological lineage. This aberrant deviation of the normal developmental program is only possible if the initial cell suffering the oncogenic insults posses enough plasticity so as to be reprogrammed by them. In this chapter we describe the nature of physiological plasticity, its biological necessity for normal development and its underlying molecular and cellular mechanisms, to put them afterwards into the context of tumor development. In order to do this, and before discussing the concepts in depth, we need to first define the terminology used and to be aware of its historical origin within the discipline of developmental biology.

Physiological plasticity is here defined as the capacity of cells (stem or differentiated) to adopt the biological properties (gene expression profile, phenotype, etc.) of other differentiated types of cells (that may belong to the same or different lineages). Competence (potency) would therefore be a specific manifestation of plasticity, defined as the ability of undifferentiated cells (stem cells and progenitors) to give rise to their different descendant lineages during normal development (i.e. not pathologically- or experimentally-induced). We group both concepts under the same umbrella (plasticity) since it is increasingly clear that the same mechanisms involved in stem cell competence during normal development are involved in the plasticity of more differentiated types of cells, not only in pathological conditions like tumorigenesis, but also in experimentally-induced fate-changing processes. In the last years, many advances have been made in our understanding of the biology of cellular plasticity (Graf and Enver, 2009; Gurdon and Melton, 2008; Hochedlinger and Jaenisch, 2006; Vicente-Duenas et al., 2009a). However, the molecular bases of stem cell competence (i.e. plasticity) maintenance or entry into the differentiation programs are not yet completely understood (Niakan et al., 2010).

Competence (potency) as we have defined it above is only one of the main properties that define stem cells. The other is their self-renewal capacity, determined by their ability to undergo the asymmetric cell divisions that allow them to maintain themselves in an unchanged state and, at the same time, to generate daughter cells that enter into the differentiation/proliferation cascade (Ward and Dirks, 2007). In this way, when the stem cell divides asymmetrically, it gives rise to a new identical stem cell and a multipotential progenitor/precursor that will originate all the variety of differentiated cells. When the division is symmetrical, two identical daughter cells are created that either retain the same stem properties of the mother cell or start the differentiation program, losing the self-renewal capability and their stem cell properties.

What we have outlined are the main features of normal development of stem-cell based tissues in physiological conditions. However, these processes can be deregulated by many different mechanisms, both experimentally in the laboratory and in numerous pathologies, like cancer or developmental abnormalities. In all these cases, cellular reprogramming is the cause, but the consequences can be very different depending on the triggering mechanisms and the plasticity of the initiating cell. As we will discuss in the next section, our understanding of the biology of development has increased enormously in the last half century, and many different processes have been described in diverse organisms in different laboratories. This has also created a great deal of confusion in the scientific nomenclature, and many of the terms commonly used have different meanings for different authors in different fields (for example, researchers working in different model organisms), in some cases more restrictive, in some more wide-ranging. In this chapter, besides the terms that we have already defined, we will use the following terminology (Figure 1):

- "Dedifferentiation": the mechanism by which the normal developmental program is reverted in such a way that differentiated cells give rise to more plastic, earlier progenitors.
- "Transdifferentiation" designs the direct conversion (reprogramming) of a differentiated cell type into another different mature cell, without the need of dedifferentiating to earlier developmental stages; it usually involves the passage through cellular intermediates that are non-physiological and share markers that are normally mutually exclusive, corresponding to the initiating and the final cell. As we will discuss later, induced pluripotency would be a particular case of transdifferentiation, rather than being a dedifferentiation process, due to the existence of those non-physiological intermediates.
- "Commitment": the point of no return in physiological development, where the cell irreversibly enters a specific differentiation program. For a stem cell, it implies the loss of self-renewal.
- "Epigenetic": the inheritance of patterns of gene expression, without affecting the genetic code itself. In other words, the inheritance that is not codified in the DNA sequence. From the molecular point of view, it designs all the chromatin modifications that establish (and determine the propagation of) the different possible patterns of gene expression of a given, unique genome.
- "Reprogramming": from the cellular point of view, the natural or experimentally-induced alteration of the differentiation program of a given cell. From the molecular point of view, all the molecular changes (i.e., epigenetic) that take place in a cell that is changing its identity. Dedifferentiation and transdifferentiation are types of reprogramming, usually experimentally-induced. Oncogenesis is also a form of reprogramming, in this case one that spontaneously happens in nature.
- "Cancer Stem Cells" (CSCs): the cells responsible for the maintenance, propagation, metastasis and relapse of tumors. They posses self-renewal and differentiation capabilities and can give rise to all the cellular types that compose the tumor mass. Also named cancer-maintaining-cells.
- "Cancer cell-of-origin": the normal cell that first suffers the oncogenic hit and initiates the tumoral process. It is usually the one giving rise to the CSC. It can be either a differentiated cell or a stem/progenitor cell.

2. Historical perspective

Since the beginning of human history, men have looked for the ideal of eternal youth, and the myths about regeneration of diseased organs (or even resurrection) are among the oldest of mankind (Odelberg, 2004). The Egyptian god Osiris had his body resurrected and recomposed after having been torn into pieces and thrown in the Nile. The Hydra from the Greek mythology could regenerate its multiple heads when they were severed, and only by burning the stumps could Hercules defeat the creature. Also, as a punishment for revealing the secret of fire to the humans, Prometheus was chained to the mountain where an eagle ate his entrails, which would regenerate every new day. All these imaginary creatures have a reflection in the natural world, and this was also observed in very ancient times, and already Aristotle (384-322 BC) reported that lizards regenerated their tails. But only in the Age of Enlightenment will this aspect of the natural world become the matter of scientific study. In 1712, Réamur reports the regeneration of the limbs and claws of crayfish (Reaumur, 1712); in 1744, Trembley discovers that the two halves of the Hydra polyp can regenerate a whole new organism (hence its name) (Trembley, 1744); in 1769, Spallanzani describes how tadpoles can regenerate their tails and salamanders can regrow amputated limbs, tails and jaws (Spallanzani, 1769). During most of the 19th and first half of the 20th centuries, research was mainly focused in the description of these processes from the morphological point of view (Birnbaum and Sanchez Alvarado, 2008; Odelberg, 2004). Nevertheless, the detailed analyses performed already showed that, in order for the regenerative process to take place, the cells that are normally forming part of the organs are not enough, and a special type of cells are required: the progenitor cells. The origin of the latter was at that time unclear; in some cases, like for the regeneration of skin, blood, muscles or bones, progenitors are shown to exist in the tissues in small numbers, and to become activated as a consequence of the lesions. In other cases, the progenitors seem to arise from differentiated cells that change their developmental program and become dedifferentiated. The best example of this mechanism is observed in urodeles, a group of very primitive vertebrates (salamanders, newts, axolotls). In them, once the lesion has occurred, cells from the normal tissues form a pool of proliferative progenitors known as the regenerative blastema (Bodemer and Everett, 1959; Chalkley, 1954; Hay and Fischman, 1961). These cells will in turn give rise to all the tissues in the new limb/tail. This extraordinary example of cellular plasticity has been almost completely lost in more evolved vertebrates. Amphibians also provided the first animal model of experimentally-induced reprogramming when, in 1952, Briggs and King managed to generate frog tadpoles by transplanting the nucleus of cells from the blastula into Xenopus oocytes, reverting cellular differentiation (Briggs and King, 1952). Afterwards, Gurdon showed that also differentiated cells could be reprogrammed by using nuclei from intestinal epithelia cells as donors (Gurdon, 1962). These milestone findings clearly indicated that the genetic potential of cells did not diminish during differentiation, and that there were no genetic changes occurring during development. The final proof that this principle extends also to mammals was the cloning of Dolly the sheep by Wilmut and colleagues in 1997 (Wilmut et al., 1997). This was the definitive proof that the changes that happen during differentiation are fully reversible, demonstrating that the fate restrictions that occur during normal development are the result of epigenetic modifications. These studies also showed that there were factors in the oocyte cytoplasm capable of reverting the epigenetic program and inducing a reprogramming that led to the appearance of a totipotent phenotype.

The search for the reprogramming factors followed a parallel route. In 1987 it was shown that ectopic expression of the *Antennapedia* homeotic gene lead to changes in the body plan of *Drosophila*, that got extra legs instead of antennae (Schneuwly et al., 1987). Later it was found that the ectopic expression of *eyeless* controlled the full gene cascade responsible of eye development and could lead to the formation of ectopic eyes in *Drosophila* legs (Gehring, 1996). In mammals, the first master regulatory transcription factor identified was MyoD, which could transdifferentiate fibroblasts into the myogenic lineage (Davis et al., 1987). Other examples of these reprogramming events dependent on single factors are the transdifferentiation of mouse B cells into macrophages by C/EBPα (Xie et al., 2004) or the dedifferentiation of committed B cells by the loss of Pax5 (Cobaleda and Busslinger, 2008; Cobaleda et al., 2007a; Nutt et al., 1999). All these data proved that the alteration of the transcriptional profile by just one factor could cause stable fate changes, and provided the

rationale for the search of the factors capable of reprogramming to full pluripotency that led, in 2006, to the identification by Takahashi and Yamanaka of the four transcription factors capable of inducing pluripotency in terminally differentiated cells (Takahashi and Yamanaka, 2006), as we will describe with more detail in the following sections.
On the other side, cancer has also been known since the origins of mankind. The first references are the Edwin Smith and Ebers papyri from the 3000 BC and 1500 BC, respectively (Hajdu, 2004). The Edwin Smith papyrus contains the first description of breast cancer, with the conclusion that there is no treatment for the disease. Cancer was not so prevalent in ancient times, since life span was much shorter, but it was already clearly identified. Hippocrates (460–375 BC) noted that growing tumors occurred mostly in adults and they reminded him of a moving crab, which led to the terms *carcinos* and *cancer*. Celsus (25 BC–AD 50) also compared cancer with a crab, because it adheres to surrounding structures like if it had claws; he introduced the first classification for breast carcinoma and recommended surgical therapy. However, he already noted that tumors could only be cured if removed at early stages because, even after excision and correct healing of the scar, breast carcinomas could recur with swelling in the armpit and cause death by spreading into the body. Galen (131–AD 200) already advised surgery by cutting into healthy tissue around the border of the tumor (Hajdu, 2004). If we make a 2000-year leap to our days, it seems disappointingly surprising how little those old critical findings have been overcome by modern medicine. Indeed, for solid tumors, still today clean surgical margins and lack of lymph node invasion are the most important prognostic markers, and only if tumors are resected completely before spreading (something that it is anyway impossible to ascertain with current technologies) can curation be guaranteed. Much more is what we have learnt in the last thirty years about the molecular biology of the disease. In 1979 it was shown that the phenotype of transformed cells could be transferred to normal fibroblasts by DNA transfection (Shih et al., 1979). In 1982 the molecular cloning of the first human oncogene was reported simultaneously by several groups (Goldfarb et al., 1982; Lane et al., 1982; Parada et al., 1982; Santos et al., 1982), to be soon identified as the RAS gene. Since then, many genes have been described as oncogenes or tumor suppressors, and the molecular basis of their transforming activities have been described to great detail. A comprehensive study of this topic falls out of the scope of this chapter, but there are some aspects that must be taken into account for further posterior discussion. One of them is that, for many types of tumors, specific mutations have been described to be tightly associated to the tumor phenotype, especially in the case of mesenchymal tumors caused by chromosomal aberrations (Cobaleda et al., 1998; Sanchez-Garcia, 1997). This association already suggested that the oncogenic aberrations might be acting as new specification factors that determine the tumor appearance and/or phenotype. In 2000, Hanahan and Weinberg summarized the main features that needed to be disrupted in normal cellular behavior in order for allow a tumor to appear and progress (Hanahan and Weinberg, 2000). These main aspects are related with the survival and proliferation of cancer cells. However, much less attention has been paid to the aspects related to the differentiation. In fact, if cellular fate was carved into stone, cancer would be impossible, since no new lineages could be generated other than the normal, physiologic ones. Here is where the normal mechanisms regulating cellular identity and plasticity play an essential role in allowing cancers to arise and hopefully, as we will discuss, they might be the key to its eradication.

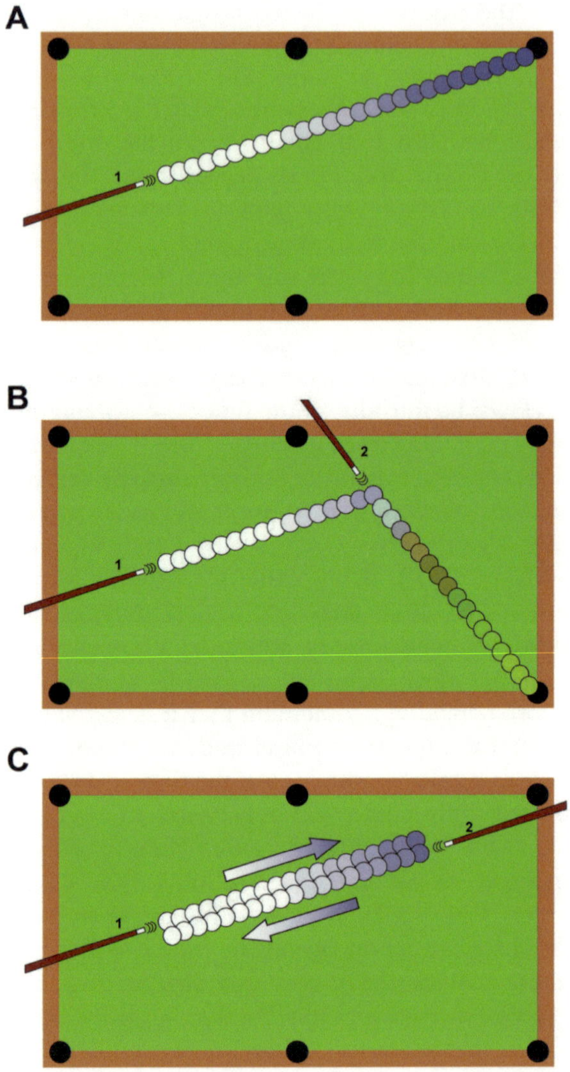

Fig. 1. The road from developmental plasticity to cancer. Development is here conceptualized as a pool ball rolling towards different directions depending on the strokes it has received. For simplicity, the pool table is flat and horizontal, but in reality the shape of the "developmental terrain" also is an essential contribution to fate determination (see text). A) In normal development, fate is established once the initial impulse has been provided by internal transcription factors or external signals, and then the cell develops "lineally" towards this fate. B) Transdifferentiation. The introduction of a new driving force (cue nº 2, for example a transcription factor) redirects the cell towards a new fate, pushing it out of its normal route. C) Dedifferentiation. An inversion of the normal process of development, following the same differentiation intermediates that were followed in the first instance, but in a reversed order. Here, an opposite driving force is depicted (cue nº 2) but this reversion could also be due to a lack of initial impulse (i.e., lack of an essential driving transcription factor).

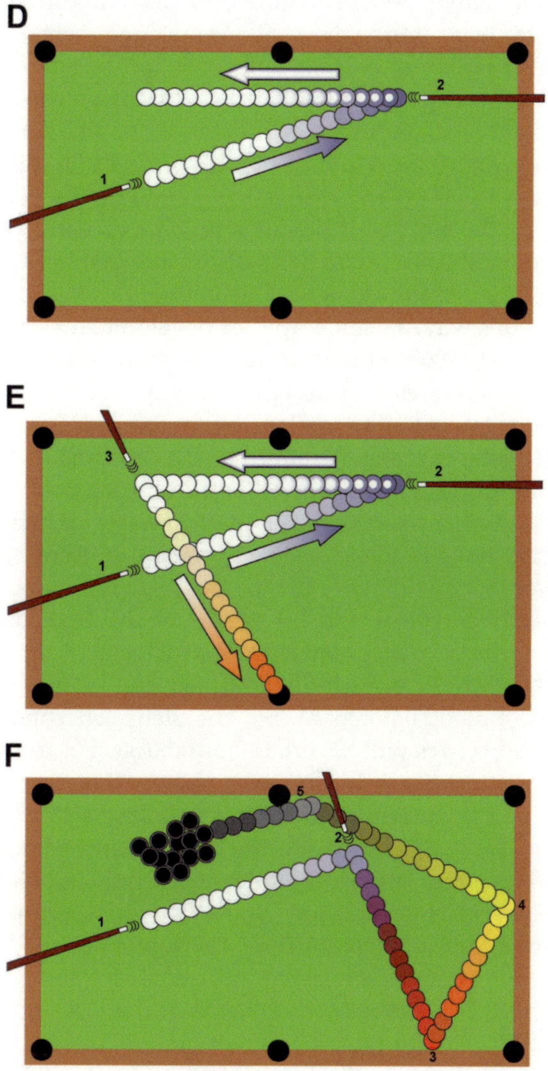

D) Induction of pluripotency. Again, an external force (Yamanaka factors, for example) counteracts programmed development and sends the cell back to a progenitor condition, but in this case going through non-physiological cellular intermediates. E) Reprogramming. After pluripotency has been induced as depicted in the previous panels, the cells can be redirected towards new fates with the help of external of internal stimuli (cue n° 3). F) Tumorigenesis. An oncogenic hit (cue n° 2), hitting the right cellular intermediate with the right strength and angle sends the cell down to a new developmental program that will lead to the development of a tumour. According to this view, many of the second hits in tumorigenesis (n° 3, 4, 5) are already implicit given the first hit and the nature of the cell.

3. Molecular bases of plasticity

As we have mentioned before, differentiation has been traditionally considered as an irreversible process. It was more than 50 years ago when Conrad Waddington conceptualized the irreversibility of cellular differentiation as marbles falling down a slope (Waddington, 1957). This conceptual and very graphical image has been afterwards widely used to visually depict the meaning of transdifferentiation, dedifferentiation or pluripotent reprogramming (Hochedlinger and Plath, 2009), all of them "uphill" processes that must overcome natural barriers to take place. Interestingly enough, this conceptual view has been given a new meaning by the studies of the gene regulatory networks (GRNs) that control differentiation; from the mathematical analysis of the interactions among all the genes that are expressed in a cell in a certain moment, a geometric description of the developmental potential is obtained. In this way, a "landscape" of developmental probabilities is generated (Enver et al., 2009; Huang, 2009; Huang et al., 2009) in which "valleys" represent the different cellular fates, connected through "slopes" or "channels", that are the differentiation routes. It is important to realize that, in this conceptualization, the landscape is in fact defined by the gene expression pattern of the cell itself, not something external to it. In this landscape, pluripotency would be a "basin of attraction" situated at the top of a peak. Pluripotency therefore behaves like a mathematical attractor, a metastable state maintained by small variations in the levels of expression of transcriptional and epigenetic regulators. The cells would slide towards the most stable configuration through the slopes, and those primed to differentiate would be located at the edge of the "attractor basin". Therefore, the stemness of a cellular population is a metastable equilibrium defined by the gene interactions at the level of each individual cell and, consequently, each cell has a different intrinsic developmental potential. So, the stem cell condition is not static, but rather is a continuum that moves within certain boundaries. For example, in the case of the established stem cell marker Sca-1 it has been shown that, in a clonal population of progenitor cells, there is a Gaussian distribution of its levels of expression (Chang et al., 2008). But these cells are not confined to a specific level of expression, as cells at both ends of the levels of expression can, with time, recapitulate the whole population with the complete range of expression levels. Furthermore, these sub-compartments present different transcriptomes that confer them distinct intrinsic developmental tendencies towards diverse lineages. These results indicate that each individual cell is an intermediate in a continuum of fluctuating transcriptomes. This range of variation is at the basis of the stochastic choice of lineage (Chang et al., 2008). The study of a different marker, Stella, in this case in embryonic stem (ES) cells, has provided similar findings (Hayashi et al., 2008). Stella is a marker of stem cell identity that shows a mixed expression in ES cells, demonstrating that they are not uniform, but rather represent a metastable state between intracellular mass- and epiblast-like states while retaining pluripotency. This equilibrium can be shifted in response to several factors, like for example epigenetic regulators (Hayashi et al., 2008).

The heterogeneous expression of phenotypic markers can be extended to the much more significant level of the transcription factors. Phenotypic heterogeneity is a known characteristic of progenitors at the population level, and it has been long known that they present a promiscuous activation of lineage-associated genes (Hu et al., 1997). Also the genes that are associated with the maintenance and specification of the pluripotent state vary in the population. In this context, recent results (Kalmar et al., 2009) show that *Nanog* levels experience random fluctuations within the ES cell population, giving rise to two different compartments: one stable, with high levels of *Nanog* expression, and another much more unstable, with low levels of *Nanog*, and much more prone to differentiate and lose pluripotentiality (Kalmar et al., 2009). With the examples that we have provided, we can see that pluripotency is a state of dynamic heterogeneity of a population, and it is at the same type maintained and driven towards differentiation by fluctuations in the levels of expression of transcriptional and epigenetic regulators. The cells that are in the centre of the attractor "basin" are less prone to differentiate than the ones approaching the "edge" of the "basin". The latter are already primed to differentiate, so that commitment is a spontaneous but rare phenomenon, unless it is elicited by external signals that disrupt the metastable equilibrium (Enver et al., 2009; Huang, 2009). This dynamic view explains the duality between the simultaneous plasticity and heterogeneity of multipotent populations, and also how the balance between instructed and stochastic cell fate decisions takes place.

4. Loss of plasticity during normal development

As we have already mentioned, through the normal developmental processes that allow stem and primitive progenitor cells to become differentiated, and as a result of physiological plasticity, the identity of the cells change and new fates are adopted. These events occur in a progressive manner, in such a way that several distinct cell intermediates are generated with more restricted potential until the final mature, specialized cell types are generated and functionally integrated into the tissues and organs. Each lineage is characterized by a defined gene expression profile, resulting of the action of transcription factors and epigenetic modifications in a certain cellular environment. We have described how the stem cell state is that of a metastable equilibrium that can be disrupted towards differentiation either by random intracellular noise variation or by the induction by extracellular signals. Once the stem cells start the differentiation process, they begin to make reciprocally excluding lineage choices controlled by cross-antagonism between competing transcription factors, in such a way that different transcription factors, controlling different subsets of genes associated with specific lineages, are also controlling their activities in a reciprocal manner, maintaining an equilibrium that can easily be skewed towards one or the other side by external signals (Loose et al., 2007; Swiers et al., 2006). With the advent of flow cytometry and its capacity to separate cells according to defined combinations of surface markers, the study of the development of the hematopoietic system has provided enormous insight into the molecular and cellular mechanisms of lineage commitment. Indeed, their peculiar characteristics have allowed the isolation and purification of many distinct differentiation intermediates, making developmental haematopoiesis the ideal field of research to explore the mechanisms of lineage commitment and plasticity. From there, the developmental models identified have been extrapolated to other experimental systems, usually with great success. The above-described cross-antagonism model can therefore also be found in the development of the haematopoietic system. For example, the interaction between the transcription factors GATA-1 and PU.1 in myeloid progenitors, where they reciprocally inhibit each other and therefore create a binary decision situation for the progenitor that must choose between erythroid/megakaryocyte or myeloid-monocytic fates (Enver et al., 2009; Laiosa et al., 2006). This equilibrium creates a third intermediate condition defined by the balance between the expressions of both factors, which would correspond to a bipotent progenitor condition. This model has also been found to apply in other systems, like the early fate choice of pancreatic progenitors between endocrine and acinar cell lineages, in this

case under the control of cross-repressive interactions between the transcription factors Nkx6 and Ptf1a (Schaffer et al., 2010). So, in non-committed progenitors there are basal levels of parallel expression of opposed transcription factors; this explains the occurrence of multilineage gene priming, initially described in haematopoietic stem and progenitor cells (Enver et al., 2009; Hu et al., 1997). However, either in *in vitro* or *in vivo* settings many different developmental intermediates have been described by different groups, and there is still a lot of controversy about the exact steps that are really followed in normal development, because all experimental systems are imperfect and, like it happens to particles in Heisenberg´s uncertainty principle, the mere isolation of the cells already affects their developmental potential, and the conditions under which this potential is studied are also to a certain degree dictating the possible outcomes. Nevertheless, it is generally accepted that there is a hierarchical loss of developmental potential in a gradual progression through many serial differentiation options in such a way that, at any point, a progenitor would only have to choose between two mutually exclusive options (Brown et al., 2007; Ceredig et al., 2009). Afterwards, and to mature towards terminally differentiated cells, the progenitors will have to interact with the suitable extrinsic signals (like the cytokines, for example) that would for that reason carry out a more permissive than instructive function.
Although this process is mainly governed by transcription factors, epigenetic modifications occur in a progressive manner that modify the chromatin in different ways and help in stabilizing expression patterns and their transmission to daughter cells. These epigenetic memory systems involve mainly chromatin regulators of the Trithorax and Polycomb group proteins, and are in charge of maintaining cell-type-specific expression patterns in many developmental systems (Ringrose and Paro, 2004, 2007). For many years these epigenetic marks were considered irreversible (in parallel with differentiation), but the most recent findings are revealing that they are much more dynamic than initially thought and that they contribute greatly to the competence of progenitors. Along these lines, the so-called bivalent chromatin regions have been found in embryonic stem (ES) cells, that correspond to genome sections simultaneously marked by H3K27me3 (a repressive mark) and H3K4me3 (an activating one), and it has been proposed that these domains work by controlling developmental genes in these cells while keeping them poised for activation or deactivation, suggesting a chromatin-based mechanism for pluripotency maintenance (Bernstein et al., 2006; Mikkelsen et al., 2007; Sharov and Ko, 2007). The resolution of the bivalent domains into either a permanent 'on' or 'off' state is closely related to the commitment of the cell. Initially it was thought to be restricted only to progenitors and only related with genes that had to be kept silent and then activated. However, it seems that bivalent domains also can appear in differentiated cells like T cells (Roh et al., 2006) and seem to provide a way to postpone either the activation or the repression of a functionally distinct group of genes, mainly developmental transcription factors (Pietersen and van Lohuizen, 2008). The fact that epigenetic modifications themselves are much more flexible than previously thought fits very well with the increasing examples of plasticity during development. Indeed, a rigid model based on irreversible molecular modifications of the chromatin cannot accommodate all the different processes of differentiation, and it is especially difficult to reconcile with developmental systems in which terminal differentiation steps require an extensive reprogramming of the gene expression profiles with respect to the ones existing in previous partially differentiated cellular intermediates. In these systems in which the so-called mature cells should still maintain a high degree of plasticity (i.e., a certain degree of "stemness") a different molecular mechanism must exist to make such quick reprogramming possible.

As a way of an example to illustrate the above-mentioned points, and how developmental plasticity plays a role in both normal and pathological differentiation we are going to describe the development of a system that has been very well characterized: B cells in the hematopoietic system. In the adult, the generation of mature B cells begins with the hematopoietic stem cells (HSCs) in the bone marrow (BM). HSCs will be gradually restricted towards the B lymphocyte lineage through several stages of differentiation. Initially they give rise to multipotent progenitors (MPPs), which have lost the self-renewal capacity but retain multilineage differentiation potential. After that, they generate lymphoid-primed multipotent progenitors (LMPPs) that already lack erythroid and megakaryocyte potential (Adolfsson et al., 2005). LMMPs give rise to early lymphocyte progenitors (ELPs) characterised by the activation of recombination-activating genes (Igarashi et al., 2002); these will afterwards differentiate into common lymphoid progenitors (CLPs) with potential already restricted to B, T and NK pathways (Hardy et al., 2007; Kondo et al., 1997). The expression of the transcription factor Pax5 determines definitive commitment to the B cell lineage at the pro-B cell developmental stage (see below). Rearrangements of immunoglobulin heavy and light chain genes lead to the generation of immature B cells in the bone marrow, expressing a functional B cell receptor (BCR) in their surface (IgM) (Jung et al., 2006). These immature B cells leave the bone marrow and travel to the peripheral lymphoid organs where they become mature B cells (Hardy and Hayakawa, 2001). However, mature B cells in the periphery are not in fact, regardless of their name, the last differentiation stage of their lineage, because they are in fact waiting for an external signal (the antigen recognition) to experience the terminal differentiation process that will result in the generation of antibody-producing plasma cells. So, in response to T cell-dependent antigens, a dedicated structure, the germinal centre (GC) is formed, where B cells undergo several cycles of proliferation, somatic hypermutation, immunoglobulin class switching and selection. Positively selected GC B cells can then either become terminally differentiated plasma cells or memory cells (Klein and Dalla-Favera, 2008). However, the gene expression program of plasma cells is very different to the one of B cells and, in fact, for many genes it shows similarities with the expression profile of progenitors (Delogu et al., 2006; Shaffer et al., 2002; Shapiro-Shelef and Calame, 2005). So this is an example of a case where the terminal differentiation involves a complete reprogramming of the transcriptional profile of the previous developmental stage. Clearly, in a system like this plasticity must be guaranteed in the late differentiation stages to allow for the last reprogramming step to occur, even if a progressive limitation of developmental options takes place together with differentiation. This last step of terminal differentiation to plasma cells would not be possible if the epigenetic marking of activated and repressed genes that have been established during lineage specification was irreversible. Therefore, a mechanism must exist for the maintenance of B cell identity that allows this identity to be lost for terminal differentiation. In order to understand the molecular basis for this process we must first describe the mechanisms that establish and maintain B cell characteristics.

In uncommitted hematopoietic progenitors, as we have described, plasticity (competence) is based on their capacity to maintain a promiscuous level of basal expression of lineage-specific genes in the process of multilineage priming (Akashi et al., 2003; Hu et al., 1997). This promiscuous gene expression pattern allows the progenitors to respond to environmental signals that, in combination with the right transcription factors, will lead them into the different specific lineages. In the case of B cells, this signalling is provided by IL7, in combination with the transcription factors E2A, EBF1 and PAX5 (Cobaleda and

Busslinger, 2008; Cobaleda et al., 2007b; Miller et al., 2002; Nutt and Kee, 2007). Although the precise roles of this transcription factors in these very early stages is still the subject of active investigation, it seems that E2A and EBF1 are in charge of activating the expression of B lymphoid genes at the beginning of B cell development. However, the real commitment to the lineage is controlled by PAX5. PAX5 is a transcription factor whose expression within the haematopoietic system is restricted to B cells. Due to its protein structure it has the dual capacity of acting either as a transcriptional activator or as a repressor, depending on the interacting partners (Czerny et al., 1993; Dorfler and Busslinger, 1996; Eberhard and Busslinger, 1999; Eberhard et al., 2000). Induced by Ebf, Pax5 commits cells to the B cell lineage and maintains B cell identity by concurrently repressing B-lineage-inappropriate genes and activating B-cell specific genes (Delogu et al., 2006; Schebesta et al., 2007). Once Pax5 expression has been initiated, progenitors lose their potential and are only able to differentiate along a unidirectional path towards mature B cells. In *Pax5* knockout mice (Nutt et al., 1999; Urbanek et al., 1994) B cell development cannot progress beyond the pro-B cell stage. However, since they are not yet committed, *Pax5*$^{-/-}$ proB cells behave as multipotent progenitors, because they express multilineage genes (that would have been otherwise repressed by Pax5 in normal conditions), and this allows them to be programmed into most of the haematopoietic lineages under the right conditions. All these developmental options are shut down by the reintroduction of Pax5, which actively represses all non-B cell genes (Nutt et al., 1999).

But the role of Pax5 is not over once commitment has taken place; quite the opposite, it is continuously required to maintain B cell identity and function all the way through the life of the B cell (Cobaleda et al., 2007b). Actually, deletion of *Pax5* at different B cell developmental stages by using a conditional *Pax5* allele has shown that its loss leads to the loss of B cell identity and commitment. In proB cells, loss of *Pax5* causes committed B cells to recover the capacity to differentiate into macrophages and T cells, proving that Pax5 is required not only to initiate the B cell program, but also to maintain it in early B cell development (Mikkola et al., 2002). Deletion of *Pax5* at later stages of B cell development results in the loss of mature B cells, inefficient lymphoblast formation, and reduced IgG formation. Most B cell membrane antigens are downregulated, and the transcription of B cell-specific genes is decreased, whereas the expression of non-B cell-specific genes is activated (Horcher et al., 2001; Schebesta et al., 2007). Thus, mature B cells radically change their gene expression pattern in response to *Pax5* inactivation. These effects can be easily understood when considering that Pax5 activates at least 170 genes that are essential for B cell signalling, adhesion, migration, antigen presentation, and germinal-centre B cell formation (Schebesta et al., 2007), indicating that Pax5 controls in a direct manner both B cell development and function. In the absence of Pax5, all this network collapses and the cells lose their B cell identity. The loss of B-cell specific genes upon *Pax5* deletion goes together with the loss of Pax5-dependent repression of non-B cell genes. Derepression of these genes (around 110 genes controlling functions such as receptor signalling, cell adhesion, migration, transcriptional control, and cellular metabolism (Delogu et al., 2006)) unveils a new plasticity for peripheral *Pax5*-deleted mature B cells: they can dedifferentiate *in vivo* back to early uncommitted multipotent progenitors in the bone marrow, which can afterwards give rise to other haematopoietic cell types like macrophages or T cells (Cobaleda et al., 2007a).

This Pax5-dependent plasticity has a biological reason and is directly related with the physiology of B cells. As we already mentioned, the final function of mature B cells is to become plasma cells. For this terminal differentiation to take place, *Pax5* must be downregulated, to permit the closing down of all the B cell transcriptional program (Delogu et al., 2006; Schebesta et al., 2007; Shapiro-Shelef and Calame, 2005) and allow the transition to the plasma cell stage. The process starts with the binding of the membrane BCR to its cognate specific antigen. This activates a signalling cascade that leads to the upregulation of *Blimp1*, the master regulator of the plasma cell transcriptional program and identity (Kallies and Nutt, 2007; Martins and Calame, 2008). Mature B cells and plasma cells have very different gene expression programs, which are controlled in a mutually exclusive manner by Pax5 and Blimp1, respectively. In fact, *Pax5* is directly repressed by Blimp1, as a way of eliminating B cell identity and allowing for plasma cell differentiation to proceed (Lin et al., 2002). The expression of many Pax5-activated genes is either absent or considerably reduced upon Pax5 loss in plasma cells, and Pax5-repressed genes are reexpressed in plasma cells (Delogu et al., 2006). Many of the genes that are expressed in plasma cells are also expressed in uncommitted lymphoid progenitors (Delogu et al., 2006). But, since these genes are not compatible with B cell development or function they must be silenced to maintain B cell identity. However, as they will be required for terminal differentiation into plasma cells, they cannot be irreversibly repressed in B cells by stable epigenetic modifications. The molecular mechanism underlying this versatility is based on the function of Pax5: first, it preserves B cell identity, and afterwards it allows for a simple mechanism (repression of *Pax5*) of eliminating this identity when reprogramming becomes necessary to generate a plasma cell. This is the reason why mature B cells retain such a high degree of plasticity dependent on a single gene.

This mechanism that we have outlined for B-cell differentiation is present in other systems and can explain the existence of plasticity in many other developmental models. For instance, in the process of melanocyte differentiation from adult melanocyte stem cells, the transcription factor Pax3 initiates a melanogenic program and, simultaneously, prevents downstream terminal differentiation (Lang et al., 2005). Pax3-expressing melanoblasts are therefore committed, but remain undifferentiated until Pax3-mediated repression is relieved. Hence, also in this example a transcription factor can simultaneously determine cell fate and maintain an undifferentiated state, leaving a cell poised to differentiate in response to external stimuli. This molecular mechanism implies a high degree of cellular plasticity, since the elimination of the factor(s) responsible allows the cells to readily differentiate to other lineages. Perhaps the most striking example of this plasticity is the reprogramming of adult mouse ovaries into testes induced by the removal of transcription factor Foxl2 (Uhlenhaut et al., 2009). In a fascinating result, the deletion of this single, organ-identity-maintaining gene leads to the full conversion of all the female ovary tissues into their male ontological equivalents, showing that cellular (and even organ) plasticity can be much less hidden than we think, and that cell (and organ) identity can be maintained by just a single gene (Uhlenhaut et al., 2009).

5. Experimental control of plasticity: reprogramming

In the previous sections we have described the different levels of physiological plasticity that can be found during normal development, and shown that they are in fact necessary for differentiation to occur. However, we have also seen that this plasticity is usually not manifested spontaneously, but is rather something latent in the cells that we can only reveal in an artificial way. As a general rule, the ultimate cellular identity of any particular differentiation pathway is stable and typically corresponds to a very specialized cellular type with a highly specific physiological function. Therefore, on paper, plasticity, from the point of view of normal development, is a property that should in principle be limited to stem cells and progenitors (i.e. cells that require this competence for their function). This could be called the physiological plasticity, that is, the normal competence of progenitors that we have previously discussed. All other types of cells should remain stable and maintain their identity. Indeed, most reprogramming cases occur either "on purpose" in the lab (experimental reprogramming for regenerative medicine) or in an "accidental" manner in nature (reprogramming in tumorigenesis, see below). However, this notion of stability was seriously challenged by the results for Yamanaka´s group showing that, and least in an experimental setting in the laboratory, reprogramming specialized cells to pluripotency only required the action of four factors (or even less): the 4 transcription factors from Yamanaka: Oct4, Sox2, c-Myc and Klf4 (Takahashi and Yamanaka, 2006). This finding showed in a definitive manner that there is a latent developmental potential retained in the cell, and what are the factors required to unleash it. The knowledge of reprogramming as a reality was already present, as we have mentioned before, in the results from the seminal nuclear reprogramming from the 1950-60s (Briggs and King, 1952; Gurdon, 1962). However, even though it was since then obvious that a cell nucleus could be converted from the program of a differentiated cell into that of a pluripotent progenitor just by being transferred into the right cytoplasmic environment, it was difficult to imagine that only a few of factors were really required to make the entire process possible. We have also seen that the gain and/or loss of single, essential, factors can alter the whole developmental program of a cell.

In the laboratory, there are several experimental approaches to achieve cellular reprogramming that might lead to pluripotency. On one side, there is nuclear transfer, where the whole nucleus is taken away from one cell and transferred into a new one, a previously enucleated oocyte whose cytoplasms contains all the factors required to impose an multipotential state. Although this method does not involve the acquisition of genetic changes, obviously the whole nuclear environment is changed, with all the possible consequences that this may have (Byrne et al., 2007; Gurdon and Melton, 2008; Hochedlinger and Jaenisch, 2006). Another possibility for reprogramming is cellular fusion, which allows the nuclei of a cell to act over that of another cell and therefore, under the appropriate circumstances, alter fate (Yamanaka and Blau, 2010). Exogenous expression of transcription factors was one of the first ways of demonstrating how reprogramming could take place (see Section 2), in this case without reverting cells back to a pluripotent stage (Zhou and Melton, 2008a). Some examples include transdifferentiation of adult pancreatic exocrine cells to β cells after expression of the transcription factors Ngn3, Pdx1 and Mafa (Zhou et al., 2008; Zhou and Melton, 2008a, b), the conversion of fibroblasts into myogenic cells by the myogenic factor MyoD (Davis et al., 1987) and the transdifferentiation of committed B lymphocytes to macrophages by expression of C/EBPα (Xie et al., 2004). The identification of the right cocktail of factors led to the reprogramming to pluripotency (induced-pluripotency stem cells, iPSCs) by the introduction of stem cell-specific genes into a differentiated cell (Maherali et al., 2007; Okita et al., 2007; Takahashi and Yamanaka, 2006; Wernig et al., 2007). This can be done by introducing genetic changes in the treated cells or in a less invasive, transient way, using specific drugs or transient vectors (Abujarour and Ding, 2009; Mikkelsen et al., 2008; Stadtfeld et al., 2008a; Stadtfeld et al., 2008b).

Another possibility of exploiting physiological plasticity for experimentally-induced reprogramming is to eliminate the specific transcription factors (usually master regulators) responsible for maintaining the identity and function of the differentiated cell and for keeping its epigenetic state. This, as we have seen, leads to a lineage reprogramming into new cell types like in the case of the conversion of mature B cells into T cells (Cobaleda and Busslinger, 2008; Cobaleda et al., 2007a).

Of all these methods, nuclear transfer is empirical, but all the other ones require a precise knowledge of the transcriptional and epigenetic machineries that control the identities of the starting cellular material and the final desired product. It is very clear now that, together with the specific activation or repression of transcription factors (usually master regulators of specific lineages), the epigenetic modifications are an indispensable part of the process, since they are the ones that define the "flexibility" of the cell to be reprogrammed. As we have mentioned before, in general, differentiated cells correspond to a highly specialized compartment with no plasticity. According to this fact, it has been recently described that in the haematopoietic system the HSCs are 300 times more prone to reprogramming than B or T cells (Eminli et al., 2009).

Since the differentiated state is the more stable one, a certain level of "activation energy" is required to move the cells "uphill" to become again pluripotent. From this point of view of inducing pluripotency, there are two possibilities (Yamanaka, 2009): i) either only some cells in the population can be reprogrammed, because they are the ones that are responsive to the reprogramming factors (elite model), or ii) all the cells are equally susceptible to reprogramming (stochastic model). The latest evidences indicate that the second possibility happens to be true and that, given the appropriate combination of stimuli (in this case, the reprogramming factors), any cell can be reprogrammed to change fate (Hanna et al., 2009), and that the process can be accelerated either by interfering with the DNA damage checkpoint (see below) or by increasing the expression of some of the reprogramming factors, like Nanog (Hanna et al., 2009). The global inefficiency of the reprogramming process, even in the most favourable conditions, clearly suggests that, independently of the initial number of cells that are actually responsive to the reprogramming factors, very few of them can finally achieve full reprogramming. It has been shown that factor-induced reprogramming is a gradual process with several more or less defined cellular intermediates (Stadtfeld et al., 2008a). Some of these non-physiological reprogramming intermediates (remember our definition of transdifferentiation) can be isolated as cell lines stuck at some point of the conversion process (Mikkelsen et al., 2008). The study of these incompletely reprogrammed intermediates shows that they have re-activated stem cell renewal and maintenance genes, but those genes in charge of pluripotency are still repressed. Also, the cells have not been able of completely repressing the expression of lineage-specific transcription factors. On top of that, these cells have failed in completing epigenetic remodelling and still retain persistent DNA hypermethylation marks (Mikkelsen et al., 2008).

6. Cancer: the dark side of plasticity

We have shown that plasticity is an essential feature of development. However, as all aspects of normal physiology, it also represents a "weakness" that can give rise to the origin of diseases. As we have mentioned, cancer is a differentiation disease, and tumorigenesis represent the outcome of a deviation of the normal process of differentiation in which a new lineage, the tumour, is created, with new properties and characteristics, but still similar in some ways to normal lineages. In other words, cancer could be considered as a particular case of "wrong" reprogramming.

In the last decade great advances have been made in our understanding of the cellular origin of cancer. Many of these findings have been driven by the postulation and final coming of age of the theory of the cancer stem cells (CSCs). It is beyond of the scope of this chapter to detail all the aspects and implications of this theory, which have been previously discussed to great extent (Cobaleda et al., 2008; Cobaleda and Sanchez-Garcia, 2009; Lobo et al., 2007; Reya et al., 2001; Sanchez-Garcia et al., 2007; Vicente-Duenas et al., 2009a), so here we will limit our discussion to the aspects related to cellular plasticity and differentiation. The CSC theory proposes that tumours are heterogeneous tissues, maintained by tissue-specific stem cells, in a manner very similar to any other stem cell-based tissue in the organism. Therefore in any tumour, different types of cells coexist: some of them are differentiated cells, lacking the possibility of propagating cancer, and that normally constitute the main mass of the tumour. However, there is also a variable, but generally small, percentage of cancer stem cells (CSCs), which are defined by the fact that they are the only ones that posses the capacity of replenishing the tumour mass and of transplanting the cancer (Castellanos et al., 2010; Greaves, 2010; Hermann et al., 2010; Lane and Gilliland, 2010; Sanchez-Garcia, 2010; Shackleton, 2010; Vicente-Duenas et al., 2010). Therefore, if cancer is a stem-cell driven tissue, it becomes crucial to identify the first cell suffering the oncogenic alteration(s) i.e., the normal cell that will give rise to the cancer stem cell, and the mechanisms that are behind this fate reprogramming. This first cell, as previously defined, would be the cancer cell-of-origin. What is clear is that the initiating cell's intrinsic plasticity must allow the cell to be reprogrammed into the new tumoral type(s). So cellular plasticity and the responsiveness of the cell to the reprogramming effects of the oncogene are therefore critical factors in the tumorigenesis process, and this implies that specific cancer-inducing alterations happen in particular cells (stem or differentiated, see below), and that it is the reciprocal interaction between the cellular plasticity and the differentiating capabilities of the oncogenic event(s) what determines the final resultant tumor phenotype.
From the point of view of the nature of the oncogenic alteration(s) and its potential reprogramming capabilities, traditionally in the field of cancer research it was assumed that more than one hit was required to switch from a normal healthy cell into a tumoral one, implying that many different aspects of cellular biology must be altered in the progress to final tumorigenesis (Hanahan and Weinberg, 2000). Also in the field of plasticity it was consequently assumed that, to convert a certain cell into a different one, more than one single alteration was required. This was partially supported for a long time by the fact that the only way to achieve full reprogramming to pluripotency was nuclear transplantation, a purely empirical method in which it was impossible to isolate or identify the factors responsible for the stem state. This seemed to suggest that many elements were necessary for reprogramming to occur. In fact, as we have discussed before, for "simple" changes in identity, like it could be a transdifferentiation process, a single, transcription factor could be all that is required to induce the reprogramming, as long as it is the right factor for the right type of cell (Cobaleda et al., 2007a; Davis et al., 1987; Nutt et al., 1999; Xie et al., 2004). This was similar as how a single initial oncogenic lesion may only cause an alteration in proliferation, or a partial block in differentiation. The breakthrough of Takahashi and Yamanaka (Takahashi and Yamanaka, 2006) showed that only 4 transcription factors ("four hits") were necessary for induction of pluripotency. Of note, the 4 transcription factors have been shown to play an oncogenic role in different contexts, and both *c-Myc* and *Klf4* are well-known oncogenes (Chen et al., 2008; Okita et al., 2007; Rowland et al., 2005; Tanaka et al., 2007). This is a clear evidence of the essential mechanistic link between reprogramming

and cancer, and illustrates the fact that there are a certain number of genes/proteins that are strong enough so as to induce the change of expression patterns in a global manner affecting cellular identity. Only strong regulators of the transcriptional and/or epigenetic machineries can reprogram. Therefore, the multistep nature of tumorigenesis can be compared with the series of developmentally unfavoured "uphill" steps required for full reprogramming to pluripotency. All these barriers are biologically designed to protect cells from transformation, that is, to prevent cells from changing their identity. There are many articles and reviews describing the capacity that the different oncogenes have for blocking or interfering with essential cellular functions (Hanahan and Weinberg, 2000). In the case of the reprogramming factors our knowledge is still incomplete, but the answers are gradually arising from the study of partially reprogrammed states and also by introducing the different factors at different times during the process of induction of pluripotency, starting from mouse fibroblasts (Sridharan et al., 2009). This kind of experiments has allowed showing that the different factors have temporal and separable contributions during the reprogramming process. In the initial stages, and previously to the induction of the ES-cell-like gene expression program, silencing of the somatic cell gene expression program takes place, mainly due to the action of c-Myc, although it is not yet clear how this gene mediates repressive effects in this context. Nevertheless, it has previously been shown that histone deacetylase inhibitors like valproic acid (VPA) can partially substitute for c-Myc in the reprogramming process (Huangfu et al., 2008) (see below) collaborating in the repression of the differentiated cells' gene program. Therefore, it would seem that c-Myc mostly acts before the pluripotency regulators are activated and, consequently, ectopic expression of c-Myc is only required for the first few days of reprogramming (Sridharan et al., 2009). Actually, it seems that c-Myc could be dispensable for reprogramming, but in its absence there is a massive decrease in the efficiency of the process (Nakagawa et al., 2008; Wernig et al., 2008). It seems that the other factors, Oct4, Sox2, and Klf4, need to act together in establishing the pluripotent condition, since they cannot associate with their target genes in cells that are only partially reprogrammed, most probably because the histone methylation pattern does not allow their binding (Sridharan et al., 2009). This correlates with our knowledge about the function of these factors in ES cells, were they bind cooperatively to hundred of genes in overlapping genomic sites (Boyer et al., 2005; Loh et al., 2006), acting in a coordinated manner to maintain the transcriptional program required for pluripotency.

However, even though the four Yamanaka factors can be sufficient for reprogramming most cell types, there are cases where they are not enough. One of the most striking examples is precisely that of B cells. In mature B lymphocytes, the four factors cannot achieve full reprogramming, and another molecular manipulation is required: the extinction of Pax5 expression (Hanna et al., 2008). As we have mentioned before, the elimination of Pax5 by itself is all what is required for mature B cells to dedifferentiate to early multipotential progenitors, since Pax5 is the responsible for the initiation and maintenance of B-cell identity and function (Cobaleda et al., 2007a). So the presence of such a strong factor requires its specific elimination in order to achieve reprogramming. These results also connect reprogramming to tumorigenesis, since it had previously been described that the loss of cellular identity induced by the absence of Pax5 led to the development of tumours or an early-B cell progenitor phenotype (Cobaleda et al., 2007a), indicating that the loss of the identity of the initial cell is an essential step in tumorigenesis. In fact, a very similar observation has been made in human patients with the uncommon transdifferentiation of follicular B cell lymphoma (FL) into a myeloid histiocytic/dendritic cell (H/DC) sarcoma

(Feldman et al., 2008). The FL and H/DC tumors of each patient are clonally related, since they contain the same immunoglobulin rearrangements and an identical IgH-BCL2 translocation breakpoint. It has been suggested that the translocation-induced overexpression of BCL2 leads to a prolonged survival of FL B that can facilitate their loss of B-lineage identity and subsequent reprogramming into H/DC tumor cells (Feldman et al., 2008). There are more examples corroborating the fact that loss of cell identity is essential for tumoral reprogramming. For example, in human Hodking lymphomas the inactivation of the B cell factor E2A by overexpression of its specific antagonists activated B cell factor 1 (ABF-1) and inhibitor of differentiation 2 (Id2) leads to the loss of B cell markers and expression of lineage-inappropriate genes that characterizes the tumour pathognomonic Reed-Sternberg cells (Mathas et al., 2006). Another aspect worth mentioning is the fact that, in contrast to mature B cells, earlier B cell developmental stages could be reprogrammed to pluripotency just with the four Yamanaka factors (Hanna et al., 2008), again underscoring the idea that the degree of differentiation of the target cell impacts directly in the reprogramming efficiency.

An essential component of both the reprogramming process and tumoral progression are epigenetic changes. It is clear that cancer does not only depend on genetic mutations, but also on epigenetic changes that establish a new pattern of heritability, providing a cellular memory by which the new tumoral cellular identity can be maintained, and that these alterations constitute an essential part of cancer initiation and progression (Ting et al., 2006). The role of epigenetic alterations in tumour origin and progression is well known and it has been comprehensively reviewed elsewhere (Esteller, 2007, 2008; Esteller and Herman, 2002). All epigenetic marks become altered in tumours, leading to changes in gene expression. These changes have been very well described to affect many specific genes in charge of controlling cellular functions, which therefore become altered in cancer. But these changes are in fact global and affect the whole cellular identity. The tumour-related epigenetic alterations can either be independent from the initiating oncogenic mutation and simply due to tumour progression, or they can be directly linked to the first oncogenic event, like it happens in the case of chromosomal translocations that affect histone-modification genes (Esteller, 2008). In the case of reprogramming to pluripotency, something similar happens, since epigenetic modifications are an intrinsic part of the process and they need to take place in a global manner, not just by the specific regulation of some individual genes that is mainly accomplished by the transcription factors. This explains why the efficiency of reprogramming increases greatly in the presence of chemicals interfering with epigenetic marks in an unspecific (i.e., not locus-restricted) manner. For example, treatment with 5-aza-cytidine (AZA), a DNA methyltransferase inhibitor, induces a rapid transition to fully reprogrammed iPSCs (Huangfu et al., 2008; Mikkelsen et al., 2008), and the use of valproic acid (VPA), a histone deacetylase (HDAC) inhibitor, greatly improves the induction to pluripotency (Huangfu et al., 2008). Treatment with the inhibitor of the G9a methyltransferase named BIX-01294 increases the efficiency of reprogramming using just two factors, Oct4 and Klf4, to levels similar to the ones achieved when using the four factors (Shi et al., 2008). G9a methyltransferase is essential for the extinction of the pluripotency program upon exit to differentiation because, by means of its histone methylation activity, it blocks target-gene reactivation in the absence of transcriptional repressors, and this leads to the silencing of embryonic genes like Oct4 (Feldman et al., 2006). Also, simultaneously, G9a promotes DNA methylation, and therefore prevents the reprogramming to the undifferentiated state (Epsztejn-Litman et al., 2008; Feldman et al., 2006). All these facts support the idea that global epigenetic changes affecting a large and unknown number of genes are a critical selective component of the reprogramming process, and that the addition of chemicals that facilitate these molecular changes helps the process by lowering the activation energy barrier for this "uphill" process. A very important practical consequence of these findings is the fact that epigenetic therapies are already in use or in very advanced clinical trials against cancer. Their mechanisms of action are based on the assumption that, by globally affecting epigenetic patters of tumoral cells, they can restore the normal levels of expression of genes that are required for the normal control of cellular proliferation and/or differentiation. Like for any other chemotherapy, the effects are systemic, but it is likely to affect primarily the tumoral cells and leave non-proliferative cells relatively unaffected. Since 2004, AZA is FDA-approved as the first drug of the new class of demethylating agents for the treatment of myelodysplastic syndromes (Kaminskas et al., 2005), and there are many other clinical trials evaluating the effects of AZA in other cancer types (Sacchi et al., 1999). Something similar happens with HDAC inhibitors (Dey, 2006; Lane and Chabner, 2009). All these findings emphasize once more the nature of cancer as a pathological case of "wrong" reprogramming, as a differentiation disease.

As we have seen, both the changes in the epigenetic patterns and the gain or loss of transcriptional regulators are essential components of the tumour generation and of the experimentally-induced reprogramming processes. It is clear that these alterations, although based in mechanisms normally existing in the cells, are undesirable for normal cellular development and functioning, so the cells have evolved a series of safety mechanisms to avoid these alterations or their effects and maintain their identity and function. In the context of cancer there have been many studies in the last decades describing how all these safety mechanisms are bent, broken or bypassed to allow tumour generation and progression (Hanahan and Weinberg, 2000). The most recent results in the less advanced field of reprogramming seem to indicate that, also in this experimentally-induced "progression to pluripotency" (in analogy to tumoral progression) exactly as it happens in tumour progression, the elimination of the DNA damage control checkpoint tremendously increases the efficiency of the reprogramming process. Thus, the inactivation of the p53-p21 axis by different approaches allows a much higher percentage of the starting cells to successfully complete the process to full pluripotency (Banito et al., 2009; Hong et al., 2009; Kawamura et al., 2009; Krizhanovsky and Lowe, 2009; Li et al., 2009; Marion et al., 2009; Utikal et al., 2009; Zhao et al., 2008) . However, this enhanced efficiency is achieved at the price of a much higher genetic instability, and the iPSCs generated in this way carry many genetic aberrations of different types. This is corresponding to the facts that we have previously mentioned showing that reprogramming is an "uphill", developmentally unfavourable process that imposes a great stress to the cells and that most of the cells therefore, in normal conditions, fail to complete (Mikkelsen et al., 2008). These results do not only further support the idea of cancer as a disease of cellular differentiation but, furthermore, indicate that indeed, the aberrant transcription factors, deregulated signalling molecules and epigenetic regulators are the main dynamic forces behind the tumoral process, and that many of the other alterations (for example, loss of p53) play just a permissive role for tumoral progression.

We have until now examined the processes of reprogramming and tumorigenesis mainly from a molecular point of view. The inclusion of epigenetics in our description encompasses to a certain degree cellular identity, since the epigenetic pattern of chromatin modifications can be broadly assimilated to cellular identity. However, in the next final paragraphs we are going to discuss the tumoral reprogramming phenomenon from a more classical cellular point of view. In the field of cancer research it has conventionally been assumed that the phenotype of the tumoral cell was a mirror of the one of the normal cell from which it arose. Most tumour cells present the characteristics of differentiated cell types (more or less aberrant). Therefore, for every type of tumour, the cell of origin had to be found in its closest relative in the normal tissue. However, the solidification of the cancer stem cell (CSC) theory has led to a re-thinking of these concepts (Cobaleda and Sanchez-Garcia, 2009; Vicente-Duenas et al., 2009b). First, since tumours are postulated to be stem cell-based tissues, not all the tumoral cells are equally capable of regenerating the tumour, but only those cells with CSC properties. Most of the cells lack this capacity, although there can be great variations in the percentage of CSCs within a tumour. This has important repercussions for our understanding of tumour origin. If tumours are maintained by aberrant cells with the characteristics of stem cells, then where do these cells come from? The cancer cell-of-origin would therefore be a normal cell that has undergone reprogramming by the oncogenic events to give rise to a CSC, a new pathological cell with stem cell properties. One possibility is that the oncogenic mutations take place in a normal stem cell that, in this way, becomes reprogrammed to originate the new pathological tissue. This has been long known to be the case for chronic myelogenous leukaemia (CML), where the causing chromosomal translocation t(9;22) is present in most lineages of differentiated haematopoietic cells, thus indicating that an early progenitor is the cell of origin (Melo and Barnes, 2007). Recent advances in modelling human diseases in the mouse have allowed us to prove this fact experimentally; indeed, restricting the oncogenic alteration to the stem cell compartment in the mouse is all that is required to generate a full CML with the whole variety of differentiated cells (Perez-Caro et al., 2009; Vicente-Duenas et al., 2009b). Also for intestinal cancers it has been proven in mice that they have their origin in the crypt stem cells, by activating the Wnt signalling pathway specifically in the stem cell compartment. This leads to the generation of adenomas where a differentiation hierarchy is maintained. On the contrary, if the oncogenic lesions are targeted to the non-stem, more differentiated intestinal epithelial cells, only small, short-lived microadenomas appear (Barker et al., 2008; Zhu et al., 2008). In other tissular context, targeting astrocytoma-associated oncogenic lesions to the nervous system progenitors results in tumour development, whereas targeting them to the zone containing just differentiated cells only gives rise to local astrogliosis (Alcantara Llaguno et al., 2009). In all these and other similar cases (Dirks, 2008; Joseph et al., 2008; Zheng et al., 2008) it is therefore clear that the initiating event must take place in a stem cell, even if, afterwards, the macroscopic tumour is composed by differentiated cells. This indicates a pathological direct reprogramming mediated by the oncogenic lesions.

The other alternative is that of the cancer cell-of-origin being a differentiated cell type. In this case the cells must be reprogrammed not only towards a new fate, but also to regain stem cell characteristics in a process of tumoral reprogramming to pluripotency. For this to occur, two aspects have to come together: first, the oncogenic alteration must be capable of conferring the stem properties and, second, the cell must have a degree of plasticity that allows the reprogramming mediated for this specific alteration to take place. It has been shown that some oncogenes, like MOZ-TIF2 (Huntly et al., 2004), MLL-AF9 (Krivtsov et al., 2006; Somervaille and Cleary, 2006), MLL-ENL (Cozzio et al., 2003), MLL-GAS (So et al., 2003) or PML-RARα (Guibal et al., 2009; Wojiski et al., 2009) can generate CSCs when they are introduced into target cells that were already committed. Some of these genes, like MLL-AF9, have been shown to be able of activating a stem cell-like self-renewal program in already committed progenitors (Krivtsov et al., 2006). A somewhat comparable situation happens with c-Myc, which can induce some parts of the transcriptional program of an embryonic stem cell in differentiated epithelial cells, thus giving rise to epithelial CSCs (Wong et al., 2008). Other oncogenes, like BCR-ABLp190, are however unable of conferring self-renewal properties (Huntly et al., 2004). In these cases, self-renewal must be provided by the target cell or by additional alterations, so that the oncogene does not immediately generates a CSC, but rather originates a precancerous cell that can afterwards give rise to a *true* CSC (Chen et al., 2007). In any case, the exact cellular origin of the initiating lesions is very difficult to determine, especially since, in many cases, the functional impact of the lesion, the clonal expansion, can become apparent only by the generation of cells that can be either upstream or downstream of the initiating cell, at least in terms of phenotypic markers. For example, in several childhood B acute lymphoblastic leukaemias (ALL) the initiating translocations originate prenatally *in utero* and act in partially committed cells as a first-hit capable of conferring this preleukaemic cell with aberrant self-renewal and survival properties (Hong et al., 2008). In AML1-ETO leukaemias, the translocation can still be detected in patients in remission, indicating that the cells can remain latent and some of their descendants can become tumorigenic with time (Miyamoto et al., 2000). In children's B-ALLs, the CSC properties can be found in blasts of more than one different developmental stage, which can also interconvert among themselves (le Viseur et al., 2008). This obviously makes the determination of the nature of the cancer-cell of origin even more difficult. Also in ALLs, the comparison of relapsed patient samples with the samples obtained from the same patients at their diagnosis by means of genomic analysis has shown that both initial and relapsed tumours share the same ancestral clone (Mullighan et al., 2008) that had diverted in different manners during the different stages of the disease. So, the nature of the CSC evolves over time with disease progression, treatment and relapse, in such a way that the properties of the CSC population in a certain moment do not necessarily reflect the nature of the initial cancer cell-of-origin (Barabe et al., 2007).

In the context of reprogramming to pluripotency, the initiating factors are not necessary anymore once the cells are already iPSCs and the process has been completed, that is to say, when the new identity has been fixed and the cell is already in a new pluripotent "attractor basin". If cancer stem cells arose through a reprogramming-like mechanism then, as a logical consequence, maybe the oncogenes initiating tumour formation might be dispensable for the posterior stages of tumour development (Krizhanovsky and Lowe, 2009). This fact correlates well with the examples of the subsistence of a pre-cancerous lesion in a stable population of cells that are already aberrant, but need secondary hits to initiate the openly tumoral differentiation program. In this way, the initiating lesion would have an active function in the reprogramming process, but afterwards it would become just a passenger mutation, or even perform a different function in tumour development that could very well be independent from its initial reprogramming activity. This could clarify the lack of success of some current targeted therapies, like the anti-BCR-ABL kinase drug imatinib which, although successfully eliminates differentiated tumour cells, fails to kill the BCR-ABL^+ CSCs (Barnes and Melo, 2006; Graham et al., 2002; Perez-Caro et al., 2009; Vicente-Duenas et al., 2009b). From a mathematical modeling point of view and consistent with the gene regulatory network (GRN) approaches, the oncogenic mutations alter one of the nodes and therefore change the architecture of the network, thus leading to a change in the landscape topography and giving rise to new abnormal attractors (new "valleys") where cancer stem cells are trapped (Huang et al., 2009). This modeling also fits with the above-discussed postulate that a cell can stay in the new attractor even after the stimulus that triggered the transition has already disappeared, implying that the transient expression of an oncogene can be enough to trigger a lasting malignant phenotype that can become independent for its maintenance on the originating mutation (Huang et al., 2009).

7. Future prospects

Cancer is the second cause of mortality in the developed countries and its incidence is quickly rising in the Third World too. Current treatments for cancer are still focused in the idea of tumours as diseases in which the normal processes of proliferation are altered and consequently, therapies are targeted against proliferating cells. All these treatments are therefore unspecific and highly toxic, particularly for the non-cancerous cells in the organism with highly proliferation rates (epithelia, hair...). The most recent research advances have shown that cancer must be considered to a great degree as a disease of differentiation in which a new tissue, the tumour, emerges from cells that, following an oncogenic event, acquire new pathological fates. So it follows that cancer is a disease that, at least in its initial stages, is closely linked to reprogramming. Therefore, the research in reprogramming is intimately tied to that in cancer.

Considering cancer as a reprogramming disease gives us a new point of view over the disease in our search for new therapeutic strategies. Differentiation therapies are already in use for some very specific cases of cancer (e.g., differentiation of PML-RARα-positive acute promyelocytic leukaemias with the use of retinoic acid). Reprogramming to pluripotency also gets stuck at in the "uphill" way to pluripotency (Mikkelsen et al., 2008) and it is very probable that tumoral cells are very similar to these partially reprogrammed intermediates, whose study should help us to learn how to force tumour cells out of their blocked condition. This is in fact what is planned to achieve with the use of the newest epigenetic drugs that are already approved or close to approval for treatment of specific tumours. Along the way we are also progressively learning more about the molecular mechanisms that govern epigenetic marks, and this knowledge about the epigenetic control of self-renewal, differentiation and maintenance of identity should help us to obtain more specifically targeted epigenetic therapies (Jones, 2007).

Our increasing knowledge and control over the mechanisms programming cellular identity should make us able of developing strategies to reprogram cancer cells in different ways. It has already been shown that it is possible to use nuclear transplantation approaches to reprogram melanoma cells (Hochedlinger et al., 2004) embryonal carcinomas (Blelloch et al., 2004) and even to clone mouse embryos from brain tumours (Li et al., 2003). All these findings indicate that it can be perfectly feasible to reprogram tumour cells. Hopefully in a near future we will possess the scientific and technological knowledge so as to be able of modifying tumoral cell fate at will to reprogram them either by forcing them to differentiate and disappear or to become susceptible to new therapies.

8. Acknowledgements

We thank all members of labs 13 at IBMCC and B-15 and B-16 at the Department of Physiology and Pharmacology for their helpful comments and constructive discussions. Research in the group is supported partially by FEDER (Fondo de Investigaciones Sanitarias PI080164), Proyectos Intramurales Especiales (CSIC) and Junta de Castilla y León (SA060A09 and Proyecto Biomedicina 2009-2010). F.A.J. is the recipient of an FPU fellowship from Ministerio de Ciencia e Innovación. E.C.S. is the recipient of a JAE-predoc fellowship from the CSIC.

9. References

Abujarour, R., and Ding, S. (2009). Induced pluripotent stem cells free of exogenous reprogramming factors. *Genome Biol* 10, 220.

Adolfsson, J., Mansson, R., Buza-Vidas, N., Hultquist, A., Liuba, K., Jensen, C.T., Bryder, D., Yang, L., Borge, O.J., Thoren, L.A., *et al.* (2005). Identification of Flt3+ lympho-myeloid stem cells lacking erythro-megakaryocytic potential a revised road map for adult blood lineage commitment. *Cell* 121, 295-306.

Akashi, K., He, X., Chen, J., Iwasaki, H., Niu, C., Steenhard, B., Zhang, J., Haug, J., and Li, L. (2003). Transcriptional accessibility for genes of multiple tissues and hematopoietic lineages is hierarchically controlled during early hematopoiesis. *Blood* 101, 383-389.

Alcantara Llaguno, S., Chen, J., Kwon, C.H., Jackson, E.L., Li, Y., Burns, D.K., Alvarez-Buylla, A., and Parada, L.F. (2009). Malignant astrocytomas originate from neural stem/progenitor cells in a somatic tumor suppressor mouse model. *Cancer Cell* 15, 45-56.

Banito, A., Rashid, S.T., Acosta, J.C., Li, S., Pereira, C.F., Geti, I., Pinho, S., Silva, J.C., Azuara, V., Walsh, M., *et al.* (2009). Senescence impairs successful reprogramming to pluripotent stem cells. *Genes Dev* 23, 2134-2139.

Barabe, F., Kennedy, J.A., Hope, K.J., and Dick, J.E. (2007). Modeling the initiation and progression of human acute leukemia in mice. *Science* 316, 600-604.

Barker, N., Ridgway, R.A., van Es, J.H., van de Wetering, M., Begthel, H., van den Born, M., Danenberg, E., Clarke, A.R., Sansom, O.J., and Clevers, H. (2008). Crypt stem cells as the cells-of-origin of intestinal cancer. *Nature*.

Barnes, D.J., and Melo, J.V. (2006). Primitive, quiescent and difficult to kill: the role of non-proliferating stem cells in chronic myeloid leukemia. *Cell Cycle* 5, 2862-2866.

Bernstein, B.E., Mikkelsen, T.S., Xie, X., Kamal, M., Huebert, D.J., Cuff, J., Fry, B., Meissner, A., Wernig, M., Plath, K., *et al.* (2006). A bivalent chromatin structure marks key developmental genes in embryonic stem cells. *Cell* 125, 315-326.

Birnbaum, K.D., and Sanchez Alvarado, A. (2008). Slicing across kingdoms: regeneration in plants and animals. *Cell* 132, 697-710.

Blelloch, R.H., Hochedlinger, K., Yamada, Y., Brennan, C., Kim, M., Mintz, B., Chin, L., and Jaenisch, R. (2004). Nuclear cloning of embryonal carcinoma cells. *Proc Natl Acad Sci U S A* 101, 13985-13990.

Bodemer, C.W., and Everett, N.V. (1959). Localization of newly synthesized proteins in regenerating newt limbs as determined by radioautographic localization of injected methionine-S35. *Dev Biol* 1, 327-342.

Boyer, L.A., Lee, T.I., Cole, M.F., Johnstone, S.E., Levine, S.S., Zucker, J.P., Guenther, M.G., Kumar, R.M., Murray, H.L., Jenner, R.G., *et al.* (2005). Core transcriptional regulatory circuitry in human embryonic stem cells. *Cell* 122, 947-956.

Briggs, R., and King, T.J. (1952). Transplantation of Living Nuclei From Blastula Cells into Enucleated Frogs' Eggs. *Proc Natl Acad Sci U S A* 38, 455-463.

Brown, G., Hughes, P.J., Michell, R.H., Rolink, A.G., and Ceredig, R. (2007). The sequential determination model of hematopoiesis. *Trends Immunol* 28, 442-448.

Byrne, J.A., Pedersen, D.A., Clepper, L.L., Nelson, M., Sanger, W.G., Gokhale, S., Wolf, D.P., and Mitalipov, S.M. (2007). Producing primate embryonic stem cells by somatic cell nuclear transfer. *Nature* 450, 497-502.

Castellanos, A., Vicente-Duenas, C., Campos-Sanchez, E., Cruz, J.J., Garcia-Cenador, M.B., Lazo, P.A., Perez-Losada, J., and Sanchez-Garcia, I. (2010). Cancer as a reprogramming-like disease: implications in tumor development and treatment. *Semin Cancer Biol* 20, 93-97.

Ceredig, R., Rolink, A.G., and Brown, G. (2009). Models of haematopoiesis: seeing the wood for the trees. *Nat Rev Immunol* 9, 293-300.

Cobaleda, C., and Busslinger, M. (2008). Developmental plasticity of lymphocytes. *Curr Opin Immunol* 20, 139-148.

Cobaleda, C., Cruz, J.J., Gonzalez-Sarmiento, R., Sanchez-Garcia, I., and Perez-Losada, J. (2008). The Emerging Picture of Human Breast Cancer as a Stem Cell-based Disease. *Stem Cell Rev* 4, 67-79.

Cobaleda, C., Jochum, W., and Busslinger, M. (2007a). Conversion of mature B cells into T cells by dedifferentiation to uncommitted progenitors. *Nature* 449, 473-477.

Cobaleda, C., Perez-Losada, J., and Sanchez-Garcia, I. (1998). Chromosomal abnormalities and tumor development: from genes to therapeutic mechanisms. *Bioessays* 20, 922-930.

Cobaleda, C., and Sanchez-Garcia, I. (2009). B-cell acute lymphoblastic leukaemia: towards understanding its cellular origin. *Bioessays* 31, 600-609.

Cobaleda, C., Schebesta, A., Delogu, A., and Busslinger, M. (2007b). Pax5: the guardian of B cell identity and function. *Nat Immunol* 8, 463-470.

Cozzio, A., Passegue, E., Ayton, P.M., Karsunky, H., Cleary, M.L., and Weissman, I.L. (2003). Similar MLL-associated leukemias arising from self-renewing stem cells and short-lived myeloid progenitors. *Genes Dev* 17, 3029-3035.

Czerny, T., Schaffner, G., and Busslinger, M. (1993). DNA sequence recognition by Pax proteins: bipartite structure of the paired domain and its binding site. *Genes Dev* 7, 2048-2061.

Chalkley, D.T. (1954). A quantitative histological analysis of forelimb regeneration in Triturus viridescens. *J Morphol* 94, 21-70.

Chang, H.H., Hemberg, M., Barahona, M., Ingber, D.E., and Huang, S. (2008). Transcriptome-wide noise controls lineage choice in mammalian progenitor cells. *Nature* 453, 544-547.

Chen, L., Shen, R., Ye, Y., Pu, X.A., Liu, X., Duan, W., Wen, J., Zimmerer, J., Wang, Y., Liu, Y., *et al.* (2007). Precancerous stem cells have the potential for both benign and malignant differentiation. *PLoS ONE* 2, e293.

Chen, Y., Shi, L., Zhang, L., Li, R., Liang, J., Yu, W., Sun, L., Yang, X., Wang, Y., Zhang, Y., and Shang, Y. (2008). The molecular mechanism governing the oncogenic potential of SOX2 in breast cancer. *J Biol Chem* 283, 17969-17978.

Davis, R.L., Weintraub, H., and Lassar, A.B. (1987). Expression of a single transfected cDNA converts fibroblasts to myoblasts. *Cell* 51, 987-1000.

Delogu, A., Schebesta, A., Sun, Q., Aschenbrenner, K., Perlot, T., and Busslinger, M. (2006). Gene repression by Pax5 in B cells is essential for blood cell homeostasis and is reversed in plasma cells. *Immunity* 24, 269-281.

Dey, P. (2006). Chromatin remodeling, cancer and chemotherapy. *Curr Med Chem* 13, 2909-2919.

Dirks, P.B. (2008). Cancer's source in the peripheral nervous system. *Nat Med* 14, 373-375.

Dorfler, P., and Busslinger, M. (1996). C-terminal activating and inhibitory domains determine the transactivation potential of BSAP (Pax-5), Pax-2 and Pax-8. *Embo J* 15, 1971-1982.

Eberhard, D., and Busslinger, M. (1999). The partial homeodomain of the transcription factor Pax-5 (BSAP) is an interaction motif for the retinoblastoma and TATA-binding proteins. *Cancer Res* 59, 1716s-1724s; discussion 1724s-1725s.

Eberhard, D., Jimenez, G., Heavey, B., and Busslinger, M. (2000). Transcriptional repression by Pax5 (BSAP) through interaction with corepressors of the Groucho family. *Embo J* 19, 2292-2303.

Eminli, S., Foudi, A., Stadtfeld, M., Maherali, N., Ahfeldt, T., Mostoslavsky, G., Hock, H., and Hochedlinger, K. (2009). Differentiation stage determines potential of hematopoietic cells for reprogramming into induced pluripotent stem cells. *Nat Genet* 41, 968-976.

Enver, T., Pera, M., Peterson, C., and Andrews, P.W. (2009). Stem cell states, fates, and the rules of attraction. *Cell Stem Cell* 4, 387-397.

Epsztejn-Litman, S., Feldman, N., Abu-Remaileh, M., Shufaro, Y., Gerson, A., Ueda, J., Deplus, R., Fuks, F., Shinkai, Y., Cedar, H., and Bergman, Y. (2008). De novo DNA methylation promoted by G9a prevents reprogramming of embryonically silenced genes. *Nat Struct Mol Biol* 15, 1176-1183.

Esteller, M. (2007). Cancer epigenomics: DNA methylomes and histone-modification maps. *Nat Rev Genet* 8, 286-298.

Esteller, M. (2008). Epigenetics in cancer. *N Engl J Med* 358, 1148-1159.

Esteller, M., and Herman, J.G. (2002). Cancer as an epigenetic disease: DNA methylation and chromatin alterations in human tumours. *J Pathol* 196, 1-7.

Feldman, A.L., Arber, D.A., Pittaluga, S., Martinez, A., Burke, J.S., Raffeld, M., Camos, M., Warnke, R., and Jaffe, E.S. (2008). Clonally related follicular lymphomas and histiocytic/dendritic cell sarcomas: evidence for transdifferentiation of the follicular lymphoma clone. *Blood* 111, 5433-5439.

Feldman, N., Gerson, A., Fang, J., Li, E., Zhang, Y., Shinkai, Y., Cedar, H., and Bergman, Y. (2006). G9a-mediated irreversible epigenetic inactivation of Oct-3/4 during early embryogenesis. *Nat Cell Biol* 8, 188-194.

Gehring, W.J. (1996). The master control gene for morphogenesis and evolution of the eye. *Genes Cells* 1, 11-15.

Goldfarb, M., Shimizu, K., Perucho, M., and Wigler, M. (1982). Isolation and preliminary characterization of a human transforming gene from T24 bladder carcinoma cells. *Nature* 296, 404-409.

Graf, T., and Enver, T. (2009). Forcing cells to change lineages. *Nature* 462, 587-594.

Graham, S.M., Jorgensen, H.G., Allan, E., Pearson, C., Alcorn, M.J., Richmond, L., and Holyoake, T.L. (2002). Primitive, quiescent, Philadelphia-positive stem cells from patients with chronic myeloid leukemia are insensitive to STI571 in vitro. *Blood* 99, 319-325.

Greaves, M. (2010). Cancer stem cells: back to Darwin? *Semin Cancer Biol* 20, 65-70.

Guibal, F.C., Alberich-Jorda, M., Hirai, H., Ebralidze, A., Levantini, E., Di Ruscio, A., Zhang, P., Santana-Lemos, B.A., Neuberg, D., Wagers, A.J., *et al.* (2009). Identification of a myeloid committed progenitor as the cancer-initiating cell in acute promyelocytic leukemia. *Blood* 114, 5415-5425.

Gurdon, J.B. (1962). The developmental capacity of nuclei taken from intestinal epithelium cells of feeding tadpoles. *J Embryol Exp Morphol* 10, 622-640.

Gurdon, J.B., and Melton, D.A. (2008). Nuclear reprogramming in cells. *Science* 322, 1811-1815.

Hajdu, S.I. (2004). A note from History: Greco-Roman Thought about Cancer. *Cancer* 100, 3.

Hanahan, D., and Weinberg, R.A. (2000). The hallmarks of cancer. *Cell* 100, 57-70.

Hanna, J., Markoulaki, S., Schorderet, P., Carey, B.W., Beard, C., Wernig, M., Creyghton, M.P., Steine, E.J., Cassady, J.P., Foreman, R., *et al.* (2008). Direct reprogramming of terminally differentiated mature B lymphocytes to pluripotency. *Cell* 133, 250-264.

Hanna, J., Saha, K., Pando, B., van Zon, J., Lengner, C.J., Creyghton, M.P., van Oudenaarden, A., and Jaenisch, R. (2009). Direct cell reprogramming is a stochastic process amenable to acceleration. *Nature* 462, 595-601.

Hardy, R.R., and Hayakawa, K. (2001). B cell development pathways. *Annu Rev Immunol* 19, 595-621.

Hardy, R.R., Kincade, P.W., and Dorshkind, K. (2007). The protean nature of cells in the B lymphocyte lineage. *Immunity* 26, 703-714.

Hay, E.D., and Fischman, D.A. (1961). Origin of the blastema in regenerating limbs of the newt Triturus viridescens. An autoradiographic study using tritiated thymidine to follow cell proliferation and migration. *Dev Biol* 3, 26-59.

Hayashi, K., Lopes, S.M., Tang, F., and Surani, M.A. (2008). Dynamic equilibrium and heterogeneity of mouse pluripotent stem cells with distinct functional and epigenetic states. *Cell Stem Cell* 3, 391-401.

Hermann, P.C., Bhaskar, S., Cioffi, M., and Heeschen, C. (2010). Cancer stem cells in solid tumors. *Semin Cancer Biol* 20, 77-84.

Hochedlinger, K., Blelloch, R., Brennan, C., Yamada, Y., Kim, M., Chin, L., and Jaenisch, R. (2004). Reprogramming of a melanoma genome by nuclear transplantation. *Genes Dev* 18, 1875-1885.

Hochedlinger, K., and Jaenisch, R. (2006). Nuclear reprogramming and pluripotency. *Nature* 441, 1061-1067.

Hochedlinger, K., and Plath, K. (2009). Epigenetic reprogramming and induced pluripotency. *Development* 136, 509-523.

Hong, D., Gupta, R., Ancliff, P., Atzberger, A., Brown, J., Soneji, S., Green, J., Colman, S., Piacibello, W., Buckle, V., *et al.* (2008). Initiating and cancer-propagating cells in TEL-AML1-associated childhood leukemia. *Science* 319, 336-339.

Hong, H., Takahashi, K., Ichisaka, T., Aoi, T., Kanagawa, O., Nakagawa, M., Okita, K., and Yamanaka, S. (2009). Suppression of induced pluripotent stem cell generation by the p53-p21 pathway. *Nature* 460, 1132-1135.

Horcher, M., Souabni, A., and Busslinger, M. (2001). Pax5/BSAP maintains the identity of B cells in late B lymphopoiesis. *Immunity* 14, 779-790.

Hu, M., Krause, D., Greaves, M., Sharkis, S., Dexter, M., Heyworth, C., and Enver, T. (1997). Multilineage gene expression precedes commitment in the hemopoietic system. *Genes Dev* 11, 774-785.

Huang, S. (2009). Reprogramming cell fates: reconciling rarity with robustness. *Bioessays* 31, 546-560.

Huang, S., Ernberg, I., and Kauffman, S. (2009). Cancer attractors: a systems view of tumors from a gene network dynamics and developmental perspective. *Semin Cell Dev Biol* 20, 869-876.

Huangfu, D., Maehr, R., Guo, W., Eijkelenboom, A., Snitow, M., Chen, A.E., and Melton, D.A. (2008). Induction of pluripotent stem cells by defined factors is greatly improved by small-molecule compounds. *Nat Biotechnol* 26, 795-797.

Huntly, B.J., Shigematsu, H., Deguchi, K., Lee, B.H., Mizuno, S., Duclos, N., Rowan, R., Amaral, S., Curley, D., Williams, I.R., *et al.* (2004). MOZ-TIF2, but not BCR-ABL, confers properties of leukemic stem cells to committed murine hematopoietic progenitors. *Cancer Cell* 6, 587-596.

Igarashi, H., Gregory, S.C., Yokota, T., Sakaguchi, N., and Kincade, P.W. (2002). Transcription from the RAG1 locus marks the earliest lymphocyte progenitors in bone marrow. *Immunity* 17, 117-130.

Jones, R.S. (2007). Epigenetics: reversing the 'irreversible'. *Nature* 450, 357-359.

Joseph, N.M., Mosher, J.T., Buchstaller, J., Snider, P., McKeever, P.E., Lim, M., Conway, S.J., Parada, L.F., Zhu, Y., and Morrison, S.J. (2008). The loss of Nf1 transiently promotes self-renewal but not tumorigenesis by neural crest stem cells. *Cancer Cell* 13, 129-140.

Jung, D., Giallourakis, C., Mostoslavsky, R., and Alt, F.W. (2006). Mechanism and control of V(D)J recombination at the immunoglobulin heavy chain locus. *Annu Rev Immunol* 24, 541-570.

Kalmar, T., Lim, C., Hayward, P., Munoz-Descalzo, S., Nichols, J., Garcia-Ojalvo, J., and Martinez Arias, A. (2009). Regulated fluctuations in nanog expression mediate cell fate decisions in embryonic stem cells. *PLoS Biol* 7, e1000149.

Kallies, A., and Nutt, S.L. (2007). Terminal differentiation of lymphocytes depends on Blimp-1. *Curr Opin Immunol* 19, 156-162.

Kaminskas, E., Farrell, A., Abraham, S., Baird, A., Hsieh, L.S., Lee, S.L., Leighton, J.K., Patel, H., Rahman, A., Sridhara, R., *et al.* (2005). Approval summary: azacitidine for treatment of myelodysplastic syndrome subtypes. *Clin Cancer Res* 11, 3604-3608.

Kawamura, T., Suzuki, J., Wang, Y.V., Menendez, S., Morera, L.B., Raya, A., Wahl, G.M., and Belmonte, J.C. (2009). Linking the p53 tumour suppressor pathway to somatic cell reprogramming. *Nature* 460, 1140-1144.

Klein, U., and Dalla-Favera, R. (2008). Germinal centres: role in B-cell physiology and malignancy. *Nat Rev Immunol* 8, 22-33.

Kondo, M., Weissman, I.L., and Akashi, K. (1997). Identification of clonogenic common lymphoid progenitors in mouse bone marrow. *Cell* 91, 661-672.

Krivtsov, A.V., Twomey, D., Feng, Z., Stubbs, M.C., Wang, Y., Faber, J., Levine, J.E., Wang, J., Hahn, W.C., Gilliland, D.G., *et al.* (2006). Transformation from committed progenitor to leukaemia stem cell initiated by MLL-AF9. *Nature* 442, 818-822.

Krizhanovsky, V., and Lowe, S.W. (2009). Stem cells: The promises and perils of p53. *Nature* 460, 1085-1086.

Laiosa, C.V., Stadtfeld, M., and Graf, T. (2006). Determinants of lymphoid-myeloid lineage diversification. *Annu Rev Immunol* 24, 705-738.

Lane, A.A., and Chabner, B.A. (2009). Histone deacetylase inhibitors in cancer therapy. *J Clin Oncol* 27, 5459-5468.

Lane, M.A., Sainten, A., and Cooper, G.M. (1982). Stage-specific transforming genes of human and mouse B- and T-lymphocyte neoplasms. *Cell* 28, 873-880.

Lane, S.W., and Gilliland, D.G. (2010). Leukemia stem cells. *Semin Cancer Biol* 20, 71-76.

Lang, D., Lu, M.M., Huang, L., Engleka, K.A., Zhang, M., Chu, E.Y., Lipner, S., Skoultchi, A., Millar, S.E., and Epstein, J.A. (2005). Pax3 functions at a nodal point in melanocyte stem cell differentiation. *Nature* 433, 884-887.

le Viseur, C., Hotfilder, M., Bomken, S., Wilson, K., Rottgers, S., Schrauder, A., Rosemann, A., Irving, J., Stam, R.W., Shultz, L.D., *et al.* (2008). In childhood acute lymphoblastic leukemia, blasts at different stages of immunophenotypic maturation have stem cell properties. *Cancer Cell* 14, 47-58.

Li, H., Collado, M., Villasante, A., Strati, K., Ortega, S., Canamero, M., Blasco, M.A., and Serrano, M. (2009). The Ink4/Arf locus is a barrier for iPS cell reprogramming. *Nature* 460, 1136-1139.

Li, L., Connelly, M.C., Wetmore, C., Curran, T., and Morgan, J.I. (2003). Mouse embryos cloned from brain tumors. *Cancer Res* 63, 2733-2736.

Lin, K.I., Angelin-Duclos, C., Kuo, T.C., and Calame, K. (2002). Blimp-1-dependent repression of Pax-5 is required for differentiation of B cells to immunoglobulin M-secreting plasma cells. *Mol Cell Biol* 22, 4771-4780.

Lobo, N.A., Shimono, Y., Qian, D., and Clarke, M.F. (2007). The biology of cancer stem cells. *Annu Rev Cell Dev Biol* 23, 675-699.

Loh, Y.H., Wu, Q., Chew, J.L., Vega, V.B., Zhang, W., Chen, X., Bourque, G., George, J., Leong, B., Liu, J., *et al.* (2006). The Oct4 and Nanog transcription network regulates pluripotency in mouse embryonic stem cells. *Nat Genet* 38, 431-440.

Loose, M., Swiers, G., and Patient, R. (2007). Transcriptional networks regulating hematopoietic cell fate decisions. *Curr Opin Hematol* 14, 307-314.

Maherali, N., Sridharan, R., Xie, W., Utikal, J., Eminli, S., Arnold, K., Stadtfeld, M., Yachechko, R., Tchieu, J., Jaenisch, R., *et al.* (2007). Directly reprogrammed fibroblasts show global epigenetic remodeling and widespread tissue contribution. *Cell Stem Cell* 1, 55-70.

Marion, R.M., Strati, K., Li, H., Murga, M., Blanco, R., Ortega, S., Fernandez-Capetillo, O., Serrano, M., and Blasco, M.A. (2009). A p53-mediated DNA damage response limits reprogramming to ensure iPS cell genomic integrity. *Nature* 460, 1149-1153.

Martins, G., and Calame, K. (2008). Regulation and functions of Blimp-1 in T and B lymphocytes. *Annu Rev Immunol* 26, 133-169.

Mathas, S., Janz, M., Hummel, F., Hummel, M., Wollert-Wulf, B., Lusatis, S., Anagnostopoulos, I., Lietz, A., Sigvardsson, M., Jundt, F., *et al.* (2006). Intrinsic inhibition of transcription factor E2A by HLH proteins ABF-1 and Id2 mediates reprogramming of neoplastic B cells in Hodgkin lymphoma. *Nat Immunol* 7, 207-215.

Melo, J.V., and Barnes, D.J. (2007). Chronic myeloid leukaemia as a model of disease evolution in human cancer. *Nat Rev Cancer* 7, 441-453.

Mikkelsen, T.S., Hanna, J., Zhang, X., Ku, M., Wernig, M., Schorderet, P., Bernstein, B.E., Jaenisch, R., Lander, E.S., and Meissner, A. (2008). Dissecting direct reprogramming through integrative genomic analysis. *Nature* 454, 49-55.

Mikkelsen, T.S., Ku, M., Jaffe, D.B., Issac, B., Lieberman, E., Giannoukos, G., Alvarez, P., Brockman, W., Kim, T.K., Koche, R.P., *et al.* (2007). Genome-wide maps of chromatin state in pluripotent and lineage-committed cells. *Nature* 448, 553-560.

Mikkola, I., Heavey, B., Horcher, M., and Busslinger, M. (2002). Reversion of B cell commitment upon loss of Pax5 expression. *Science* 297, 110-113.

Miller, J.P., Izon, D., DeMuth, W., Gerstein, R., Bhandoola, A., and Allman, D. (2002). The earliest step in B lineage differentiation from common lymphoid progenitors is critically dependent upon interleukin 7. *J Exp Med* 196, 705-711.

Miyamoto, T., Weissman, I.L., and Akashi, K. (2000). AML1/ETO-expressing nonleukemic stem cells in acute myelogenous leukemia with 8;21 chromosomal translocation. *Proc Natl Acad Sci U S A* 97, 7521-7526.

Mullighan, C.G., Phillips, L.A., Su, X., Ma, J., Miller, C.B., Shurtleff, S.A., and Downing, J.R. (2008). Genomic analysis of the clonal origins of relapsed acute lymphoblastic leukemia. *Science* 322, 1377-1380.

Nakagawa, M., Koyanagi, M., Tanabe, K., Takahashi, K., Ichisaka, T., Aoi, T., Okita, K., Mochiduki, Y., Takizawa, N., and Yamanaka, S. (2008). Generation of induced pluripotent stem cells without Myc from mouse and human fibroblasts. *Nat Biotechnol* 26, 101-106.

Niakan, K.K., Ji, H., Maehr, R., Vokes, S.A., Rodolfa, K.T., Sherwood, R.I., Yamaki, M., Dimos, J.T., Chen, A.E., Melton, D.A., *et al.* (2010). Sox17 promotes differentiation in mouse embryonic stem cells by directly regulating extraembryonic gene expression and indirectly antagonizing self-renewal. *Genes Dev* 24, 312-326.

Nutt, S.L., Heavey, B., Rolink, A.G., and Busslinger, M. (1999). Commitment to the B-lymphoid lineage depends on the transcription factor Pax5. *Nature* 401, 556-562.

Nutt, S.L., and Kee, B.L. (2007). The transcriptional regulation of B cell lineage commitment. *Immunity* 26, 715-725.

Odelberg, S.J. (2004). Unraveling the molecular basis for regenerative cellular plasticity. *PLoS Biol* 2, E232.

Okita, K., Ichisaka, T., and Yamanaka, S. (2007). Generation of germline-competent induced pluripotent stem cells. *Nature* 448, 313-317.

Parada, L.F., Tabin, C.J., Shih, C., and Weinberg, R.A. (1982). Human EJ bladder carcinoma oncogene is homologue of Harvey sarcoma virus ras gene. *Nature* 297, 474-478.

Perez-Caro, M., Cobaleda, C., Gonzalez-Herrero, I., Vicente-Duenas, C., Bermejo-Rodriguez, C., Sanchez-Beato, M., Orfao, A., Pintado, B., Flores, T., Sanchez-Martin, M., *et al.* (2009). Cancer induction by restriction of oncogene expression to the stem cell compartment. *Embo J* 28, 8-20.

Pietersen, A.M., and van Lohuizen, M. (2008). Stem cell regulation by polycomb repressors: postponing commitment. *Curr Opin Cell Biol* 20, 201-207.

Reaumur, R.A.F. (1712). Sur les diverses reproductions qui se font dans les écrevisses, les omars, les crabes, etc. et entr'autres sur celles de leurs jambes et de leurs écailles. *Mém Acad Roy Sci*, 223-245.

Reya, T., Morrison, S.J., Clarke, M.F., and Weissman, I.L. (2001). Stem cells, cancer, and cancer stem cells. *Nature* 414, 105-111.

Ringrose, L., and Paro, R. (2004). Epigenetic regulation of cellular memory by the Polycomb and Trithorax group proteins. *Annu Rev Genet* 38, 413-443.

Ringrose, L., and Paro, R. (2007). Polycomb/Trithorax response elements and epigenetic memory of cell identity. *Development* 134, 223-232.

Roh, T.Y., Cuddapah, S., Cui, K., and Zhao, K. (2006). The genomic landscape of histone modifications in human T cells. *Proc Natl Acad Sci U S A* 103, 15782-15787.

Rowland, B.D., Bernards, R., and Peeper, D.S. (2005). The KLF4 tumour suppressor is a transcriptional repressor of p53 that acts as a context-dependent oncogene. *Nat Cell Biol* 7, 1074-1082.

Sacchi, S., Kantarjian, H.M., O'Brien, S., Cortes, J., Rios, M.B., Giles, F.J., Beran, M., Koller, C.A., Keating, M.J., and Talpaz, M. (1999). Chronic myelogenous leukemia in nonlymphoid blastic phase: analysis of the results of first salvage therapy with three different treatment approaches for 162 patients. *Cancer* 86, 2632-2641.

Sanchez-Garcia, I. (2010). Getting to the stem of cancer. *Semin Cancer Biol* 20, 63-64.

Sanchez-Garcia, I. (1997). Consequences of chromosomal abnormalities in tumor development. *Annu Rev Genet* 31, 429-453.

Sanchez-Garcia, I., Vicente-Duenas, C., and Cobaleda, C. (2007). The theoretical basis of cancer-stem-cell-based therapeutics of cancer: can it be put into practice? *Bioessays* 29, 1269-1280.

Santos, E., Tronick, S.R., Aaronson, S.A., Pulciani, S., and Barbacid, M. (1982). T24 human bladder carcinoma oncogene is an activated form of the normal human homologue of BALB- and Harvey-MSV transforming genes. *Nature* 298, 343-347.

Schaffer, A.E., Freude, K.K., Nelson, S.B., and Sander, M. (2010). Nkx6 transcription factors and Ptf1a function as antagonistic lineage determinants in multipotent pancreatic progenitors. *Dev Cell* 18, 1022-1029.

Schebesta, A., McManus, S., Salvagiotto, G., Delogu, A., Busslinger, G.A., and Busslinger, M. (2007). Transcription factor Pax5 activates the chromatin of key genes involved in B cell signaling, adhesion, migration, and immune function. *Immunity* 27, 49-63.

Schneuwly, S., Klemenz, R., and Gehring, W.J. (1987). Redesigning the body plan of Drosophila by ectopic expression of the homoeotic gene Antennapedia. *Nature* 325, 816-818.

Shackleton, M. Normal stem cells and cancer stem cells: similar and different. *Semin Cancer Biol* 20, 85-92.

Shaffer, A.L., Lin, K.I., Kuo, T.C., Yu, X., Hurt, E.M., Rosenwald, A., Giltnane, J.M., Yang, L., Zhao, H., Calame, K., and Staudt, L.M. (2002). Blimp-1 orchestrates plasma cell differentiation by extinguishing the mature B cell gene expression program. *Immunity* 17, 51-62.

Shapiro-Shelef, M., and Calame, K. (2005). Regulation of plasma-cell development. *Nat Rev Immunol* 5, 230-242.

Sharov, A.A., and Ko, M.S. (2007). Human ES cell profiling broadens the reach of bivalent domains. *Cell Stem Cell* 1, 237-238.

Shi, Y., Desponts, C., Do, J.T., Hahm, H.S., Scholer, H.R., and Ding, S. (2008). Induction of pluripotent stem cells from mouse embryonic fibroblasts by Oct4 and Klf4 with small-molecule compounds. *Cell Stem Cell* 3, 568-574.

Shih, C., Shilo, B.Z., Goldfarb, M.P., Dannenberg, A., and Weinberg, R.A. (1979). Passage of phenotypes of chemically transformed cells via transfection of DNA and chromatin. *Proc Natl Acad Sci U S A* 76, 5714-5718.

So, C.W., Karsunky, H., Passegue, E., Cozzio, A., Weissman, I.L., and Cleary, M.L. (2003). MLL-GAS7 transforms multipotent hematopoietic progenitors and induces mixed lineage leukemias in mice. *Cancer Cell* 3, 161-171.

Somervaille, T.C., and Cleary, M.L. (2006). Identification and characterization of leukemia stem cells in murine MLL-AF9 acute myeloid leukemia. *Cancer Cell* 10, 257-268.

Spallanzani, L. (1769). Prodromo di un opera da imprimersi sopra la riproduzioni animali (An Essay on Animal Reproduction). T.B.d. Hondt, ed. (London).

Sridharan, R., Tchieu, J., Mason, M.J., Yachechko, R., Kuoy, E., Horvath, S., Zhou, Q., and Plath, K. (2009). Role of the murine reprogramming factors in the induction of pluripotency. *Cell* 136, 364-377.

Stadtfeld, M., Maherali, N., Breault, D.T., and Hochedlinger, K. (2008a). Defining molecular cornerstones during fibroblast to iPS cell reprogramming in mouse. *Cell Stem Cell* 2, 230-240.

Stadtfeld, M., Nagaya, M., Utikal, J., Weir, G., and Hochedlinger, K. (2008b). Induced pluripotent stem cells generated without viral integration. *Science* 322, 945-949.

Swiers, G., Patient, R., and Loose, M. (2006). Genetic regulatory networks programming hematopoietic stem cells and erythroid lineage specification. *Dev Biol* 294, 525-540.

Takahashi, K., and Yamanaka, S. (2006). Induction of pluripotent stem cells from mouse embryonic and adult fibroblast cultures by defined factors. *Cell* 126, 663-676.

Tanaka, Y., Era, T., Nishikawa, S., and Kawamata, S. (2007). Forced expression of Nanog in hematopoietic stem cells results in a gammadeltaT-cell disorder. *Blood* 110, 107-115.

Ting, A.H., McGarvey, K.M., and Baylin, S.B. (2006). The cancer epigenome--components and functional correlates. *Genes Dev* 20, 3215-3231.

Trembley, A. (1744). Memoires pour Servir a L'histoire d'un Genre de Polypes d'eau Douce, a Bras en Forme de Cornes (Leiden: Jean and Herman Verbeek).

Uhlenhaut, N.H., Jakob, S., Anlag, K., Eisenberger, T., Sekido, R., Kress, J., Treier, A.C., Klugmann, C., Klasen, C., Holter, N.I., *et al.* (2009). Somatic sex reprogramming of adult ovaries to testes by FOXL2 ablation. *Cell* 139, 1130-1142.

Urbanek, P., Wang, Z.Q., Fetka, I., Wagner, E.F., and Busslinger, M. (1994). Complete block of early B cell differentiation and altered patterning of the posterior midbrain in mice lacking Pax5/BSAP. *Cell* 79, 901-912.

Utikal, J., Polo, J.M., Stadtfeld, M., Maherali, N., Kulalert, W., Walsh, R.M., Khalil, A., Rheinwald, J.G., and Hochedlinger, K. (2009). Immortalization eliminates a roadblock during cellular reprogramming into iPS cells. *Nature* 460, 1145-1148.

Vicente-Duenas, C., Cobaleda, C., Perez-Losada, J., and Sanchez-Garcia, I. (2010). The evolution of cancer modeling: the shadow of stem cells. *Dis Model Mech* 3, 149-155.

Vicente-Duenas, C., de Diego, J.G., Rodriguez, F.D., Jimenez, R., and Cobaleda, C. (2009a). The Role of Cellular Plasticity in Cancer Development. *Curr Med Chem.*

Vicente-Duenas, C., Perez-Caro, M., Abollo-Jimenez, F., Cobaleda, C., and Sanchez-Garcia, I. (2009b). Stem-cell driven cancer: "hands-off" regulation of cancer development. *Cell Cycle* 8, 1314-1318.

Waddington, C.H. (1957). The Strategy of the Genes (London).

Ward, R.J., and Dirks, P.B. (2007). Cancer stem cells: at the headwaters of tumor development. *Annu Rev Pathol* 2, 175-189.

Wernig, M., Meissner, A., Cassady, J.P., and Jaenisch, R. (2008). c-Myc is dispensable for direct reprogramming of mouse fibroblasts. *Cell Stem Cell* 2, 10-12.

Wernig, M., Meissner, A., Foreman, R., Brambrink, T., Ku, M., Hochedlinger, K., Bernstein, B.E., and Jaenisch, R. (2007). In vitro reprogramming of fibroblasts into a pluripotent ES-cell-like state. *Nature* 448, 318-324.

Wilmut, I., Schnieke, A.E., McWhir, J., Kind, A.J., and Campbell, K.H. (1997). Viable offspring derived from fetal and adult mammalian cells. *Nature* 385, 810-813.

Wojiski, S., Guibal, F.C., Kindler, T., Lee, B.H., Jesneck, J.L., Fabian, A., Tenen, D.G., and Gilliland, D.G. (2009). PML-RARalpha initiates leukemia by conferring properties of self-renewal to committed promyelocytic progenitors. *Leukemia* 23, 1462-1471.

Wong, D.J., Liu, H., Ridky, T.W., Cassarino, D., Segal, E., and Chang, H.Y. (2008). Module map of stem cell genes guides creation of epithelial cancer stem cells. *Cell Stem Cell* 2, 333-344.

Xie, H., Ye, M., Feng, R., and Graf, T. (2004). Stepwise reprogramming of B cells into macrophages. *Cell* 117, 663-676.

Yamanaka, S. (2009). Elite and stochastic models for induced pluripotent stem cell generation. *Nature* 460, 49-52.

Yamanaka, S., and Blau, H.M. (2010). Nuclear reprogramming to a pluripotent state by three approaches. *Nature* 465, 704-712.

Zhao, Y., Yin, X., Qin, H., Zhu, F., Liu, H., Yang, W., Zhang, Q., Xiang, C., Hou, P., Song, Z., *et al.* (2008). Two supporting factors greatly improve the efficiency of human iPSC generation. *Cell Stem Cell* 3, 475-479.

Zheng, H., Chang, L., Patel, N., Yang, J., Lowe, L., Burns, D.K., and Zhu, Y. (2008). Induction of abnormal proliferation by nonmyelinating schwann cells triggers neurofibroma formation. *Cancer Cell* 13, 117-128.

Zhou, Q., Brown, J., Kanarek, A., Rajagopal, J., and Melton, D.A. (2008). In vivo reprogramming of adult pancreatic exocrine cells to beta-cells. *Nature* 455, 627-632.

Zhou, Q., and Melton, D.A. (2008a). Extreme makeover: converting one cell into another. *Cell Stem Cell* 3, 382-388.

Zhou, Q., and Melton, D.A. (2008b). Pathways to New {beta} Cells. *Cold Spring Harb Symp Quant Biol.*

Zhu, L., Gibson, P., Currle, D.S., Tong, Y., Richardson, R.J., Bayazitov, I.T., Poppleton, H., Zakharenko, S., Ellison, D.W., and Gilbertson, R.J. (2008). Prominin 1 marks intestinal stem cells that are susceptible to neoplastic transformation. *Nature*

2

From where do Cancer-Initiating Cells Originate?

Stéphane Ansieau[1], Anne-Pierre Morel[1,2] and Alain Puisieux[1,2,3]
[1,2,3]*Inserm, U590, Lyon, F-69008*
[2,3]*Centre Léon Bérard, Lyon, F-69008*
[3]*Université Lyon I, Lyon, F-69008*
France

1. Introduction

Cancer development is generally depicted as successive waves of Darwinian selection of cells harbouring genetic and epigenetic abnormalities, providing them with proliferative, survival and adaptive advantages. As genetic alterations preferentially operate on naked DNA, original targeted cells are presumably either proliferating or engaged in a reprogramming process, both cellular mechanisms being associated with chromatin decondensation. Taking this point in consideration, appropriate candidates include a large set of embryonic cells (or embryonic stem-cells) as well as adult stem/progenitor cells when engaged in a repopulation process, a mechanism either permanent as in regenerative tissues such as the intestine, the colon or the skin, or sporadically induced in response to insults, such as wound healings. Studies of hematopoietic cancers point out that the malignancy might originate from the alteration of a single cell displaying both self-renewal and differentiation potentials. By similarity with normal stem-cells, that are able to reconstitute a complete tissue, this observation led to the development of the "cancer stem-cell" (CSC) concept. Indeed, in chronic myeloid leukaemia (CML), several type of blood cells including their most primitive precursors display a similar chromosomal recombination (named the Philadelphia chromosome) leading to the production of the aberrant BCR-ABLp120 fusion protein. This genetic alteration was therefore likely to drive transformation of precursor cells or stem-cells, deregulating the production of mature cells without affecting their ability to execute their normal differentiation (Bonnet and Dick, 1997). Accordingly, the restricted expression of the aberrant BCR-ABLp120 fusion protein in $Sca1^+$ stem-cells was shown, in transgenic mice, to mimic human CML, characterized by a progression from chronic towards an acute phase (Perez-Caro et al., 2009). While the inhibition of the activity of the kinase by the ST1571 chemical compound, according to the resistance of the human leukaemia stem cells to the chemical (Graham et al., 2002; Hu et al., 2006; Primo et al., 2006; Jiang et al., 2007), did not modify the survival of the transgenic mice, CSC ablation eradicated tumours, demonstrating undoubtedly their role in AML development and the therapeutic interest of eradicating them (Perez-Caro et al., 2009). Since then, a large number of laboratories attempt to extend the CSC theory to solid tumours. The observation that metastases and their original primary tumour share a similar heterogeneity indeed argue in favour of the presence of a subset of CSCs displaying both self-renewing and differentiation capabilities. In such a scenario, CSCs are expected to represent a minor population of the tumour, giving rise to differentiated cells that, per definition, would have lost their self-renewal capabilities and thereby their tumour driving potential. In the last decade, based on phenotypic and/or functional similarities with their normal counterparts, CSCs have been successfully isolated form numerous cancer types, including breast tumours, gliomas and melanomas and described as displaying self-renewal and differentiation properties. Validating the concept that a limited number of cells resulting from the transformation of normal stem-cells continuously fuel the tumour has constituted a real breakthrough in the cancer field and has had major repercussions in the design of novel therapeutic approaches. Nonetheless, as discussed below, several of the experimental assays commonly used to evaluate stem-like properties are individually questionable. These doubts raise some concerns on the real biological properties of the isolated CSC subpopulations and impact on the current debate concerning their potential origin. Noticeably, even the term of "cancer stem-cells" is probably not appropriated referring to their normal counterparts. Although some adult normal stem-cells were found to be highly proliferative (Barker et al., 2009), they generally are depicted as poorly proliferating cells, able to concomitantly maintain their pool and generate their progeny through asymmetric divisions. As far as we know, if the proportion of CSC is maintained during tumour growth, this is far away of demonstrating that they actually share this same property. The potential filiation between normal stem-cells and CSCs thus remains a matter of discussion, leading to the emergence of the alternative "tumour-initiating cells" terminology.

The questionable characterisation of CSC

In this first section, we will attempt to demonstrate the limit of the techniques currently used for isolating CSCs and the conflicting results they provide. These techniques consist in identifying CSCs by exploiting expected similarities with their normal counterparts, including some phenotypic features, their ability to efflux drugs and to grow as colonospheres, when cultured in low adherent conditions. Sorting CSC from tumours or tumour cell lines, taking advantage of specific stem-cell markers, is a commonly used approach but *in fine* turned out to be more difficult as previously thought. A major reason is that this notion of "specificity" is often biased by the quality of the available antibodies used and by our current limited knowledge on normal stem cell features. A significant example is provided by the contradictory results generated by using the transmembrane protein CD133 as a stem-cell marker. In numerous studies, monoclonal antibodies to CD133 were defined as appropriate tools to isolate CSC from various tumour types (Barker et al., 2009; Yin et al., 1997; Uchida et al., 2000; Lee et al., 2005; Sagrinati et al., 2006; Richardson et al., 2004; Kordes et al., 2007; Oshima et al., 2007; Sugiyama et al., 2007; Ito et al., 2007). Nonetheless, by generating transgenic mice expressing the LacZ reporter gene under the control of the CD133 promoting sequences, the transmembrane protein was found expressed by mature luminal ductal epithelial cells in adult organs, suggesting that it is not a specific marker of stem-cells (Shmelkov et al., 2008). The interest in using CD133 was further challenged, as these authors next demonstrated, taking advantage of IL10 knock-out mice, that cancer cells in primary colon carcinomas uniformly express CD133. Evenmore, $CD133^+$ and $CD133^-$ cells isolated from secondary tumours display similar tumorigenic potential, as assessed by serial transplantations into immuno-compromised mice, and were both capable of forming colonospheres *in vitro* at a similar rate (Shmelkov et al., 2008).

The ability of stem cells to efflux drugs, due to a high expression level of transporters, was also exploited for isolating CSCs. This approach led to the detection by flow cytometry of a population of cells named side population (SP), able to efflux the DNA binding Hoechst 3342 dye. Unfortunately SP and CSC populations do not always match. In mice bone marrows, SP subpopulation was originally found to be enriched in hematopoietic stem cells (Goodell et al., 1996). Consistently, progenitor cells were restricted to the SP fraction of mammospheres (Dontu et al., 2003) and SP purified from several cancer cell lines show enhanced tumorigenicity *in vivo* relative to their non-SP cohorts (Ho et al., 2007; Patrawala et al., 2005). Nonetheless, in some tumor types, SP populations are not enriched in SSC (Mitsutake et al., 2007; Stingl et al., 2006; Burger et al., 2004) and purified mouse mammary SP cells do not efficiently repopulate the mammary gland in a reconstitution assay (Alvi et al., 2003). This discrepancy is likely to reflect the existence of various cell populations that actually share with stem-cells a set of common properties.

Enrichment in stem-cells in low adherent culture conditions is an additional commonly used approach to isolate CSC. This technology was originally performed to evaluate the self-renewal capacity of neural cells (Reynolds and Weiss, 1996), next adopted for human breast epithelial cells to form mammospheres (Dontu et al., 2003) and finally extended to various cancer types. Individual cells able to grow in low adherent conditions for up to five consecutive passages indeed display a gene expression profile consistent with progenitor properties, validating the experimental approach. These conditions might however simply select for cells displaying resistance to anoïkis. One could easily envisage that the stress conditions provided by the low adherence actually enforce cells to adapt through a genomic reprogramming, potentially a partial dedifferentiation, leading to the expression of some stem cell-associated genes. Evenmore, the function of normal stem cells is highly regulated by their niche through direct and paracrine interactions with supporting cells and the extracellular matrix. One could then wonder why in sphere cultures, in absence of this niche, cells might display stem-cell properties.

A more recent assay has consisted in purifying CSC based on the detoxifying aldehyde dehydrogenase 1 (ALDH1) enzymatic activity, previously detected in a set of normal stem-cells (Armstrong et al., 2004; Matsui et al., 2004; Hess et al., 2004). Nonetheless, attempts to isolate breast CSCs according to their antigenic phenotype or to their ALDH1 activity led again to the isolation of different cell subpopulations that at the most partially overlap, suggesting that actually any of these markers are strictly allotted to stem-cells (Al-Hajj et al., 2003; Fillmore and Kuperwasser, 2008; Ginestier et al., 2007).

The stem cell potentiality of the presumed isolated CSC subpopulations is next evaluated through various functional assays. As theoretically, a single CSC should be able to reconstitute a complete tumour, a commonly used assay consists in evaluating their tumorigenic potential when xenografted at limit dilutions in immunosuppressive mice. This assay turns out being also questionable. Considering that cells have to evade from the immune system (even in immuno-compromised hosts), their antigenic phenotype and their immunosuppressive properties might impinge on their tumorigenic potential. Moreover, their ability to interfere with the host environment is undoubtedly a limiting factor. Taking this information in consideration, optimisation of the experimental conditions, including selection of more highly immuno-compromised or humanised mice, dramatically increased the detectable frequency of tumorigenic cells (Quintana et al., 2008). One fourth of melanoma cells were thus found to display a tumorigenic potential, independently of their CD133 antigenic phenotype (Quintana et al., 2008). Consistently, a large proportion of cells isolated from primary Eμ-Myc pre-B/B lymphoma, Eμ-N-Ras thymic lymphomas and PU.1$^{-/-}$ acute myeloid leukaemia sustain tumour growth when transplanted in NOD/SCID immuno-deficient mice, challenging the concept that tumours arise from rare CSCs, at least for malignancies with substantial homogeneity (Kelly et al., 2007). Recently, the Herlyn laboratory actually demonstrated that CSCs did not contribute to tumour initiation but were rather found as essential for long term maintenance, as judged by serial transplantations in *nude* mice (Roesch et al., 2010). Finally, transplantations in mice are generally performed with individualised cells, although maintaining them in a niche has recently been shown as determinant for their tumorigenic potential (Liu et al., 2009). Conclusions based on xenograft experiments should therefore be considered with caution.

If CSCs are able to reconstitute the heterogeneous populations of a primary tumour, they are additionally suggested to display a differential potential (Dirks, 2008). As previously mentioned, CSCs are often sorted out of primary tumours/cell lines based on the expression of specific antigens. By definition, the non cancer stem-cell subpopulation that presumably represents the large pool of differentiated cells constituting the bulk of the tumour is represented by the cellular fraction lacking this specific marker. The differentiation potential of the presumed isolated CSCs often relies on their ability to evolve into their differentiated counterparts. While this shift is likely to reflect some reprogramming, these data are far away from demonstrating pluri-potentiality, with a potential to commit into various differentiation programs. At the most, transplantation of these cells in mice gives rise to tumours that display a similar heterogeneity as the primary tumours they originate from. Whether this heterogeneity reflects an adaptive partial reprogramming rather than a dedifferentiation-differentiation process is plausible.

In conclusion, various recent observations reveal the intrinsic limits of each of these experimental approaches. While combining them is probably helpful in interpreting the results, it is obviously not sufficient, implying the development of additional tools. The establishment of novel transgenic mouse models is undoubtedly a promising alternative in further exploring tumour initiation. As a first example, the activation of the Wnt pathway in LG5^{+}/CD133^{+} or Bmi1^{+} intestine stem cells was recently found to promote adenomas while it fails to do so when induced in short-lived transit amplifying cells (Barker et al., 2009; Zhu et al., 2009). These studies provide first evidences that a window of time exists for mutations in intestinal epithelial cells to initiate tumour formation. More sophisticated engineered transgenic mouse models, recapitulating the sequential accumulation of genetic alterations will probably be of further help in understanding the tumour progression process in the next future.

Origins of CSCs

While some studies suggest that CSC may arise from the transformation of their normal counterparts, recent observations rather suggest that they originate from fully differentiated cells through an adaptive transdifferentiation program (Figure 1). This hypothesis originally

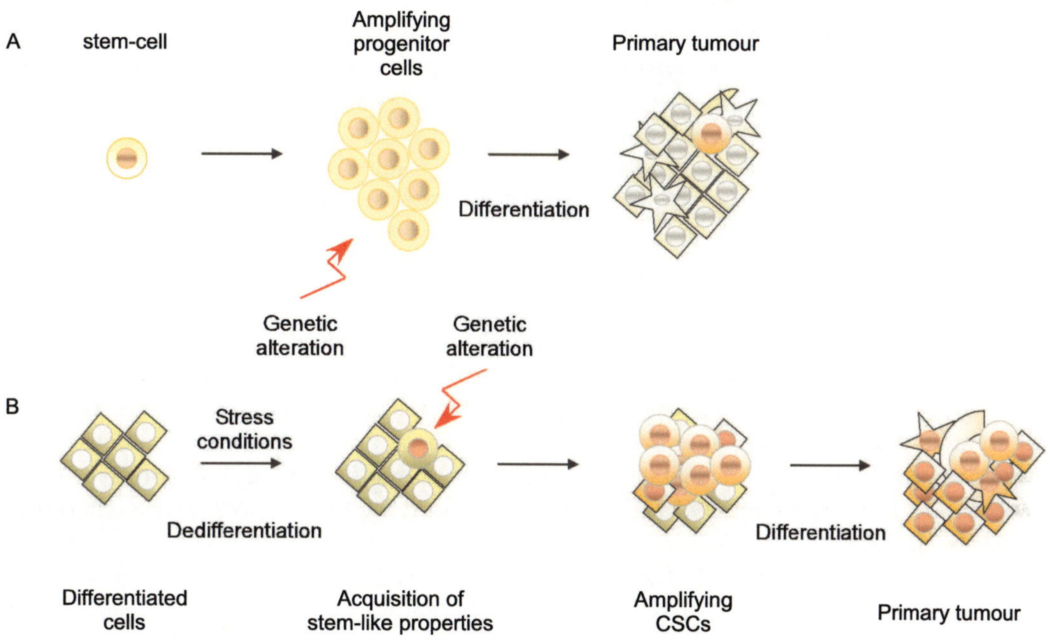

Fig. 1. The "cancer stem-cell theory" (panel A) is based on the assumption that during tissue regeneration, the amplification of progenitor cells opens a window of time suitable for accumulating genetic alterations, leading to the emergence of cancer cell-stems (CSCs). CSCs would thus initiate and sustain tumour growth.
Alternatively, under stress conditions, fully differentiated cells reacquire stem-like properties, including self-renewal properties (panel B). This gain of function is influenced by cellular intrinsic properties as well as micro-environmental conditions. These cells could potentially be prone to transformation and give rise to CSCs.
Both models are not exclusive. CSCs and cell dedifferentiation would thus constitute the initial and secondary tumour drivers, respectively.

emerges from *in vitro* cell transformation assays. Transformation of human mammary epithelial cells (HMECs) consisted in sequentially infecting cells with the catalytic sub-unit of the telomerase (immortalisation step), the SV40 T/t antigens (these viral proteins have pleiotropic effects including the neutralisation of both Rb- and p53-dependent-oncosuppressive pathways) and an activated version of the mitogenic protein Ras (H-Ras^{G12V}) (Elenbaas et al., 2001). Cell transformation was found to be invariably associated with cellular morphological changes associated with an epithelial-mesenchymal transition (EMT) (Morel et al., 2008; Mani et al., 2008). EMT is a trans-differentiation process that consists in turning polarized and adjacent epithelial cells into individual and motile mesenchymal ones. Originally identified as a biological process essential for the morphogenetic movements during the embryonic development, its aberrant reactivation in cancers is currently considered as one of the main driving cancer cell dissemination (Thiery et al., 2009). Studying the contribution of EMT in cell transformation led to the demonstration that it actually constitutes a dedifferentiation process, providing cells with some stem-like properties (Morel et al., 2008; Mani et al., 2008; Vesuna et al., 2009). Cells that have undergone an EMT were thus found to form mammospheres in low adherent conditions and to be highly tumorigenic when orthotopically xenografted at limit dilution in *nude* mice. They additionally display a $CD44^{high}$ $CD24^{low}$ antigenic phenotype that was previously allotted to mammary CSCs (Al-Hajj et al., 2003). EMT being by definition a reversible process, these cells continuously generate $CD44^{low}$ $CD24^{high}$ epithelial cells that interestingly lack a tumorigenic potential (Morel et al., 2008; Mani et al., 2008; Vesuna et al., 2009). In regards to the EMT-associated properties, the transdifferentiation process was thus considered as a biological process able to convert differentiated epithelial cells into CSCs. EMT being strongly impacted by micro-environmental conditions, the balance between differentiated cells and CSCs was then proposed to be a highly dynamic process with important repercussions on therapeutic approaches, eradication of the entire primary tumour, including differentiated cells, being henceforth a requisite to prevent recurrence (Gupta et al., 2009).

Despite the obvious interest of these works, we still can emit some reserve about their meaning. Obviously, EMT is a reversible transdifferentiation process associated with a profound genetic reprogramming and major consequent phenotypic changes. Considering that mesenchymal cells display a pluripotency based on their ability to turn into epithelial ones, is probably a miss-interpretation, rather reflecting the equilibrium between the two cell fates of this transdifferentiation process. Recently, in appropriate culture conditions, HMEC-transformed mesenchymal derivatives were found to initiate chondrocytic, adipocytic or osteoblastic differentiation programs, highlighting their pluripotency (Battula et al., 2010). Nonetheless, as previously mentioned, these cells harbour a set of genetic alterations, including the expression of viral proteins which are known to impact on multiple cellular functions. Whether similar results would be obtained in more "physiological" conditions, by combining EMT-permissive conditions with a restricted number of genetic events, is warranted to further evaluate the relevance of these observations. The CSC features of these HMEC derivatives were next supported by their tumorigenic potentials at limiting conditions. If CSCs are rather important for tumour maintenance than for tumour initiation (Roesch et al., 2010), this result would more highlight a direct role of EMT in facilitating cell transformation and tumour initiation. Finally, these cells were described as displaying a similar antigenic phenotype as the one originally attributed to mammary CSCs (Al-Hajj et al., 2003) Nonetheless, likewise the $CD133^{+}$ population, $CD44^{high}CD24^{low}$ cells might actually include much more than the CSCs, which antigenic phenotype has been restricted to $CD44^{high}CD24^{low}ESA^{+}$ or $CD44^{high}CD24^{low}ALDH1^{+}$ cells (Fillmore and Kuperwasser, 2008; Ginestier et al., 2007). Rather than providing cells with real stem-like properties, EMT might actually provide cells with some plasticity, facilitating potentially the transformation process and helping them to adapt to microenvironmental changes. In other terms, this plasticity and adaptation to microenvironmental changes implies that $CD44^{high}CD24^{low}$ mesenchymal cells constitute a pool of tumour-driving cells whereas the $CD44^{low}CD24^{high}$ epithelial counterparts behave as a latent reserve of cancer cells reactivated in hostile conditions. In line with such a model, when exposed to EGFR tyrosine kinase inhibitor (TKI), a minor subpopulation of non small cell lung cancer derived cells that express some stem-cell-associated antigens (such as CD133) adopt a quiescent phenotype and resistance. Emergence of these resistant clones is abrogated in presence of trichostatin, an inhibitor of histone deacetylases, suggesting that it reflects a transient reprogramming, involving epigenetic changes, rather than an enrichment of a pre-existing cell subpopulation. When maintained in presence of TKI, a proportion of these cells restarts proliferating, giving rise to resistant cell lines that revert to a sensitive stage when released from the drug (Sharma et al., 2010). Cell reprogramming thus provides a route for cells to adapt to hostile conditions, a mechanism that the authors interestingly compare to the antibiotic-tolerant bacterial subpopulations termed "persisters" (Sharma et al., 2010). By similarity, EMT might be an escape from hypoxic conditions and mechanical constrains and the stem-like features associated with, just be a mirror of this adaptative process. Whether these cells are particularly prone to transformation, in light of their proliferation capabilities, remains to be determined. Some genetic events might similarly favour cell dedifferentiation into CSCs. Indeed, murine fibroblasts lacking the RB proteins were found to generate colonospheres at confluency and to reconstitute monolayers when plated at lower density. Interestingly, these colonospheres were found to be tumorigenic when xenografted in mice at limit dilutions, to include a SP, to express stem-cell markers and to additionally display differentiation properties (Liu et al., 2009). In conclusion, this plasticity might provide cells with survival advantages, when placed in hostile conditions. Overall, these recent observations demonstrate that the stem-like properties harboured by numerous cancer cells do not rely on any particular relationship to normal stem-cells but rather reflect the Darwinian selection that operates within a tumour.

Evolution of the concepts and therapeutic consequences

According to the CSC theory, eradicating the rare CSCs would be sufficient to clear tumours. A selection step implying a gain in plasticity and adaptation potential rather suggests that the eradication of all cancer cells, including the differentiated ones, is actually a requisite to eliminate all risks of recurrence. Beyond the cognitive interest, the origin of CSCs might impact on the design of future therapies. If CSCs display a low proliferation potential, they are supposed to be resistant to standard radio- or chemotherapies. Evenmore, these treatments could have the noxious effect to enforce differentiated cancer cells to evolve into tumour-driving ones. Numerous studies are currently engaged to determine the relative importance of various signalling pathways in these cells. The design of additional drugs that might additionally annihilate the dedifferentiation potential of the differentiated cancer cells should also be considered. Obviously, drugs preventing transient epigenetic changes, such as the histone deacetylase (HDAC) inhibitor trichostatin (TSA) might be appropriate (Sharma et al., 2010). Recently, numerous histone deacetylase inhibitors have been identified and some were recently found as efficient in clinical trials for cancer treating (for recent reviews see Lane and Chabner, 2009; Sebova and Fridrichova, 2010). Alternatively, one could also envisage that the plasticity is maintained to some extent and engaging cells further in a differentiation program might avoid them to rescue from insults, potentially explaining the synergistic effect of some differentiation agents and radiation in eradicating xenografted tumours (Kawamata et al., 2006).

2. Conclusions

The relevance of the cancer-stem cell theory and the origin of CSCs remains currently a matter of discussion. The interpretation of the data obtained in this field is complicated by the fact that selection pressures enforce cancer cells to constantly evolve and gain in plasticity. Adaptation to hostile environment is likely driven by transient dedifferentiation processes, likely associated with the acquisition of some stem-like properties. The co-existence of various cancer cell populations within a primary tumour makes the interpretation of the results somehow difficult. Further investigations with help from novel techniques, including sophisticated transgenic mouse models, will probably clarify the current debate. Undoubtedly, these fields of research will shed light on impenetrable aspects of the tumorigenesis and open up new horizons for eradicating cancers.

3. References

Al-Hajj,M., Wicha,M.S., ito-Hernandez,A., Morrison,S.J., and Clarke,M.F. (2003). Prospective identification of tumorigenic breast cancer cells. Proc. Natl. Acad. Sci. U. S. A *100*, 3983-3988.

Alvi,A.J., Clayton,H., Joshi,C., Enver,T., Ashworth,A., Vivanco,M.M., Dale,T.C., and Smalley,M.J. (2003). Functional and molecular characterisation of mammary side population cells. Breast Cancer Res. *5*, R1-R8.

Armstrong,L., Stojkovic,M., Dimmick,I., Ahmad,S., Stojkovic,P., Hole,N., and Lako, M. (2004). Phenotypic characterization of murine primitive hematopoietic progenitor cells isolated on basis of aldehyde dehydrogenase activity. Stem Cells *22*, 1142-1151.

Barker,N., Ridgway,R.A., van Es,J.H., van de,W.M., Begthel,H., van den,B.M., Danenberg,E., Clarke,A.R., Sansom,O.J., and Clevers,H. (2009). Crypt stem cells as the cells-of-origin of intestinal cancer. Nature *457*, 608-611.

Battula,V.L., Evans,K.W., Hollier,B.G., Shi,Y., Marini,F.C., Ayyanan,A., Wang,R.Y., Brisken,C., Guerra,R., Andreeff,M., and Mani,S.A. (2010). Epithelial-Mesenchymal Transition-Derived Cells Exhibit Multi-Lineage Differentiation Potential Similar to Mesenchymal Stem Cells. Stem Cells.

Bonnet,D. and Dick,J.E. (1997). Human acute myeloid leukemia is organized as a hierarchy that originates from a primitive hematopoietic cell. Nat. Med. *3*, 730-737.

Burger,H., van,T.H., Boersma,A.W., Brok,M., Wiemer,E.A., Stoter,G., and Nooter,K. (2004). Imatinib mesylate (STI571) is a substrate for the breast cancer resistance protein (BCRP)/ABCG2 drug pump. Blood *104*, 2940-2942.

Dirks,P.B. (2008). Brain tumor stem cells: bringing order to the chaos of brain cancer. J. Clin. Oncol. *26*, 2916-2924.

Dontu,G., Abdallah,W.M., Foley,J.M., Jackson,K.W., Clarke,M.F., Kawamura,M.J., and Wicha,M.S. (2003). In vitro propagation and transcriptional profiling of human mammary stem/progenitor cells. Genes Dev. *17,* 1253-1270.

Elenbaas,B., Spirio,L., Koerner,F., Fleming,M.D., Zimonjic,D.B., Donaher,J.L., Popescu,N.C., Hahn,W.C., and Weinberg,R.A. (2001). Human breast cancer cells generated by oncogenic transformation of primary mammary epithelial cells. Genes Dev. *15,* 50-65.

Fillmore,C.M. and Kuperwasser,C. (2008). Human breast cancer cell lines contain stem-like cells that self-renew, give rise to phenotypically diverse progeny and survive chemotherapy. Breast Cancer Res. *10,* R25.

Ginestier,C., Hur,M.H., Charafe-Jauffret,E., Monville,F., Dutcher,J., Brown,M., Jacquemier,J., Viens,P., Kleer,C.G., Liu,S., Schott,A., Hayes,D., Birnbaum,D., Wicha,M.S., and Dontu,G. (2007). ALDH1 is a marker of normal and malignant human mammary stem cells and a predictor of poor clinical outcome. Cell Stem Cell *1,* 555-567.

Goodell,M.A., Brose,K., Paradis,G., Conner,A.S., and Mulligan,R.C. (1996). Isolation and functional properties of murine hematopoietic stem cells that are replicating in vivo. J. Exp. Med. *183,* 1797-1806.

Graham,S.M., Jorgensen,H.G., Allan,E., Pearson,C., Alcorn,M.J., Richmond,L., and Holyoake,T.L. (2002). Primitive, quiescent, Philadelphia-positive stem cells from patients with chronic myeloid leukemia are insensitive to STI571 in vitro . Blood *99,* 319-325.

Gupta,P.B., Chaffer,C.L., and Weinberg,R.A. (2009). Cancer stem cells: mirage or reality? Nat. Med. *15,* 1010-1012.

Hess,D.A., Meyerrose,T.E., Wirthlin,L., Craft,T.P., Herrbrich,P.E., Creer,M.H., and Nolta,J.A. (2004). Functional characterization of highly purified human hematopoietic repopulating cells isolated according to aldehyde dehydrogenase activity. Blood *104,* 1648-1655.

Ho,M.M., Ng,A.V., Lam,S., and Hung,J.Y. (2007). Side population in human lung cancer cell lines and tumors is enriched with stem-like cancer cells. Cancer Res. *67,* 4827-4833.

Hu,Y., Swerdlow,S., Duffy,T.M., Weinmann,R., Lee,F.Y., and Li,S. (2006). Targeting multiple kinase pathways in leukemic progenitors and stem cells is essential for improved treatment of Ph+ leukemia in mice. Proc. Natl. Acad. Sci. U. S. A *103,* 16870-16875.

Ito,Y., Hamazaki,T.S., Ohnuma,K., Tamaki,K., Asashima,M., and Okochi,H. (2007). Isolation of murine hair-inducing cells using the cell surface marker prominin-1/CD133. J. Invest Dermatol. *127,* 1052-1060.

Jiang,X., Zhao,Y., Smith,C., Gasparetto,M., Turhan,A., Eaves,A., and Eaves,C. (2007). Chronic myeloid leukemia stem cells possess multiple unique features of resistance to BCR-ABL targeted therapies. Leukemia *21,* 926-935.

Kawamata,H., Tachibana,M., Fujimori,T., and Imai,Y. (2006). Differentiation-inducing therapy for solid tumors. Curr. Pharm. Des *12,* 379-385.

Kelly,P.N., Dakic,A., Adams,J.M., Nutt,S.L., and Strasser,A. (2007). Tumor growth need not be driven by rare cancer stem cells. Science *317,* 337.

Kordes,C., Sawitza,I., Muller-Marbach,A., le-Agha,N., Keitel,V., Klonowski-Stumpe,H., and Haussinger,D. (2007). CD133+ hepatic stellate cells are progenitor cells. Biochem. Biophys. Res. Commun. *352*, 410-417.

Lane,A.A. and Chabner,B.A. (2009). Histone deacetylase inhibitors in cancer therapy. J. Clin. Oncol. *27*, 5459-5468.

Lee,A., Kessler,J.D., Read,T.A., Kaiser,C., Corbeil,D., Huttner,W.B., Johnson,J.E., and Wechsler-Reya,R.J. (2005). Isolation of neural stem cells from the postnatal cerebellum. Nat. Neurosci. *8*, 723-729.

Liu,Y., Clem,B., Zuba-Surma,E.K., El-Naggar,S., Telang,S., Jenson,A.B., Wang,Y., Shao,H., Ratajczak,M.Z., Chesney,J., and Dean,D.C. (2009). Mouse fibroblasts lacking RB1 function form spheres and undergo reprogramming to a cancer stem cell phenotype. Cell Stem Cell *4*, 336-347.

Mani,S.A., Guo,W., Liao,M.J., Eaton,E.N., Ayyanan,A., Zhou,A.Y., Brooks,M., Reinhard,F., Zhang,C.C., Shipitsin,M., Campbell,L.L., Polyak,K., Brisken,C., Yang,J., and Weinberg,R.A. (2008). The epithelial-mesenchymal transition generates cells with properties of stem cells. Cell *133*, 704-715.

Matsui,W., Huff,C.A., Wang,Q., Malehorn,M.T., Barber,J., Tanhehco,Y., Smith,B.D., Civin,C.I., and Jones,R.J. (2004). Characterization of clonogenic multiple myeloma cells. Blood *103*, 2332-2336.

Mitsutake,N., Iwao,A., Nagai,K., Namba,H., Ohtsuru,A., Saenko,V., and Yamashita, S. (2007). Characterization of side population in thyroid cancer cell lines: cancer stem-like cells are enriched partly but not exclusively. Endocrinology *148*, 1797-1803.

Morel,A.P., Lievre,M., Thomas,C., Hinkal,G., Ansieau,S., and Puisieux,A. (2008). Generation of breast cancer stem cells through epithelial-mesenchymal transition. PLoS. One. *3*, e2888.

Oshima,Y., Suzuki,A., Kawashimo,K., Ishikawa,M., Ohkohchi,N., and Taniguchi,H. (2007). Isolation of mouse pancreatic ductal progenitor cells expressing CD133 and c-Met by flow cytometric cell sorting. Gastroenterology *132*, 720-732.

Patrawala,L., Calhoun,T., Schneider-Broussard,R., Zhou,J., Claypool,K., and Tang,D.G. (2005). Side population is enriched in tumorigenic, stem-like cancer cells, whereas ABCG2+ and A. Cancer Res. *65*, 6207-6219.

Perez-Caro,M., Cobaleda,C., Gonzalez-Herrero,I., Vicente-Duenas,C., Bermejo-Rodriguez,C., Sanchez-Beato,M., Orfao,A., Pintado,B., Flores,T., Sanchez-Martin,M., Jimenez,R., Piris,M.A., and Sanchez-Garcia,I. (2009). Cancer induction by restriction of oncogene expression to the stem cell compartment. EMBO J. *28*, 8-20.

Primo,D., Flores,J., Quijano,S., Sanchez,M.L., Sarasquete,M.E., del Pino-Montes,J., Gaarder,P.I., Gonzalez,M., and Orfao,A. (2006). Impact of BCR/ABL gene expression on the proliferative rate of different subpopulations of haematopoietic cells in chronic myeloid leukaemia. Br. J. Haematol. *135*, 43-51.

Quintana,E., Shackleton,M., Sabel,M.S., Fullen,D.R., Johnson,T.M., and Morrison,S.J. (2008). Efficient tumour formation by single human melanoma cells. Nature *456*, 593-598.

Reynolds,B.A. and Weiss,S. (1996). Clonal and population analyses demonstrate that an EGF-responsive mammalian embryonic CNS precursor is a stem cell. Dev. Biol. *175*, 1-13.

Richardson,G.D., Robson,C.N., Lang,S.H., Neal,D.E., Maitland,N.J., and Collins,A.T. (2004). CD133, a novel marker for human prostatic epithelial stem cells. J. Cell Sci. *117*, 3539-3545.

Roesch,A., Fukunaga-Kalabis,M., Schmidt,E.C., Zabierowski,S.E., Brafford,P.A., Vultur,A., Basu,D., Gimotty,P., Vogt,T., and Herlyn,M. (2010). A temporarily distinct subpopulation of slow-cycling melanoma cells is required for continuous tumor growth. Cell *141*, 583-594.

Sagrinati,C., Netti,G.S., Mazzinghi,B., Lazzeri,E., Liotta,F., Frosali,F., Ronconi,E., Meini,C., Gacci,M., Squecco,R., Carini,M., Gesualdo,L., Francini,F., Maggi,E., Annunziato,F., Lasagni,L., Serio,M., Romagnani,S., and Romagnani,P. (2006). Isolation and characterization of multipotent progenitor cells from the Bowman's capsule of adult human kidneys. J. Am. Soc. Nephrol. *17*, 2443-2456.

Sebova,K. and Fridrichova,I. (2010). Epigenetic tools in potential anticancer therapy. Anticancer Drugs *21*, 565-577.

Sharma,S.V., Lee,D.Y., Li,B., Quinlan,M.P., Takahashi,F., Maheswaran,S., McDermott,U., Azizian,N., Zou,L., Fischbach,M.A., Wong,K.K., Brandstetter,K., Wittner,B., Ramaswamy,S., Classon,M., and Settleman,J. (2010). A chromatin-mediated reversible drug-tolerant state in cancer cell subpopulations. Cell *141*, 69-80.

Shmelkov,S.V., Butler,J.M., Hooper,A.T., Hormigo,A., Kushner,J., Milde,T., St,C.R., Baljevic,M., White,I., Jin,D.K., Chadburn,A., Murphy,A.J., Valenzuela,D.M., Gale,N.W., Thurston,G., Yancopoulos,G.D., D'Angelica,M., Kemeny,N., Lyden,D., and Rafii,S. (2008). CD133 expression is not restricted to stem cells, and both CD133+ and CD133- metastatic colon cancer cells initiate tumors. J. Clin. Invest *118*, 2111-2120.

Stingl,J., Eirew,P., Ricketson,I., Shackleton,M., Vaillant,F., Choi,D., Li,H.I., and Eaves,C.J. (2006). Purification and unique properties of mammary epithelial stem cells. Nature *439*, 993-997.

Sugiyama,T., Rodriguez,R.T., McLean,G.W., and Kim,S.K. (2007). Conserved markers of fetal pancreatic epithelium permit prospective isolation of islet progenitor cells by FACS. Proc. Natl. Acad. Sci. U. S. A *104*, 175-180.

Thiery,J.P., Acloque,H., Huang,R.Y., and Nieto,M.A. (2009). Epithelial-mesenchymal transitions in development and disease. Cell *139*, 871-890.

Uchida,N., Buck,D.W., He,D., Reitsma,M.J., Masek,M., Phan,T.V., Tsukamoto,A.S., Gage,F.H., and Weissman,I.L. (2000). Direct isolation of human central nervous system stem cells. Proc. Natl. Acad. Sci. U. S. A *97*, 14720-14725.

Vesuna,F., Lisok,A., Kimble,B., and Raman,V. (2009). Twist modulates breast cancer stem cells by transcriptional regulation of CD24 expression. Neoplasia. *11*, 1318-1328.

Yin,A.H., Miraglia,S., Zanjani,E.D., meida-Porada,G., Ogawa,M., Leary,A.G., Olweus,J., Kearney,J., and Buck,D.W. (1997). AC133, a novel marker for human hematopoietic stem and progenitor cells. Blood *90*, 5002-5012.

Zhu,L., Gibson,P., Currle,D.S., Tong,Y., Richardson,R.J., Bayazitov,I.T., Poppleton, H., Zakharenko,S., Ellison,D.W., and Gilbertson,R.J. (2009). Prominin 1 marks intestinal stem cells that are susceptible to neoplastic transformation. Nature *457*, 603-607.

3

Connections between Genomic Instability and Cancer Stem Cells

Linda Li, Laura Borodyansky and Youxin Yang
GI Cancer Laboratory, Division of Gastroenterology, Beth Israel Deaconess Medical Center, Harvard Medical School, Boston, MA 02215 USA

1. Introduction

Cancer is caused by successive gene mutations that amount to confer malignant phenotype. Genomic instability is considered a key endogenous mechanism for accumulation of mutations, and therefore, has been proposed as an engine of tumorigenesis. Recently, cancer stem cells, or tumor initiating cells, have been identified in a variety of human cancers. These cancer stem cells are believed to be responsible for the initiation of malignant growth and metastasis of some, and perhaps all cancer types. How are these two engines of tumorigenesis related to each other? Is genomic instability a driving force in the genesis of cancer stem cells? Is the genome in cancer stem cells inherently unstable? Could genomic instability in cancer stem cells be the cause of the observed cancer cell heterogeneity? In this article, we will discuss some early clues indicating that these two driving forces of tumorigenesis appear to be intimately connected.

2. Genomic instability

Genomic instability is a key hallmark of malignancy (Aguilera & Gómez-González, 2008; Jallepalli & Lengauer, 2001; Venkitaraman, 2007). Cancer cells bear numerous molecular changes encompassing nearly 10 years of genesis in vivo. The old question of whether the chicken or the egg came first comes to mind when one attempts to sort out whether a molecular change is the cause or a consequence of cancer (Venkitaraman, 2007). This question is particularly challenging since most cancer research relies on cultured cancer cells, devoid of both actual chronologic age and natural physiologic milieu. Genomic instability exemplifies the challenge of such an undertaking: is genomic instability a cause or simply a ramification of the malignant process? Many lines of evidence suggest that genomic instability is a causative factor rather than a result of cancer (Aguilera & Gómez-González, 2008; Jallepalli & Lengauer, 2001; Venkitaraman, 2007). Thus, it seems that genomic instability is intimately linked to cancer stem cells.

3. Cancer stem cell

Cancer stem cells also called tumor-initiating cells, are characterized by their self-renewal capacity and ability to initiate tumors (Ailles & Weissman, 2007; Clarke et al., 2006; Dick,

2008; Wicha et al., 2006). Cancer stem cell populations have been identified in a variety of human cancer types (Ailles & Weissman, 2007; Clarke et al., 2006; Dick, 2008; Wicha et al., 2006). Strictly speaking, some isolated cancer stem cells may be more accurately referred to as cancer stemloids (or stem cell-like cancer cells) (Blagosklonny, 2007). Although these cells may exist only as a minority within the cancer cell population, mounting evidence suggests that cancer stem cells contribute to tumor growth, metastasis, and resistance to therapy (Ailles & Weissman, 2007; Clarke et al., 2006; Dick, 2008; Wicha et al., 2006).

4. Genomic instability as a driving force for transforming normal stem cells to cancer stem cells

Adult normal stem cells represent one purported origin of cancer stem cells. What causes the transformation from normal stem cells to cancer stem cells? Is genomic instability involved in this transformation? Recent work casts insight into potential roles of GIN in the transformation of normal adult stem cells to cancer stem cells. Mirura et al. obtained cancer progenitor cells from bone marrow derived mesenchymal stem cells after long term culture (Miura et al., 2006). Interestingly, these cancer progenitor cells formed fibrosarcoma in vivo. The mechanism of transformation was found to be associated with accumulated chromosomal abnormality and increased c-Myc expression (Miura et al., 2006), suggesting an association between cancer progenitor cells and genomic instability. Such an association was also observed in non-hematopoietic stem cells. After a long term culture of human adult non-tumorigenic neural stem cells, Shiras et al. observed concurrent emergence of a high level of genomic instability and a spontaneously immortalized clone which developed into a cell line with features of cancer stem cells, including the capacity to form CD133 positive neurospheres and development into intracranial tumors (Shiras et al., 2007). Additionally, increased expression of well known developmental genes (Notch and Hes) were found both before and after cell transformation (Shiras et al., 2007). Therefore, genomic instability could be a potential driving force in the transformation of normal stem cells into cancer stem cells.
How does genomic instability contribute to the transformation of normal stem cells? It has been suggested that normal stem cells and their cellular pathways may acquire stochastic malignant ability (Lagasse, 2008). Clark and colleagues generated highly metastatic cancer stem cells by implantation of murine embryonic germ cells (EGCs) into the testes of adult severe combined immune deficiency (SCID) mice (Conway et al., 2009). Karyotype analysis showed that generation of cancer stem cells is associated with acquisition of genomic rearrangements not found in the original EGCs. Microarray-based gene expression analysis revealed similarity between EGCs and cancer stem cells, and the differentially expressed transcripts are consistent with activation of oncogene pathways. This work suggests that genomic instability may induce stochastic activation of cancer gene pathways in transformation of normal stem cells to cancer stem cells (Conway et al., 2009). Alternatively, cancer stem cells may be derived from clonal selection for resistance to growth limiting conditions imposed by mutagens or carcinogens (Blagosklonny, 2002).

5. Genomic instability in cancer stem cells

Is the genome inherently unstable in stem cells? If the answer is yes, cancer stem cells may have two reasons for having an unstable genome: being a stem cell as well as a cancer cell.

Let us first look at embryonic stem (ES) cells. Human ES (hES) cells, like other stem cells, have the capacity to self-renew without differentiation, and yet can differentiate to various tissue types upon exposure to specific differentiation cues. It has been technically challenging to propagate hES cells in vitro without allowing differentiation (Bodnar et al., 2004). Cultured hES cells have been shown to have genomic instability with frequent aneuploidy of chromosomes 12, 17q and X, suggesting that the increased dosage of chromosome 17q and 12 genes may provide a selective advantage for propagation of undifferentiated hES cells (Draper et al., 2004). Additionally, long term in vitro culture can result in almost 100% cells with genomic instability, hypothesized by the authors to possibly be an adaptation to loss of ECM support (Imreh et al., 2006). By analyzing 17 hES cell lines with comparative genomic hybridization (CGH), Spits et al. identified amplification of 20q11.21 and a derivative of chromosome 18 (Spits et al., 2008). It is unclear whether hES cells are inherently genetically unstable or if genomic instability is a strong selection factor for long term viability and establishment of hES cells.

By following five human embryonic cell lines over long term cultures, Lefort et al. identified recurrent genomic instability. An amplification of 2.5–4.6 mb at 20q11.21 was recurrent in four out five cell lines. This amplification has also been associated with oncogenic transformation. This study suggests that some genomic instability changes may be selected due to growth advantage they confer to hES cells (Lefort et al., 2008).

The next question to ask is how stable is the genome of adult stem cells? Unlike hES cells, human adult stem cells by design must be maintained for an average human life span of approximately 75 years. Arguably, genomic stability is essential for the maintenance and longevity of adult stem cells (Gerson et al., 2006). Supporting of this hypothesis is the observed premature aging and high cancer incidence in medical syndromes with genetic defects in DNA repair machinery, such as ataxia telengiectasia, xeroderma pigmentosum and Bloom syndrome, to name a few.

Why do embryonic stem cells tend to have increased genomic instability? Work by Mantel et al. suggests that there is uncoupling of apoptosis from mitotic checkpoint activation in both hES and mouse embryonic stem cells (mES) cells. The group showed that mitotic spindle checkpoint activation in somatic cells or in ESC-derived early differentiated cells resulted in robust apoptosis, yet same treatment did not trigger apoptosis in ESCs. It is therefore possible that such tolerance of ploidy changes by ESCs contribute to the karyotypic instability (Mantel et al., 2007). Aoki et al. (Aoki et al., 2007) also observed a three to nine fold increase in anaphase bridge index (ABI), a measure of chromosomal instability, in polyps and mESCs with beta-catenin/Wnt pathway activation resulting from APC/beta-catenin mutations. The WNT signal-activated ES cells produced new chromosomal aberrations at higher rate.

Gene array analysis suggests that cancer stem cells resemble embryonic rather than adult stem cells (Wong et al., 2008). It may be possible that there is similar kind of uncoupling (Bao et al., 2006) between mitotic checkpoint activation and apoptosis in cancer stem cells. Another possible reason for increased genomic instability in cancer stem cells is malignant transformation of aged stem cells. Stem cells have a lifetime exposure to various tumorigenic agents and other stress, and are therefore prime targets for malignant transformation (Ju & Rudolph, 2006).

6. Genomic instability in cancer stem cells as a potential mechanism for cancer cell heterogeneity

If cancer stem cells are genomically unstable, it is plausible to reason that genomic instability may contribute to the heterogeneity in cancer cells forming the bulk majority of the tumor (Solé et al., 2008). Wang et al. performed karyotype analysis on a melanoma patient experiencing apparent complete remission and subsequent recurrence over a 12 year period (Grichnik, 2006). Their data point to the existence of a common progenitor cancer cell that gives rise to genomically unstable progeny. Cells karyotyped from the same culture revealed chromosomal differences suggesting ongoing chromosomal instability within the cell population isolated from each metastasis (Grichnik, 2006; Wang et al., 2006).
When cancer stem cell self-renew, numerous genetic variants can be produced. Heterogeneous cancer stem cell populations may acquire drug resistant or metastatic phenotypes. According to this model, cancer stem cells with genomic instability is considered "a powerful vehicle with a powerful engine", a formidable force for generating heterogeneity and a daunting challenge for designing targeted therapy against one specific pathway (Jones et al., 2008). Initial success with targeted therapy, limited albeit unequivocally positive, suggests cancer heterogeneity is not a completely insurmountable phenotype for designing therapy. Cancer stem cells may present a relatively less heterogeneous cell population for targeting than their progeny.

7. Conclusion

Early clues have indicated that genomic instability and cancer stem cells appear to be intimately connected.
Genomic instability might be a potential driving force in the transformation of normal stem cells into cancer stem cells.
Future studies need to focus more on early detection and management of the stem cells carrying genomic instability before they undergo malignant transformation.

8. Acknowledgment

We thank Drs. Johannes Fruehauf and Shuanglin Xiang for their discussion and support.

9. References

Aguilera, A. & Gómez-González, B. (2008). Genome instability: a mechanistic view of its causes and consequences. *Nature Reviews Genetics*, Vol.9, No.3, (March 2008), pp. 204-17, ISSN 1471-0056

Ailles, L.E. & Weissman, I.L. (2007). Cancer stem cells in solid tumors. ***Current Opinion in Biotechnology***, Vol.18, No.5, (October 2007), pp. 460-6, ISSN 0958-1669

Aoki, K.; Aoki, M.; Sugai, M.; Harada, N.; Miyoshi, H.; Tsukamoto, T.; Mizoshita, T.; Tatematsu, M.; Seno, H.; Chiba, T.; Oshima, M.; Hsieh, C.L. & Taketo, M.M. (2007). Chromosomal instability by beta-catenin/TCF transcription in APC or beta-catenin mutant cells. *Oncogene*, Vol.26, No.24, (May 2007), pp. 3511-20, ISSN 0950-9232

Bao, S.; Wu, Q.; McLendon, R.E.; Hao, Y.; Shi, Q.; Hjelmeland, A.B.; Dewhirst, M.W.; Bigner, D.D. & Rich, J.N. (2006). Glioma stem cells promote radioresistance by preferential activation of the DNA damage response. *Nature*, Vol.444, No. 7120, (December 2006), pp. 756-60, ISSN 0028-0836

Blagosklonny, M.V. (2002). Oncogenic resistance to growth-limiting conditions. *Nature Reviews Cancer*, Vol.2, No.3, (March 2002), pp. 221-5, ISSN 1474-175X

Blagosklonny, M.V. (2007). Cancer stem cell and cancer stemloids: from biology to therapy. *Cancer Biology and Therapy*, Vol.6, No.11, (November 2007), pp. 1684-90, ISSN 1538-4047

Bodnar, M.S.; Meneses, J.J.; Rodriguez, R.T. & Firpo, M.T. (2004). Propagation and maintenance of undifferentiated human embryonic stem cells. *Stem Cells and Development*, Vol.13, No.3, (June 2004), pp. 243-53, ISSN 1547-3287

Clarke, M.F.; Dick, J.E.; Dirks, P.B.; Eaves, C.J.; Jamieson, C.H.; Jones, D.L.; Visvader, J.; Weissman, I.L. & Wahl, G.M. (2006). Cancer stem cells--perspectives on current status and future directions: AACR Workshop on cancer stem cells. *Cancer Research*, Vol.66, No.19, (October 2006), pp. 9339-44, ISSN 0008-5472

Conway, A.E.; Lindgren, A.; Galic, Z.; Pyle, A.D.; Wu, H.; Zack, J.A.; Pelligrini, M.; Teitell, M.A. & Clark, A.T. (2009). A pluripotency and self-renewal program controls the expansion of genetically unstable cancer stem cells in pluripotent stem cell-derived tumors. *Stem Cells*, Vol.27, No.1, (January 2009), pp. 18–28, ISSN 1066-5099

Dick, J.E. (2008). Stem cell concepts renew cancer research. *Blood*, Vol.112, No.13, (December 2008), pp. 4793-807, ISSN 0006-4971

Draper, J.S.; Smith, K.; Gokhale, P.; Moore, H.D.; Maltby, E.; Johnson, J.; Meisner, L.; Zwaka, T.P.; Thomson, J.A. & Andrews, P.W. (2004). Recurrent gain of chromosomes 17q and 12 in cultured human embryonic stem cells. *Nature Biotechnology*, Vol.22, No.1, (January 2004), pp. 53-4, ISSN 1087-0156

Gerson, S.L.; Reese, J. & Kenyon, J. (2006). DNA repair in stem cell maintenance and conversion to cancer stem cells. *Ernst Schering Foundation Symposium Proceedings*, No.5, pp. 231-44

Grichnik, J.M. (2006). Genomic instability and tumor stem cells. *The Journal of Investigative Dermatology*, Vol.126, No.6, (June 2006), pp. 1214-6, ISSN 0022-202X

Imreh, M.P.; Gertow, K.; Cedervall, J.; Unger, C.; Holmberg, K.; Szöke, K.; Csöregh, L.; Fried, G.; Dilber, S.; Blennow, E. & Ahrlund-Richter, L. (2006). In vitro culture conditions favoring selection of chromosomal abnormalities in human ES cells. *Journal of Cellular Biochemistry*, Vol.99, No.2, (October 2006), pp. 508-16, ISSN 0730-2312

Jallepalli, P.V. & Lengauer, C. (2001). Chromosome segregation and cancer: cutting through the mystery. *Nature Reviews Cancer*, Vol.1, No.2, (November 2001), pp. 109-17, ISSN 1474-175X

Jones, S.; Zhang, X.; Parsons, D.W.; Lin, J.C.; Leary, R.J.; Angenendt, P.; Mankoo, P.; Carter, H.; Kamiyama, H.; Jimeno, A.; Hong, S.M.; Fu, B.; Lin, M.T.; Calhoun, E.S.; Kamiyama, M.; Walter, K.; Nikolskaya, T.; Nikolsky, Y.; Hartigan, J.; Smith, D.R.; Hidalgo, M.; Leach, S.D.; Klein, A.P.; Jaffee, E.M.; Goggins, M.; Maitra, A.; Iacobuzio-Donahue, C.; Eshleman, J.R.; Kern, S.E.; Hruban, R.H.; Karchin, R.; Papadopoulos, N.; Parmigiani, G.; Vogelstein, B.; Velculescu, V.E. & Kinzler, K.W. (2008). Core signaling pathways in human pancreatic cancers revealed by global genomic analyses. *Science*, Vol.321, No. 5897, (September 2008), pp. 1801-6, ISSN 0036-8075

Ju, Z. & Rudolph, K.L. (2006). Telomeres and telomerase in cancer stem cells. *European Journal of Cancer*, Vol.42, No.9, (June 2006), pp. 1197-203, ISSN 0959-8049

Lagasse, E. (2008). Cancer stem cells with genetic instability: the best vehicle with the best engine for cancer. *Gene Therapy*, Vol.15, No.2, (January 2008), pp. 136-42, ISSN 0969-7128

Lefort, N.; Feyeux, M.; Bas, C.; Féraud, O.; Bennaceur-Griscelli, A.; Tachdjian, G.; Peschanski, M. & Perrier, A.L. (2008). Human embryonic stem cells reveal recurrent genomic instability at 20q11.21. *Nature Biotechnology*, Vol.26, No.12, (December 2008), pp. 1364-6, ISSN 1087-0156

Mantel, C.; Guo, Y.; Lee, M.R.; Kim, M.K.; Han, M.K.; Shibayama, H.; Fukuda, S.; Yoder, M.C.; Pelus, L.M.; Kim, K.S. & Broxmeyer, H.E. (2007). Checkpoint-apoptosis uncoupling in human and mouse embryonic stem cells: a source of karyotypic instability. *Blood*, Vol.109, No.10, (May 2007), pp. 4518-27, ISSN 0006-4971

Miura, M.; Miura, Y.; Padilla-Nash, H.M.; Molinolo, A.A.; Fu, B.; Patel, V.; Seo, B.M.; Sonoyama, W.; Zheng, J.J.; Baker, C.C.; Chen, W.; Ried, T. & Shi, S. (2006). Accumulated chromosomal instability in murine bone marrow mesenchymal stem cells leads to malignant transformation. *Stem Cells*, Vol.24, No.4, (April 2006), pp. 1095-103, ISSN 1066-5099

Shiras, A.; Chettiar, S.T.; Shepal, V.; Rajendran, G.; Prasad, G.R. & Shastry, P. (2007). Spontaneous transformation of human adult nontumorigenic stem cells to cancer stem cells is driven by genomic instability in a human model of glioblastoma. *Stem Cells*, Vol.25, No.6, (June 2007), pp. 1478-89, ISSN 1066-5099

Solé, R.V.; Rodríguez-Caso, C.; Deisboeck, T.S. & Saldaña, J. (2008). Cancer stem cells as the engine of unstable tumor progression. *Journal of Theoretical Biology*, Vol.253, No.4, (August 2008), pp. 629-37, ISSN 0022-5193

Spits, C.; Mateizel, I.; Geens, M.; Mertzanidou, A.; Staessen, C.; Vandeskelde, Y.; Van der Elst, J.; Liebaers, I. & Sermon, K. (2008). Recurrent chromosomal abnormalities in human embryonic stem cells. *Nature Biotechnology*, Vol.26, No.12, (December 2008), pp. 1361-3, ISSN 1087-0156

Venkitaraman, A.R. (2007). Chromosomal instability in cancer: causality and interdependence. *Cell Cycle*, Vol.6, No.19, (October 2007), pp. 2341-3, ISSN 1538-4101

Wang, E.; Voiculescu, S.; Le Poole, I.C.; El-Gamil, M.; Li, X.; Sabatino, M.; Robbins, P.F.; Nickoloff, B.J. & Marincola, F.M. (2006). Clonal persistence and evolution during a decade of recurrent melanoma. *The Journal of Investigative Dermatology*, Vol.126, No.6, (June 2006), pp. 1372-7, ISSN 0022-202X

Wicha, M.S.; Liu, S. & Dontu, G. (2006). Cancer stem cells: an old idea--a paradigm shift. *Cancer Research*, Vol.66, No.4, (February 2006), pp. 1883-90, ISSN 0008-5472

Wong, D.J.; Segal, E. & Chang, H.Y. (2008). Stemness, cancer and cancer stem cells. *Cell Cycle*, Vol.7, No.23, (December 2008), pp. 3622-4, ISSN 1538-4101

4

Cancer Stem Cells as a Result of a Reprogramming-Like Mechanism

Carolina Vicente-Dueñas[1], Isabel Romero-Camarero[1],
Teresa Flores[2], Juan Jesús Cruz[3] and Isidro Sanchez-Garcia[1]
*[1]Experimental Therapeutics and Translational Oncology Program,
Instituto de Biología Molecular y Celular del Cáncer,
CSIC/ Universidad de Salamanca, Campus M. de Unamuno s/n,
37007-SALAMANCA*
*[2]Departamento de Anatomía Patológica, Universidad de Salamanca,
Edificio Departamental, Campus M. de Unamuno s/n,
37007-SALAMANCA*
*[3]Cátedra-Servicio de Oncología Médica, Hospital Universitario de
Salamanca-Universidad de Salamanca, Salamanca
Spain*

1. Introduction

The treatment of cancer is generally based on histological grade, respectability and the presence or absence of metastasis. Because interventions after the manifestation of metastasis are notoriously ineffective for most cancers, great effort is invested in the development of targeted therapies to eradicate or suppress the growth of cancer. A complete understanding of the cancer process requires more detailed knowledge of the mechanisms maintaining neoplastic growth and it is is a prerequisite not only for understanding the genesis of human cancer but also for the identification of molecular events responsible for cancer maintenance. New drugs must be designed against the mechanisms that are responsible for cancer maintenance not for the initial event that transform a normal cell into cancer cell, because it is possible that the first alteration of the cancer cell will have no function in the subsequent steps of cancer development. Much effort is currently being expended to target the mutated oncogenes and tumour suppressor genes that control neoplastic cell growth directly. Inactivation of oncogene(s) can cause cancer remission, implying that oncogenes are the Achilles' heel of cancers. This current "hands on" model of cancer has kept oncogenes firmly in focus as therapeutic targets and is in agreement with the fact that in human cancers all cancerous cells, with independence of the cellular heterogeneity existing within the tumour, carry the same oncogenic genetic lesions. However, many of the new classes of agents targeting the oncogenes usually do not show a permanent clinical benefit. These clinical observations suggest that oncogene-induced tumourigenesis is not reversible through the unique inactivation of the gene defect(s) initiating cancer development. But, what are the mechanisms of tumor relapse by which tumors evolve to escape oncogene dependence? Several recent studies of the effect of oncogenes in stem cells in cancer development (Barker et al., 2009; Perez-Caro et al., 2009; Zhu et al., 2009; Bussard et al., 2010; Jacques et al., 2010; Nakagawa et al., 2010; Saring et al., 2010; Zhang et al., 2010) implicate that tumor reprogramming (where the maintenance of oncogene expression is not critical for the generation of differentiated tumor cells) might represent a potentially important mechanism of tumour development for many types of cancer and that, if this is the case, the oncogenes that initiate tumor formation might be dispensable for tumor progression and/or maintenance. The practical implications that this new point of view has for the therapy of cancer are obviously enormous (Castellanos et al., 2010). This chapter addresses the impact of these results toward a better understanding of carcinogenesis and proposes research avenues for tackling these issues in the future.

2. The cancer stem cell (CSC) concept

The cancer stem cell (CSC) theory hypothesizes that a cancer maintains a hierarchical organization similar to a normal tissue. Thus, the tumor mass is the result of differentiated progeny of rarer CSCs with self-renewal capacity (Sanchez-Garcia et al., 2007). Chronic myeloid leukemia (CML) is universally regarded as providing the strongest evidence in support of the CSC concept. Fialkow and his colleagues first suggested that CML arose from rare transformed hematopoietic stem cells (HSC) nearly 40 years ago, when they showed that both granulocytes and red blood cells from CML patients were derived from a common cell (Fialkow et al., 1977). However, the term tumor/cancer stem cell was first coined nearly 40 years ago to highlight the observation that only a minority of multiple myeloma cells were capable of clonogenic growth (Hamburger and Salmon, 1977). The last decade has witnessed an increasing re-appreciation of the role of these heterogenous cellular cues in cancer development and therapy. This re-evaluation represents a rather crucial detour from the widely held view that the neoplastic phenotype resulted from uncontrolled proliferation of tumor cells. The CSC concept would explain not only the low clonogenic capacity of most malignancies, but also why complete treatment responses translate into cures in only a minority of cancer patients. Initial responses in cancer represent therapeutic effectiveness against the bulk cancer cells, while rarer resistant CSCs could be responsible for relapse. Accordingly, improving the results of cancer therapy would require identification and better understanding of the biology of CSC (Perez-Caro et al., 2009; Saito et al., 2010) (**Figure 1**).
Within this framework, fundamental determinants of neoplastic disease are to be found within the CSC and, thus the role of CSC regarding cancer biology, management and therapy needs to be evaluated (Sanchez-Garcia, 2009). It should be noted that partial tumor responses to therapy mean little if CSCs are the major cells determining outcome (Sanchez-Garcia, 2009). Because of the difficulty of assessing the effects of therapies on the rare CSCs responsible for cancer maintenance and relapse, the development of new clinical approaches will require new clinical paradigms and methodologies that should rely heavily on preclinical modelling, using novel preclinical assays to evaluate the fate of CSC (Sanchez-Garcia et al., 2007) Preclinical studies should assess the effects of therapies on CSC and differentiated cancer cell populations. This could allow us to take directly to the patient a fully functional new approach (**Figure 1**).
A related concept is that the exact definition of "stemness" is elusive and stemness may be more of a cotinuum or a property that may be regained in cancer, which would suggest that neither the hierarchical nor the stochastic model are exclusively right.

Furthermore, we must call the attention to the fact that the fundamental concept essential to the CSC hypothesis does not have anything to do with the absolute frequency of these cells within the tumour; indeed, what the model states is that there is a functional heterogeneity within the tumor cellular components, and that there is only a defined population of cells that can initiate/maintain malignant growth in vivo while the remaining cells cannot. Thus, the therapeutic implications of the CSC concept are equally important whatever their frequency is within each tumour type: they are the cells that must be effectively targeted to achieve a definitive cure on the long round (Perez-Caro et al., 2009; Saito et al., 2010) (**Figure 1**).

3. Stem cells and cancer initiation

The nature of the cell in which the initiating mutation occurred in human cancer has received little attention during the last decades. Since the process of carcinogenesis need to accumulate a number of oncogenic events during long periods of time, only cells with self-renewal capacity, would be in the tissue enough time to accumulate the oncogenic alterations necessary for the complete cell transformation. This fact seems to be particularly evident, in tumors originated in tissues with high cellular turnover, as the skin, the intestine or the breast, where normal stem cells should be the target for the oncogenic initiation event (Al-Hajj et al., 2003; Singh et al., 2004; Wang et al., 2009; Jacques et al., 2010). For more differentiated cells to originate epithelial cancer, it would be necessary that the first oncogenic event to induce a fully tumor phenotype, or at least be able to trigger a partial stem cell-like program that permit the differentiated progenitor to acquire surviving and self-renewal capabilities, and probably new adhesion properties near the basal membrane to avoid being expelled from the tissue under the normal cellular turnover. In recent years, there is growing evidence that stem cells are the cells of origin for several types of cancer (Sanchez-Garcia et al., 2007; Vicente-Dueñas et al., 2009). An example is provided by the chronic myelogenous leukaemia (CML), a granulocytic disease (Melo and Barnes, 2007). However, the *BCR-ABL* translocation, pathognomonic of this disease, does not arise in a granulocyte, but rather in a cell at the beginning of the hematopoietic differentiation tree (Jamieson et al., 2004).

4. Caveats for identification of CSC in human cancer

In human cancer the definition of the identity of CSCs comes from experiments of serial transplantation of flow cytometry-sorted cell populations into immunocompromised mice. The CSC-containing population should recapitulate the cellular heterogeneity present in the primary human cancer and must have the capacity for self-renewal on serial passaging (Cobaleda and Sanchez-Garcia, 2009). However, there are many technical issues concerning the isolation and determination of CSC capabilities from human cancer samples, ranging from the methods of selection of the cells themselves to the choice of the recipient animals where the cells can reveal their potential and to the injection site within the recipient (Cobaleda and Sanchez-Garcia, 2009). To avoid these caveats an alternative way to study the CSC population is to use mice as a system model.

5. Identification of CSC in mouse models of human cancer

Much of our current conceptualization of how tumorigenesis occurs in humans is strongly influenced by mouse models of cancer development (Perez-Losada et al., 2002; Sanchez-

Martin et al., 2002; Perez-Mancera et al., 2005a; Perez-Mancera et al., 2005b;). But studies in mice in which the oncogenic alteration(s) is not directed to the specific cells of origin, as it normally occurs in most current mouse models, should be interpreted cautiously (Vicente-Dueñas et al., 2010)

The genetic alterations found in human cancer seem to occur during specific periods of time and restricted to a few specific cells. In several cases, like in the case of CML, the cancer cell-of-origin is a stem/progenitor cell, and this explains the stem properties that allow the CSCs to maintain the tumor mass. However there are also many cancers where most probably the cancer cell-of-origin would be a more differentiated cell (Cobaleda et al., 2007). In these cases, the combination of the reprogramming capabilities of the oncogenic alteration and the intrinsic plasticity of the target cell (i.e., its susceptibility to the reprogramming) determine the final outcome of a CSC. Since not all the cells present the same susceptibility to reprogramming, and not all the oncogenes posses the same reprogramming capacities (i.e., the ability to confer stem cell features to the target cell), the targeting of the oncogenic alteration to the wrong cellular compartment is a likely cause of failure in the generation of accurate mouse models of human cancer. Considering these facts, three independent groups have already shown that the genotype-phenotype correlations found in human cancer can be established in mice by specific targeting of stem cells (Barker et al., 2009; Perez-Caro et al., 2009; Zhu et al., 2009).

6. Cancer as a reprogramming-like disease

In a normal stem cell-driven tissue, genetic programming of stem cells is all what is required to (re)constitute all differentiated cells forming the tissue and the genetic information responsible for the stem cell programming is not anymore expressed within the differentiated cells that form the tissue. As we have mentioned before, in the last years, many evidences have been accumulated indicating that cancers are also hierarchically organized tissues which can be created and maintained like a normal stem-cell-based tissue (Etzioni et al., 2003; Sanchez-Garcia et al., 2007; Jemal et al., 2009). The most challenging arena in which to prove this concept are those tumors whose main cellular components are terminally differentiated cells. A clear example of this kind of tumors is the chronic phase of CML. To elucidate if CML is a stem cell-driven tissue, we developed mice limiting *BCR-ABL* expression to the Sca1+ cells (Sca1-BCRABL mice) (Sanchez-Garcia et al., 2009). Thus, our Sca1-BCRABL is a very suitable *in vivo* model to study the consequences of ectopic expression of *BCR-ABL* targeted to stem cells. However, in human CML and in most animal models of cancer, the oncogenic alteration(s) is(are) present in all the cellular types that compose the tumoral tissue, from the cancer cell-of-origin to the terminal differentiated granulocytes. In our stem cell-driven Sca1-BCRABL model, the expression of the oncogene is restricted to the stem/progenitor compartment but is nevertheless capable of generating a full-blown CML with all its differentiated cellular components. Of course, the demonstration that CML development can be established in mice by limiting oncogene expression to Sca1^{+} cells implies that abolishing oncogene function does not interfere with the formation of differentiated tumor cells, and suggest that the oncogene imposes a gene regulatory state in stem cells that somehow persists during hematopoiesis and which imposes a tumor phenotype reflective of the usual CML, an observation that seems to apply to other cancer-initiating gene defects (Sanchez-Garcia et al., 2009). Therefore, we hypothesize that the oncogene mediates tumorigenesis through epigenetic/genetic modification of target genes that remain in this modified state in the mature tumor even in the absence of *BCR-ABL* in agreement with a reprogramming role for *BCR-ABL* in regulating CML formation. Supporting these observations, it has been recently shown that only stem cells, but not astrocytes, gave rise to brain tumors, independently of their location. This suggests a cell-autonomous mechanism that enables stem cells to generate brain tumors, underlining an important role of stem cells and the relevance of initial genetic mutations in the pathogenesis and phenotype of brain tumors.

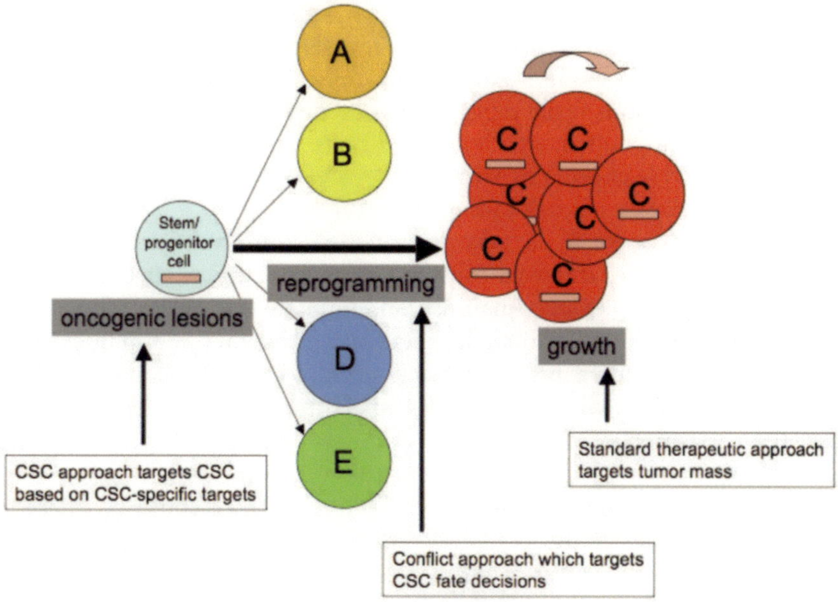

Fig. 1. Approaches to target CSC.

Recent breakthroughs have shown that reprogramming of differentiated cells can be achieved by the transient expression of a limited number of transcription factors that can "reset" the epigenetic status of the cells and allow them to adopt a new plethora of possible fates. Several of these reprogramming factors were previously known for their oncogenic activity, already connecting the role of oncogenes with tumoral cell fate reprogramming. Furthermore, it has recently been shown that the elimination of p53, whose function is to prevent the survival and expansion of cells with genetic damage, greatly enhances the reprogramming efficiency in the generation of induced pluripotent cells (iPS) (Castellanos et al., 2010). These p53-null reprogrammed cells carry, however, several types of mutations (Castellanos et al., 2010). These results confirm the fact that the absence of the tumor suppressor does not have an instructive role in tumorigenesis, but just a permissive one, so p53 would prevent cells with damage from being successfully terminally reprogrammed. This indicates that the driving force of the reprogramming process are the reprogramming factors themselves, and that just the necessity of maintaining genetic integrity prevents the reprogrammed cells with any kind of damage to progress along the newly programmed pathway. As a logical consequence, it has recently been proposed that cancer stem cells might arise through a reprogramming-like mechanism and that, if this is the case, perhaps the oncogenes that initiate tumor formation might be dispensable for tumor progression

(Castellanos et al., 2010). Further to this, it has also been shown in the haematopoietic and nervous systems that the susceptibility of cells to reprogramming is inversely proportional to their degree of differentiation, and that hematopoietic stem cells (HSC) are 300 times more prone to be reprogrammed than B or T cells (Castellanos et al., 2010). Our results show that this stem cell reprogramming is indeed possible in the case of *BCR-ABL*. But perhaps the most crucial question is whether these hands-off regulation mechanisms can be found in other cancer types, especially tumors of epithelial origin, which represent the bulk of human cancers. Importantly, a small subset of *Sca1-BCR-ABL* mice develops additional solid tumors. Considering that Sca1 has been identified as a almost universal stem cell marker in many different tissues, these data would suggest that the view of cancer as a reprogramming-like disease is not specific to only hematopietic tissues, but rather represents a broader mechanism for deregulation of stem cell differentiation, providing a paradigm that can be applied to solid-organ cancers and, together with all the above discussed findings, provide enough experimental evidence to support the view of cancer as a reprogramming-like disease (Castellanos et al., 2010).

This model of cancer (**Figure 1**) is very informative with respect to the fact that the oncogenic mutations can have different roles in CSC versus differentiated cancer cells, and explains why targeted therapies like imatinib can eliminate the latter without affecting the former. However, we should be cautious in interpreting the data as a mimicking of human disease as mouse cells are more prone of transformation than human cells and thus one mutation can lead to full blown cancer in the mouse transgenic model but not in human. Furthermore, the regulation of certain genes/pathways might differ between mouse and human.

There are many evidences now suggesting that human cancer could be considered as a reprogramming-like disease. If the potential growth of cancer depends on CSCs and on oncogenes that can function in a hands-off manner, it would be important to know how to eradicate these cells and/or inactivate the reprogramming mechanism (Castellanos et al., 2010) (**Figure 1**).

7. Conclusions

There are many evidences now suggesting that human cancer could be considered as a reprogramming-like disease (Castellanos et al., 2010). If the potential growth of cancer depends on CSCs and on oncogenes that can function in a hands-off manner, it would be important to know how to eradicate these cells and/or inactivate the reprogramming mechanism (**Figure 1**). The coming years will show whether this optimism is well founded, or whether the immense complexity of this disease will continue to confound our best endeavours to tackle cancer.

8. Acknowledgements

Research in our groups is partially supported by FEDER and by MICINN (SAF2009-08803 to ISG), by Junta de Castilla y León (Proyecto Biomedicina 2009-2010 to ISG, and Proyecto Biomedicina 2010-2011 to CVD), by MEC OncoBIO Consolider-Ingenio 2010 (Ref. CSD2007-0017) to ISG, by NIH grant (R01 CA109335-04A1) to ISG, by Sandra Ibarra Foundation to ISG, and by Group of Excellence Grant (GR15) from Junta de Castilla y Leon to ISG and JJC.

9. References

Al-Hajj, M.; Wicha, M. S.; Benito-Hernandez, A.; Morrison, S. J. & Clarke M. F. (2003). Prospective identification of tumorigenic breast cancer cells. *Proc Natl Acad Sci U S A* 100:3983-3988.

Barker, N.; Ridgway, R.A.; van Es, J.H.; van de Wetering, M.; Begthel, H.; van den Born, M.; Danenberg, E.; Clarke, A.R.; Sansom, O.J. & Clevers, H. (2009). Crypt stem cells as the cells-of-origin of intestinal cancer. *Nature*. 457(7229):608-611.

Bonnet, D. & Dick, J. E. (1997). Human acute myeloid leukemia is organized as a hierarchy that originates from a primitive hematopoietic cell. *Nat Med* 3:730-737.

Bussard, K,M.; Boulanger, C.A.; Booth, B.W.; Bruno, R.D. & Smith, G.H. (2010). Reprogramming human cancer cells in the mouse mammary gland. *Cancer Res*. 70(15):6336-6343.

Castellanos, A.; Vicente-Dueñas, C.; Campos-Sánchez, E.; Cruz, J.J.; García-Criado, F.J.; García-Cenador, M.B.; Lazo, P.A.; Pérez-Losada, J. & Sánchez-García, I. (2010). Cancer as a reprogramming-like disease: implications in tumor development and treatment. *Semin Cancer Biol*. 20(2):93-97.

Cobaleda, C.; Jochum, W. & Busslinger, M. (2007). Conversion of mature B cells into T cells by dedifferentiation to uncommitted progenitors. *Nature* 449:473-477.

Cobaleda, C. & Sanchez-Garcia, I. (2009). B-cell acute lymphoblastic leukaemia: towards understanding its cellular origin. *Bioessays* 31:600-609.

Etzioni, R.; Urban, N.; Ramsey, S.; McIntosh, M.; Schwartz, S.; Reid, B.; et al. (2003). The case for early detection. *Nat Rev Cancer* 3:243-252.

Fialkow, P. J.; Jacobson, R. J. & Papayannopoulou, T. (1977). Chronic myelocytic leukemia: clonal origin in a stem cell common to the granulocyte, erythrocyte, platelet and monocyte/macrophage. *Am. J. Med.* 63, 125–130.

Hamburger, A. & Salmon, S. E. (1977). Primary bioassay of human myeloma stem cells. *J Clin Invest* 60:846-854.

Jacques, T.S.; Swales, A.; Brzozowski, M. J.; Henriquez, N. V.; Linehan, J. M.; Mirzadeh, Z.; et al., (2010). Combinations of genetic mutations in the adult neural stem cell compartment determine brain tumour phenotypes. *EMBO J* 29:222-235.

Jamieson, C. H.; Ailles, L. E.; Dylla, S. J.; Muijtjens, M.; Jones, C.; Zehnder, J. L. et al. (2004). Granulocyte-macrophage progenitors as candidate leukemic stem cells in blast-crisis CML. *N Engl J Med* 351:657-667.

Jemal, A.; Siegel, R.; Ward, E.; Hao, Y.; Xu, J.; Thun, M. J. (2009). Cancer statistics, 2009. *CA Cancer J Clin* 59:225-49.

Melo, J. V. & Barnes, D. J. (2007) Chronic myeloid leukaemia as a model of disease evolution in human cancer. *Nat Rev Cancer* 7:441-453

Nakagawa, M.; Takizawa, N.; Narita, M.; Ichisaka, T. & Yamanaka, S. (2010) Promotion of direct reprogramming by transformation-deficient Myc. *Proc Natl Acad Sci U S A*. 107(32):14152-14157.

Pérez-Caro, M.; Cobaleda, C.; González-Herrero, I.; Vicente-Dueñas, C.; Bermejo-Rodríguez, C.; Sánchez-Beato, M., Orfao, A.; Pintado, B.; Flores, T.; Sánchez-Martín, M.; Jiménez, R.; Piris; M.A. & Sánchez-García; I. (2009) Cancer induction by restriction of oncogene expression to the stem cell compartment. *EMBO J*. 28(1):8-20.

Perez-Losada, J.; Sanchez-Martin, M.; Rodriguez-Garcia, A.; Sanchez, M. L.; Orfao, A.; Flores. T. et al. (2002). Zinc-finger transcription factor Slug contributes to the function of the stem cell factor c-kit signaling pathway. *Blood* 100:1274-286.

Perez-Mancera, P. A.; Perez-Caro, M. ; Gonzalez-Herrero, I.; Flores, T.; Orfao, A.; de Herreros, A. G. et al. (2005a). Cancer development induced by graded expression of Snail in mice. *Hum Mol Genet*

Perez-Mancera, P. A.; Gonzalez-Herrero, I.; Perez-Caro, M.; Gutierrez-Cianca, N.; Flores, T.; Gutierrez-Adan, A. et al. (2005b). SLUG in cancer development. *Oncogene* 24:3073-3082.

Saito, Y.; Uchida, N.; Tanaka, S.; Suzuki, N.; Tomizawa-Murasawa, M.; Sone, A. et al. (2010) Induction of cell cycle entry eliminates human leukemia stem cells in a mouse model of AML. *Nat Biotechnol*. 28:275-280.

Sánchez-García, I.; Vicente-Dueñas, C. & Cobaleda, C. (2007)The theoretical basis of cancer-stem-cell-based therapeutics of cancer: Can it be put into practice?. *BioEssays* 29: 1269-1280.

Sánchez-García, I. (2009). The crossroads of oncogenesis and metastasis. *New England Journal of Medicine* 2009; 360: 297-299.

Sanchez-Martin, M.; Rodriguez-Garcia, A.; Perez-Losada, J.; Sagrera, A.; Read, A. P. & Sanchez-Garcia, I. (2002). SLUG (SNAI2) deletions in patients with Waardenburg disease. *Hum Mol Genet* 11:3231-3236.

Sarig, R.; Rivlin, N.; Brosh, R.; Bornstein, C.; Kamer, I.; Ezra, O.; Molchadsky, A.; Goldfinger, N.; Brenner, O. & Rotter, V. (2010). Mutant p53 facilitates somatic cell reprogramming and augments the malignant potential of reprogrammed cells. *J Exp Med*. Aug 9. [Epub ahead of print].

Singh, S. K.; Clarke, I. D.; Hide, T. & Dirks, P. B. (2004) Cancer stem cells in nervous system tumors. *Oncogene* 23:7267-73.

Vicente-Duenas, C., Perez-Caro, M., Abollo-Jimenez, F., Cobaleda, C. & Sanchez-Garcia, I. (2009). Stem-cell driven cancer: "hands-off" regulation of cancer development. *Cell Cycle* 8:1314-1318.

Vicente-Duenas, C.; Cobaleda, C.; Perez-Losada, J. & Sanchez-Garcia, I. (2010). The evolution of cancer modeling: the shadow of stem cells. *Dis Model Mech*. 3(3-4):149-155.

Wang, X.; Kruithof-de Julio, M.; Economides, K. D.; Walker, D.; Yu, H.; Halili, M. V. et al. (2009). A luminal epithelial stem cell that is a cell of origin for prostate cancer. *Nature* 461:495-500.

Zhang, B.; Strauss, A.C; Chu, S.; Li, M.; Ho, Y.; Shiang, K.D.; Zinder, D.S.; Huettner, C.S.; Shultz, L.; Holyoake, T. & Bhatia, R. (2010). Effective targeting of quiescent chronic myelogenous leukemia stem cells by histone deacetylase inhibitors in combination with imatinib mesylate. *Cancer Cell*. 17(5):427-442.

Zhu, L.; Gibson, P.; Currle, D.S.; Tong, Y.; Richardson, R.J.; Bayazitov, I.T.; Poppleton, H.; Zakharenko, S.; Ellison, D.W. & Gilbertson, R.J. (2009). Prominin 1 marks intestinal stem cells that are susceptible to neoplastic transformation. *Nature*. 457(7229):603-607.

Part 2

Stem Cells in Specific Tumors

5

Breast Cancer Stem Cells

Marco A. Velasco-Velázquez[1,2],
Xuanmao Jiao[1] and Richard G. Pestell[1]
[1]*Kimmel Cancer Center, Thomas Jefferson University*
[2]*Facultad de Medicina, Universidad Nacional Autónoma de México*
[1]*USA*
[2]*México*

1. Introduction

Breast cancer is the most common non-cutaneous type of cancer in women and the most common cause of cancer-related mortality among women worldwide, with more than 1,000,000 new cases and more than 410,000 deaths each year (Parkin et al., 2005; Anderson et al., 2006; Parkin & Fernandez, 2006). Even when breast cancer mortality is decreasing in developed countries due to primary prevention, screening, and improved therapies, there were still 130,000 deaths in europe (Boyle & Ferlay, 2005) and 40,000 deaths in US (Ries et al., 2008) during 2004. Moreover, in less developed countries breast cancer patients show poorer treatment outcomes and increased mortality rates as result of diagnosis at a more advanced stage (Boyle, 2005).

Therapy for breast cancer includes cytotoxic, hormonal, and immunotherapeutic agents. In general, these agents induce response rates ranging from 60% to 80% for primary breast cancers and about 50% of metastases (Guarneri & Conte, 2004; Gonzalez-Angulo et al., 2007). However, despite the frecuency of primary responses, the median duration of response to chemotherapy is 8 to 14 months (Pusztai & Hortobagyi, 1998). Consequently, 20% to 70% of patients show recurrent disease within 5 years (Pusztai & Hortobagyi, 1998; Pisani et al., 2002; Colleoni et al., 2004). The use of local radiotherapy in addition to chemotherapy reduces mortality by 17 to 30% and is particularly beneficial for patients with extensive nodal metastasis, which tend to contain a higher absolute number of chemotherapy resistant cells (Ragaz, 2009).

These data indicate that even though current treatments are active at the beginning of therapy, progression still occurs in the majority of patients. Furthermore, when recurrence appears, resistance to therapy is common increasing the risk of death (Gonzalez-Angulo et al., 2007). The failure of current treatments necessitates new approaches. Such approaches must consider the potential role of cancer stem cells (CSCs) in the initiation, maintenance, and clinical outcome of breast cancers.

2. Breast cancer stem cells

The cells within a tumor display functional heterogeneity, with different morphology, differentiation grade, proliferation rate, and invasiveness (Heppner & Miller, 1983). Recent studies suggest that the ability of a tumor to proliferate and propagate relies on a small population of stem-like cells, called cancer stem cells (CSCs). CSCs share fundamental characteristics with normal adult stem cells: they divide asymmetrically producing one stem cell and one progenitor cell. In normal stem cells, this allows the continuation of the stem cell compartment and starts the production of cells that undergoes multilineage differentiation. Similarly, CSCs have the ability to perpetually self-renew and to produce tumors comprised of cells with different phenotypes. Since their discovery in leukaemia (Bonnet & Dick, 1997), the existence of a subpopulation of CSCs has been corroborated in several solid tumours, including breast, brain, colon, pancreas, prostate, lung, and head and neck tumors (Glinsky, 2007; Li et al., 2007; Prince et al., 2007; Eramo et al., 2008).

2.1 Identification and isolation of breast CSCs

The discovery of CSCs in human breast tumors was reported in 2003 by Al-Hajj and collaborators. They discovered a cellular population characterized by cell-surface $CD44^{+}/CD24^{-/low}/ESA^{+}$ markers, and lineage^{-} (lack of expression of CD2, CD3, CD10, CD 16, CD18, CD31, CD64, and CD140b). As few as 200 of these cells were able to form tumors when injected into NOD/SCID mice while tens of thousands of other cells could not (Al-Hajj et al., 2003). The tumors that were generated recapitulated the phenotypic heterogeneity of the initial tumor, containing a minority of $CD44^{+}/CD24^{-/low}$/lineage^{-} cells that can be serially passaged to form new tumors (Al-Hajj et al., 2003). The $CD44^{+}/CD24^{-}$ phenotype has been used extensively to identify and isolate cancer cells with increased tumorigenicity (Fig. 1).

Breast CSCs have also been isolated from patient samples after *in vitro* propagation (Ponti et al., 2005) and from breast cancer cell lines (Fillmore & Kuperwasser, 2008). The breast CSCs convey an ability to form mammospheres in culture. Mammosphere culture is a system that allows the propagation of mammary epithelial cells in an undifferentiated state, based on their ability to proliferate in suspension as non-adherent spheres (Dontu et al., 2003; Dontu et al., 2004). Accordingly, the capacity to form mammospheres is increased in early progenitor/stem cells. These cells have the ability to differentiate along all three mammary epithelial lineages and to generate complex functional structures in reconstituted 3D culture systems (Dontu et al., 2003; Dontu et al., 2004). The mammospheres from breast cancer cells are enriched in cells with the $CD44^{+}/CD24^{-/low}$ phenotype, and these cells retain tumor-initiating capability when injected into NOD/SCID mice (Fig. 1). However, only a fraction of $CD44^{+}/CD24^{-/low}$ cells is able to form secondary mammospheres (Ponti et al., 2005). Consistent with these findings, cancer cell lines that are enriched (90%) in $CD44^{+}/CD24^{-/low}$ cells are not more tumorigenic than cell lines that contain only 5% of cells with the same phenotype (Fillmore & Kuperwasser, 2008), indicating that only a subgroup within the $CD44^{+}/CD24^{-/low}$ cells are self-renewing.

As only a subpopulation of $CD44^{+}/CD24^{-}$ cells form tumors, additional markers have been investigated. Aldehyde dehydrogenase (ALDH) family of cytosolic isoenzymes are responsible for oxidizing intracellular aldehydes, leading to the oxidation of retinol to retinoic acid, an event that ocurrs in early stem cell differentiation. ALDH1 is the predominant ALDH isoform in mammalian cells. Increased ALDH activity has been described in human hematopoietic stem cells as well as in cancer stem cells of multiple tissues (Hess et al., 2004; Corti et al., 2006). Aldefluor staining for the identification of breast CSCs uses an uncharged ALDH substrate, BAAA (BODIPY-aminoacetaldehyde). BAAA is

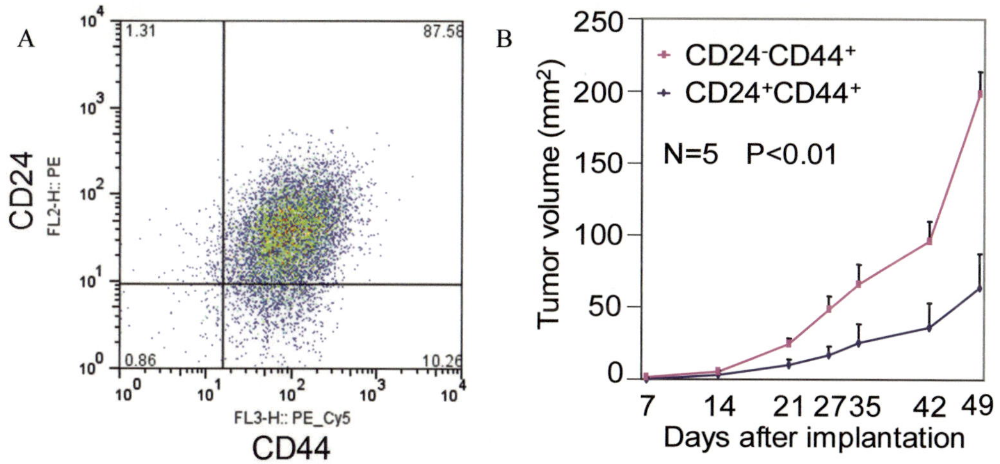

Fig. 1. Increased tumorigenicity of $CD44^+/CD24^-$ Met-1 mouse breast cancer cells (from Wu et al., 2010 J Biol Chem, in press). A) Met-1 cells were separated by immunosorting based on the phenotypes CD44+/CD24- or CD44+/CD24+. B) Tumor regeneration after after subcutaneous implantation of 1000 sorted cells per mouse.

taken up by living cells through passive diffusion and converted by intracellular ALDH into a negatively charged reaction product BAA^- (BODIPY-aminoacetate). BAA^- is retained inside cells expressing high levels of ALDH, causing them to become brightly fluorescent (Christ et al., 2007). Thus, the ALDH-expressing cells can be detected in the green fluorescence channel (520-540 nm) of a standard flow cytometer (Fig. 2). Breast tumor cells positive for ALDH activity are able to generate tumors in NOD/SCID mice with phenotypic characteristics resembling the parental tumor, suggesting that the $ALDH^+$ pool contain the CSC population (Ginestier et al., 2007). The cell selection using the $CD44^+/CD24^-/ALDH^+$ phenotype increases the tumorigenicity of breast cancer cells in comparision with $CD44^+/CD24^-$ or $ALDH^+$ cells (Ginestier et al., 2007).

New strategies to improve the identification and isolation efficiency of breast CSCs have been recently reported (Cicalese et al., 2009; Pece et al., 2010; Sajithlal et al., 2010). The fluorescent dye PKH26 has been used to identify the fraction of stem cells in normal human mammary cells. Briefly, the method consists of labelling the cell membrane with PKH26 and then culturing the mammary cells in suspension to form mammospheres. After 7-10 days only the slow cycling cells retain the dye and can be sorted based on their PKH26 fluorescence intensity. The $PKH26^{hi}$ cells (0.2-0.4% of the total cell population) are able to form secondary mammospheres, divide asymetrically, express markers of pluripotentiality, and can reconstitute a normal mammary epithelium when transplanted into NOD/SCID mice, indicating that this population is highly enriched in stem cells (Pece et al., 2010). The same strategy has been successfully used to enrich breast CSCs in ErbB2 transgenic mice (Cicalese et al., 2009) and from human cancer cell lines (Fig. 3). Furthermore, analysis of the expression profile of $PKH26^{hi}$ cells allowed the identification of the $CD49f^+/DLL1^{hi}/DNER^{hi}$ phenotype as prospective markers of human breast CSCs (Pece et al., 2010). $CD49f^+/DLL1^{hi}/DNER^{hi}$ cells are present in human breast tumor samples, corresponding to 1.5-6% of the cancer cells. The $CD49f^+/DLL1^{hi}/DNER^{hi}$ fraction is enriched in CSCs, since the injection of only 500 of those cells was sufficient to produce tumors in NOD/SCID mice (Pece et al., 2010).

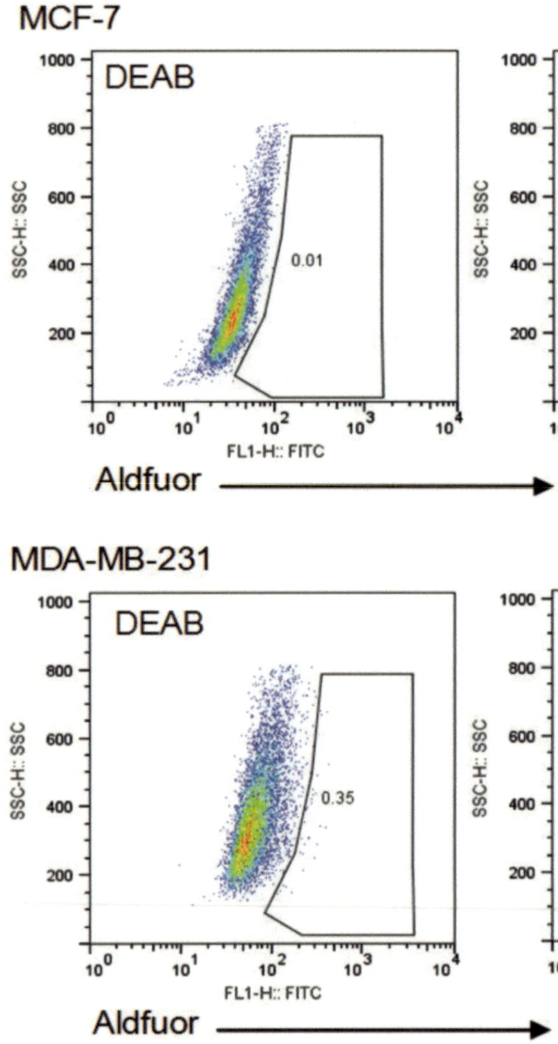

Fig. 2. Aldefluor assay of MCF-7 and MDA-MB-231 breast cancer cells (Jiao et al., unpublished). This assay allows the identification and separation of CSCs based on the activity of ALDH. DEAB is an inhibitor of ALDH used to increase specificity of the assay. Note that the ALDH+ fraction in MCF-7 cells is almost undetectable.

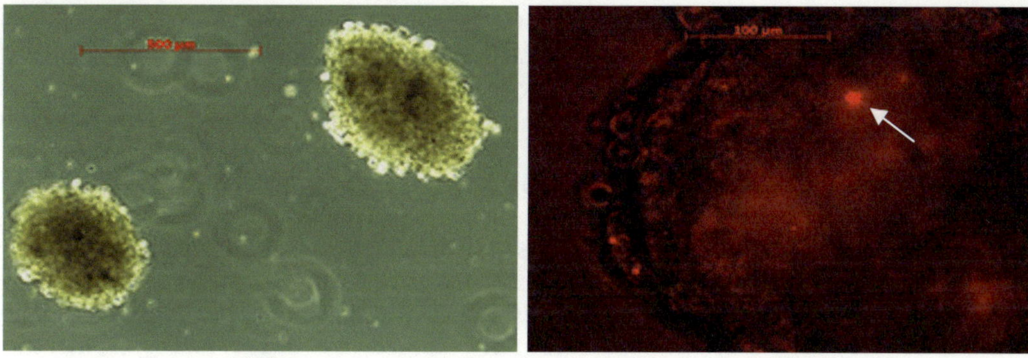

(A) (B)

Fig. 3. PKH26 retention during mammosphere culture (Velasco-Velazquez et al., unpublished). A) Hs578T human breast cancer cells cultured in non-adherent conditions for 7 days (bright field). B) Fluorescence microscopy shows that only a few cells retain a high level of PKH26 (arrow). Those cells have properties of CSCs.

A different approach was recently reported by Sajithlal and collaborators (Sajithlal et al., 2010). They tagged the CSC population from human cancer cell lines with green fluorescent protein (GFP) under the control of the Oct3/4 promoter. In MCF-7 cells only 1% of the population expressed GFP, and the large majority of those cells were $CD44^+/CD24^-$. GFP^+ cells were sorted and maintained in culture. Unexpectedly, the $CD44^+/CD24^-/GFP^+$ phenotype remained stable for more than one year, suggesting that the incorporation of the promoter blocks CSC differentiation. As predicted, the GFP+ cells were 100-300 times more tumorigenic that the rest of tumor cells and displayed an increased resistance to cytotoxic drugs. Similar results were found when other breast cancer cell lines were stably transfected with the Oct3/4 promoter (Sajithlal et al., 2010). These cell lines may become valuable models in the study of CSC biology.

Other stem cell markers have been used to identify breast CSCs in murine models, including CD133 and the β1 integrin subunit (CD29). In tumor cell lines generated form Brca1 deficient mice, Wright and collaborators found two different populations of potential CSCs: one with the previously reported $CD44^+/CD24^-$ phenotype and the other being $CD133^+$ (Wright et al., 2008). Both subpopulations were able to repopulate cell fractions found in the parental cell lines, formed *in vitro* mammospheres, generated tumors in NOD/SCID mice, and expressed Oct4, a marker of pluripotency. In a similar manner, subpopulations of $CD24^{hi}CD29^{low}$ cells isolated from tumor cell lines exhibit the capacity of self-renewal, differentiation and tumorigenicity (Vassilopoulos et al., 2008). One possibility is that these cells with different immunophenotypes represent different origins of breast cancer stem cells. The $CD44^+/CD24^-$ population most likely represent basal breast cancer stem cells and cells with the $CD24^{hi}CD29^{low}$ signature most likely originate from the mammary luminal progenitor cells. These data, together with the fact that CD133 and CD29 have been used in the identification of normal and cancer stem cells from different tissues, indicate that CD133 and CD29 could be used as a marker of mouse breast CSCs. The diversity of mouse breast cancer stem cells may provide a tool to elucidate the hierarchy of breast cancer stem cells.

3. Therapeutic resistance in breast CSCs

Whether breast CSCs arise from normal stem cells or from progenitor cells that have gained the ability for self-renewal remains unclear. However, both of these hypotheses consider that the different phenotypic characteristics of normal and cancerous stem cells are caused by genetic alterations that promote changes in the signalling pathways controlling the cell cycle, differentiation, and survival. These alterations promote changes in key CSC functions that are directly related to the clinical outcome of the tumor. In the case of breast cancer, a growing body of evidence indicates that CSCs are more resistant to chemo- and radiotherapy than the non-stem tumor cells. Accordingly with the cancer stem cell hypothesis, the surviving CSCs will be capable to repopulate treated-tumors and produce relapse. Moreover, since mutations can be passed on to all the stem cell's progeny, it is likely that the new tumor will display increased resistance to therapeutic regimens, allowing evolution towards malignancy over time. Elucidation of the molecular mechanisms by which CSCs survive therapy may identify new targets for breast cancer therapeutic intervention.

3.1 Chemoresistance and mechanisms involved

The role of chemotherapy in the selection and expansion of breast CSCs has been studied using different strategies. The proportion of *in vitro* self-renewing cancer cells from patients who received neoadjuvant chemotherapy has been compared with that of cells isolated from chemotherapy-naive patients. Mammosphere formation was 14-fold higher in tumor cells from the patients that had received chemotherapy (Yu et al., 2007). Enrichment of CSCs by chemotherapy was confirmed by studying paired specimens from patients obtained by biopsy prior to chemotherapy and at surgery following neoadjuvant chemotherapy. Mammosphere formation and the proportion of $CD44^{+}/CD24^{-/low}$ cells were increased approximately 10-fold after chemotherapy (Yu et al., 2007).

Additional evidence from mouse models supports that exposure to chemotherapeutic agents elicits a selective pressure and prevents differentiation of CSCs, increasing the proportion of CSC in the tumors. Yu and collaborators studied the properties of tumors generated by SKBR3 breast cancer cells after consecutive passage in mice receiving epirubicin. Those tumors were highly enriched in $CD44^{+}/CD24^{-}/lineage^{-}$ cells, and were able to form 20-fold more mammospheres than cells isolated from tumors generated with the parental cell line (Yu et al., 2007). The expansion of the CSC population after drug treatment contributes to drug resistance. Mammary tumors from Brca1/p53-mutated mice are sensitive to cisplatin, but a few months after treatment, tumors relapse at the same site. The proportion of $CD29^{hi}/CD24^{med}$ cells (tumorigenic cells) in tumors that arise after cisplatin treatment was 4-fold greater than in untreated primary tumors (Shafee et al., 2008). Interestingly, when $CD29^{hi}/CD24^{med}$ cells from relapse tumors were injected into $Rag1^{-/-}$ mice, they formed tumors that were only partially sensitive to cisplatin. A second round of selection and transplantation further increased the $CD29^{hi}/CD24^{med}$ fraction and generated tumors that were completely refractory to cisplatin (Shafee et al., 2008), indicating the appearance of cisplatin-resistant progenitor cells.

3.1.1 Multidrug resistance transporters

The chemoresistance in breast CSCs is caused partially by the expression of ABC (ATP-Binding Cassette) transporters. A subpopulation of breast cancer cells with the capability to extrude the dye Hoechst 33342 (a measurement of ABC transporters activity) is enriched in CSCs (Patrawala et al., 2005; Christgen et al., 2007; Woodward et al., 2007). This subpopulation, called "side population" (SP), isolated from Cal-51 cells exhibited a 30-fold increased in ABCG2 mRNA expression in comparison to unsorted cells (Christgen et al.,

2007). After isolation and expansion, cells from the Cal-51 SP gave rise to a heterogeneous mix of SP and non SP cells in a proportion similar to the original cell line, in which the non SP cells lacked expression of ABCG2. Similarly, ABCG2 expression declined with *in vitro* differentiation of SKBR3 cells isolated from mouse xenotransplants (Yu et al., 2007). Thus, the expression of ABCG2 and the ability to efflux drugs is lost during differentiation of CSCs to cancer cells. These data partially explain why primary chemotherapy produces responses in the large majority of tumors but is ineffective in eradicating the cells that express ABC transporters and CSC properties.

3.1.2 Stem cell signalling pathways

Alterations in signalling pathways controlling self-renewal and cell fate, such as HER-2, Notch, Wnt, and Hedgehog, also contribute to drug resistance in breast CSCs (see (Charafe-Jauffret et al., 2008; Kakarala & Wicha, 2008) for recent reviews). For example, HER-2 may play a role in regulating breast CSC population. HER2 overexpression in breast cancer cell lines increased the CSC population as demonstrated by increased ALDH activity, mammosphere formation, tumorigenesis, and expression of stem cell related genes (Korkaya et al., 2008). ALDH1 has been reported as a major mediator of resistance to cyclophosphamide in CSCs (Dylla et al., 2008), suggesting that HER-2-medited signaling may favor resistance. Correspondingly, HER-2 inhibition with trastuzumab reduced by 50% the recurrence rate after conventional adjuvant chemotherapy (Slamon & Pegram, 2001).

HER-2-mediated CSC expansion may involve the activation of the Notch pathway, which regulates self-renewal of normal mammary stem cells (Dontu et al., 2004). Notch is aberrantly activated in human breast carcinomas (Pece et al., 2004; Stylianou et al., 2006) correlating with cyclin D1 overexpression. Notch directly induces cyclin D1 expression and Notch correlates with cyclin D1 expression during development (Stahl et al., 2006). HER-2 induced Notch-1 activation in breast cancer cells by increasing the expression of cyclin D1. In turn, cyclin D1 inhibited the expression of the Notch-1 negative regulator Numb (Lindsay et al., 2008). In ER-negative breast cancer cells, Notch-1 activation directly promoted the transcription of the antiapoptotic gene Survivin (Lee et al., 2008). In turn, increased survivin levels may deregulate multiple mitotic checkpoints, contributing to genetic instability (Lens et al., 2006) and inhibiting radiation- and drug-induced apoptosis (O'Connor et al., 2002; Ghosh et al., 2006). Additional evidence of the role of a Notch/survivin axis in breast CSCs survival and resistance include that: i) Notch-1 protects $CD44^{+}/CD24^{-/low}$ breast cancer-initiating cells from radiation (Phillips et al., 2006); ii) a neutralizing antibody against Notch-4 reduced mammosphere viability in primary cultures of ductal carcinoma *in situ* of the breast (Farnie et al., 2007); iii) the antiapoptotic protein survivin is overexpressed in breast CSC cultures (Ponti et al., 2005); and iv) chemoresitance displayed in CSCs isolated from MCF-7 cells is associated with increased expression of Notch-1 (Sajithlal et al., 2010). These data suggest that survivin and cyclin D1 may operate as a Notch-regulated cytoprotective factors that promote persistence of breast CSCs.

4. Role of CSCs in breast tumor metastasis

Metastasis is a highly complex process that comprises several sequential steps, that include escape from the primary tumor (intravasation), survival within the circulation, extravasation into a secondary site, and sustained growth in a distinct microenvironment (Woodhouse et al., 1997; Chambers et al., 2002; Pantel & Brakenhoff, 2004). Several lines of evidence indicate that metastasis is a highly inefficient process. Depending on the experimental model, 0.02-0.1% of the cancer cells that reach the circulation can develop macrometastases (Weiss, 1990; MacDonald et al., 2002; Allan et al., 2006). Recently, CSCs capable of seeding distant metastasis have been identified (Li et al., 2007) supporting the model in which CSCs initiate and sustain secondary tumor growth. Accordingly, several authors have proposed a model in which CSCs appear as the active source of metastatic spread (Wicha, 2006; Li et al., 2007; Goss et al., 2008; Visvader & Lindeman, 2008).

In agreement with that model, a subpopulation of circulating tumor cells that express stem cell markers has been identified in metastatic breast cancer patients and a high percentage of $CD44^{+}/CD24^{-}$ tumor cells have been found in metastases. (Balic et al., 2006; Aktas et al., 2009; Theodoropoulos et al., 2010). Additionally, a gene signature of invasiveness (IGS), generated by comparing the gene-expression profile of $CD44^{+}/CD24^{-}$ tumorigenic breast cancer cells with that of normal breast epithelium, is strongly associated with metastasis-free survival (Liu et al., 2007). Finally, expression of the stem cell marker ALDH in samples of inflammatory breast cancer (IBC) correlates with the development of distant metastasis and decreased survival (Charafe-Jauffret et al., 2010).

The ability of breast CSCs to invade and proliferate at the metastatic sites has been studied both *in vitro* and *in vivo*. CSCs isolated from cancer cell lines exhibited increased invasiveness and elevated expression of genes involved in invasion (IL-1α, IL-6, IL-8, CXCR4, MMP-1, and UPA) (Sheridan et al., 2006). Accordingly, $ALDH^{+}$ cells isolated from breast cancer cell lines were more migratory and invasive than the $ALDH^{-}$ cells (Charafe-Jauffret et al., 2009; Croker et al., 2009). Intracardiac injection of $ALDH^{+}$ cells isolated from human breast cancer cell lines to NOD/SCID mice generated metastases at distinct organs; in contrast, $ALDH^{-}$ cells produced only occasional metastases limited to lymph nodes (Charafe-Jauffret et al., 2009; Charafe-Jauffret et al., 2010).

Molecular genetic analysis has identified key regulators of the breast cancer stem cell phenotype using knockout and transgenic mice including c-Jun (Jiao et al., 2010) , $p21^{CIP}$ (Liu et al., 2009), NFκB (Liu et al., 2010 Cancer Res, in press) and the retinal determination gene network (RDGN) (Micalizzi et al., 2009); Wu et al., 2010 J Biol Chem, in press).

Our group has shown that molecular signals that promote "stemness" in cancer cells also promote the acquisition of metastatic ability. Using bitransgenic mice encoding a floxed c-Jun allele and mammary targeted ErbB2 we have reported that the proto-oncogene c-Jun

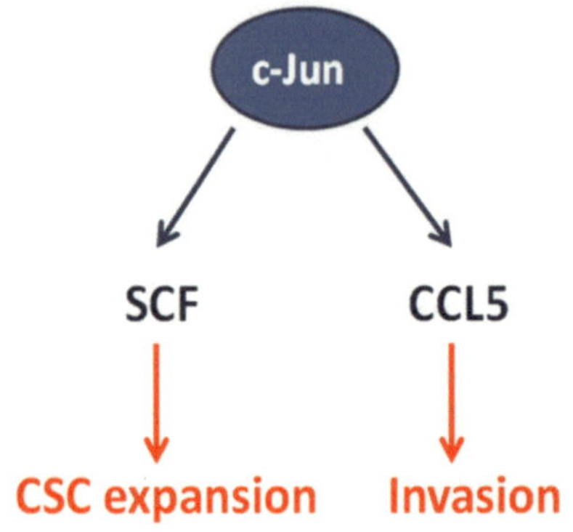

Fig. 4. Schematic representation of c-Jun-mediated cellular migration and CSC expansion via induction of SCF and CCL5 (RANTES) production (adapted from Jiao et al. 2010).

controls the transcriptional expression of SCF (Stem Cell Factor) and CCL5 (RANTES). Reduction in SCF causes a decrease in the proportion of cells expressing breast CSC markers and in CSC self-renewal, while c-Jun-mediated expression of CCL5 plays a key role in the autocrine control of the migration and invasion of breast cancer cells (Jiao et al., 2010). These studies demonstrated that a single cellular proto-oncogene is necessary to both, activate signaling pathways that promote features of CSC and maintain the invasive phenotype of mammary tumors (Fig. 4).

5. Targeting CSCs

The key roles of CSCs in breast cancer biology suggest that new therapies must target these cells. The main objective of those therapies would be the eradication of the CSC compartment with no harm to other cell types. Eradication of breast CSCs may include different strategies as summarized in Table 1.

Different approaches have been used to overcome ABC transporter-mediated chemoresistance. The anthracycline modified drug annamycin, which is not extruded by ABC transporters, was toxic to the resistant cell line MCF-7/VP (Perez-Soler et al., 1997). The plant alkaloid berberine decreased the expression of the ABCG2 transporter and reduced the "side population" of the MCF-7 cell line (Kim et al., 2008), suggesting that downregulation of ABC transporters may be useful for targeting breast CSCs. However, the ability to target drug transport in CSCs may be difficult since these cells express multiple ABC transporters (de Grouw et al., 2006). The use of inhibitors of ABC transporters simultaneously with anticancer drugs is an efficient approach to overcome resistance *in vitro* and in animal models (Ozben, 2006). However, clinical trials with this kind of inhibitors have shown that they produce serious side effects (Ozben, 2006). High-throughput screening identified the ionophore salinomycin as toxic to breast CSCs (Gupta et al., 2009). Salinomycin induced capase-independent apoptosis in human cancer cells of different origins that display multiple mechanisms of drug resistance, at concentrations that did not affected normal cell viability (Fuchs et al., 2009). Subsequent studies showed that salinomycin induces a conformational change of the ABC transporter MDR1/ABCB1 that reduces its activity (Riccioni et al., 2010). Therefore, salinomycin is particularly effective at inducing apoptosis in leukemia cells that display ABC transporter-mediated drug-resistance (Fuchs et al., 2010).

Targeting CSCs through their specific markers was partially succesful in acute myeloid leukemia (AML) (Sperr et al., 2005; Tsimberidou et al., 2006). Cytotoxic antibodies directed against CD33 (a common marker in leukemic stem cells) induced remission in some patients. However, the antibody produced cytopenia due to its effects on normal hematopoietic stem cells (Sperr et al., 2005; Tsimberidou et al., 2006). Similarly, a monoclonal antibody against CD44 induced terminal differentiation and apoptosis of AML cells in engrafted mice (Jin et al., 2006). Anti-CD44 antibodies conjugated with cytotoxic drugs or radiolabels have shown to reduce disease progression in breast cancer patients and animal models (reviewed by (Platt & Szoka, 2008)).

Other potential targets in breast CSC therapy include molecules that participate in self-renewal and cell fate. Inhibition of Hedgehog signaling in xenografts established from pancreatic cancer cell lines reduced the number of ALDH-overexpressing cells (Feldmann et al., 2008). The promoters of the MDR, hTERT, and Cox-2 genes are active in breast CSCs. Oncolytic adenoviruses driven by these promoters were effective in killing $CD44^{+}/CD24^{-/low}$ cells *in vitro*, and reducing tumor growth *in vivo* (Bauerschmitz et al., 2008).

Interruption of signals generated in the CSC microenvironment using antibodies or soluble ligands against adhesion receptors may be useful in CSC targeting. α6-integrin inactivation with antibodies or siRNA abrogated mammosphere-forming ability and tumorigenicity of breast cancer cells (Cariati et al., 2008). The IL-8 receptor CXCR1 inhibitor repertaxin reduced the breast CSC population, producing apoptosis in the tumor population, and reduced metastasis (Ginestier et al., 2010).

Target in breast CSCs	Strategy	Example
ABC transporters	Cytotoxic drugs that cannot be extruded by ABC transporters	Annamycin
	Reduce expression	Berberine siRNAs
	ABC transporters inhibitors	Salinomycin
Membrane markers	Antibodies conjugated with drugs or radioligands	Anti-CD44
Intracellular signalling molecules	Small molecule inhibitors	---
	Reduce expression	siRNAs
	Oncolytic virus activated by specific promoters	MDR promoter
Signals from the microenvironment	Small molecule receptor antagonists	Repertaxin
	Blocking antibodies	Anti-α6 integrin
	Blocking soluble ligands	Soluble HA
Others	Metabolic alteration?	Metformin

Table 1. Strategies for the eradication of CSCs.

Metformin is an anti-diabetic drug that has found to reduce breast cancer incidence and improve survival of breast cancer patients with type 2 diabetics (Vazquez-Martin et al., 2010a). Recent studies showed that the drug metformin selectively reduces the breast CSC population. In human breast cancer cell lines, metformin reduced the $CD44^{+}/CD24^{-}$ population and their ability to form mammospheres (Hirsch et al., 2009). In a xenograft mice model, concurrent treatment with metformin and doxorubicin reduced tumor mass much more effectively than either drug alone (Hirsch et al., 2009). Metformin also targeted traztasumab-resistant CSCs that overexpress HER-2 (Vazquez-Martin et al., 2010b). The mechanism involved in the metformin effects on CSCs is unclear, but seem to be associated with its activator effect on AMP-activated kinase (AMPK) (Vazquez-Martin et al., 2010a). AMPK phosphorylates and inhibits Acetyl CoA carboxylase (ACACA), the limiting enzyme of the fatty acid synthesis. Thus, metformin may be affecting cancer cell metabolism and functioning of lipid raft platforms (Vazquez-Martin et al., 2010a).

6. Conclusions

CSCs have a central role in breast cancer progression since they are involved in tumorigenesis, therapy response, and metastasis formation. Diverse methodologies based on their phenotype or specific cellular functions have been described to isolate mouse and human breast CSCs. Combinations of these methodologies improve the efficiency of purification.

Development of new therapies for targeting and eradication of breast CSCs must consider both, the differences between CSCs cells and the rest of the tumor cells and the pathways shared between CSCs and normal stem cells. Elucidation of the specific mechanisms by which CSCs survive chemotherapy, regulate self-renewal, and interact with their primary and metastatic niches will be useful for the design of new therapeutic alternatives. Such approaches may become the basis for the generation of effective and clinically applicable therapies that prevent disease relapse, metastasis and enhance patient survival.

7. References

Aktas, B., Tewes, M., Fehm, T., Hauch, S., Kimmig, R. & Kasimir-Bauer, S. (2009). Stem cell and epithelial-mesenchymal transition markers are frequently overexpressed in circulating tumor cells of metastatic breast cancer patients, *Breast Cancer Res* 11(4): R46.

Al-Hajj, M., Wicha, M.S., Benito-Hernandez, A., Morrison, S.J. & Clarke, M.F. (2003). Prospective identification of tumorigenic breast cancer cells, *Proc Natl Acad Sci U S A* 100(7): 3983-8.

Allan, A.L., Vantyghem, S.A., Tuck, A.B. & Chambers, A.F. (2006). Tumor dormancy and cancer stem cells: implications for the biology and treatment of breast cancer metastasis, *Breast Dis* 26: 87-98.

Anderson, B.O., Yip, C.H., Ramsey, S.D., Bengoa, R., Braun, S., Fitch, M., Groot, M., Sancho-Garnier, H. & Tsu, V.D. (2006). Breast cancer in limited-resource countries: health care systems and public policy, *Breast J* 12 Suppl 1: S54-69.

Balic, M., Lin, H., Young, L., Hawes, D., Giuliano, A., McNamara, G., Datar, R.H. & Cote, R.J. (2006). Most early disseminated cancer cells detected in bone marrow of breast cancer patients have a putative breast cancer stem cell phenotype, *Clin Cancer Res* 12(19): 5615-21.

Bauerschmitz, G.J., Ranki, T., Kangasniemi, L., Ribacka, C., Eriksson, M., Porten, M., Herrmann, I., Ristimaki, A., Virkkunen, P., Tarkkanen, M., Hakkarainen, T., Kanerva, A., Rein, D., Pesonen, S. & Hemminki, A. (2008). Tissue-specific promoters active in CD44+CD24-/low breast cancer cells, *Cancer Res* 68(14): 5533-9.

Bonnet, D. & Dick, J.E. (1997). Human acute myeloid leukemia is organized as a hierarchy that originates from a primitive hematopoietic cell, *Nat Med* 3(7): 730-7.

Boyle, P. (2005). Breast cancer control: signs of progress, but more work required, *Breast* 14(6): 429-38.

Boyle, P. & Ferlay, J. (2005). Cancer incidence and mortality in Europe, 2004, *Ann Oncol* 16(3): 481-8.

Cariati, M., Naderi, A., Brown, J.P., Smalley, M.J., Pinder, S.E., Caldas, C. & Purushotham, A.D. (2008). Alpha-6 integrin is necessary for the tumourigenicity of a stem cell-like subpopulation within the MCF7 breast cancer cell line, *Int J Cancer* 122(2): 298-304.

Chambers, A.F., Groom, A.C. & MacDonald, I.C. (2002). Dissemination and growth of cancer cells in metastatic sites, *Nat Rev Cancer* 2(8): 563-72.

Charafe-Jauffret, E., Ginestier, C., Iovino, F., Tarpin, C., Diebel, M., Esterni, B., Houvenaeghel, G., Extra, J.M., Bertucci, F., Jacquemier, J., Xerri, L., Dontu, G., Stassi, G., Xiao, Y., Barsky, S.H., Birnbaum, D., Viens, P. & Wicha, M.S. (2010). Aldehyde dehydrogenase 1-positive cancer stem cells mediate metastasis and poor clinical outcome in inflammatory breast cancer, *Clin Cancer Res* 16(1): 45-55.

Charafe-Jauffret, E., Ginestier, C., Iovino, F., Wicinski, J., Cervera, N., Finetti, P., Hur, M.H., Diebel, M.E., Monville, F., Dutcher, J., Brown, M., Viens, P., Xerri, L., Bertucci, F., Stassi, G., Dontu, G., Birnbaum, D. & Wicha, M.S. (2009). Breast cancer cell lines contain functional cancer stem cells with metastatic capacity and a distinct molecular signature, *Cancer Res* 69(4): 1302-13.

Charafe-Jauffret, E., Monville, F., Ginestier, C., Dontu, G., Birnbaum, D. & Wicha, M.S. (2008). Cancer stem cells in breast: current opinion and future challenges, *Pathobiology* 75(2): 75-84.

Christ, O., Lucke, K., Imren, S., Leung, K., Hamilton, M., Eaves, A., Smith, C. & Eaves, C. (2007). Improved purification of hematopoietic stem cells based on their elevated aldehyde dehydrogenase activity, *Haematologica* 92(9): 1165-72.

Christgen, M., Ballmaier, M., Bruchhardt, H., von Wasielewski, R., Kreipe, H. & Lehmann, U. (2007). Identification of a distinct side population of cancer cells in the Cal-51 human breast carcinoma cell line, *Mol Cell Biochem* 306(1-2): 201-12.

Cicalese, A., Bonizzi, G., Pasi, C.E., Faretta, M., Ronzoni, S., Giulini, B., Brisken, C., Minucci, S., Di Fiore, P.P. & Pelicci, P.G. (2009). The tumor suppressor p53 regulates polarity of self-renewing divisions in mammary stem cells, *Cell* 138(6): 1083-95.

Colleoni, M., Viale, G., Zahrieh, D., Pruneri, G., Gentilini, O., Veronesi, P., Gelber, R.D., Curigliano, G., Torrisi, R., Luini, A., Intra, M., Galimberti, V., Renne, G., Nole, F., Peruzzotti, G. & Goldhirsch, A. (2004). Chemotherapy is more effective in patients with breast cancer not expressing steroid hormone receptors: a study of preoperative treatment, *Clin Cancer Res* 10(19): 6622-8.

Corti, S., Locatelli, F., Papadimitriou, D., Donadoni, C., Salani, S., Del Bo, R., Strazzer, S., Bresolin, N. & Comi, G.P. (2006). Identification of a primitive brain-derived neural stem cell population based on aldehyde dehydrogenase activity, *Stem Cells* 24(4): 975-85.

Croker, A.K., Goodale, D., Chu, J., Postenka, C., Hedley, B.D., Hess, D.A. & Allan, A.L. (2009). High aldehyde dehydrogenase and expression of cancer stem cell markers selects for breast cancer cells with enhanced malignant and metastatic ability, *J Cell Mol Med* 13(8B): 2236-52.

de Grouw, E.P., Raaijmakers, M.H., Boezeman, J.B., van der Reijden, B.A., van de Locht, L.T., de Witte, T.J., Jansen, J.H. & Raymakers, R.A. (2006). Preferential expression of a high number of ATP binding cassette transporters in both normal and leukemic CD34+CD38- cells, *Leukemia* 20(4): 750-4.

Dontu, G., Abdallah, W.M., Foley, J.M., Jackson, K.W., Clarke, M.F., Kawamura, M.J. & Wicha, M.S. (2003). In vitro propagation and transcriptional profiling of human mammary stem/progenitor cells, *Genes Dev* 17(10): 1253-70.

Dontu, G., Jackson, K.W., McNicholas, E., Kawamura, M.J., Abdallah, W.M. & Wicha, M.S. (2004). Role of Notch signaling in cell-fate determination of human mammary stem/progenitor cells, *Breast Cancer Res* 6(6): R605-15.

Dylla, S.J., Beviglia, L., Park, I.K., Chartier, C., Raval, J., Ngan, L., Pickell, K., Aguilar, J., Lazetic, S., Smith-Berdan, S., Clarke, M.F., Hoey, T., Lewicki, J. & Gurney, A.L. (2008). Colorectal cancer stem cells are enriched in xenogeneic tumors following chemotherapy, *PLoS ONE* 3(6): e2428.

Eramo, A., Lotti, F., Sette, G., Pilozzi, E., Biffoni, M., Di Virgilio, A., Conticello, C., Ruco, L., Peschle, C. & De Maria, R. (2008). Identification and expansion of the tumorigenic lung cancer stem cell population, *Cell Death Differ* 15(3): 504-14.

Farnie, G., Clarke, R.B., Spence, K., Pinnock, N., Brennan, K., Anderson, N.G. & Bundred, N.J. (2007). Novel cell culture technique for primary ductal carcinoma in situ: role of Notch and epidermal growth factor receptor signaling pathways, *J Natl Cancer Inst* 99(8): 616-27.

Feldmann, G., Fendrich, V., McGovern, K., Bedja, D., Bisht, S., Alvarez, H., Koorstra, J.B., Habbe, N., Karikari, C., Mullendore, M., Gabrielson, K.L., Sharma, R., Matsui, W. &

Maitra, A. (2008). An orally bioavailable small-molecule inhibitor of Hedgehog signaling inhibits tumor initiation and metastasis in pancreatic cancer, *Mol Cancer Ther* 7(9): 2725-35.

Fillmore, C.M. & Kuperwasser, C. (2008). Human breast cancer cell lines contain stem-like cells that self-renew, give rise to phenotypically diverse progeny and survive chemotherapy, *Breast Cancer Res* 10(2): R25.

Fuchs, D., Daniel, V., Sadeghi, M., Opelz, G. & Naujokat, C. (2010). Salinomycin overcomes ABC transporter-mediated multidrug and apoptosis resistance in human leukemia stem cell-like KG-1a cells, *Biochem Biophys Res Commun* 394(4): 1098-104.

Fuchs, D., Heinold, A., Opelz, G., Daniel, V. & Naujokat, C. (2009). Salinomycin induces apoptosis and overcomes apoptosis resistance in human cancer cells, *Biochem Biophys Res Commun* 390(3): 743-9.

Ghosh, J.C., Dohi, T., Raskett, C.M., Kowalik, T.F. & Altieri, D.C. (2006). Activated checkpoint kinase 2 provides a survival signal for tumor cells, *Cancer Res* 66(24): 11576-9.

Ginestier, C., Hur, M.H., Charafe-Jauffret, E., Monville, F., Dutcher, J., Brown, M., Jacquemier, J., Viens, P., Kleer, C.G., Liu, S., Schott, A., Hayes, D., Birnbaum, D., Wicha, M.S. & Dontu, G. (2007). ALDH1 is a marker of normal and malignant human mammary stem cells and a predictor of poor clinical outcome, *Cell Stem Cell* 1(5): 555-67.

Ginestier, C., Liu, S., Diebel, M.E., Korkaya, H., Luo, M., Brown, M., Wicinski, J., Cabaud, O., Charafe-Jauffret, E., Birnbaum, D., Guan, J.L., Dontu, G. & Wicha, M.S. (2010). CXCR1 blockade selectively targets human breast cancer stem cells in vitro and in xenografts, *J Clin Invest* 120(2): 485-97.

Glinsky, G.V. (2007). Stem cell origin of death-from-cancer phenotypes of human prostate and breast cancers, *Stem Cell Rev* 3(1): 79-93.

Gonzalez-Angulo, A.M., Morales-Vasquez, F. & Hortobagyi, G.N. (2007). Overview of resistance to systemic therapy in patients with breast cancer, *Adv Exp Med Biol* 608: 1-22.

Goss, P., Allan, A.L., Rodenhiser, D.I., Foster, P.J. & Chambers, A.F. (2008). New clinical and experimental approaches for studying tumor dormancy: does tumor dormancy offer a therapeutic target?, *APMIS* 116(7-8): 552-68.

Guarneri, V. & Conte, P.F. (2004). The curability of breast cancer and the treatment of advanced disease, *Eur J Nucl Med Mol Imaging* 31 Suppl 1: S149-61.

Gupta, P.B., Onder, T.T., Jiang, G., Tao, K., Kuperwasser, C., Weinberg, R.A. & Lander, E.S. (2009). Identification of selective inhibitors of cancer stem cells by high-throughput screening, *Cell* 138(4): 645-59.

Heppner, G.H. & Miller, B.E. (1983). Tumor heterogeneity: biological implications and therapeutic consequences, *Cancer Metastasis Rev* 2(1): 5-23.

Hess, D.A., Meyerrose, T.E., Wirthlin, L., Craft, T.P., Herrbrich, P.E., Creer, M.H. & Nolta, J.A. (2004). Functional characterization of highly purified human hematopoietic repopulating cells isolated according to aldehyde dehydrogenase activity, *Blood* 104(6): 1648-55.

Hirsch, H.A., Iliopoulos, D., Tsichlis, P.N. & Struhl, K. (2009). Metformin selectively targets cancer stem cells, and acts together with chemotherapy to block tumor growth and prolong remission, *Cancer Res* 69(19): 7507-11.

Jiao, X., Katiyar, S., Willmarth, N.E., Liu, M., Ma, X., Flomenberg, N., Lisanti, M.P. & Pestell, R.G. (2010). c-Jun induces mammary epithelial cellular invasion and breast cancer stem cell expansion, *J Biol Chem* 285(11): 8218-26.

Jin, L., Hope, K.J., Zhai, Q., Smadja-Joffe, F. & Dick, J.E. (2006). Targeting of CD44 eradicates human acute myeloid leukemic stem cells, *Nat Med* 12(10): 1167-74.

Kakarala, M. & Wicha, M.S. (2008). Implications of the cancer stem-cell hypothesis for breast cancer prevention and therapy, *J Clin Oncol* 26(17): 2813-20.

Kim, J.B., Ko, E., Han, W., Shin, I., Park, S.Y. & Noh, D.Y. (2008). Berberine Diminishes the Side Population and ABCG2 Transporter Expression in MCF-7 Breast Cancer Cells, *Planta Med.*

Korkaya, H., Paulson, A., Iovino, F. & Wicha, M.S. (2008). HER2 regulates the mammary stem/progenitor cell population driving tumorigenesis and invasion, *Oncogene* 27(47): 6120-30.

Lee, C.W., Raskett, C.M., Prudovsky, I. & Altieri, D.C. (2008). Molecular dependence of estrogen receptor-negative breast cancer on a notch-survivin signaling axis, *Cancer Res* 68(13): 5273-81.

Lens, S.M., Vader, G. & Medema, R.H. (2006). The case for Survivin as mitotic regulator, *Curr Opin Cell Biol* 18(6): 616-22.

Li, C., Heidt, D.G., Dalerba, P., Burant, C.F., Zhang, L., Adsay, V., Wicha, M., Clarke, M.F. & Simeone, D.M. (2007). Identification of pancreatic cancer stem cells, *Cancer Res* 67(3): 1030-7.

Li, F., Tiede, B., Massague, J. & Kang, Y. (2007). Beyond tumorigenesis: cancer stem cells in metastasis, *Cell Res* 17(1): 3-14.

Lindsay, J., Jiao, X., Sakamaki, T., Casimiro, M.C., Shirley, L.A., Tran, T.H., Ju, X., Liu, M., Li, Z., Wang, C., Katiyar, S., Rao, M., Allen, K.G., Glazer, R.I., Ge, C., Stanley, P., Lisanti, M.P., Rui, H. & Pestell, R.G. (2008). ErbB2 induces Notch1 activity and function in breast cancer cells, *Clin Transl Sci* 1(2): 107-15.

Liu, M., Casimiro, M.C., Wang, C., Shirley, L.A., Jiao, X., Katiyar, S., Ju, X., Li, Z., Yu, Z., Zhou, J., Johnson, M., Fortina, P., Hyslop, T., Windle, J.J. & Pestell, R.G. (2009). p21CIP1 attenuates Ras- and c-Myc-dependent breast tumor epithelial mesenchymal transition and cancer stem cell-like gene expression in vivo, *Proc Natl Acad Sci U S A* 106(45): 19035-9.

Liu, R., Wang, X., Chen, G.Y., Dalerba, P., Gurney, A., Hoey, T., Sherlock, G., Lewicki, J., Shedden, K. & Clarke, M.F. (2007). The prognostic role of a gene signature from tumorigenic breast-cancer cells, *N Engl J Med* 356(3): 217-26.

MacDonald, I.C., Groom, A.C. & Chambers, A.F. (2002). Cancer spread and micrometastasis development: quantitative approaches for in vivo models, *Bioessays* 24(10): 885-93.

Micalizzi, D.S., Christensen, K.L., Jedlicka, P., Coletta, R.D., Baron, A.E., Harrell, J.C., Horwitz, K.B., Billheimer, D., Heichman, K.A., Welm, A.L., Schiemann, W.P. & Ford, H.L. (2009). The Six1 homeoprotein induces human mammary carcinoma cells to undergo epithelial-mesenchymal transition and metastasis in mice through increasing TGF-beta signaling, *J Clin Invest* 119(9): 2678-90.

O'Connor, D.S., Wall, N.R., Porter, A.C. & Altieri, D.C. (2002). A p34(cdc2) survival checkpoint in cancer, *Cancer Cell* 2(1): 43-54.

Ozben, T. (2006). Mechanisms and strategies to overcome multiple drug resistance in cancer, *FEBS Lett* 580(12): 2903-9.

Pantel, K. & Brakenhoff, R.H. (2004). Dissecting the metastatic cascade, *Nat Rev Cancer* 4(6): 448-56.

Parkin, D.M., Bray, F., Ferlay, J. & Pisani, P. (2005). Global cancer statistics, 2002, *CA Cancer J Clin* 55(2): 74-108.

Parkin, D.M. & Fernandez, L.M. (2006). Use of statistics to assess the global burden of breast cancer, *Breast J* 12 Suppl 1: S70-80.

Patrawala, L., Calhoun, T., Schneider-Broussard, R., Zhou, J., Claypool, K. & Tang, D.G. (2005). Side population is enriched in tumorigenic, stem-like cancer cells, whereas ABCG2+ and ABCG2- cancer cells are similarly tumorigenic, *Cancer Res* 65(14): 6207-19.

Pece, S., Serresi, M., Santolini, E., Capra, M., Hulleman, E., Galimberti, V., Zurrida, S., Maisonneuve, P., Viale, G. & Di Fiore, P.P. (2004). Loss of negative regulation by Numb over Notch is relevant to human breast carcinogenesis, *J Cell Biol* 167(2): 215-21.

Pece, S., Tosoni, D., Confalonieri, S., Mazzarol, G., Vecchi, M., Ronzoni, S., Bernard, L., Viale, G., Pelicci, P.G. & Di Fiore, P.P. (2010). Biological and molecular heterogeneity of breast cancers correlates with their cancer stem cell content, *Cell* 140(1): 62-73.

Perez-Soler, R., Neamati, N., Zou, Y., Schneider, E., Doyle, L.A., Andreeff, M., Priebe, W. & Ling, Y.H. (1997). Annamycin circumvents resistance mediated by the multidrug resistance-associated protein (MRP) in breast MCF-7 and small-cell lung UMCC-1 cancer cell lines selected for resistance to etoposide, *Int J Cancer* 71(1): 35-41.

Phillips, T.M., McBride, W.H. & Pajonk, F. (2006). The response of CD24(-/low)/CD44+ breast cancer-initiating cells to radiation, *J Natl Cancer Inst* 98(24): 1777-85.

Pisani, P., Bray, F. & Parkin, D.M. (2002). Estimates of the world-wide prevalence of cancer for 25 sites in the adult population, *Int J Cancer* 97(1): 72-81.

Platt, V.M. & Szoka, F.C., Jr. (2008). Anticancer therapeutics: targeting macromolecules and nanocarriers to hyaluronan or CD44, a hyaluronan receptor, *Mol Pharm* 5(4): 474-86.

Ponti, D., Costa, A., Zaffaroni, N., Pratesi, G., Petrangolini, G., Coradini, D., Pilotti, S., Pierotti, M.A. & Daidone, M.G. (2005). Isolation and in vitro propagation of tumorigenic breast cancer cells with stem/progenitor cell properties, *Cancer Res* 65(13): 5506-11.

Prince, M.E., Sivanandan, R., Kaczorowski, A., Wolf, G.T., Kaplan, M.J., Dalerba, P., Weissman, I.L., Clarke, M.F. & Ailles, L.E. (2007). Identification of a subpopulation of cells with cancer stem cell properties in head and neck squamous cell carcinoma, *Proc Natl Acad Sci U S A* 104(3): 973-8.

Pusztai, L. & Hortobagyi, G.N. (1998). High-dose chemotherapy: how resistant is breast cancer?, *Drug Resist Updat* 1(1): 62-72.

Ragaz, J. (2009). Radiation impact in breast cancer, *Breast Cancer Res* 11 Suppl 3: S14.

Riccioni, R., Dupuis, M.L., Bernabei, M., Petrucci, E., Pasquini, L., Mariani, G., Cianfriglia, M. & Testa, U. (2010). The cancer stem cell selective inhibitor salinomycin is a p-glycoprotein inhibitor, *Blood Cells Mol Dis* 45(1): 86-92.

Ries, L.A.G., Melbert, D., Krapcho, M., Stinchcomb, D.G., Howlader, N., Horner, M.J., Mariotto, A., Miller, B.A., Feuer, E.J., Altekruse, S.F., Lewis, D.R., Clegg, L., Eisner, M.P., Reichman, M. & Edwards, B.K. (2008). *SEER Cancer Statistics Review, 1975-2005*. Bethesda, MD, National Cancer Institute.

Sajithlal, G.B., Rothermund, K., Zhang, F., Dabbs, D.J., Latimer, J.J., Grant, S.G. & Prochownik, E.V. (2010). Permanently blocked stem cells derived from breast cancer cell lines, *Stem Cells* 28(6): 1008-18.

Shafee, N., Smith, C.R., Wei, S., Kim, Y., Mills, G.B., Hortobagyi, G.N., Stanbridge, E.J. & Lee, E.Y. (2008). Cancer stem cells contribute to cisplatin resistance in Brca1/p53-mediated mouse mammary tumors, *Cancer Res* 68(9): 3243-50.

Sheridan, C., Kishimoto, H., Fuchs, R.K., Mehrotra, S., Bhat-Nakshatri, P., Turner, C.H., Goulet, R., Jr., Badve, S. & Nakshatri, H. (2006). CD44+/CD24- breast cancer cells exhibit enhanced invasive properties: an early step necessary for metastasis, *Breast Cancer Res* 8(5): R59.

Slamon, D. & Pegram, M. (2001). Rationale for trastuzumab (Herceptin) in adjuvant breast cancer trials, *Semin Oncol* 28(1 Suppl 3): 13-9.

Sperr, W.R., Florian, S., Hauswirth, A.W. & Valent, P. (2005). CD 33 as a target of therapy in acute myeloid leukemia: current status and future perspectives, *Leuk Lymphoma* 46(8): 1115-20.

Stahl, M., Ge, C., Shi, S., Pestell, R.G. & Stanley, P. (2006). Notch1-induced transformation of RKE-1 cells requires up-regulation of cyclin D1, *Cancer Res* 66(15): 7562-70.

Stylianou, S., Clarke, R.B. & Brennan, K. (2006). Aberrant activation of notch signaling in human breast cancer, *Cancer Res* 66(3): 1517-25.

Theodoropoulos, P.A., Polioudaki, H., Agelaki, S., Kallergi, G., Saridaki, Z., Mavroudis, D. & Georgoulias, V. (2010). Circulating tumor cells with a putative stem cell phenotype in peripheral blood of patients with breast cancer, *Cancer Lett* 288(1): 99-106.

Tsimberidou, A.M., Giles, F.J., Estey, E., O'Brien, S., Keating, M.J. & Kantarjian, H.M. (2006). The role of gemtuzumab ozogamicin in acute leukaemia therapy, *Br J Haematol* 132(4): 398-409.

Vassilopoulos, A., Wang, R.H., Petrovas, C., Ambrozak, D., Koup, R. & Deng, C.X. (2008). Identification and characterization of cancer initiating cells from BRCA1 related mammary tumors using markers for normal mammary stem cells, *Int J Biol Sci* 4(3): 133-42.

Vazquez-Martin, A., Oliveras-Ferraros, C., Barco, S.D., Martin-Castillo, B. & Menendez, J.A. (2010b). The anti-diabetic drug metformin suppresses self-renewal and proliferation of trastuzumab-resistant tumor-initiating breast cancer stem cells, *Breast Cancer Res Treat*.

Vazquez-Martin, A., Oliveras-Ferraros, C., Cufi, S., Martin-Castillo, B. & Menendez, J.A. (2010a). Metformin and Energy Metabolism in Breast Cancer: From Insulin Physiology to Tumour-initiating Stem Cells, *Curr Mol Med* 10(7): 674-91.

Visvader, J.E. & Lindeman, G.J. (2008). Cancer stem cells in solid tumours: accumulating evidence and unresolved questions, *Nat Rev Cancer* 8(10): 755-68.

Weiss, L. (1990). Metastatic inefficiency, *Adv Cancer Res* 54: 159-211.

Wicha, M.S. (2006). Cancer stem cells and metastasis: lethal seeds, *Clin Cancer Res* 12(19): 5606-7.

Woodhouse, E.C., Chuaqui, R.F. & Liotta, L.A. (1997). General mechanisms of metastasis, *Cancer* 80(8 Suppl): 1529-37.

Woodward, W.A., Chen, M.S., Behbod, F., Alfaro, M.P., Buchholz, T.A. & Rosen, J.M. (2007). WNT/beta-catenin mediates radiation resistance of mouse mammary progenitor cells, *Proc Natl Acad Sci U S A* 104(2): 618-23.

Wright, M.H., Calcagno, A.M., Salcido, C.D., Carlson, M.D., Ambudkar, S.V. & Varticovski, L. (2008). Brca1 breast tumors contain distinct CD44+/CD24- and CD133+ cells with cancer stem cell characteristics, *Breast Cancer Res* 10(1): R10.

Wu, K., Jiao, X., Li, Z., Katiyar, S., Casimiro, M.C., Yang, W., Zhang, Q., Willmarth, N.E., Chepelev, I., Crosariol, M., Wei, Z., Li, A., Zhao, J., & Pestell, R.G. (2010). The cell fate determination factor dachshund reprograms breast cancer stem cell function. *J Biol Chem* in press.

Yu, F., Yao, H., Zhu, P., Zhang, X., Pan, Q., Gong, C., Huang, Y., Hu, X., Su, F., Lieberman, J. & Song, E. (2007). let-7 regulates self renewal and tumorigenicity of breast cancer cells, *Cell* 131(6): 1109-23.

6

Glioma Stem Cells: Cell Culture, Markers and Targets for New Combination Therapies

Candace A. Gilbert and Alonzo H. Ross
University of Massachusetts Medical School
United States

1. Introduction

Gliomas are brain tumors with glial cell characteristics, and are composed of a heterogeneous mix of cells, which includes glioma stem cells. Gliomas include astrocytomas, oligodendrogliomas, ependymoma, and mixed gliomas. Gliomas account for 32% of all brain and central nervous system tumors (CNS) and 80% of all malignant brain and CNS tumors (CBTRUS, 2010). The WHO grade III anaplastic astrocytomas (AAs) and grade IV glioblastoma multiforme (GBMs) are highly invasive tumors and make up approximately three-quarters of all gliomas (CBTRUS, 2010). GBM is the most common and malignant form of brain tumor. GBMs make up 17% of all primary brain tumors in the United States, with an incidence of 3.17 cases per 100,000 persons per year (CBTRUS, 2010). Although both the knowledge of glioma biology and the available resources for treatment have greatly increased over the past decade, the expected survival of malignant glioma patients remains dismal. For AA patients, the current five-year and ten-year survival rates are 27.4% and 21.3%, respectively (CBTRUS, 2010). GBM patients have a much lower survival. The current five-year and ten-year survival rates for GBM patients are 4.5% and 2.7%, respectively (CBTRUS, 2010). Clinical treatment for gliomas consists of a combination of surgical resection, radiotherapy and chemotherapy. Due to the infiltrative nature of GBMs, complete removal of the tumor by surgery is not possible. Following surgery, the conventional radiation dosage of up to 60 Gy is given daily in 2 Gy fractions (Buatti et al 2008). The commonly used chemotherapy drug, temozolomide (Temodar®), is an alkylating agent that is taken orally and readily penetrates the blood-brain barrier (Ostermann *et al.*, 2004). 1,3-bis(2-chloroethyl)-1-nitrosourea (BCNU) is an older drug that surgeons deposit in the tumor bed as dissolvable wafers (Grossman *et al.*, 1992). Both of these drugs alkylate DNA at multiple sites, including the O^6 position of guanine, which can result in futile cycles of DNA repair and, ultimately, cell death (Sarkaria *et al.*, 2008). These alkylating agents can also induce senescence (Gunther *et al.*, 2003). Temozolomide is administered as both concomitant and adjuvant treatments to radiotherapy. This aggressive treatment increases the two-year survival rate for GBM patients from 10.4%, with radiotherapy alone, to 26.5% (Stupp *et al.*, 2005). Cells that escape radiotherapy- and chemotherapy-induced cell death eventually re-enter the cell cycle and contribute to local tumor recurrence. Despite advances in chemotherapy regimens, the median progression free survival in AA and GBM patients is, 15.2 months (Chamberlain *et al.*, 2008) and 6.9 months (Stupp *et al.*, 2005), respectively. The median overall survival time for GBMs is 14.6 months (Stupp *et al.*, 2005).

2. Discovery of neural and glioma stem cells

The discovery of adult neural stem cells paved the way for the glioma stem cell field. Until the mid-20th century, the consensus in the neuroscience field was that adult neural stem cells did not exist. The former dogma was that the brain contained mitotic cells only during development. It is now known that neurogenesis persists throughout life. In the adult brain, neural stem cells are located primarily in the subventricular zone (Altman, 1963) and the dentate gyrus (Altman and Das, 1965). In the subventricular zone, adult neural stem cells are termed type B cells and the transit-amplifying cells are type C cells (Kriegstein and Alvarez-Buylla, 2009) (FIG 1a). The type B neural stem cells are mostly quiescent and are derived from embryonic and neonatal radial glial cells. Type B cells structurally resemble astroglial cells (Doetsch *et al.*, 1997). The adult neural stem cells and transit-amplifying cells are closely associated with blood vessels in the subventricular zone (Tavazoie et al., 2008). In the dentate gyrus of the hippocampus, the radial astrocytes are neural stem cells of the subgranular zone of the dentate gyrus (Seri et al., 2004). These cells are also referred to as type I progenitors in the subgranular zone (Fukuda et al., 2003). The subgranular zone is also located next to a vascular network, suggesting a niche for adult neural stem cells (Palmer et al., 2000). Adult neural stem cells from both the subventricular and subgranular zones express the embryonic neural stem cell markers nestin and Sox2, in addition to the astrocytic marker, glial fibrillary acidic protein (GFAP) (Doetsch et al., 1999; Seri et al., 2004; Suh et al., 2007). Unlike their differentiated progeny, these cells possess the ability to form neurospheres in serum-free cultures supplemented with growth factors (Reynolds et al., 1992). Neurospheres are heterogeneous aggregates derived from a single cell. These single cells would be plated at low densities for neurosphere assays, which were originally used to determine the percentage of neural stem cells in a culture or tissue. It is now known that both neural stem cells and transit amplifying cells can form neurospheres; however, neural stem cells are believed to have a greater, long-term proliferation potential than the transit-amplifying cells, and can therefore maintain neurosphere cultures through a large number of serial dissociations (Reynolds and Weiss, 1996). Neural stem cells have been associated with repair after strokes and severe injuries, and have been suggested as means for treatment of neurological disorders, such as Alzheimer's Disease (Gage, 2000; Zhongling et al., 2009).

While neural stem cells are necessary for normal neurological development and activity, cells with aberrant neural stem cell characteristics have been attributed to brain tumors. Glioma stem cells have many characteristics shared with adult neural stem cells, such as self-renewal, neurosphere formation, marker expression, multilineage differentiation, high motility, and localization to stem cell microenvironment niches (Sanai et al., 2005). Normal neural stem cells and glioma stem cells also share similar undifferentiated gene expression profiles, including nestin, EGF receptor, and PTEN. However, the nomenclature 'stem cell' in gliomas refers to their function and not their origin. It is currently unknown what is the cell of origin for glioma stem cells. Glioma stem cells may originate from normal neural stem cells that have undergone tumorigenic mutations or from more differentiated transit-amplifying or terminally differentiated neural cells that have undergone multiple mutations that allow the cells to be tumorigenic and revert to stemness properties (FIG 1b). Neural stem cells are probably target cells for malignant transformation. When rodent brains were exposed to avian sarcoma virus or carcinogens, tumors formed in the subventricular zone, where normal neural stem cells are believed to reside (Sanai et al., 2005). In addition, expression of Akt and K-ras in progenitor cells led to tumorigenesis (Holland et al., 2000). Conversely, several laboratories have demonstrated that genetic alterations can

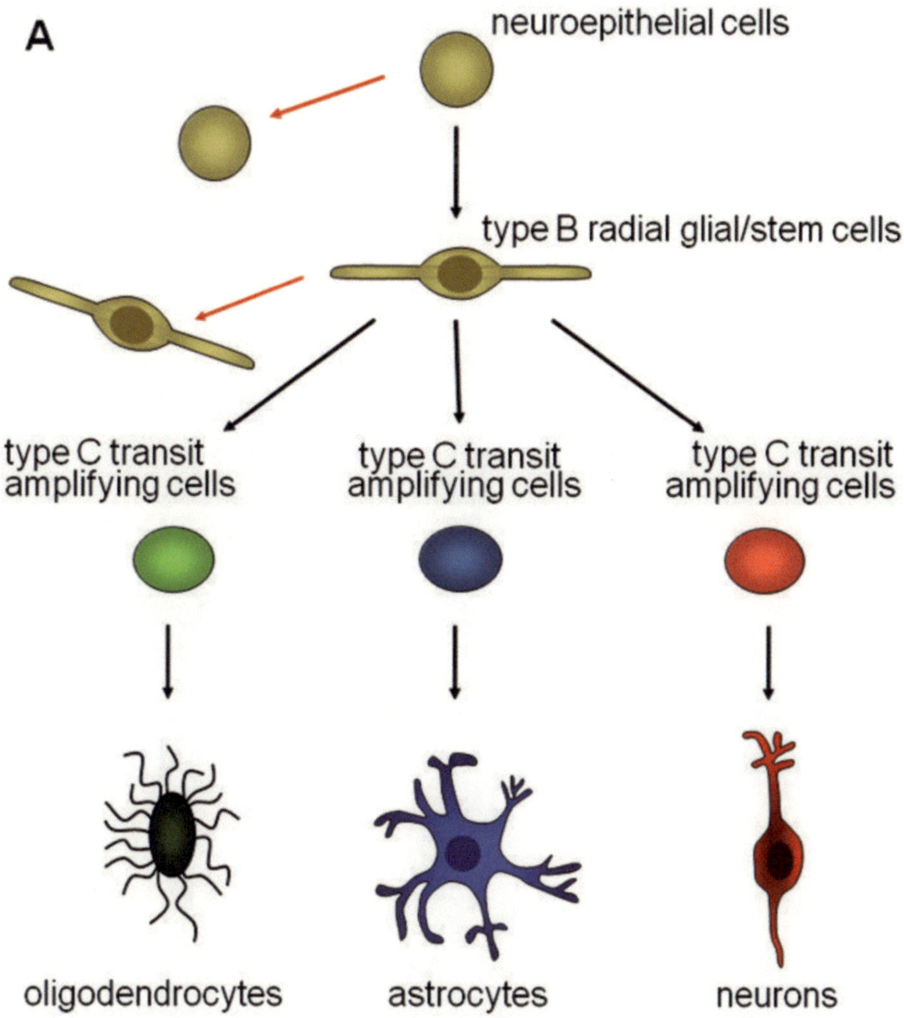

Fig. 1. A comparison of the hierarchies for normal neural stem cells and GBM CSCs. (A) NSC can either self-renew or differentiate to type B radial glia-like progenitor cells. They can then irreversibly differentiate to oligodendrocytes, astrocytes or neurons. (B) For GBM CSCs, the stem-like cells self-renew or differentiate to progenitor cells and then to more differentiated GFAP+ cells. Unlike the NSC, the differentiated cells may in some cases dedifferentiate.

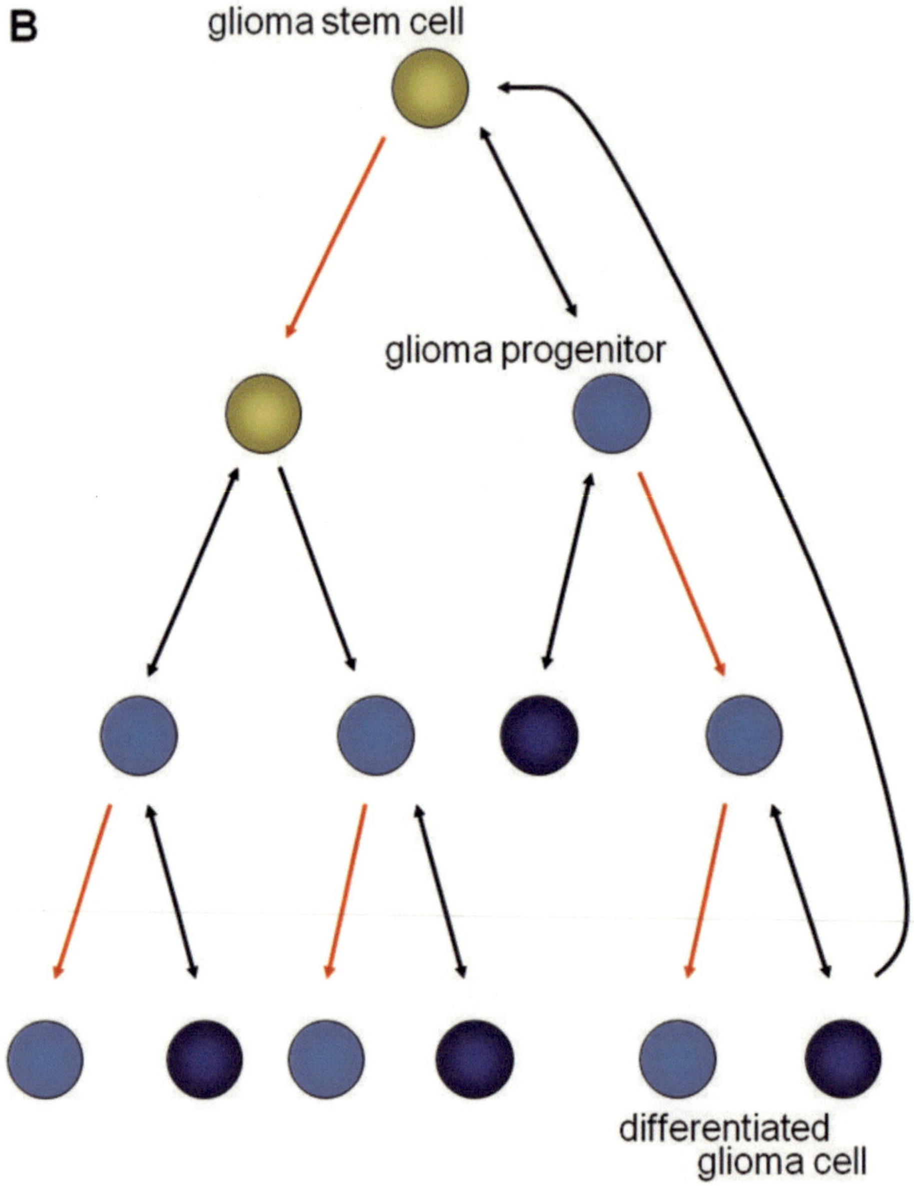

Continuation of Fig. 1.

dedifferentiated terminally differentiated astrocytes and induce tumorigenesis.(Bachoo et al., 2002; Holland et al., 1998) Due to the substantial heterogeneity among gliomas, it is likely that tumors from different patients originate from different stages of the adult neural hierarchy. This is an explanation for the distinct molecular subclasses of gliomas (Phillips et al., 2006). Regardless of the cell of origin, there are three properties that are considered essential for a cell to be universally accepted as a glioma stem cell (Rich, 2008). First, the cell must be capable of self-renewal; second, the cell should possess high proliferative potential; and third, the glioma stem cell must be capable of tumor initiation. There are additional characteristics used to define, but are not required of, glioma stem cells, because they can vary among different glioma grades and individual patients' tumors. Glioma stem cells may make up a rare population of the tumor or glioma culture; however, recent publications find that the percent of stem cells in different cancers can vary greatly, depending on tumor type and possibly the tumor environment (Eaves, 2008). Many laboratories have used the expression of stem cell markers to identify and isolate glioma stem cells, although there is no single marker that is consistent for all patients, specific to glioma stem cells, and definitely includes all glioma stem cells in a tissue. Finally, similar to neural stem cells, glioma stem cells are capable of multilineage differentiation, albeit aberrant, and the ratio of the differentiated progeny as well as progeny that express markers from multiple lineages can be varied between tumors (FIG 1b and c) (Varghese et al., 2008). However, as it is rare for an individual glioma to exhibit the full hierarchy see in normal brain tissue from neural stem cell differentiation, it is not expected that each glioma stem cell can differentiate into all lineages (Sanai et al., 2005). Therefore, one would expect the differentiation of a glioma stem cell to mimic the lineage composition of the parent tumor.

3. Glioma stem cell cultures

Traditionally, glioma cells were grown in the presence of serum as adherent cultures (FIG 2). The serum-grown cultures are tumorigenic, but unlike the invasive phenotype seen in patient gliomas, serum cultures commonly yield circumscribed tumors in intracranial xenograft models (Radaelli et al., 2009). Gene expression in serum cultures can be drastically different from the original tumor (Lee et al., 2006). Like neural stem cells, glioma stem cells can be grown in serum-free media with the growth factors EGF and FGF (Galli et al., 2004). Neurosphere cultures are currently the most common method used to propagate glioma stem cells, but a new *in vitro* technique to grow glioma stem cells is emerging, which utilizes laminin-coated plates with serum-free media.

3.1 Neurosphere cultures

The presence of self-renewing glioma stem cells was first demonstrated in 2003. Two laboratories demonstrated that glioma tissue cultured in serum-free media supplemented with growth factors form non-adherent spheroids with an enhanced glioma stem cell population (FIG 2 and 3). The glioma neurosphere cultures maintain genetic profiles similar to the original patients' tumors and form invasive tumors in intracranial xenografts (Ernst et al., 2009; Lee et al., 2006; Singh et al., 2004). When plated at clonal density, each neurosphere arises from an individual glioma stem cell or transit-amplifying cell. Despite their clonal origin, neurospheres are heterogeneous aggregates that consist of glioma stem cells, transit-amplifying cells, and more differentiated glioma cells. The percentage of neurosphere-initiating can vary greatly among glioma cultures, and neurosphere formation has been demonstrated to increase when neural stem cells are transformed (Li et al., 2009). The majority of cells in a neurosphere are transit-amplifying cells (Ahmed, 2009). When these neurosphere cultures are dissociated to single cells, a small percentage of the cells can form secondary and tertiary neurospheres for many passages (Chen et al., 2010; Reynolds and Weiss, 1996). Glioma stem cells have a high capacity to proliferate and self-renew and robustly form secondary neurospheres.

When exposed to fetal bovine serum, neurosphere cells differentiate down the lineage of the parent tumor (Singh et al., 2003). Therefore, gliomas preferentially differentiate to astrocytes, but multilineage differentiation can occasionally be observed with neuronal lineages, and some abnormal cells with mixed phenotypes. It should be noted that these lineages are based on markers but not function. For example, the crucial test for a neuron is an action potential, which is not tested. Also, a significant difference between neural stem cell and glioma stem cell cultures is that serum differentiation of normal neural stem cells is permanent (Lee et al., 2006), while glioma lines established as serum cultures can be converted to neurospheres in serum-free media (Gilbert et al., 2010; Qiang et al., 2009).

Neurosphere cultures express known neural stem cell genes, such as Musashi-1, Sox2, and Bmi-1 (Hemmati et al., 2003) (FIG 2). Stem cell membrane markers, such as CD133 and CD15, are also expressed in neurosphere cultures and are discussed in further detail in subsequent sections. Using neurosphere assays to analyze glioma stem cell content can be complicated. As mentioned above, both glioma stem cells and transit amplifying cells are capable of neurosphere formation. In addition, neurospheres aggregate and fuse with one another when the cells are plated at higher densities (Singec et al., 2006). Therefore, the number of neurospheres is a measure of the number of both glioma stem cells and transit amplifying cells and is accurate only when the cells are plated at low densities. Despite these concerns, neurosphere cultures remain a valuable tool in glioma stem cell research.

3.2 Laminin-coated cultures

A key aspect of the neurosphere culture system is that the serum-free, defined media maintains the glioma stem cell phenotype of the cells. However, in addition to glioma stem cells, neurospheres contain more differentiated progeny and regions of cell death. This is thought to be caused by the condensed structure of the neurosphere, which hinders the diffusion of the growth factors to the innermost cells (Woolard and Fine, 2009). Differentiation and cell death could be limited if glioma cultures were grown in a monolayer in the presence of serum-free, defined medium. This can be achieved by culturing glioma samples in the serum-free, defined medium on laminin-coated cell culture plates (Pollard et al., 2009). When cultured on laminin-coated plates, cells that would normally form neurospheres grow as an adherent culture, which allows all of the cells equal access to growth factors. The adherent glioma stem cell lines are less heterogeneous than neurosphere cultures, and almost all of the cells express glioma stem cell genes, such as Sox2, Nestin, CD133 and CD44 (FIG 2). There is minimal expression of differentiation markers. The adherent, laminin cultures are capable of tumor formation when as few as 100 cells were intracranially injected into immunocompromised mice, demonstrating the high percentage of tumor-initiating glioma stem cells. An additional benefit of the laminin glioma stem cell culture system is that all gliomas with good cell viability formed long-term cell lines.

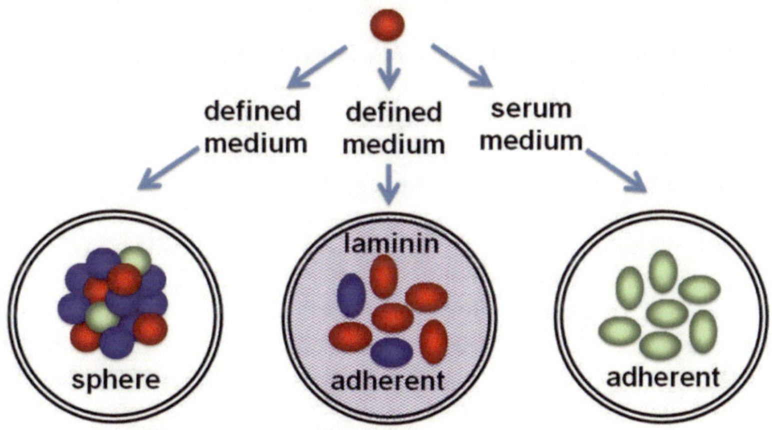

CSC	Transit-amplifying	Astrocytic
CD133, A2B5, SSEA-1, Sox2, BMI1, integrin alpha 6, podoplanin	TBR2, DLX2 and decreased stem cell markers,	GFAP

Fig. 2. Proposed lineages and culture methods for GBM CSCs. The CSCs (red circles) are cultured in defined medium to enhance stem cell properties. They express stem cell markers, listed below. CSCs are likely heterogeneous and may not express all of these markers, and may show additional tumor-to-tumor variation. CSCs differentiate to transit-amplifying cells (blue circles). The transit-amplifying cells show decreased expression of stem cell markers, and Chen et al (2010) recently suggested that TBR2 and DLX2 are markers for these cells. In mature spheres, a few of the transit-amplifying cells differentiate to astrocytic cells and, to a lesser degree, neuronal and oligodendrocytic cells (astrocytic cells shown as green circles). For cells adhering to laminin-coated substratum, stem cell marker expression is enhances, suggesting that the fraction of CSCs is increased. In addition, there are very few astrocytic cells. Serum treatment rapidly induces astrocytic differentiation.

4. Glioma stem cell markers

Markers are commonly used to identify and isolate different cells types. The most commonly used cell surface markers for glioma stem cells are CD133, CD15, and A2B5. New, less characterized markers are also being tested for glioma stem cells. When cells are isolated from tumors or glioma cultures with these markers, their stem cell characteristics can be analyzed based on stem cell gene expression, multilineage differentiation capabilities and neurosphere formation; however, tumor formation in xenograft models is the most important method to confirm that a marker identifies the glioma stem cell population. Despite many successes using cell surface markers such as CD133, it has become increasingly clear that individual gliomas are very heterogeneous and in addition, tumors vary greatly from patient to patient (Phillips et al., 2006). There is currently no universally accepted collection of markers for isolation of a pure population of glioma stem cells (Gilbert and Ross, 2009). In addition, to complicate the glioma stem cell field, some of the markers used appear to only be relevant when the cells are isolated directly from the tumor tissue. The heterogeneity of malignant gliomas may make it difficult to use a single set of markers to identify and purify glioma stem cells in every glioma.

4.1 CD133

CD133 (also known as Prominin-1) was first discovered as a cell surface marker for hematopoietic stem cells (Miraglia *et al.*, 1997). In the human fetal brain, CD133 is a marker for neural stem cells (Uchida *et al.*, 2000). CD133 expression has also been observed in intermediate radial glial cells in the early postnatal brain, and in ependymal cells in the adult brain (Coskun et al., 2008; Pfenninger et al., 2007). Neurogenic astrocytes in the neural stem cell region of the subventricular zone do not express CD133. Despite its inconsistent expression in adult neural stem cells, CD133 has been used to isolate populations of cancer stem cells from multiple types of brain tumors (Singh *et al.*, 2003; Singh *et al.*, 2004). Expression of CD133 in anaplastic astrocytomas and glioblastoma multiforme varies among patients and tumor grade, with reports of 0 – 64% (Ogden et al., 2008; Singh et al., 2003; Singh et al., 2004; Son et al., 2009). $CD133^+$ cells from gliomas are capable of multilineage differentiation and have a high capacity for neurosphere formation. The corresponding $CD133^-$ cells did not proliferate in neurosphere cultures. Furthermore, $CD133^+$ glioma cells express significantly higher levels of neural stem cell genes, such as nestin, Msi-1, maternal embryonic leucine zipper kinase (MELK) and CXCR4 (Liu *et al.*, 2006). These data support the stem cell genotype of $CD133^+$ glioma stem cells and suggests that similar signaling pathways may be involved in normal neural stem cells and brain cancers. The gold standard to classify a cell as a glioma stem cell is that it can form a xenograft tumor that is capable of serial transplantations in immunodeficient mice. $CD133^+$ glioma cells have an increased capacity for tumor initiation after intracranial transplantation into mice (Singh *et al.*, 2004). Injection of only 100 $CD133^+$ cells results in tumors capable of serial transplantation, while 100,000 $CD133^-$ injected cells do not form tumors. It is important to note that the laboratories that have had the most success studying glioma stem cells based on CD133 expression have isolated the cells from primary patient tissue and fresh xenograft samples (Bao et al., 2006a; Singh et al., 2004; Wang et al., 2010).

CD133 knockout mice manifest with a progressive photoreceptor degeneration that leads to total vision loss (Zacchigna et al., 2009). It is surprising that with the wide range of expression of cells expressing CD133 throughout the body and its link to stem cells that there are not more developmental defects. However, the authors suggest that further studies to characterize the mice under stressed conditions may uncover other defects in the CD133 -/- mouse model. An additional explanation is that the family member Prominin-2, which may provide redundant functions, is co-expressed in most tissues, excluding the retina (Fargeas et al., 2003). Other than its involvement in retinal development, little is known about CD133 function. Recent reports demonstrate that its expression may be cell cycle-dependent (Beier et al., 2007; Jaksch et al., 2008) or regulated by hypoxic environments (Griguer et al., 2008). In addition, in the small intestines and the prostate, CD133 marks both the transit-amplifying population and the stem cells (Grey et al., 2009; Snippert et al., 2009). These data imply that CD133 may only identify a subset of glioma stem cells that are actively proliferating, and $CD133^+$ populations may include progenitor cells.

A rising concern for CD133 as a glioma stem cell marker is that up to 40% of freshly isolated glioma tumors do not express CD133 (Son et al., 2009). Tumors negative for CD133 expression still included cells with stem cell-like properties of self-renewal, multilineage differentiation, and xenograft tumor formation (Beier et al., 2007). Differences in CD133 expression among gliomas may be result from the origin of the tumor-initiating cell (Lottaz et al., 2010). Cells isolated from $CD133^+$ tumors express a "proneural" gene signature and resemble fetal neural stem cells, while cells from $CD133^-$ tumors have "mesenchymal" genes and resemble adult neural stem cells. The gene profile differences of the cells from $CD133^+$ and $CD133^-$ tumors are not an artifact of neurosphere cultures, because the tumor types are still grouped together when cells are grown as laminin cultures. Further complicating the use of CD133 as a glioma stem cell marker, many glioma cells express a truncated form of CD133 that is not recognized by commonly used antibodies (Osmond et al., 2010). Collectively, these data demonstrate that CD133 is not a universal stem cell marker for GBMs and highlight the limits of selecting for glioma stem cells using CD133.

4.2 A2B5

A2B5 is a cell surface ganglioside expressed on neural precursor cells in the adult human brain (Nunes et al., 2003), and on neural stem cells isolated from the subventricular zone of human embryos (Tchoghandjian et al., 2010). Neural stem cells derived from human embryonic stem cells also express A2B5 (Pruszak et al., 2007). In anaplastic astrocytomas and glioblastoma multiforme, 33 - 90% of the cells express A2B5 (Ogden et al., 2008). A2B5+ cells are capable of intracranial tumor formation, while $A2B5^-$ cells do not initiate tumors (Ogden et al., 2008; Tchoghandjian et al., 2010). Co-expression of A2B5 and CD133 was observed in glioma cells. However, $A2B5^+/CD133^+$ and the $A2B5^+/CD133^-$ populations were capable of neurosphere formation and tumor initiation. Xenograft tumors from the $A2B5^+/CD133^-$ population were highly infiltrative, while tumors originating from $A2B5^+/CD133^+$ cells were more circumscribed (Tchoghandjian et al., 2010). Since glioma

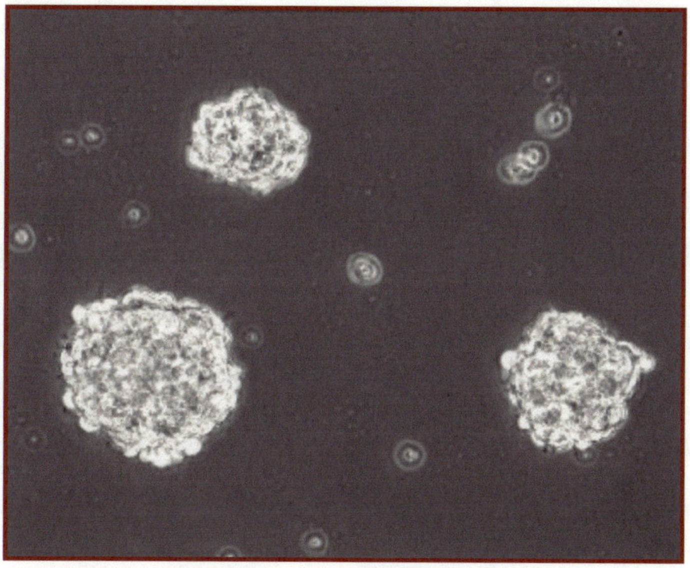

Fig. 3. Micrograph of neurosphere. Glioblastoma cells grown in defined medium form neurospheres. Each sphere contains a mix of cells, including stem-like cells with high capacity of self-renewal, progenitor and differentiated cells (Fig. 1B).

cells expressing A2B5 form tumors regardless of their CD133 status, A2B5 appears to identify an additional glioma stem cell population. Ogden et al., state that the A2B5 data do not diminish the utility of CD133 as a glioma stem cell marker, but rather demonstrates a broader population of cells capable of tumor formation. Contrarily, the very high percentage of A2B5$^+$ cells brings up the question of the rarity of the tumor initiating, cancer stem cell in some tissues. It will be interesting to see in the future if additional markers can identify a purer subset of glioma stem cells from the A2B5$^+$ population, or if like observed in melanomas (Quintana et al., 2008), the glioma stem cell population could make up a very large percent of the tumor.

4.3 CD15

CD15 (also known as SSEA-1 and Lewis-X Antigen) is a carbohydrate adhesion molecule associated with glycolipids and glycoproteins. CD15 expression has been shown on neural stem cells derived from human embryonic stem cells and embryonic neural stem cells (Barraud et al., 2007; Pruszak et al., 2007). In freshly isolated GBMs, distinct populations of CD15 varied from 2.4 – 70% (Son et al., 2009). CD15$^+$ cells had increased expression of stem cell genes, such as Sox2 and Bmi1, and were capable of self-renewal and multilineage differentiation. CD15$^+$ cells also form neurospheres in serum-free, defined medium, while CD15$^-$ cells had minimal neurosphere formation (Mao et al., 2009). A large percent of CD133$^+$ cells co-expressed CD15, but there was also a unique population of CD15$^+$/CD133$^-$ cells. Additionally, tumors negative for CD133 possessed CD15$^+$ cells (Son et al., 2009). CD15$^+$ cells isolated from GBMs were highly tumorigenic, while SSEA-1$^-$ cells displayed limited tumor formation in mouse intracranial xenografts. Importantly, 23 out of 24 primary GBMs analyzed contained a subpopulation of CD15$^+$ cells. Cells expressing CD15 that were isolated from CD15$^+$/CD133$^-$ neurospheres were capable of forming intracranial tumors in mice (Mao et al., 2009). These results together suggest that CD15 is a useful marker for both normal neural stem cells and glioma stem cells, and may identify new CD133$^-$ glioma stem cells.

4.4 New markers: Podoplanin and Integrin Alpha 6

There are two new promising cancer stem cell markers. The first, podoplanin, is a mucin-type transmembrane glycoprotein. It is over expressed in a variety of cancers, including squamous cell carcinomas, colorectal carcinomas and brain tumors (Cortez et al., 2010). For glioblastomas, podoplanin is expressed both in tumors and primary neurospheres in culture (Christensen Neurosurgery 2010). Elevated levels of podoplanin are associated with invasiveness, but the mechanism is not known (Cortez et al., 2010; Shen et al., 2010). The second new marker, integrin alpha 6, plays an important role in normal neural stem cells (Lathia et al., 2010). Integrin alpha 6 binds laminin and plays a role in maintaining the stem cells in the subventricular zone. Lathia et al. provided strong evidence that integrin alpha 6-positive cells have cancer stem cell characteristics. These cells are more proliferative and potent for neurosphere and tumor formation.

5. Glioma stem cell protection mechanisms

5.1 Immunosuppression

The capacity to evade tumor surveillance by the immune system may be a key step in the development of cancer and may involve cancer stem cells (Jaiswal *et al.*, 2010). The immune responses to GBMs can be potent (Di Tomaso *et al.*, 2010; Lichtor and Glick, 2003). For example, dendritic cells loaded with glioma cancer stem cells and then injected subcutaneously substantially suppress intracranial tumor growth (Pellegatta *et al.*, 2006). Ironically, antigens associated with glioma cancer stem cells may activate the immune system, and by an independent mechanism, GBM cells may suppress the immune system. GBMs secrete immunosuppressive factors, including TGF-β, VEGF, PGE_2, B7-H1, galectin-3 and CCL-2 (Wei *et al.*, 2010). Conditioned medium from GBMs inhibits T-cell proliferation and induces T regulatory cells (Tregs), which can suppress the functions of T-cells, B-cells, dendritic cells, monocytes, macrophages and natural killer (NK) cells (Humphries *et al.*, 2010; Wei *et al.*, 2010). Di Tomaso and colleagues (2010) found that glioma stem cells were particularly effective for inhibition of T-cell proliferation. In addition, phagocytic cells can play an important role in clearing tumor cells (Jaiswal *et al.*, 2010), and high-grade GBMs may include up to 30% microglia cells (Hanisch and Kettenmann, 2007). Rodrigues et al. (2010) concluded that GBMs suppress activation of microglial cells, and the GBM-suppressed microglial cells, in turn, suppress T-cell activity by secreting immunosuppressive factors, IL-10 and Fas-ligand. The multiple immunosuppressive mechanisms are consistent with our view that interactions with the immune system play a major role in the development of GBMs.

It has been suggested that cancer is a result of malignant cells evading the body's immune system. Glioma stem cells disrupt tumor immunosurveillance and result in both ineffective adaptive and innate immune responses. This is another mechanism that glioma stem cells help protect the tumor, which results in high rates of tumor recurrence and patient death. Theoretically, targeting the glioma stem cell-induced immunosuppression can enhance the survival of glioma patients.

5.2 Chemoresistance and radioresistance

By several mechanisms, the stem cell character of glioma stem cells may also contribute to resistance of tumor cells to therapy (FIG 4). First, normal stem cells can assume a quiescent state that is regulated by the stem cell niche. Cells that are not proliferating or stop after DNA damage have an enhanced chance of survival. Several groups have proposed that cancer stem cells readily assume a quiescent state and later, following DNA repair, repopulate the tumor (Mellor et al., 2005; Scopelliti et al., 2009). Our laboratory recently demonstrated that even low doses of temozolomide can induce quiescence followed by a robust recovery of the culture (Mihaliak *et al.*, 2010). The neurosphere recovery assay provides a quantitative cell culture assay to test the efficacy of drug combinations at inhibiting repopulation. We demonstrated that temozolomide drastically diminished initial neurosphere formation in many glioma cultures; however, these cultures eventually recovered and formed a robust number of secondary neurospheres (Mihaliak *et al.*, 2010). The ability of temozolomide treated neurospheres to recover and repopulate the culture suggests that some cells undergo a transient cell cycle arrest, allowing them to evade cell death and eventually resume proliferation. $CD133^+$ cells were more resistant to multiple chemotherapeutic agents, including temozolomide, compared to $CD133^-$ cells from the same primary glioma cultures (Liu et al., 2006). Glioma cells that survived after 1,3-bis(2-chloroethyl)-1-nitrosourea (BCNU) treatment expressed high levels of $CD133^+$ and retained their tumorigenic potential in intracranial mouse xenografts (Kang and Kang, 2007). In addition, ionizing radiation enriched the $CD133^+$ population of human glioma cultures

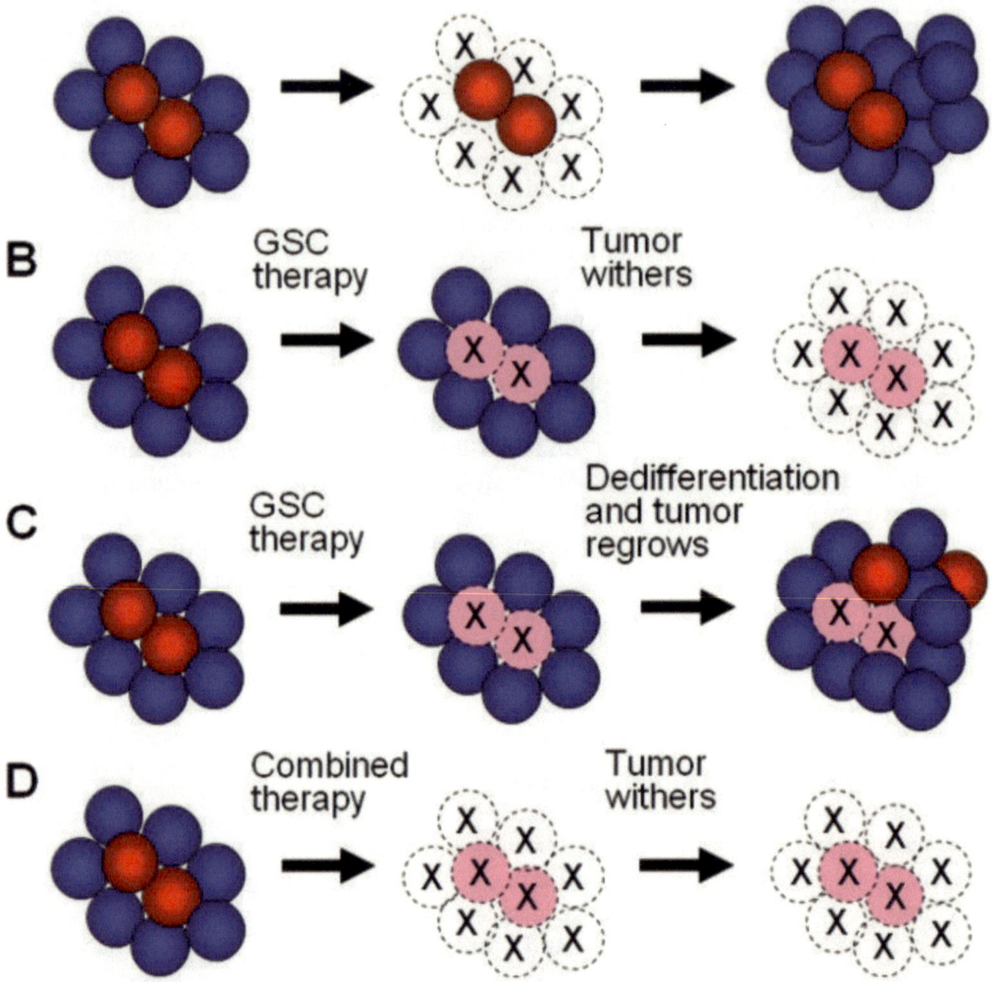

Fig. 4. CSCs and cancer therapy. The CSC model helps us to understand why current cancer therapies fail and aids development of novel, more effective approaches. (A) It has been proposed that CSCs (red circles) are resistant to current cancer therapy, survive even the most rigorous therapies that kill the more differentiated cells (blue circles) and allow tumor repopulation. (B) One of the most appealing aspects of the CSC model is that therapies directed against CSCs might eliminate the cells with long-term self-renewal potential, and the more differentiated cells, which lack self-renewal potential, will eventually cease cell proliferation and die. (C) In a more recent CSC model (Chen et al and Fig. 1), some differentiated cells can revert to CSCs. If this model is correct, then a therapy exclusively directed against the CSCs would allow creation of new CSCs and repopulation of the tumor. (D) A new approach that takes into account dedifferentiation is to combine CSC directed therapy to decrease the number of the most important cells and a nonspecific therapy to clear the differentiated cells and, thereby, reduce the chance of dedifferentiation.

derived from xenografts and GBM patient samples (Bao et al., 2006a). Based on these data, $CD133^+$ populations were more resistant to ionizing radiation in colony formation assays compared to the corresponding $CD133^-$ populations. On the other hand, it has been shown that number of $CD133^+$ glioma cells can decrease or show no significant change after chemotherapy treatment (Beier et al., 2008; Mihaliak et al., 2010). There may be several explanations for these inconsistent results. First, these differences could support the issue that CD133 is not a universal stem cell marker for all gliomas. Second, they could be due to different sources of the glioma stem cells, for example neurosphere cultures, versus xenografts, versus fresh patient tissue. Finally, the disparate results may be on account of the time points that the data are analyzed after treatments and the concentrations of the drug treatments. Mihaliak et al. (2010) demonstrated that the chemotherapy treatments induced a cell cycle arrest in the neurosphere initiating cells at clinically relevant doses, but required higher concentrations to induce cell death in the bulk of the cells. The drug concentrations to achieve this cell cycle arrest varied both by cell line and by the chemotherapy drug used. Therefore, depending on the time point that the culture is analyzed, the ratios of glioma stem cells to the total bulk cells can greatly vary.

Another feature that normal stem cells and glioma stem cells share is expression of drug efflux pumps. Adenosine triphosphate-binding cassette (ABC) pumps, ABCG2 and P-glycoprotein are expressed on glioma stem cells and are responsible for efflux of the fluorescent Hoechst 33342 dye, leading to the side population, which is enriched in glioma stem cells (Lu and Shervington, 2008). However, in a model system, ABCG2-positive and -negative cells showed no difference in tumor formation in mice (Patrawala *et al.*, 2005). The ABC transporters are often proposed to enhance survival of glioma stem cells by efflux of chemotherapy drugs, but temozolomide is not a substrate for ABCG2, and expression of ABCG2 did not provide resistance to temozolomide treatment (Bleau *et al.*, 2009).

Glioma stem cells express a variety of proteins that promote survival following cancer treatment. The major drug resistance protein, MGMT, and anti-apoptotic genes such as FLIP, BCL-2, BCL-XL, cIAP1 and survivin were upregulated in CD133+ glioma cells (Ghods et al., 2007; Liu et al., 2006). Ionizing radiation resulted in a greater activation of DNA checkpoint responses in $CD133^+$ cells by phosphorylation of Rad15, ATM, Chk1 and Chk2 than in the autologous $CD133^-$ cells (Bao et al., 2006a). This indicates that $CD133^+$ glioma stem cells resistance to radiotherapy is partially due to enhanced DNA repair. As a result, pathways related to glioma stem cell functions and resistance to therapy will be promising targets for novel therapies.

6. Therapeutic targets

Current glioma treatments target the bulk of the tumor, but are insufficient (FIG 4). Since tumor recurrence is attributed to glioma stem cell therapy resistance, treatments that directly target glioma stem cells could yield long-term cures. Many have hypothesized that once the glioma stem cells have been eliminated, the bulk tumor would not be able to sustain itself and would disseminate; however, in gliomas, it has been hypothesized that some differentiated tumor cells have the ability to revert to stem cell-like cells (FIG 2 and 4) (Chen et al., 2010; Gupta et al., 2009). The most affective treatments would consist of radiation and chemotherapy against the bulk tumor combined with direct-targeted against the glioma stem cell population. Signaling pathways associated with either mechanisms of resistance or pathways required for the function of glioma stem cells could be targeted to enhance therapy.

6.1 Notch pathway

The Notch signaling pathway is an important regulator in normal development, adult stem cell maintenance, and tumorigenesis in multiple organs, including the brain (Koch and Radtke, 2007). Notch signaling is a promising pathway to target glioma cells, since the Notch receptors, their ligands, and downstream targets are commonly over-expressed in glioma tissue and cell lines (Fischer and Gessler, 2007; Kanamori *et al.*, 2007; Shih and Holland, 2006). The Notch gene mutation was first discovered in flies with 'notched' wings (Radtke and Raj, 2003). There are four mammalian Notch receptors (Notch1 through 4) and five membrane-associated ligands in the Delta and Jagged families. Activation of the Notch pathway through cell-cell interactions initiates a signaling cascade (Pannuti et al., 2010). When a ligand binds to a Notch receptor, the metalloprotease ADAM protein cleaves the extracellular domain of Notch, which initiates intracellular cleavage by the gamma secretase complex (Stockhausen et al., 2010). The gamma-secretase cleavage releases the Notch intracellular domain (NICD), which facilitates its translocation into the nucleus (Miele, 2006). The NICD forms a complex with CSL (CBF1/Suppressor of Hairless/Lag1) and drives transcription of downstream targets, including members of the Hairy enhancer of split (Hes) and Hes-related repressor protein (HERP/Hey) families (Iso et al., 2003), cyclin D (Ronchini and Capobianco, 2001), and c-myc (Sharma et al., 2006), and p21 (Guo et al., 2009). Notch signaling is a promising target for directed therapy since it can be blocked at multiple stages of the pathway (Rizzo et al., 2008). The most common approach to block the Notch pathway in basic research, and in Phase I and Phase II clinical trials, is via small molecule inhibitors of gamma-secretase (Miele, 2006). Administration of gamma-secretase inhibitors blocks the cleavage of the Notch receptor, and the intracellular domain remains bound to the cellular membrane, halting the Notch signaling cascade. Treatment with gamma-secretase inhibitors can lead to gastrointestinal tract cytotoxicity (Barten et al., 2006); however, intermittent treatment schedules can to diminish these side effects (Rizzo et al., 2008).

Inhibiting the Notch signaling pathway can target the glioma stem cell population. Notch signaling directly activates transcription of the stem cell marker, nestin (Shih and Holland, 2006). Expression of nestin in a murine K-ras glioma model was demonstrated to correlate specifically with Notch activation. Likewise, knockdown of Notch by shRNAs or γ-secretase inhibitors decreased the expression of stem cell markers nestin and CD133 and decreased neurosphere formation (Jeon et al., 2008). Inhibiting the Notch pathway through gamma-secretase inhibitors or shRNAs against Notch1, both led to suppression of cell growth and increased differentiation (Kanamori et al., 2007). In glioma cultures, GSI treatment suppressed cell growth and decreased neurosphere formation and tumor growth of CD133+ cells (Fan et al., 2010). Correspondingly, increased Notch signaling enhanced glioma cell survival (Purow *et al.*, 2005). Gamma-secretase inhibitors were also shown to sensitize glioma neurosphere cultures to radiation, thereby, increasing the efficacy of radiotherapy (Wang et al., 2010). The combination of temozolomide chemotherapy with gamma-secretase inhibitor treatment also decreased neurosphere formation and inhibited neurosphere recovery (Gilbert et al., 2010). *Ex vivo* treatment of glioma xenografts with temozolomide and gamma-secretase inhibitors extended tumor latency and survival, and *in vivo* temozolomide and gamma-secretase inhibitor treatment blocked tumor progression in 50% of mice with pre-existing tumors. These results suggest that an active Notch pathway maintains the glioma stem cell population and provides protection from chemotherapy and radiation treatments. Therefore, therapies targeting Notch receptors, ligands and downstream targets may enhance current glioma treatments.

6.2 Hedgehog pathway

The Hedgehog gene was first discovered in flies due to a mutation in the gene that caused Drosophila larvae to possess hedgehog-like spines (Mohler, 1988). The Hedgehog pathway is vital for normal brain development and neural stem cell survival (Ahn and Joyner, 2005; Wechsler-Reya and Scott, 1999). There are three mammalian Hedgehog homologues, the most studied being Sonic Hedgehog (Marti and Bovolenta, 2002). Sonic Hedgehog is the ligand that activates the pathway, and when it is not present, the Patched receptor inhibits the Smoothed membrane-bound protein. When the ligand binds to Patched, Smoothened is activated, which in turn activates the downstream targets of the Gli transcription factors (Gli1 through 3), which were first discovered in human glioma (Kinzler et al., 1987). Glioma cell lines and primary glioma tissues commonly express Patched, Sonic Hedgehog and Gli (Clement et al., 2007; Dahmane et al., 2001). The Hedgehog pathway can be blocked with steroidal alkaloid, Smoothened inhibitor, cyclopamine (Chen et al., 2002). Cyclopamine is a naturally occurring compound that was discovered in a fascinating manner. The compound was named after a group of lambs that were born with one eye in the center of their forehead, imitating a Cyclops (Binns et al., 1964). The parental sheep had grazed on wild corn lilies that produced the cyclopamine, leading to incomplete developmental growth, which was later attributed to the inhibition of the Hedgehog pathway (Cooper et al., 1998).

The Hedgehog pathway plays an important role in glioma tumorigenesis. Treatment of neurosphere cultures with cyclopamine, inhibited sphere formation, and enhanced radiation treatment (Bar et al., 2007) and temozolomide chemotherapy (Clement et al., 2007). Cyclopamine treatment also depleted the number of nestin$^+$ cells, CD133$^+$ cells, and the Hoechst 33342 side population, suggesting that inhibition of the Hedgehog pathway decreases the glioma stem cells (Bar et al., 2007). *In vivo* cyclopamine treatment reduced tumor volume intracranial neurosphere xenografts (Clement et al., 2007). Active Hedgehog signaling in glioma cultures increased survival after chemotherapy and Gli1 expression in patient tissues is associated with glioma recurrence after chemotherapy (Cui et al., 2010). Treatment with cyclopamine to block the Hedgehog pathway increased the cytotoxicity in chemotherapy treated cultures. These data suggest that inhibiting the Hedgehog pathway enhances the sensitivity to current GBM radiation and chemotherapy treatments by targeting the glioma stem cell population.

6.3 VEGF, Angiogenesis, and Bevacizumab

Aberrant, inordinate angiogenesis is a hallmark of malignant gliomas. This abnormal angiogenesis supports tumor growth and has been considered a target for glioma therapy. Glioma stem cells have been associated with a vascular stem cell niche. Nestin$^+$ and CD133$^+$ brain tumor cells were consistently located in the proximity of the tumor's vascular system (Calabrese et al., 2007). It has been demonstrated that xenografts from CD133$^+$ glioma cells form highly vascular tumors compared to xenografts from CD133$^-$ cells (Bao et al., 2006b). In addition, secretion of vascular endothelial growth factor (VEGF) from CD133$^+$ cells was consistently upregulated. The VEGF family and the tyrosine kinase VEGF receptors are important in glioma angiogenesis. When VEGF binds to the receptor, the MAP kinase pathway, the Raf-MEK-Erk pathway, and the PI3K-Akt pathway are activated (Korpanty et al., 2010). The VEGF pathway can be blocked with the FDA-approved bevacizumab (Avastin™), a neutralizing monoclonal antibody against free VEGF. Bevacizumab *in vivo* treatment inhibited the growth of subcutaneous and intracranial CD133$^+$ glioma xenografts (Bao et al., 2006b). Anti-angiogenesis treatments have been demonstrated to decrease glioma growth. The vascular niche may regulate glioma stem cell proliferation and provide a protective shield for glioma stem cells against treatment. Therefore, therapies targeting the fundamental angiogenic factors could simultaneously be a treatment against glioma stem cells. Early results from clinical trials with bevacizumab have proved hopeful (Desjardins et al., 2008; Friedman et al., 2009; Kreisl et al., 2009). Although there have been only minimal, well-tolerated side effects (Rahman et al., 2010), the gliomas that recur after bevacizumab treatment are diffuse tumors that are unusually distant from the primary glioma (Zuniga et al., 2009).

Current glioma therapies may fail to cure patients because glioma stem cells possess mechanisms to evade treatments and enhance survival. The remaining cells promote tumor regrowth. To circumvent the many protective features of glioma stem cells, such as chemoresistance, radioresistance, and immunosuppression, therapies for glioma stem cells must target the vital pathways for glioma stem cell function and their vascular niche. Combining drugs that target glioma stem cells with surgery, current chemotherapies, and radiation will enhance the overall survival for glioma treatment and decrease tumor recurrence.

7. Summary and future directions of the glioma stem cell field

In our view, the cancer stem cell model has had a positive effect on cancer research, leading to a close examination of tumor cell heterogeneity brought about by differentiation, as well as other causes (Shackleton et al., 2009). However, the model has also led to a series of new questions and controversies. First, is this model applicable to all gliomas? Ogden et al. (2008) found that CD133 only identifies cancer stem cells in a small subset of GBMs (1/6 tumors). In addition, there are CD133- GBMs that are still aggressive tumors (Beier et al., 2007). If CD133 does not select for cancer stem cells in every glioma, is there a better, more universal marker available? As noted in this review, other markers are being tested, but right now there is no agreement in the field. Second, perhaps, the markers are not working because the cancer stem cell model is too simple. Chen et al. (2010) proposed that there is no single marker signature for the cancer stem cell. Instead, they proposed that there are at least three cell types with varying degrees of stemness. An intriguing aspect of this model is the hierarchy. In most models, the cancer stem cells irreversibly differentiate to cells with less potential for self-renewal and tumor formation. In some cases, the more differentiated cells may be able to dedifferentiate back to a stem-like cells (Chen et al., 2010; Gupta et al., 2009). Third, what is the best source of cells for glioma stem cell studies, and what is the best method to culture these cells? Some of the most thorough studies utilize cells shortly after removal of tumors from patients or immunodeficient mice and not cells maintained in culture for many passages (Bao et al., 2006a; Singh et al., 2004; Wang et al., 2010). To enhance stem cell properties, glioma cells are commonly grown as neurospheres in defined medium. A newer method is to grow adherent cells on laminin-coated plastic (Pollard et al., 2009), and there are critics and advocates for this method (Reynolds and Vescovi, 2009; Woolard and Fine, 2009). Fourth, the most important question for the clinic is whether the glioma stem cells are the cells in the tumor that are most resistant to therapy and hence, lead to repopulation of the tumor? The disagreements on this point may relate to the preceding questions and inconsistencies about glioma stem cell markers and methods to culture these cells. Until we agree on what is a glioma stem cell and how to prepare them, disagreements between different groups and studies will continue. Given this complexity, what is the best strategy for cancer therapy? Advocates for the cancer stem cell model suggested that therapy be directed against glioma stem cells, and the remainder of the tumor cells will eventually wither away (Cheng et al., 2010). However, since it has been proposed that the differentiated cells can dedifferentiate into stem cell-like cancer cells (Chen et al., 2010; Gupta et al., 2009), only targeting the glioma stem cells could lead to tumor recurrence. This suggests that to have successful long-term cures of gliomas, combined therapy targeting both the bulk of the tumor and the glioma stem cells will be necessary (Cheng et al., 2010). Promising research has recently taken this novel approach combining a directed therapy against the Notch pathway either with chemotherapy (Gilbert et al., 2010) or radiotherapy (Wang et al., 2010). These studies demonstrate the proof-of-principle for the enhancement of current therapies with new cancer stem cell directed drugs. The glioma stem cell field is continuously growing and it will be exciting to see these translational studies tested in the clinical setting.

8. References

Ahmed, S. (2009). The culture of neural stem cells. J Cell Biochem *106*, 1-6.

Ahn, S., and Joyner, A.L. (2005). In vivo analysis of quiescent adult neural stem cells responding to Sonic hedgehog. Nature *437*, 894-897.

Altman, J. (1963). Autoradiographic investigation of cell proliferation in the brains of rats and cats. Anat Rec *145*, 573-591.

Altman, J., and Das, G.D. (1965). Autoradiographic and histological evidence of postnatal hippocampal neurogenesis in rats. J Comp Neurol *124*, 319-335.

Bachoo, R.M., Maher, E.A., Ligon, K.L., Sharpless, N.E., Chan, S.S., You, M.J., Tang, Y., DeFrances, J., Stover, E., Weissleder, R., *et al.* (2002). Epidermal growth factor receptor and Ink4a/Arf: convergent mechanisms governing terminal differentiation and transformation along the neural stem cell to astrocyte axis. Cancer Cell *1*, 269-277.

Bao, S., Wu, Q., McLendon, R.E., Hao, Y., Shi, Q., Hjelmeland, A.B., Dewhirst, M.W., Bigner, D.D., and Rich, J.N. (2006a). Glioma stem cells promote radioresistance by preferential activation of the DNA damage response. Nature *444*, 756-760.

Bao, S., Wu, Q., Sathornsumetee, S., Hao, Y., Li, Z., Hjelmeland, A.B., Shi, Q., McLendon, R.E., Bigner, D.D., and Rich, J.N. (2006b). Stem cell-like glioma cells promote tumor angiogenesis through vascular endothelial growth factor. Cancer Res *66*, 7843-7848.

Bar, E.E., Chaudhry, A., Lin, A., Fan, X., Schreck, K., Matsui, W., Piccirillo, S., Vescovi, A.L., DiMeco, F., Olivi, A., *et al.* (2007). Cyclopamine-mediated hedgehog pathway inhibition depletes stem-like cancer cells in glioblastoma. Stem Cells *25*, 2524-2533.

Barraud, P., Stott, S., Mollgard, K., Parmar, M., and Bjorklund, A. (2007). In vitro characterization of a human neural progenitor cell coexpressing SSEA4 and CD133. J Neurosci Res *85*, 250-259.

Barten, D.M., Meredith, J.E., Jr., Zaczek, R., Houston, J.G., and Albright, C.F. (2006). Gamma-secretase inhibitors for Alzheimer's disease: balancing efficacy and toxicity. Drugs R D *7*, 87-97.

Beier, D., Hau, P., Proescholdt, M., Lohmeier, A., Wischhusen, J., Oefner, P.J., Aigner, L., Brawanski, A., Bogdahn, U., and Beier, C.P. (2007). CD133(+) and CD133(-) glioblastoma-derived cancer stem cells show differential growth characteristics and molecular profiles. Cancer Res *67*, 4010-4015.

Beier, D., Rohrl, S., Pillai, D.R., Schwarz, S., Kunz-Schughart, L.A., Leukel, P., Proescholdt, M., Brawanski, A., Bogdahn, U., Trampe-Kieslich, A., *et al.* (2008). Temozolomide preferentially depletes cancer stem cells in glioblastoma. Cancer Res *68*, 5706-5715.

Binns, W., James, L.F., and Shupe, J.L. (1964). Toxicosis of Veratrum Californicum in Ewes and Its Relationship to a Congenital Deformity in Lambs. Ann N Y Acad Sci *111*, 571-576.

Bleau, A.M., Hambardzumyan, D., Ozawa, T., Fomchenko, E.I., Huse, J.T., Brennan, C.W., and Holland, E.C. (2009). PTEN/PI3K/Akt pathway regulates the side population phenotype and ABCG2 activity in glioma tumor stem-like cells. Cell Stem Cell *4*, 226-235.

Calabrese, C., Poppleton, H., Kocak, M., Hogg, T.L., Fuller, C., Hamner, B., Oh, E.Y., Gaber, M.W., Finklestein, D., Allen, M., *et al.* (2007). A perivascular niche for brain tumor stem cells. Cancer Cell *11*, 69-82.

CBTRUS (2010). CBTRUS Statistical Report: Primary Brain and Central Nervous

System Tumors Diagnosed in the United States in 2004-2006. (Hinsdale, IL, Central Brain Tumor Registry of the United States).

Chamberlain, M.C., Wei-Tsao, D.D., Blumenthal, D.T., and Glantz, M.J. (2008). Salvage chemotherapy with CPT-11 for recurrent temozolomide-refractory anaplastic astrocytoma. Cancer *112*, 2038-2045.

Chen, J.K., Taipale, J., Cooper, M.K., and Beachy, P.A. (2002). Inhibition of Hedgehog signaling by direct binding of cyclopamine to Smoothened. Genes Dev *16*, 2743-2748.

Chen, R., Nishimura, M.C., Bumbaca, S.M., Kharbanda, S., Forrest, W.F., Kasman, I.M., Greve, J.M., Soriano, R.H., Gilmour, L.L., Rivers, C.S., *et al.* (2010). A hierarchy of self-renewing tumor-initiating cell types in glioblastoma. Cancer Cell *17*, 362-375.

Cheng, L., Bao, S., and Rich, J.N. (2010). Potential therapeutic implications of cancer stem cells in glioblastoma. Biochem Pharmacol *80*, 654-665.

Clement, V., Sanchez, P., de Tribolet, N., Radovanovic, I., and Ruiz i Altaba, A. (2007). HEDGEHOG-GLI1 signaling regulates human glioma growth, cancer stem cell self-renewal, and tumorigenicity. Curr Biol *17*, 165-172.

Cooper, M.K., Porter, J.A., Young, K.E., and Beachy, P.A. (1998). Teratogen-mediated inhibition of target tissue response to Shh signaling. Science *280*, 1603-1607.

Cortez, M.A., Nicoloso, M.S., Shimizu, M., Rossi, S., Gopisetty, G., Molina, J.R., Carlotti, C., Jr., Tirapelli, D., Neder, L., Brassesco, M.S., *et al.* (2010). miR-29b and miR-125a regulate podoplanin and suppress invasion in glioblastoma. Genes Chromosomes Cancer.

Coskun, V., Wu, H., Blanchi, B., Tsao, S., Kim, K., Zhao, J., Biancotti, J.C., Hutnick, L., Krueger, R.C., Jr., Fan, G., *et al.* (2008). CD133+ neural stem cells in the ependyma of mammalian postnatal forebrain. Proc Natl Acad Sci U S A *105*, 1026-1031.

Cui, D., Xu, Q., Wang, K., and Che, X. (2010). Gli1 is a potential target for alleviating multidrug resistance of gliomas. J Neurol Sci *288*, 156-166.

Dahmane, N., Sanchez, P., Gitton, Y., Palma, V., Sun, T., Beyna, M., Weiner, H., and Ruiz i Altaba, A. (2001). The Sonic Hedgehog-Gli pathway regulates dorsal brain growth and tumorigenesis. Development *128*, 5201-5212.

Desjardins, A., Reardon, D.A., Herndon, J.E., 2nd, Marcello, J., Quinn, J.A., Rich, J.N., Sathornsumetee, S., Gururangan, S., Sampson, J., Bailey, L., *et al.* (2008). Bevacizumab plus irinotecan in recurrent WHO grade 3 malignant gliomas. Clin Cancer Res *14*, 7068-7073.

Di Tomaso, T., Mazzoleni, S., Wang, E., Sovena, G., Clavenna, D., Franzin, A., Mortini, P., Ferrone, S., Doglioni, C., Marincola, F.M., *et al.* (2010). Immunobiological characterization of cancer stem cells isolated from glioblastoma patients. Clin Cancer Res *16*, 800-813.

Doetsch, F., Caille, I., Lim, D.A., Garcia-Verdugo, J.M., and Alvarez-Buylla, A. (1999). Subventricular zone astrocytes are neural stem cells in the adult mammalian brain. Cell *97*, 703-716.

Doetsch, F., Garcia-Verdugo, J.M., and Alvarez-Buylla, A. (1997). Cellular composition and three-dimensional organization of the subventricular germinal zone in the adult mammalian brain. J Neurosci *17*, 5046-5061.

Eaves, C.J. (2008). Cancer stem cells: Here, there, everywhere? Nature *456*, 581-582.

Ernst, A., Hofmann, S., Ahmadi, R., Becker, N., Korshunov, A., Engel, F., Hartmann, C., Felsberg, J., Sabel, M., Peterziel, H., *et al.* (2009). Genomic and expression profiling of glioblastoma stem cell-like spheroid cultures identifies novel tumor-relevant genes associated with survival. Clin Cancer Res *15*, 6541-6550.

Fan, X., Khaki, L., Zhu, T.S., Soules, M.E., Talsma, C.E., Gul, N., Koh, C., Zhang, J., Li, Y.M., Maciaczyk, J., *et al.* (2010). NOTCH pathway blockade depletes CD133-positive glioblastoma cells and inhibits growth of tumor neurospheres and xenografts. Stem Cells *28*, 5-16.

Fargeas, C.A., Florek, M., Huttner, W.B., and Corbeil, D. (2003). Characterization of prominin-2, a new member of the prominin family of pentaspan membrane glycoproteins. J Biol Chem *278*, 8586-8596.

Fischer, A., and Gessler, M. (2007). Delta-Notch--and then? Protein interactions and proposed modes of repression by Hes and Hey bHLH factors. Nucleic Acids Res *35*, 4583-4596.

Friedman, H.S., Prados, M.D., Wen, P.Y., Mikkelsen, T., Schiff, D., Abrey, L.E., Yung, W.K., Paleologos, N., Nicholas, M.K., Jensen, R., *et al.* (2009). Bevacizumab alone and in combination with irinotecan in recurrent glioblastoma. J Clin Oncol *27*, 4733-4740.

Fukuda, S., Kato, F., Tozuka, Y., Yamaguchi, M., Miyamoto, Y., and Hisatsune, T. (2003). Two distinct subpopulations of nestin-positive cells in adult mouse dentate gyrus. J Neurosci *23*, 9357-9366.

Gage, F.H. (2000). Mammalian neural stem cells. Science *287*, 1433-1438.
Galli, R., Binda, E., Orfanelli, U., Cipelletti, B., Gritti, A., De Vitis, S., Fiocco, R., Foroni, C., Dimeco, F., and Vescovi, A. (2004). Isolation and characterization of tumorigenic, stem-like neural precursors from human glioblastoma. Cancer Res *64*, 7011-7021.
Ghods, A.J., Irvin, D., Liu, G., Yuan, X., Abdulkadir, I.R., Tunici, P., Konda, B., Wachsmann-Hogiu, S., Black, K.L., and Yu, J.S. (2007). Spheres isolated from 9L gliosarcoma rat cell line possess chemoresistant and aggressive cancer stem-like cells. Stem Cells *25*, 1645-1653.
Gilbert, C.A., Daou, M., Moser, R.P., and Ross, A.H. (2010). γ-Secretase Inhibitors Enhance Temozolomide Treatment of Human Gliomas by Inhibiting Neurosphere Repopulation and Xenograft Recurrence. Cancer Res *70*, 6870-6879.
Gilbert, C.A., and Ross, A.H. (2009). Cancer stem cells: cell culture, markers, and targets for new therapies. J Cell Biochem *108*, 1031-1038.
Grey, B.R., Oates, J.E., Brown, M.D., and Clarke, N.W. (2009). Cd133: a marker of transit amplification rather than stem cell phenotype in the prostate? BJU Int *103*, 856-858.
Griguer, C.E., Oliva, C.R., Gobin, E., Marcorelles, P., Benos, D.J., Lancaster, J.R., Jr., and Gillespie, G.Y. (2008). CD133 is a marker of bioenergetic stress in human glioma. PLoS One *3*, e3655.
Grossman, S.A., Reinhard, C., Colvin, O.M., Chasin, M., Brundrett, R., Tamargo, R.J., and Brem, H. (1992). The intracerebral distribution of BCNU delivered by surgically implanted biodegradable polymers. J Neurosurg *76*, 640-647.
Gunther, W., Pawlak, E., Damasceno, R., Arnold, H., and Terzis, A.J. (2003). Temozolomide induces apoptosis and senescence in glioma cells cultured as multicellular spheroids. Br J Cancer *88*, 463-469.
Guo, D., Ye, J., Dai, J., Li, L., Chen, F., Ma, D., and Ji, C. (2009). Notch-1 regulates Akt signaling pathway and the expression of cell cycle regulatory proteins cyclin D1, CDK2 and p21 in T-ALL cell lines. Leuk Res *33*, 678-685.
Gupta, P.B., Chaffer, C.L., and Weinberg, R.A. (2009). Cancer stem cells: mirage or reality? Nat Med *15*, 1010-1012.
Hanisch, U.K., and Kettenmann, H. (2007). Microglia: active sensor and versatile effector cells in the normal and pathologic brain. Nat Neurosci *10*, 1387-1394.
Hemmati, H.D., Nakano, I., Lazareff, J.A., Masterman-Smith, M., Geschwind, D.H., Bronner-Fraser, M., and Kornblum, H.I. (2003). Cancerous stem cells can arise from pediatric brain tumors. Proc Natl Acad Sci U S A *100*, 15178-15183.
Holland, E.C., Celestino, J., Dai, C., Schaefer, L., Sawaya, R.E., and Fuller, G.N. (2000). Combined activation of Ras and Akt in neural progenitors induces glioblastoma formation in mice. Nat Genet *25*, 55-57.
Holland, E.C., Hively, W.P., DePinho, R.A., and Varmus, H.E. (1998). A constitutively active epidermal growth factor receptor cooperates with disruption of G1 cell-cycle arrest pathways to induce glioma-like lesions in mice. Genes Dev *12*, 3675-3685.
Humphries, W., Wei, J., Sampson, J.H., and Heimberger, A.B. (2010). The role of tregs in glioma-mediated immunosuppression: potential target for intervention. Neurosurg Clin N Am *21*, 125-137.

Iso, T., Kedes, L., and Hamamori, Y. (2003). HES and HERP families: multiple effectors of the Notch signaling pathway. J Cell Physiol *194*, 237-255.

Jaiswal, S., Chao, M.P., Majeti, R., and Weissman, I.L. (2010). Macrophages as mediators of tumor immunosurveillance. Trends Immunol *31*, 212-219.

Jaksch, M., Munera, J., Bajpai, R., Terskikh, A., and Oshima, R.G. (2008). Cell cycle-dependent variation of a CD133 epitope in human embryonic stem cell, colon cancer, and melanoma cell lines. Cancer Res *68*, 7882-7886.

Jeon, H.M., Jin, X., Lee, J.S., Oh, S.Y., Sohn, Y.W., Park, H.J., Joo, K.M., Park, W.Y., Nam, D.H., DePinho, R.A., *et al.* (2008). Inhibitor of differentiation 4 drives brain tumor-initiating cell genesis through cyclin E and notch signaling. Genes Dev *22*, 2028-2033.

Kanamori, M., Kawaguchi, T., Nigro, J.M., Feuerstein, B.G., Berger, M.S., Miele, L., and Pieper, R.O. (2007). Contribution of Notch signaling activation to human glioblastoma multiforme. J Neurosurg *106*, 417-427.

Kang, M.K., and Kang, S.K. (2007). Tumorigenesis of chemotherapeutic drug-resistant cancer stem-like cells in brain glioma. Stem Cells Dev *16*, 837-847.

Kinzler, K.W., Bigner, S.H., Bigner, D.D., Trent, J.M., Law, M.L., O'Brien, S.J., Wong, A.J., and Vogelstein, B. (1987). Identification of an amplified, highly expressed gene in a human glioma. Science *236*, 70-73.

Koch, U., and Radtke, F. (2007). Notch and cancer: a double-edged sword. Cell Mol Life Sci *64*, 2746-2762.

Korpanty, G., Sullivan, L.A., Smyth, E., Carney, D.N., and Brekken, R.A. (2010). Molecular and clinical aspects of targeting the VEGF pathway in tumors. J Oncol *2010*, 652320.

Kreisl, T.N., Kim, L., Moore, K., Duic, P., Royce, C., Stroud, I., Garren, N., Mackey, M., Butman, J.A., Camphausen, K., *et al.* (2009). Phase II trial of single-agent bevacizumab followed by bevacizumab plus irinotecan at tumor progression in recurrent glioblastoma. J Clin Oncol *27*, 740-745.

Kriegstein, A., and Alvarez-Buylla, A. (2009). The glial nature of embryonic and adult neural stem cells. Annu Rev Neurosci *32*, 149-184.

Lathia, J.D., Gallagher, J., Heddleston, J.M., Wang, J., Eyler, C.E., Macswords, J., Wu, Q., Vasanji, A., McLendon, R.E., Hjelmeland, A.B., *et al.* (2010). Integrin alpha 6 regulates glioblastoma stem cells. Cell Stem Cell *6*, 421-432.

Lee, J., Kotliarova, S., Kotliarov, Y., Li, A., Su, Q., Donin, N.M., Pastorino, S., Purow, B.W., Christopher, N., Zhang, W., *et al.* (2006). Tumor stem cells derived from glioblastomas cultured in bFGF and EGF more closely mirror the phenotype and genotype of primary tumors than do serum-cultured cell lines. Cancer Cell *9*, 391-403.

Li, L., Dutra, A., Pak, E., Labrie, J.E., 3rd, Gerstein, R.M., Pandolfi, P.P., Recht, L.D., and Ross, A.H. (2009). EGFRvIII expression and PTEN loss synergistically induce chromosomal instability and glial tumors. Neuro Oncol *11*, 9-21.

Lichtor, T., and Glick, R.P. (2003). Cytokine immuno-gene therapy for treatment of brain tumors. J Neurooncol *65*, 247-259.

Liu, G., Yuan, X., Zeng, Z., Tunici, P., Ng, H., Abdulkadir, I.R., Lu, L., Irvin, D., Black, K.L., and Yu, J.S. (2006). Analysis of gene expression and chemoresistance of CD133+ cancer stem cells in glioblastoma. Mol Cancer *5*, 67.

Lottaz, C., Beier, D., Meyer, K., Kumar, P., Hermann, A., Schwarz, J., Junker, M., Oefner, P.J., Bogdahn, U., Wischhusen, J., *et al.* (2010). Transcriptional profiles of CD133+ and CD133- glioblastoma-derived cancer stem cell lines suggest different cells of origin. Cancer Res *70*, 2030-2040.

Lu, C., and Shervington, A. (2008). Chemoresistance in gliomas. Mol Cell Biochem *312*, 71-80.

Mao, X.G., Zhang, X., Xue, X.Y., Guo, G., Wang, P., Zhang, W., Fei, Z., Zhen, H.N., You, S.W., and Yang, H. (2009). Brain Tumor Stem-Like Cells Identified by Neural Stem Cell Marker CD15. Transl Oncol *2*, 247-257.

Marti, E., and Bovolenta, P. (2002). Sonic hedgehog in CNS development: one signal, multiple outputs. Trends Neurosci *25*, 89-96.

Mellor, H.R., Ferguson, D.J., and Callaghan, R. (2005). A model of quiescent tumour microregions for evaluating multicellular resistance to chemotherapeutic drugs. Br J Cancer *93*, 302-309.

Miele, L. (2006). Notch signaling. Clin Cancer Res *12*, 1074-1079.

Mihaliak, A.M., Gilbert, C.A., Li, L., Daou, M., Moser, R.P., Reeves, A., Cochran, B.H., and Ross, A.H. (2010). Clinically relevant doses of chemotherapy agents reversibly block formation of glioblastoma neurospheres. Cancer Lett *296*, 168-177.

Miraglia, S., Godfrey, W., Yin, A.H., Atkins, K., Warnke, R., Holden, J.T., Bray, R.A., Waller, E.K., and Buck, D.W. (1997). A novel five-transmembrane hematopoietic stem cell antigen: isolation, characterization, and molecular cloning. Blood *90*, 5013-5021.

Mohler, J. (1988). Requirements for hedgehog, a segmental polarity gene, in patterning larval and adult cuticle of Drosophila. Genetics *120*, 1061-1072.

Nunes, M.C., Roy, N.S., Keyoung, H.M., Goodman, R.R., McKhann, G., 2nd, Jiang, L., Kang, J., Nedergaard, M., and Goldman, S.A. (2003). Identification and isolation of multipotential neural progenitor cells from the subcortical white matter of the adult human brain. Nat Med *9*, 439-447.

Ogden, A.T., Waziri, A.E., Lochhead, R.A., Fusco, D., Lopez, K., Ellis, J.A., Kang, J., Assanah, M., McKhann, G.M., Sisti, M.B., *et al.* (2008). Identification of A2B5+CD133- tumor-initiating cells in adult human gliomas. Neurosurgery *62*, 505-514; discussion 514-515.

Osmond, T.L., Broadley, K.W., and McConnell, M.J. (2010). Glioblastoma cells negative for the anti-CD133 antibody AC133 express a truncated variant of the CD133 protein. Int J Mol Med *25*, 883-888.

Ostermann, S., Csajka, C., Buclin, T., Leyvraz, S., Lejeune, F., Decosterd, L.A., and Stupp, R. (2004). Plasma and cerebrospinal fluid population pharmacokinetics of temozolomide in malignant glioma patients. Clin Cancer Res *10*, 3728-3736.

Palmer, T.D., Willhoite, A.R., and Gage, F.H. (2000). Vascular niche for adult hippocampal neurogenesis. J Comp Neurol *425*, 479-494.

Pannuti, A., Foreman, K., Rizzo, P., Osipo, C., Golde, T., Osborne, B., and Miele, L. (2010). Targeting Notch to target cancer stem cells. Clin Cancer Res *16*, 3141-3152.

Patrawala, L., Calhoun, T., Schneider-Broussard, R., Zhou, J., Claypool, K., and Tang, D.G. (2005). Side population is enriched in tumorigenic, stem-like cancer cells, whereas ABCG2+ and ABCG2- cancer cells are similarly tumorigenic. Cancer Res *65*, 6207-6219.

Pellegatta, S., Poliani, P.L., Corno, D., Menghi, F., Ghielmetti, F., Suarez-Merino, B., Caldera, V., Nava, S., Ravanini, M., Facchetti, F., *et al.* (2006). Neurospheres enriched in cancer stem-like cells are highly effective in eliciting a dendritic cell-mediated immune response against malignant gliomas. Cancer Res *66*, 10247-10252.

Pfenninger, C.V., Roschupkina, T., Hertwig, F., Kottwitz, D., Englund, E., Bengzon, J., Jacobsen, S.E., and Nuber, U.A. (2007). CD133 is not present on neurogenic astrocytes in the adult subventricular zone, but on embryonic neural stem cells, ependymal cells, and glioblastoma cells. Cancer Res *67*, 5727-5736.

Phillips, H.S., Kharbanda, S., Chen, R., Forrest, W.F., Soriano, R.H., Wu, T.D., Misra, A., Nigro, J.M., Colman, H., Soroceanu, L., *et al.* (2006). Molecular subclasses of high-grade glioma predict prognosis, delineate a pattern of disease progression, and resemble stages in neurogenesis. Cancer Cell *9*, 157-173.

Pollard, S.M., Yoshikawa, K., Clarke, I.D., Danovi, D., Stricker, S., Russell, R., Bayani, J., Head, R., Lee, M., Bernstein, M., *et al.* (2009). Glioma stem cell lines expanded in adherent culture have tumor-specific phenotypes and are suitable for chemical and genetic screens. Cell Stem Cell *4*, 568-580.

Pruszak, J., Sonntag, K.C., Aung, M.H., Sanchez-Pernaute, R., and Isacson, O. (2007). Markers and methods for cell sorting of human embryonic stem cell-derived neural cell populations. Stem Cells *25*, 2257-2268.

Purow, B.W., Haque, R.M., Noel, M.W., Su, Q., Burdick, M.J., Lee, J., Sundaresan, T., Pastorino, S., Park, J.K., Mikolaenko, I., *et al.* (2005). Expression of Notch-1 and its ligands, Delta-like-1 and Jagged-1, is critical for glioma cell survival and proliferation. Cancer Res *65*, 2353-2363.

Qiang, L., Yang, Y., Ma, Y.J., Chen, F.H., Zhang, L.B., Liu, W., Qi, Q., Lu, N., Tao, L., Wang, X.T., *et al.* (2009). Isolation and characterization of cancer stem like cells in human glioblastoma cell lines. Cancer Lett *279*, 13-21.

Quintana, E., Shackleton, M., Sabel, M.S., Fullen, D.R., Johnson, T.M., and Morrison, S.J. (2008). Efficient tumour formation by single human melanoma cells. Nature *456*, 593-598.

Radaelli, E., Ceruti, R., Patton, V., Russo, M., Degrassi, A., Croci, V., Caprera, F., Stortini, G., Scanziani, E., Pesenti, E., *et al.* (2009). Immunohistopathological and neuroimaging characterization of murine orthotopic xenograft models of glioblastoma multiforme recapitulating the most salient features of human disease. Histol Histopathol *24*, 879-891.

Radtke, F., and Raj, K. (2003). The role of Notch in tumorigenesis: oncogene or tumour suppressor? Nat Rev Cancer *3*, 756-767.

Rahman, R., Smith, S., Rahman, C., and Grundy, R. (2010). Antiangiogenic therapy and mechanisms of tumor resistance in malignant glioma. J Oncol *2010*, 251231.

Reynolds, B.A., Tetzlaff, W., and Weiss, S. (1992). A multipotent EGF-responsive striatal embryonic progenitor cell produces neurons and astrocytes. J Neurosci *12*, 4565-4574.

Reynolds, B.A., and Vescovi, A.L. (2009). Brain cancer stem cells: Think twice before going flat. Cell Stem Cell *5*, 466-467; author reply 468-469.

Reynolds, B.A., and Weiss, S. (1996). Clonal and population analyses demonstrate that an EGF-responsive mammalian embryonic CNS precursor is a stem cell. Dev Biol *175*, 1-13.

Rich, J.N. (2008). The Implications of the Cancer Stem Cell Hypothesis for Neuro-Oncology and Neurology. Future Neurol *3*, 265-273.

Rizzo, P., Osipo, C., Foreman, K., Golde, T., Osborne, B., and Miele, L. (2008). Rational targeting of Notch signaling in cancer. Oncogene *27*, 5124-5131.

Rodrigues, J.C., Gonzalez, G.C., Zhang, L., Ibrahim, G., Kelly, J.J., Gustafson, M.P., Lin, Y., Dietz, A.B., Forsyth, P.A., Yong, V.W., *et al.* (2010). Normal human monocytes exposed to glioma cells acquire myeloid-derived suppressor cell-like properties. Neuro Oncol *12*, 351-365.

Ronchini, C., and Capobianco, A.J. (2001). Induction of cyclin D1 transcription and CDK2 activity by Notch(ic): implication for cell cycle disruption in transformation by Notch(ic). Mol Cell Biol *21*, 5925-5934.

Sanai, N., Alvarez-Buylla, A., and Berger, M.S. (2005). Neural stem cells and the origin of gliomas. N Engl J Med *353*, 811-822.

Sarkaria, J.N., Kitange, G.J., James, C.D., Plummer, R., Calvert, H., Weller, M., and Wick, W. (2008). Mechanisms of chemoresistance to alkylating agents in malignant glioma. Clin Cancer Res *14*, 2900-2908.

Scopelliti, A., Cammareri, P., Catalano, V., Saladino, V., Todaro, M., and Stassi, G. (2009). Therapeutic implications of Cancer Initiating Cells. Expert Opin Biol Ther *9*, 1005-1016.

Seri, B., Garcia-Verdugo, J.M., Collado-Morente, L., McEwen, B.S., and Alvarez-Buylla, A. (2004). Cell types, lineage, and architecture of the germinal zone in the adult dentate gyrus. J Comp Neurol *478*, 359-378.

Shackleton, M., Quintana, E., Fearon, E.R., and Morrison, S.J. (2009). Heterogeneity in cancer: cancer stem cells versus clonal evolution. Cell *138*, 822-829.

Sharma, V.M., Calvo, J.A., Draheim, K.M., Cunningham, L.A., Hermance, N., Beverly, L., Krishnamoorthy, V., Bhasin, M., Capobianco, A.J., and Kelliher, M.A. (2006). Notch1 contributes to mouse T-cell leukemia by directly inducing the expression of c-myc. Mol Cell Biol *26*, 8022-8031.

Shen, Y., Chen, C.S., Ichikawa, H., and Goldberg, G.S. (2010). SRC induces podoplanin expression to promote cell migration. J Biol Chem *285*, 9649-9656.

Shih, A.H., and Holland, E.C. (2006). Notch signaling enhances nestin expression in gliomas. Neoplasia *8*, 1072-1082.

Singec, I., Knoth, R., Meyer, R.P., Maciaczyk, J., Volk, B., Nikkhah, G., Frotscher, M., and Snyder, E.Y. (2006). Defining the actual sensitivity and specificity of the neurosphere assay in stem cell biology. Nat Methods *3*, 801-806.

Singh, S.K., Clarke, I.D., Terasaki, M., Bonn, V.E., Hawkins, C., Squire, J., and Dirks, P.B. (2003). Identification of a cancer stem cell in human brain tumors. Cancer Res *63*, 5821-5828.

Singh, S.K., Hawkins, C., Clarke, I.D., Squire, J.A., Bayani, J., Hide, T., Henkelman, R.M., Cusimano, M.D., and Dirks, P.B. (2004). Identification of human brain tumour initiating cells. Nature *432*, 396-401.

Snippert, H.J., van Es, J.H., van den Born, M., Begthel, H., Stange, D.E., Barker, N., and Clevers, H. (2009). Prominin-1/CD133 marks stem cells and early progenitors in mouse small intestine. Gastroenterology *136*, 2187-2194 e2181.

Son, M.J., Woolard, K., Nam, D.H., Lee, J., and Fine, H.A. (2009). SSEA-1 is an enrichment marker for tumor-initiating cells in human glioblastoma. Cell Stem Cell *4*, 440-452.

Stockhausen, M.T., Kristoffersen, K., and Poulsen, H.S. (2010). The functional role of Notch signaling in human gliomas. Neuro Oncol *12*, 199-211.

Stupp, R., Mason, W.P., van den Bent, M.J., Weller, M., Fisher, B., Taphoorn, M.J., Belanger, K., Brandes, A.A., Marosi, C., Bogdahn, U., *et al.* (2005). Radiotherapy plus concomitant and adjuvant temozolomide for glioblastoma. N Engl J Med *352*, 987-996.

Suh, H., Consiglio, A., Ray, J., Sawai, T., D'Amour, K.A., and Gage, F.H. (2007). In vivo fate analysis reveals the multipotent and self-renewal capacities of Sox2+ neural stem cells in the adult hippocampus. Cell Stem Cell *1*, 515-528.

Tavazoie, M., Van der Veken, L., Silva-Vargas, V., Louissaint, M., Colonna, L., Zaidi, B., Garcia-Verdugo, J.M., and Doetsch, F. (2008). A specialized vascular niche for adult neural stem cells. Cell Stem Cell *3*, 279-288.

Tchoghandjian, A., Baeza, N., Colin, C., Cayre, M., Metellus, P., Beclin, C., Ouafik, L., and Figarella-Branger, D. (2010). A2B5 Cells from Human Glioblastoma have Cancer Stem Cell Properties. Brain Pathol *20*, 211-221.

Uchida, N., Buck, D.W., He, D., Reitsma, M.J., Masek, M., Phan, T.V., Tsukamoto, A.S., Gage, F.H., and Weissman, I.L. (2000). Direct isolation of human central nervous system stem cells. Proc Natl Acad Sci U S A *97*, 14720-14725.

Varghese, M., Olstorn, H., Sandberg, C., Vik-Mo, E.O., Noordhuis, P., Nister, M., Berg-Johnsen, J., Moe, M.C., and Langmoen, I.A. (2008). A comparison between stem cells from the adult human brain and from brain tumors. Neurosurgery *63*, 1022-1033; discussion 1033-1034.

Wang, J., Wakeman, T.P., Lathia, J.D., Hjelmeland, A.B., Wang, X.F., White, R.R., Rich, J.N., and Sullenger, B.A. (2010). Notch promotes radioresistance of glioma stem cells. Stem Cells *28*, 17-28.

Wechsler-Reya, R.J., and Scott, M.P. (1999). Control of neuronal precursor proliferation in the cerebellum by Sonic Hedgehog. Neuron *22*, 103-114.

Wei, J., Barr, J., Kong, L.Y., Wang, Y., Wu, A., Sharma, A.K., Gumin, J., Henry, V., Colman, H., Sawaya, R., *et al.* (2010). Glioma-associated cancer-initiating cells induce immunosuppression. Clin Cancer Res *16*, 461-473.

Woolard, K., and Fine, H.A. (2009). Glioma stem cells: better flat than round. Cell Stem Cell *4*, 466-467.

Zacchigna, S., Oh, H., Wilsch-Brauninger, M., Missol-Kolka, E., Jaszai, J., Jansen, S., Tanimoto, N., Tonagel, F., Seeliger, M., Huttner, W.B., *et al.* (2009). Loss of the cholesterol-binding protein prominin-1/CD133 causes disk dysmorphogenesis and photoreceptor degeneration. J Neurosci *29*, 2297-2308.

Zhongling, F., Gang, Z., and Lei, Y. (2009). Neural stem cells and Alzheimer's disease: challenges and hope. Am J Alzheimers Dis Other Demen *24*, 52-57.

Zuniga, R.M., Torcuator, R., Jain, R., Anderson, J., Doyle, T., Ellika, S., Schultz, L., and Mikkelsen, T. (2009). Efficacy, safety and patterns of response and recurrence in patients with recurrent high-grade gliomas treated with bevacizumab plus irinotecan. J Neurooncol *91*, 329-336.

Cancer Stem Cells in Lung Cancer: Distinct Differences between Small Cell and Non-Small Cell Lung Carcinomas

Koji Okudela, M.D., Ph.D.[1], Noriyuki Nagahara, M.D., Ph.D.[2], Akira Katayama, Ph.D.[3], Hitoshi Kitamura, M.D., Ph.D.[1]
[1]Department of Pathology, Graduate School of Medicine, Yokohama City University, 3-9 Fukuura, Kanazawa-ku, Yokohama 236-0004
Departments of [2]Environmental Medicine and [3]Biological Chemistry and Molecular Biology, Graduate School of Medicine, Nippon Medical School 1-1-5 Sendagi, Bunkyo-ku, Tokyo 113-8602
Japan

1. Introduction

Lung cancer is one of the most common malignancies worldwide and a leading cause of cancer-related deaths. It is increasing year by year in almost all areas of the world, except for a slight decrease in certain countries [1]. Lung cancer consists of heterogeneous groups in terms of pathological features and is commonly classified into the following two major types, small cell lung carcinoma (SCLC) and non-small cell lung carcinoma (NSCLC). NSCLC also is a group of heterogeneous histological types, the majority of which are squamous cell carcinoma (SQC) and adenocarcinoma (ADC) with roughly similar frequencies (30-40% each), and large cell carcinoma (LCC) with a lower frequency (< 10%). SCLC comprises nearly 20% of lung cancer. ADC and LCC are further sub-classified into several categories, respectively. The classification of lung cancer is not only of academic interest but also of practical necessity, because the biological aggressiveness, responsiveness to therapeutic intervention and patients' prognosis are greatly different among the respective types [2].

Lung cancer originates from the airway epithelia of larger and smaller bronchi as well as of alveoli. While it is generally accepted that cancer cells are derived from progenitor or tissue stem cells, relatively little has been elucidated with regard to the identification of airway stem cells and the molecular mechanisms underlying their self-renewal and differentiation abilities [3-5], in contrast to other epithelial tissues such as the intestine, mammary gland, and skin [6].

The heterogeneity of lung cancer likely reflects differences in the site of origin (proximal versus peripheral), and, more importantly, in the type of cell of origin, i.e., progenitor (tissue stem) cells. The diversity of etiologic factors and target genes, the types of genetic insults, and the ensuing effects, activation or inactivation, on the genes involved, would also be responsible for the heterogeneity of lung cancer. In fact, tobacco smoke, containing more than 60 carcinogens, is generally accepted as the most important cause of almost all types of lung cancer, among which the genetic and molecular mechanisms of carcinogenesis differ considerably. The ensuing genetic alteration and epigenetic changes as well, could lead to dysfunction of molecular signal transduction pathways, which relate directly or indirectly to proliferation, differentiation, and death of the cell.

In our recent review article, we underscored that silencing alterations of both the *RB* and *TP53* genes are most likely to be important and early events in the development of SCLC, whereas alterations of the epidermal growth factor receptor (EGFR) signaling pathway play significant and important roles in NSCLC carcinogenesis [7]. We also emphasized that alterations of both the *RB* and *TP53* genes are central to the carcinogenesis of SCLC, while many other factors including achaete-scute complex homolog 1 (ASCL1) and thyroid transcription factor-1 (TTF-1) contribute to the development and biological behavior of SCLC [8].

The cancer stem cell (CSC) theory has proposed that a tumor cell subpopulation possessing self-renewal capacity which forms only a small fraction of tumor tissue is central in sustaining neoplastic lesions and is a potentially crucial target of cancer therapy [9-23]. The CSCs are possibly produced by either transformation of normal stem cells or multistep dedifferentiation of specialized progenitor cells through a progressive accumulation of genetic aberrations. Rapp, *et al.* [12] proposed a model of oncogene-induced plasticity for CSC origin by demonstrating reprogramming events triggered by a specific combination of oncogenes. Li, *et al.* [16] suggested that genomic instability is a driving force for transforming normal stem cells into CSCs and, in CSCs, a potential mechanism for cancer cell heterogeneity. The origin of CSCs and this mechanism are discussed in more detail in other chapters [The publisher may modify this part].

The CSCs of lung cancers can be considered to originate from either airway stem cells, which have not been identified yet, or respective committed progenitor cells, such as bronchioloalveolar progenitor cells, basal/mucous secretory bronchial progenitor cells, and neuroendocrine progenitor cells (see the section Origin of CSCs in lung cancer).

The CSC theory is tremendously attractive to both researchers and physicians, because the CSC is central to cancer cell biology and cancer therapy. The discovery of specific markers of CSCs in the respective types of cancers is particularly important. Furthermore, it is necessary to clarify the function of these molecules, as the disruption of the signaling pathways and gene transcriptions that control the activity of CSCs is the final goal of CSC-targeting therapy. We emphasized that a knowledge of CSC signaling pathways may lead to new treatment that kill or induce differentiation of CSCs and could better contribute to cures [24]. These treatments could be designed to target CSCs in order to induce the differentiation of CSCs, or eliminate CSCs by inhibiting the maintenance of the stem-cell state. For instance, side population (SP) cells that are considered to represent CSCs (see below), of a human lung cancer cell line (A549) totally disappeared after treatment with the selective ATP-binding cassette transporter G2 (ABCG2) inhibitor fumitremorgin C [25]. As another example, a Hedgehog signaling inhibitor cyclopamine strikingly reduced the *in vitro* invasive capacity of pancreatic cancer cell lines and also profoundly inhibited metastatic spread in an orthotopic xenograft model [26].

In regard to lung cancer, we also stressed the extreme importance of identifying specific CSC markers for the respective subtypes of lung cancer, for instance SCLC and NSCLC (ADC, SQC, LCC, and others), since they are quite different not only in phenotype but also in pathogenesis and biological behavior. In particular, SCLC is highly metastatic, drug-resistant, and rapidly fatal. The aggressiveness of SCLC may be attributable to an abundance of CSCs, as CSCs are drug-resistant and play a crucial role in cancer recurrence and metastasis. Alternatively, it is also possible that the CSCs of SCLC are endowed with specific biological properties, for instance niche-independency or strong drug-resistance, or both. If SCLC-specific CSC markers were discovered, they would be extremely useful as targets of chemotherapy, for the establishment of therapeutic regimens, and for predictions of the prognosis (outcome) of patients.

In this chapter, we discuss the characteristics of normal airway stem/progenitor cells and CSCs in lung cancer by reviewing hitherto described study results. In addition, we demonstrate the potentially distinct differences in the mechanism of maintenance of CSCs between SCLC and NSCLC, primarily focusing upon aldehyde dehydrogenase (ALDH) based on our own experiments currently underway.

2. Stem cells in healthy and injured lung

Although the airway stem cell in a strict sense has not been identified yet, several lines of evidence support the existence of regional progenitors cells, such as bronchioloalveolar progenitor cells, basal/mucous secretory bronchial progenitor cells, and neuroendocrine progenitor cells, which maintain normal homeostasis as well as play roles in repair [3-5]. These progenitor cells expand their populations in response to various insults including toxic substances, but do not become tumorigenic unless at least one genetic or epigenetic event occurs, for instance by tobacco smoke carcinogens [4,27].

3. Origin of CSCs in lung cancers

As in hematological malignancies and other solid cancers, the presence of subpopulations of cells endowed with CSC properties has been recognized in lung cancers. Like CSCs in other tissues, the CSCs of lung cancers can be considered to originate from either airway stem cells, which have not been identified yet, or respective committed progenitor cells, such as bronchioloalveolar progenitor cells, basal/mucous secretory bronchial progenitor cells, and neuroendocrine progenitor cells [3-5], resulting in the initiation of region-specific lung cancers [4].

4. Cell markers for CSCs in lung cancers

CSC markers for lung cancer are a matter of some controversy, probably reflecting the tremendous heterogeneity of lung cancers in terms of cell of origin, etiology, pathology, biology, and molecular/genetic pathogenesis [2,7]. We herein briefly discuss these markers, paying special attention to the differences between SCLC and NSCLC; representative lung CSC markers reported to date are listed in Table 1.

5. CD133

CD133 was first reported as a novel marker for human hematopoietic stem and progenitor cells [28], and later found in some types of leukemic cells [29]. Prominin-1, which was identified on neuroepithelial stem cells in mice in 1997, is a mouse homolog of the human CD133 antigen [30]. The expression of CD133 has been detected in human central nervous system stem cells [31], human trophoblasts [32], human lymphatic/vascular endothelial precursor cells [33], and human prostatic epithelial stem cells [34]. The CD133 antigen is a 120kDa five-transmembrane domain glycoprotein, and its chromosomal location (4p16.2-p12) and amino acid sequence have been clarified [35]. Although its function is still unknown, CD133 may have a role in stem cell activation/maintenance, as shown by its coexpression with β1-integrin in the epidermal basal cells [36], release of CD133-carrying membrane particles into the extracellular space from neural progenitors and some epithelial cells [37], and potential regulatory activity of cell-cell contacts [38].

Recent studies have demonstrated that CD133 is a specific marker of CSCs in a wide spectrum of malignant tumors including brain tumors, colorectal cancers, pancreatic cancers, breast cancers, prostate cancers, ovarian cancers [39-41], and some lung cancers [42]. In contrast to the general consensus that CD133 is a ubiquitous CSC marker, several studies demonstrated that CD133-negative cells in certain human tumors also possess tumorigenic activity upon xenotransplantation into immunocompromised rodents [43-45]. These results imply that the CD133-negative subpopulation also contains cells with cancer initiating cell (CIC) activity. Mizrak, *et al.* [46] pointed out that CD133 is actually detected by its glycosylated epitope, AC133, and it is likely that AC133, but not CD133, is a more reliable CSC marker. Bidlingmaier, *et al.* [47] also suggested that the use of CD133 expression as a marker for CSC should be critically evaluated. These reports may explain the discrepancy observed in the results from different studies.

In regard to lung cancers, Eramo, *et al.* [42] reported that CD133 is a useful CSC marker in both SCLC and NSCLC. In contrast, Meng, *et al.* [48] reported more than 45% of A549 (NSCLC) and H446 (SCLC) cells to be CICs regardless of CD133 expression based on the results of cloning and tumorigenic analyses. Jiang, *et al.* [49] reported that, in NSCLC, cancer cells with strong ALDH activity (see below), showed CSC features and CD133 expression. Levina, *et al.* [50] demonstrated that NSCLC cells (H460) propagated a CD133-positive CSC-like cell population, in association with the expression of Oct-4 and high nuclear β-catenin (see below), after an *in vitro* treatment with anti-cancer drugs. Chen, *et al.* [51] reported that CD133-positive NSCLC cell lines display self-renewal and chemo-radio-resistant properties. Intriguingly, in SCLC, Jiang, *et al.* [52] demonstrated that achaete-scute complex homolog 1 (ASCL1) directly regulates ALDH1A1 and CD133 and that the CD133^{high}-ALDH1A1^{high}-ASCL1^{high} subpopulation exhibits the features of CSCs both *in vitro* and *in vivo*. ASCL1 is a specific marker of SCLC and thought to play important roles in its phenotypic expression and biological aggressiveness [8,53].

6. Side population

Hoechst 33342 dye-efflux side population (SP) bone marrow cells were first discovered as hematopoietic stem cells in mice [54]. Since then, SP cells with stem-cell-like capabilities have been found in a variety of human hematologic and solid malignancies. These cells show the features of CSCs characterized by self-renewal activity, differentiated progeny production, tumorigenicity, as well as the expression of CSC markers and stem cell genes [55]. Thus, SP cells can be assumed to be CSCs. Importantly, SP cells are highly resistant to chemotherapeutic agents and crucial in therapy resistance and tumor recurrence [55-57]. Zhou, *et al.* [58] showed that expression of the *ATP binding cassette transporter superfamily member G2* (*ABCG2*) gene is an important determinant of the SP phenotype, and that it might serve as a marker for stem cells from various sources. SP cells are usually isolated and purified by fluorescence activating cell sorting (FACS) using an ultraviolet (UV) laser.

Recently, a new technique using a Violet-excited cell-permeable DNA-binding dye has been reported [59]. This method is inexpensive and yields the same results as UV-excited FACS [59]. In contrast, Wu, *et al.* [55] pointed out the following problems in using the SP phenotype as a CSC marker: 1) cells resistant to the Hoechst dye's toxicity do not consist only of stem-like cells, 2) variables in staining times, dye concentrations, and cellular concentrations can greatly affect the SP phenotype, and 3) cytometric gating strategies used to isolate SP cells lack the consistency of gating strategies used when staining with markers. These problems potentially lead to cross contamination of the SP and the non-SP fractions ultimately resulting in the production of confounding data. They emphasized that more stringent gating strategies are necessary and that a combination of isolation methods are required to enhance the purity of CSCs.

In lung cancers, Ho, *et al.* [60] reported that the SP cells in NSCLC cell lines were an enriched source of tumor-initiating cells with stem cell properties. Sung, *et al.* [25] suggested that ABCG2 played an important role in the multidrug resistance phenotype of SP cells in a NSCLC cell line, A549. In contrast, Meng, *et al.* [48] reported more than 45% of A549 (NSCLC) and H446 (SCLC) cells to be CICs regardless of SP features based on the results of cloning and tumorigenic analyses.

7. Aldehyde dehydrogenase

The ALDH superfamily represents a divergently related group of enzymes that metabolize a wide variety of endogenous and exogenous aldehydes. In the human genome, at least 19 functional genes and 3 pseudogenes have been identified [61]. ALDH also contributes to the oxidation of retinol to retinoic acid, a modulator of cell proliferation, which may also modulate stem cell proliferation [62]. Murine and human hematopoietic stem cells [63-64], murine neural stem cells [65], normal and malignant human mammary stem cells [66], and normal and malignant human colorectal stem cells [62,67] exhibit ALDH activity and express this enzyme, strongly suggesting that strong ALDH activity and/or antigen expression can be used as a marker for stem cells in a variety of cancers. ALDH activity has been measured as substrate-oxidizing activity in whole cell lysate, and the expression of the enzyme has been detected by immunoreactions with specific antibodies, such as Western blot and immunohistochemical analyses. Since the development of a new method using an ALDH-activated fluorescent substrate as a marker for the isolation of human hematopoietic stem cells [68], the so-called Aldefluor assay has been widely applied to the measurement and isolation of normal and malignant stem-cell-like cells in a variety of tissues [49,64-67]. This method is useful for isolating and purifying viable cells with high levels of ALDH activity for assays of the CSC properties of these cell populations.

8. Other lung CSC markers

Koch, *et al.* [69] demonstrated that a majority of SCLC were immunohistochemically positive for the antibody against podocalyxin-like protein 1 (PODXL-1) and hypothesized that PODXL-1 is a potential CSC marker of SCLC. PODXL-1, belonging to a large family of cell surface sialomucins and being most closely related to CD34 and endoglycan [33,70,71], is expressed in primitive hematopoietic progenitors and thought to be a marker of embryonic and hematopoietic stem cells [72].

Gutova, *et al.* [73] found that SCLC cells positive for urokinase plasminogen activator receptor (uPAR) were resistant to traditional chemotherapies and speculated that they contain a putative CSC population. Urokinase plasminogen activator (uPA) and its receptor uPAR are instrumental in controlling membrane-associated extracellular proteolysis and transmembranous signaling, thus affecting cell migration and invasion [74]. uPAR is up-regulated by several oncogenic pathways including mutations of multiple oncogenes. Alfano, *et al.* [74] underlined the importance of uPAR signaling in the prevention of apoptosis.

9. Signaling pathways in CSCs of lung cancers

Sonic hedgehog

Sonic hedgehog (Shh) is expressed by the epithelial cells, and binds and signals to Patched1/2 receptors in the underlying mesenchyme [6,75,76].
Watkins, *et al.* [77] reported the significance of Hedgehog signaling in a subset of SCLCs. Yagui-Beltrán, *et al.* [78] and Peacock, *et al.* [79] reviewed the results of studies on CSC markers and signaling pathways in pulmonary carcinogenesis with special attention to the differences between SCLC and NSCLC. Both papers emphasized the potential importance of the Hedgehog and Wnt signaling pathways in SCLC and NSCLC (see below). Interestingly, human primary or immortalized bronchial epithelial cells exposed to cigarette smoke for only eight days in culture became tumorigenic in nude mice, in association with the activation of the Hedgehog and Wnt signaling pathways [80].

Wnt signaling pathway and nuclear β-catenin

For the maintenance and activation of normal stem cells, the Wnt/β-catenin signaling pathway is crucial, as distinctly demonstrated in the intestinal mucosa epithelia, epidermis, mammary gland [6], and other tissue [81]. The importance of Wnt signaling in cancer cells has been emphasized [82], and the Wnt/β-catenin signaling cascade is a critical regulator not only of normal stem cells but also of CSCs [83]. Disruption of this signaling pathway at any step potentially causes disorders of stem cell activity and plays a crucial role in the development of cancer. For instance, sustained Wnt signaling mediated by the membrane receptor Frizzled stimulates the release of β-catenin from a cytoplasmic degradation complex composed of APC, Axin, GSK3-β and Dsh, resulting in its movement into the nucleus and activation of Lef/Tcf transcription factors for c-Myc and cyclin D1 [82]. As another example, inactivation of APC due to a gene mutation also results in the release of β-catenin from the degradation complex, leading to the neoplastic transformation of colonic epithelial stem cells [11]. Thus, nuclear β-catenin is a hallmark for active Wnt signaling [75].
As described above, Yagui-Beltrán, *et al.* [87] and Peacock, *et al.* [79] emphasized the potential importance of the Wnt signaling pathway in SCLC and NSCLC in addition to the Hedgehog signaling pathway. Also as described above, human primary or immortalized bronchial epithelial cells exposed to cigarette smoke became tumorigenic in nude mice, being associated with the activation of not only the Hedgehog signaling pathway but also the Wnt signaling pathway [80].

Other signaling pathways and transcription factors in lung CSCs

While the Wnt/β-catenin signaling pathway has been extensively investigated in many tissues including the lung, other signaling pathways are also important for controlling stem cell activity, including transmembranous Notch signaling and bone morphogenetic protein (BMP) signaling mediated by the cell membrane receptor Bmpr1a [8,75]. However, we are only beginning to understand the roles these pathways play in CSC populations of lung cancers.

B cell-specific Mo-MuLV integration site 1 (Bmi1) is a member of the Polycomb group family of proteins and a downstream effector of the extracellular signaling molecule Shh. Bmi1 is implicated in the self-renewal of multiple stem cells including hematopoietic and neural stem cells [84]. Dovey, *et al.* [85] suggested that Bmi1 is critical for both normal and tumor bronchioloalveolar stem cell expansion in mice. Koch, *et al.* [69] demonstrated that a majority of SCLCs were immunohistochemically positive for antibodies against Bmi1. From these results, they hypothesized that Bmi1 is a potential CSC marker of SCLC.

A couple of studies suggest that Oct-4 is a potential CSC marker for lung cancers. Levina, *et al.* [50] demonstrated that a human large cell cancer cell line (H460) propagated a CSC-like cell population that showed CD133, Oct-4, and high nuclear β-catenin expression after an *in vitro* treatment with anti-cancer drugs. Chen, *et al.* [51] reported that Oct-4 expression plays a crucial role in maintaining the self-renewing, CSC-like, and chemo-radio-resistant properties of CD133-positive NSCLC cell lines. Oct-4 is a member of the POU transcription factor family known to be expressed in pluripotent stem cells and to function as a transcriptional regulator of multiple genes related to stemness [86].

In vitro assay

Several *in vitro* assays have been used to identify CSCs, including sphere-formation assays, serial colony-forming unit assays (re-plating assays), and label-retention assays [10,14]. Among them, sphere-formation assays are utilized in a wide range of tissue systems including lung cancers [42,87]. However, each of these methods has potential pitfalls that complicate interpretation of the results. For instance, difficulty in confirming clonality (single cell origin) has been pointed out [10]. In addition, the culture conditions used for these assays potentially exert selection pressures upon the cultured cells, resulting in the selection of only cell populations that are able to survive and proliferate under such specific conditions. The limitations of these *in vitro* assays should be kept in mind, and a combination of methods including *in vivo* assays is necessary for the identification and isolation of CSCs.

CSC niche

The microenvironment surrounding normal and cancer stem cells, which provides the stem cell niche, plays multiple roles including as a mechanical anchorage for the stem cells and in cross-talk communication mediated by direct contact and/or indirect extracellular factors. For instance, Wnt ligands are produced and released from both stem cells and niche cells, BMP and Shh are released from niche cells and epithelial cells respectively, and Notch signaling is transmembranously transmitted between neighboring cells. The microenvironment may also provide signaling via the cell receptor integrin as suggested by its expression in prostatic CSCs [88] and its co-expression with AC133 (CD133) in the epidermal basal cells [36], as well as through metalloprotease-mediated lysophopholipid signaling [89].

The concept of a CSC niche is a matter of debate [90]. Two fundamental questions need to be answered: 1) Does a specific CSC niche exist? 2) If it does, what are the differences between the normal stem cell niche and CSC niche? Sneddon, *et al.* [23] removed some of the confusion regarding the CSC niche by proposing several possible models (Figure 1): 1) CSCs are capable of surviving in the normal stem cell niche, 2) a distinct CSC niche is necessary for activation, 3) CSCs may be capable of providing signals that instruct an otherwise quiescent niche to become activated ("hijacking the niche"), 4) CSCs could amplify an already existent activated niche, 5) CSCs may be niche-independent, that is, they themselves acquire the ability to maintain activity, and 6) there may be a discrete niche that is inhibitory for CSC maintenance. Accumulating evidence suggests that no single model fits all the diverse types of cancer. Further study is required to establish a universally acceptable CSC niche theory.

While the niche may also play an important role in the maintenance of CSCs from lung cancers, little has been elucidated yet. Hilbe, *et al.* [91] demonstrated by immunohistochemistry a significant increase in CD133-positive vascular endothelial cells in patients with NSCLC and suggested an involvement of endothelial progenitor cells in the tumor vasculature and tumor growth, as well as possibly the maintenance and activation of CSCs. More studies of the lung CSC niche are required not only to understand the biological relationship between lung CSCs and their niche but also for the development of therapeutic strategies for lung cancers.

Brief summary of lung CSC markers and potential problems

While investigations into the CSC markers of lung cancer are insufficient at this time, as discussed above and summarized in Table 1, we tentatively summarize the findings to date as follows: 1) CD133 expression and the SP phenotype are common CSC markers for SCLC and NSCLC. 2) The Wnt/β-catenin signaling pathway is also important in the maintenance and activation of CSCs in SCLC and NSCLC. 3) PODXL-1 and uPAR are potential CSC markers for SCLC, but their expression has not been well examined in NSCLC. 4) In regard to ALDH, results reported to date appear to be complicated. Its enzymatic activity has been demonstrated in SCLC and NSCLC cells by the Aldefluor assay, as well as by a spectrophotometrical assay [92-97]. On the other hand, an immunohistochemical analysis using antibodies against ALDH1A1 and ALDH3A1 in tissue sections of surgical specimens of lung cancer demonstrated the expression of these ALDH isozymes in NSCLC cases, but not in SCLC cases, suggesting that the ALDH protein expression was limited to CSCs in NSCLC [96]. In contrast, Moreb, *et al.* [93] reported that in their studies using several SCLC and NSCLC cell lines there were good correlations between the results of a Western blot analysis, a spectrophotometrical analysis, and the Aldefluor assay, in spite of a few exceptions (see below). The discrepancy among these results may be attributable to the difference in the antibodies used, and the difference between the *in vitro* and *in vivo* conditions as well.

Though evidence is still poor, it is supposed that distinct differences in the mechanism of ALDH expression and activity, as well as the role of ALDH in the maintenance/activation of CSCs, exist between SCLC and NSCLC. Furthermore, the exact mechanism and role of ALDH in the maintenance of the stemness of normal stem cells and CSCs are still unknown. To try to resolve these issues, we have carried out investigations, which are described in the following section.

Recent findings in ALDH and CSC of the lung

As described above, ALDH activity and its protein expression have been reported to be useful normal stem cell and CSC markers in a wide range of tissues [66,92,96-98]. These

ALDHs play pluripotent roles in endobiotic and xenobiotic metabolism through specific metabolic pathways. One important issue to be addressed is which ALDH isozymes are responsible for the ALDH activity used to identify stem cell progenitors. Several studies have demonstrated that ALDH activity is needed for the differentiation of primitive progenitors into mature cells, thus fulfilling one of the defining characteristics of multipotent stem cells, and some lines of evidence suggest that ALDH1A1 is an important marker of hematopoietic stem cell progenitors [92]. In fact, ALDH1A1 is one of the enzymes involved in the production of retinoic acid from retinol, and retinoic acid is considered significantly important in maintaining a balance between hematopoietic stem cell self-renewal and differentiation [92].

Moreb, *et al.* [93] systemically evaluated ALDH expression in several lung cancer cells lines (SCLC and NSCLC cell lines) utilizing the Aldefluor assay, a Western blotting, and a spectrophotometry and found a very good correlation between the results of all three. They concluded that the Aldefluor assay can be adapted successfully to measure ALDH activity in lung cancer cells, providing real time changes in ALDH activity in viable cells treated with chemotherapy or siRNA. They emphasized the importance of the use of mixed populations of cells with high ALDH levels and cells lacking ALDH activity when ALDH activity is measured by the Aldefluor assay in cells known to have high ALDH levels. Importantly, they carried out double Aldefluor and propidium iodide (PI) staining to delineate dead cells. According to their results, while ALDH expression levels were heterogeneous among the cell lines examined, overall findings revealed low levels of ALDH activity in SCLC cell lines, while higher levels were detected in some, but not all, NSCLC cell lines. The results correlated very well with protein and enzymatic activity as measured by the Western blot analysis and the spectrophotometrical assay, respectively. Intriguingly, there was one exception: The SW210.5 (SCLC) cell line registered only a small amount of ALDH activity in the spectrophotometrical assay and expressed only small amounts of ALDH1A1 and ALDH3A1 proteins in the Western blot analysis, whereas the Aldefluor assay showed high levels of ALDH activity (50% of the cells). This SCLC cell line (SW210.5) was shown to express mRNA for ALDH1A1 and ALDH2, but not ALDH3A1, by the semi-quantitative reverse transcription polymerase chain reaction (RT-PCR) assay.

Our preliminary experiments revealed very high levels of ALDH1A1 mRNA expression in some SCLC and NSCLC cell lines. We also observed considerable discrepancies between mRNA levels detected by the quantitative RT-PCR assay, protein levels analyzed by Western blotting, and the proportion of cells with enzymatic activity measured by the Aldefluor assay in several SCLC and NSCLC cell lines.

Aiming to elucidate the mechanism underlying the discrepancies observed in preliminary experiments and the previous study, we carried out the following experiments.

ALDH mRNA expression - its correlation with the most common CSC marker CD133 -

The quantitative RT-PCR assay revealed that ALDH1A1 mRNA was expressed at detectable levels in seven out of nine SCLC cell lines (77.8%), three of which expressed it at unequivocally high levels (33.3%), while it was expressed in four of the 18 NSCLC cell lines, two of which expressed it at high levels (11.1%)(Figure 2). On the other hand, ALDH2 was expressed in eight of the nine SCLC cell lines and 17 of the 18 NSCLC cell lines. The levels were lower on the whole than those of ALDH1A1 and did not remarkably differ among the cell lines. mRNA of CD133, most commonly used CSC marker, was expressed only in SCLC cell lines (66.7%, six out of nine cell lines), and its level in SCLC cell lines tended to be associated with the level of ALDH1A1, but not ALDH2. The findings suggested ALDH1A1 to have an important significance in the maintenance of stemness in lung cancer cells, and might account for the highly malignant activity of SCLCs.

ALDH protein expression in lung cancer cell lines

ALDH protein was detected by Western blotting using a non-selective antibody, which binds both ALDH1A1 and ALDH2 proteins (clone 44, BD transduction, Palo Alto, CA). The protein was expressed at high levels in two of the nine SCLC cell lines (22.2%), and two of the 18 NSCLC cell lines (11.1%)(Figure 3). The level of protein paralleled well the level of ALDH1A1 mRNA, but not ALDH2 mRNA, in NSCLC cell lines, suggesting that the protein detected by the Western blot analysis was ALDH1A1 rather than ALDH2 (Figure 2 and Figure 3). Thus, we describe the protein detected here by the Western blot analysis as ALDH1A1. Interestingly, one SCLC cell line (Lu134) with a high level of ALDH1A1 mRNA did not express ALDH1A1 (either ALDH1A1 or ALDH2) (Figure 2). This result is similar to a previous observation that a SCLC cell line, SW210.5, expressed ALDH1 mRNA, but only a very small amount of protein [93]. These findings suggest a potential post-translational mechanism to be involved in ALDH1A1 protein expression in some SCLC cells.

ALDH activity in lung cancer cell lines

The fraction of cells with ALDH activity was measured with the Aldefluor assay. The two SCLC cell lines with high ALDH1A1 protein levels (H1688 and H1618) had fractions of cells with strong ALDH activity (Figure 4). All of the SCLC cell lines with very weak ALDH protein expression (the faint bands detected by Western blotting in these cell lines were presumably ALDH2, because these cell lines expressed only ALDH2, not ALDH1A1, mRNA) had only a small fraction (less than 10%) of cells with ALDH activity. On the other hand, among NSCLC cell lines examined (A549, PC1, H441, H2087 and H1299) (not all data shown), only one (PC1) had fraction of cells with strong ALDH activity (Figure 4). One cell line with high ALDH1A1 protein levels (A549) unexpectedly had only a very small fraction of cells with strong ALDH activity. Summarizing the findings, ALDH1A1 protein expression was closely associated with ALDH activity in SCLC cells, but not necessarily in NSCLC cells, suggesting the potential post-translational mechanism to be involved in activation of ALDH1A1 protein in NSCLCs.

Primary structure of ALDH1A1 mRNA

To elucidate the possible involvement of a mutation (or polymorphism) or splicing disorder in the difference among the levels of mRNA, protein and activity, which was observed in Lu134 SCLC and A549 NSCLC cells, the nucleotide sequence of open reading frames of cDNA were analyzed. No mutation (or polymorphism) causing an amino acid substitution was found in either cell line (data not shown). However, interestingly, short mRNA variant (258 base pairs in the open reading frame, encoding 86 amino acids: see Figure 5) was found in the Lu134A cell line. This variant was found in three of eight sub-clones (37.5%) in our sub-cloning experiment (part of the result is shown in Figure 5). The result suggested the possible involvement of such a variant in the post-transcriptional regulation of ALHD1A1 expression, and also implied a potential difference between SCLC and NSCLC, although further screening of a larger number of cell lines and primary lung cancers is required to test this idea.

Post-translational modification of ALDH1A1 protein

Since no mutation was found in the cell line with the lag between ALDH1/2 protein expression and ALDH activity (A549 cells), we next verified the possible involvement of a post-translational modification. To screen for such a modification, two-dimensional Western blot analysis was performed with A549 (NSCLC) and H1688 (SCLC) cells (Figure 6). While the results did not reveal unequivocal evidence of a modification, the ALDH1A1 protein migrated slightly faster in A549 cells (Figure 6). To elucidate the mechanism underlying the lag between ALDH1A1 protein expression and ALDH activity, further investigations of protein structure and modifications such as glycosylation, phosphorylation and acetylation status, are required.

ALDH protein expression in primary lung cancers

ALDH protein expression in primary lung tumors was examined by immunohistochemistry using a non-selective antibody (clone 44, BD transduction, Palo Alto, CA), which binds both ALDH1A1 and ALHD2 proteins (ALDH1/2). The protein expression was detected in three of nine SCLCs (33.3%) and in 41 of 70 NSCLCs (58.6%)(Table 2). The levels tended to be higher in NSCLC, especially SQC, than in SCLC (Figure 5). The results were similar to those reported by Patel, *et al.* [96], who found in their immunohistochemical analysis that the ALDH isozymes 1A1 and 1A3 were expressed at significantly higher levels in NSCLC than in SCLC [96]. However, we have found that there is a discrepancy between the results of Western blotting for cancer cell lines and immunohistochemistry for primary lung cancers. The frequency of ALDH1/2 protein expression was considerably higher in primary cancers than in cell lines among NSCLCs, whereas it was similar between the two among SCLCs (Figure 3 and Table 2). Moreover, non-cancerous airway cells *in vivo*, i.e., both the bronchial, bronchiole and alveolar epithelial cells, exhibited high levels of immunohistochemical expression of ALHD1/2 protein compared to cancer cells in all cases examined (Figure 7 and Table 2). Interestingly, the two non-cancerous immortalized airway epithelial cell lines (NHBE-T and HPL1D) showed very weak expression of ALDH1/2 protein *in vitro*. The ALDH family is expressed in response to toxic stress [99-101]. The marked expression of ALDH1/2 protein in non-cancerous airway epithelial cells *in vivo* is supposed to be induced by external stimuli such as dust, cigarette smoke and so on. In NSCLCs, ALDH1/2 protein tended to be expressed more strongly among *in situ* parts than invasive parts (data not shown), in support of our supposition. Furthermore ALDH1/2 protein expression tended to decrease in parallel with the dedifferentiation process, as a large proportion of poorly differentiated NSCLCs expressed the protein only faintly (data not shown). In well-differentiated and *in situ* NSCLCs, ALDH1/2 expression may still be regulated by the physiological system (it may be lost during progression process to develop poorly differentiated ones). Although further investigation is required to elucidate the mechanism and significance of such a downregulation of ALDH1/2 protein expression in primary lung cancers, the results obtained here imply that ALDH1/2 protein plays diverse roles in different situations is not a universal stem cell marker. The mechanism to induce ALDH1/2 protein expression and its significance are likely to differ among the non-cancerous airway epithelia, NSCLCs and SCLCs.

10. Conclusion

As is widely accepted, among lung cancers, SCLC and NSCLC are distinctly different in terms of biological behavior and pathogenesis. We have hypothesized that the CSCs of these two major subtypes of lung cancer possess different biological properties and that the abundance of CSCs population differs between the two. We have here focused upon ALDH to confirm such a potential difference.

The proportion of cells with strong ALDH activity tended to be associated with the CD133 mRNA level especially in SCLC cell lines (Figure 2). Recently, Jiang, *et al.* [52] demonstrated, in SCLC cell lines, that the $ALDH1A1^{high}$-$CD133^{high}$-$ASCL1^{high}$ subpopulation exhibits the features of CSCs and that ASCL1 directly regulates ALDH1A1 and CD133 both *in vitro* and *in vivo*. Previous observations [60] are consistent with our results and also support the hypothesis that the size of the CSC fraction (population) could be one causes of highly malignant activity of SCLC. Importantly, however, not all SCLCs among cell lines and primary tumors were found to have either protein expression or a fraction of cells with high ALDH activity (Figure 4, Figure 7 and Table 2). We thus speculate that the ALDH activity is only one of the factors determining the stemness of CSCs in SCLCs. Alternatively, ALDH1A1 protein expression or ALDH activity is just part of the machinery to maintain stemness and might have significance only in some fractions of SCLCs. On the other hand, Ucar, *et al.* [95] proposed ALDH activity to be a CSC marker in a NSCLC cell line (NIH-H522 LCC cell line). Moreover, Jiang, *et al.* [49] reported that, in NSCLCs, cancer cells with strong ALDH1A1 activity, which were isolated using the Aldefluor assay followed by fluorescence-activated cell sorting, showed CSC features and CD133 expression. They proposed that ALDH1A1 is a lung cancer stem cell-associated marker, being a potential prognostic factor and therapeutic target for the treatment of patients with lung cancer. In our experiments, one NSCLC cell line (PC1 [SQC]) had a high ALDH1A1 protein level and a large fraction of cells with strong ALDH activity (Figure 3 and Figure 5), but did not express CD133 mRNA. Taken together, it is supposed that there is considerable heterogeneity in the mechanism maintaining the stemness of CSCs of SCLCs and NSCLCs.

Aside from the maintenance of stemness, another interesting finding of our experiments was that the level of ALDH1A1 mRNA did not always parallel the level of protein in SCLC cell lines, whereas, in NSCLC cell lines (Figure 3 and Figure 4), the level of protein was not always consistent with that of activity. Furthermore, the *in vivo* findings revealed that either non-cancerous airway epithelia or low-grade neoplasms such as well-differentiated or *in situ* NSCLCs showed stronger immunohistochemical expression of ALDH1A1 (possibly ALDH2 too) protein than less-differentiated cancer cells.

From the current findings, the mechanism and pathway which regulate the expression of ALDH1A1 mRNA and its protein as well as its enzymatic activity, and its role vary in different situations and among non-cancerous airway cells, NSCLCs and SCLCs, as well as among individual tumors. We speculate that ALDH1A1, its expression and/or activity, is only one of the factors determining the stemness in lung cancers.

In conclusion, the CSCs in SCLC and NSCLC differ distinctly from each other in terms not only of their abundance (suggested by CD133 mRNA levels) but also of the regulatory mechanism of ALDH1A1 expression and its activity, as well as its role in the maintenance/activation of stemness. The investigation of the mechanism of ALDH activation and its role in the maintenance of the stemness not only of CSCs but also of normal stem cells would provide a novel paradigm for stem cell biology and the development of a molecular targeting therapy for lung cancer.

11. Acknowledgments

This work was supported by the Japanese Ministry of Education, Culture, Sports, and Science (Tokyo Japan), Smoking Research Foundation (Tokyo, Japan), and by a grant from

Yokohama Medical Facility (Yokohama, Japan). We especially thank Hideaki Mitsui (Department of Pathology, Yokohama City University Graduate School of Medicine, Yokohama, Japan), Shigeko Iwanade (Division of Pathology, Kanagawa Prefectural Cardiovascular and Respiratory Center Hospital, Yokohama, Japan), and Tetsukan Woo (Department of General Thoracic Surgery, Kanagawa Prefectural Cardiovascular and Respiratory Center Hospital, Yokohama, Japan) for assistance.

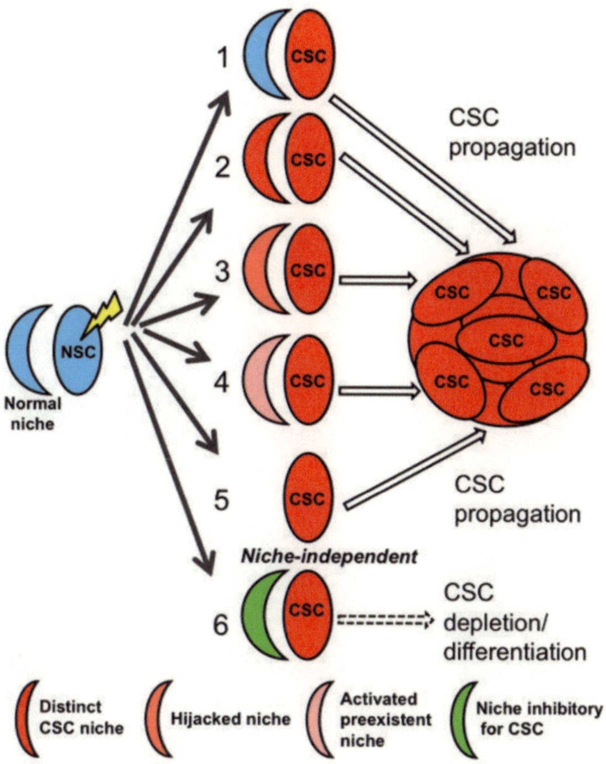

Fig. 1. Hypothesis for the relationship between cancer stem cells (CSCs) and their niche. At least one genetic or epigenetic event (yellow arrow) is required to occur in a normal stem cell (NSC; or progenitor cell, not shown here) for a CSC initiation to develop (closed arrows). The CSCs may utilize the normal niche (1), require the distinct CSC niche (2), instruct an otherwise quiescent niche to become activated by providing signals ("hijacking the niche") (3), amplify an already existent activated niche (4), or become niche-independent (5). Furthermore, there may be a discrete niche that is inhibitory for CSC maintenance (6). (Modified from [24]).

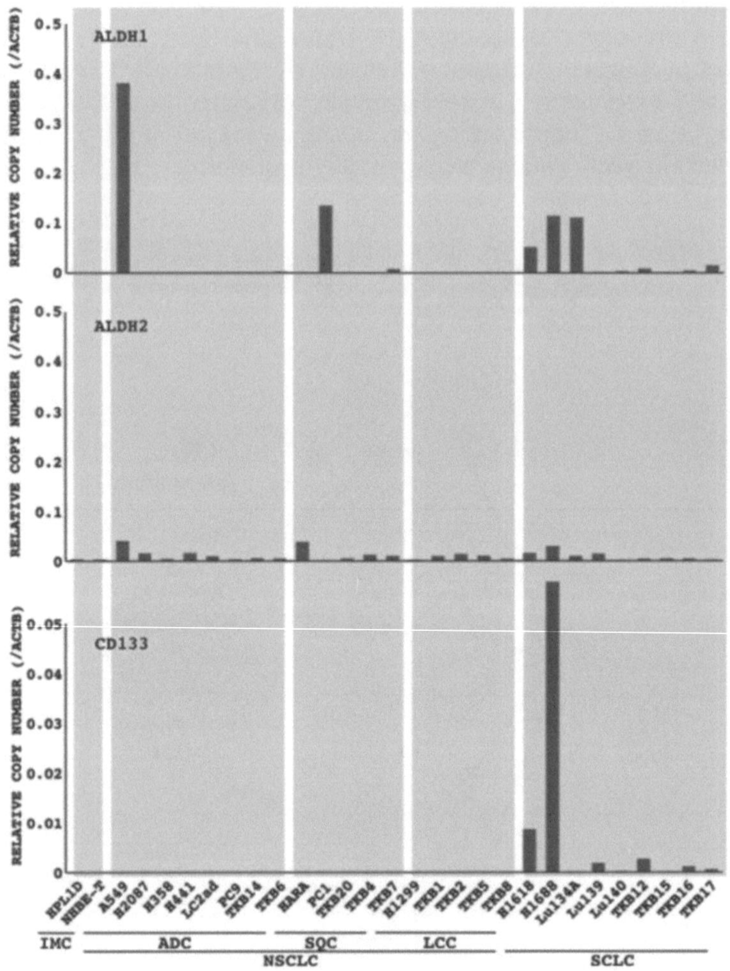

Fig. 2. Expression of ALDH1, ALDH2 and CD133 mRNA in immortalized human airway cell and lung cancer cell lines. Levels of mRNA of ALDH1, ALDH2 and CD133 and β-actin (ACTB) were measured by quantitative RT-PCR. The mRNA levels of ALDH1 (upper panel), ALDH2 (second panel) and CD133 (lower panel) relative to that of ACTB in immortalized human airway cells and lung cancer cells are presented. IMC, immortalized human airway cell lines; ADC, adenocarcinoma cell lines; SQC, squamous cell carcinoma cell lines; LCC, large cell carcinoma cell lines; NSCLC, non-small cell lung carcinoma cell lines; SCLC, small cell lung carcinoma cell lines. The experimental materials and methods are as follows. An immortalized human airway epithelial cell line (16HBE14o, Simian virus 40 (SV40)-transformed human bronchial epithelial cells) described by Cozens AL, *et al.* [102] was kindly provided by Gruenert DC (California Pacific Medical Center Research Institute, CA) via Kaneko T (Division of Respiratory Disease Center, Yokohama City Medical Center Hospital, Yokohama, Japan). A sub-clone of 16HBE14o cells, described as NHBE-T in this chapter, was used. An immortalized airway epithelial cell line (HPL1D, SV40-transformed human small airway epithelial cells) established by Masuda A, *et al.* [103], was provided by Takahashi T (Division of Molecular Carcinogenesis, Center for Neurological Disease and

Cancer, Nagoya University Graduate School of Medicine, Nagoya, Japan). Human lung cancer cell lines (A549, H358, H2087, H1618, H1688 and H1299) were purchased from American Type Culture Collection (ATCC, Manassas, VA). Human lung cancer cell lines, LC2/ad, Lu134A and Lu140 were obtained form Riken Cell Bank (Tsukuba, Japan), and PC9, PC1 and HARA from Immuno-Biological Laboratories Co. (Gunma, Japan). Human lung cancer cell lines, TKB1, TKB2, TKB4, TKB5, TKB6, TKB7, TKB8, TKB12, TKB15, TKB16, TKB17 and TKB20, were kindly provided by Kamma H (Department of Pathology, Kyorin University School of Medicine, Tokyo, Japan) via Yazawa T (Department of Pathology, Yokohama City University School of Medicine, Yokohama Japan). The cells were cultured and grown in DEMEM (Sigma Aldrich, St. Louis, MO) (NHBE-T, HPL1D, A549, H358, H2087, PC9, PC1, HARA, LC2/ad, TKB1, TKB2, TKB4, TKB5, TKB6, TKB7, TKB8, TKB20 and H1299) or RPMI1640 medium (Sigma) (H1618, H1688, Lu130, Lu134A, Lu140, TKB12, TKB15, TKB16 and TKB17) supplemented with 10% heat-inactivated fetal bovine serum (FBS) (Sigma), 100 units/ml of penicillin (Sigma), and 100 μg/ml of streptomycin (Sigma). Total RNA was extracted from the cells with Isogen reagents (NIPPON GENE, Tokyo, Japan). First-strand cDNA was synthesized from total RNA using the SuperScript First-Strand Synthesis System according to the protocols of the manufacturer (Invitrogen, Carlsbad, CA). The cDNA generated was used as a template in real-time PCR with SYBR Premix EXTaq (Takara, Kyoto, Japan). The primer set used for ALDH1A1 was forward (F), 5′- agtgcccctttggtggattc; reverse (R), 5′- aagagcttctctccactcttg. That for ALDH2 was, F, 5′- ctacacacgccatgaacctg; R, 5′- caaccacgtttccagttg. That for CD133 was, F, 5′- ttgtggcaaatcaccaggta; R, 5′- gatgttgggtctcagtcggt. That for ACTB was, F, 5′- tggcacccagcacaatgaa; R, 5′- ctaagtcatagtccgcctagaagca. The mean of the copy number of ALDH1A1, ALDH2 or CD133 normalized to the value for ACTB mRNA was obtained from triplicate reactions.

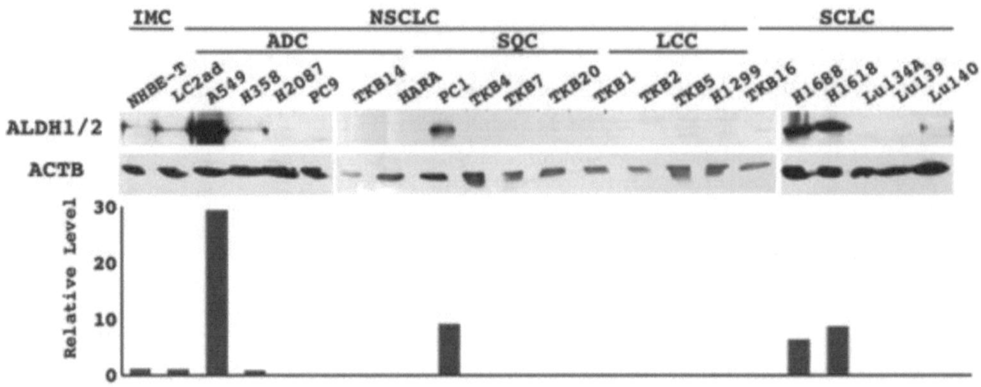

Fig. 3. Expression of ALDH1A1/ALDH2 (ALDH1/2) protein in lung cancer cell lines. ALDH1/2 (top panel) and β-actin (ACTB) (second panel) protein expressions were analyzed by Western blotting. Levels of ALDH1/2 and ACTB protein were semi-quantified with a densitometer (NIH Image; National Institute of Mental Health at Bethesda, MD). The level of ALDH1/2 normalized to that of ACTB is presented in a graph (third panel). IMC, immortalized human airway epithelial cell lines; ADC, adenocarcinoma cell lines; SQC, squamous cell carcinoma cell lines; LCC, large cell carcinoma cell lines; NSCLC, non-small cell lung carcinoma cell lines; SCLC, small cell lung carcinoma cell lines. The experimental materials and methods are as follows. The cell lines (the details of the experimental materials are described in the legend for Figure 2) grown to sub-confluence were solved with extraction buffer, as described elsewhere [104]. After centrifugation, supernatants were recovered as protein extracts. The extracts were mixed with equal volumes of 2×sample buffer [104], and then boiled. The samples were subjected to sodium dodecyl sulfate-polyacrylamide gel electrophoresis, and transferred onto PVDF membranes (Amersham, Arlington Heights, IL). The membranes were incubated with nonfat dry milk in 0.01 M Tris-buffered saline containing 0.1% Tween-20 (TBS-T) to block non-immunospecific protein binding, and then with 0.1 μg/ml of a primary antibody which non-selectively binds to both ALDH1A1 and ALDH2 (clone 44, BD Transduction, San Jones, CA) or a primary antibody against ACTB (Sigma). After washing with TBS-T, the membranes were incubated with animal-matched horseradish peroxidase-conjugated secondary antibodies (Amersham). Immunoreactivity was visualized with the enhanced chemiluminescence system (ECL, Amersham).

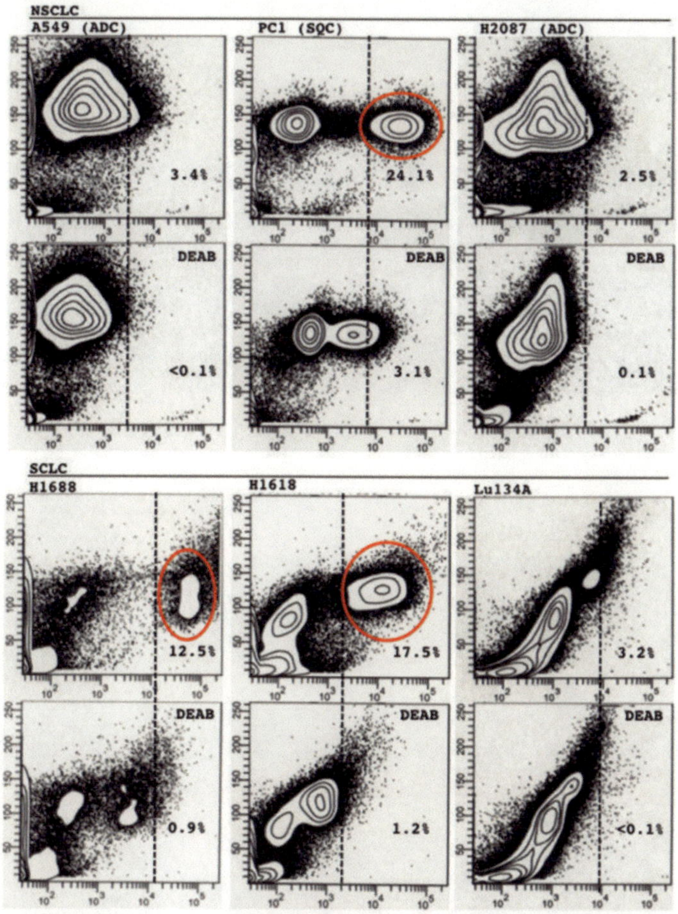

Fig. 4. Measurement of fraction of cells with ALDH activity (Aldefluor assay) in lung cancer cell lines. Cells were labeled with Aldefluor (BODIPY-aminoacetaldehyde [BAAA]) (Stem cell technology Inc., Vancouver, Canada) with or without the ALDH inhibitor diethylaminobenzaldehyde (DEAB) (Stem cell technology). The proportion of fraction of cells with ALDH activity was measured by flow cytometer. The X-axis is fluorescence intensity (log scale), and the Y-axis is forward scatter level (linear scale). The fraction of cells with strong ALDH activity is shown (red circle). NSCLC, non-small cell lung carcinoma cell lines; ADC, adenocarcinoma cell lines; SQC, squamous cell carcinoma cell lines; SCLC, small cell lung carcinoma cell lines. The experimental materials and methods are as follows. The details of the cell lines examined are described in the legend for Figure 1. Cells with ALDH activity was labeled using Aldefluor assay kit (Stem cell technology) according to the manufacturer's instructions. Briefly, 1.0×10^6 cells in 1 ml of Aldefluor assay buffer with BAAA at a concentration of 1.5 mM were incubated for 45 min at 37C. In each experiment, a sample of cells was treated under identical conditions with 50 mM of a specific ALDH inhibitor (DEAB) to serve as a negative control. The fraction of cells with ALDH activity labeled by Aldefluor was measured with a flow cytometer (BD Science, San Jose, CA) (excitation wave length 488 nm and emission wave length 525 nm (green fluorescence)). Data for 1.0×10^5 cells were collected.

A

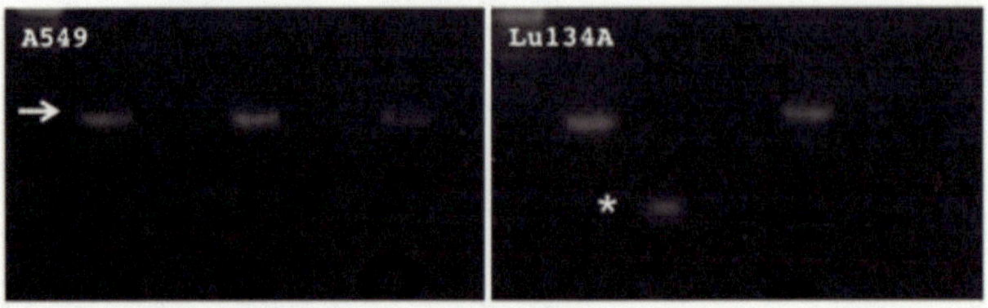

B

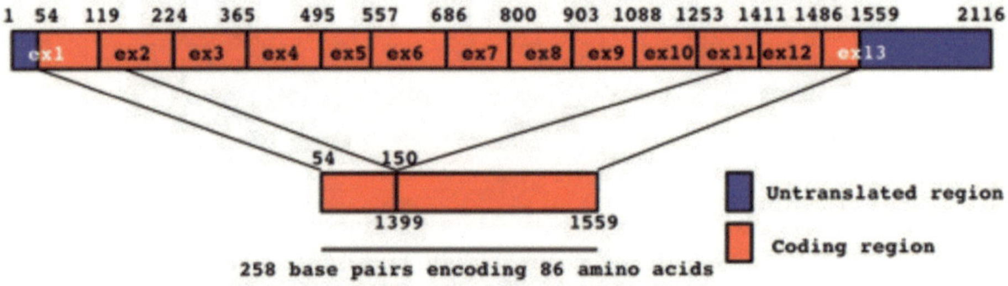

Fig. 5. Analysis of primary structure of mRNA of ALDH1A1. The protein-coding sequence in ALDH1A1 mRNA was amplified by RT-PCR using primers, forward, 5'-aggagccgaatcagaaatgtc; reverse, 5'-aagagcttctctccactcttg, according to the method descried in the legend for Figure 2. The PCR product was sub-cloned into the plasmid vector pT7Blue (Novagen, Darmstadt, Germany), and then its size was checked by PCR using universal primers (T7 promoter primer and M13M4 primer (Novagen)). (A) A representative result from A549 (ADC) and Lu134A (SCLC) cells is shown. Shorter PCR products (faster migrating band (asterisk)) were found in some sub-clones from Lu134A. Bands of expected size with a full-length coding region of ALDH1A1 (NCBI accession # NM_000689) are indicated with an arrow. (B) Schema of the primary structure of the consensus mRNA and the shorter variant with their mRNA spliced sites in the *ALDH1A1* gene, is shown. The shorter novel variant consists of parts of exon 1, exon2, exon 11, exon 12, and exon 13. "ex" in figure means exon.

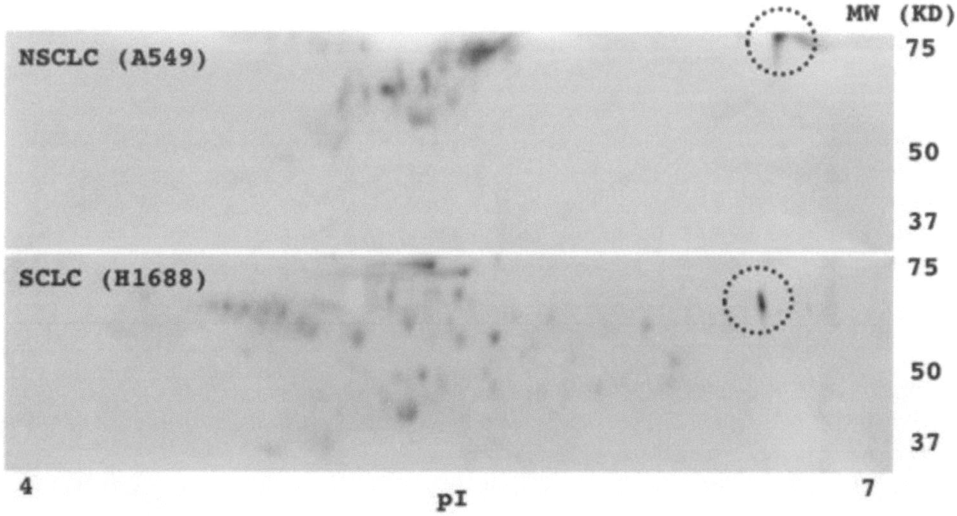

Fig. 6. Two-dimensional Western blotting analysis of ALDH1A1/ALDH2 (ALDH1/2) protein in a NSCLC cell line (top panel; A549) and SCLC cell line (Bottom panel; H1688). Spots of ALDH1/2 protein were circulated with dashed lines. MW, molecular weight; KD, kilo-dalton; pI, isoelectric point plugin. The experimental materials and methods are as follows. Two-dimensional electrophoresis (2-DE) was carried out using a horizontal electrophoresis system (Maltiphor II; Amersham) according to the manufacture's instruction. Briefly, equal amount of protein sample was subjected to the first-dimensional isoelectric focusing, and followed by the second dimensional sodium dodecyl sulfate-polyacrylamide gel electrophoresis. The details of method are described elsewhere [105,106]. The separated proteins on the 2-DE gels were transferred onto a polyvinylidene difluoride membrane (FluoroTrans® PVDF Membrane, Nippon Genetics, Tokyo, Japan). The membranes were incubated with nonfat dry milk in 0.01 M Tris-buffered saline containing 0.1% Tween-20 (TBS-T) to block non-immunospecific protein binding, and then with 0.1 μg/ml of a primary antibody, which non-selectively binds to both ALDH1A1 and ALDH2 (clone 44, BD Transduction). After washing with TBS-T, the membranes were incubated with animal-matched horseradish peroxidase-conjugated secondary antibodies (Amersham). Immunoreactivity was visualized with the enhanced chemiluminescence system (ECL, Amersham).

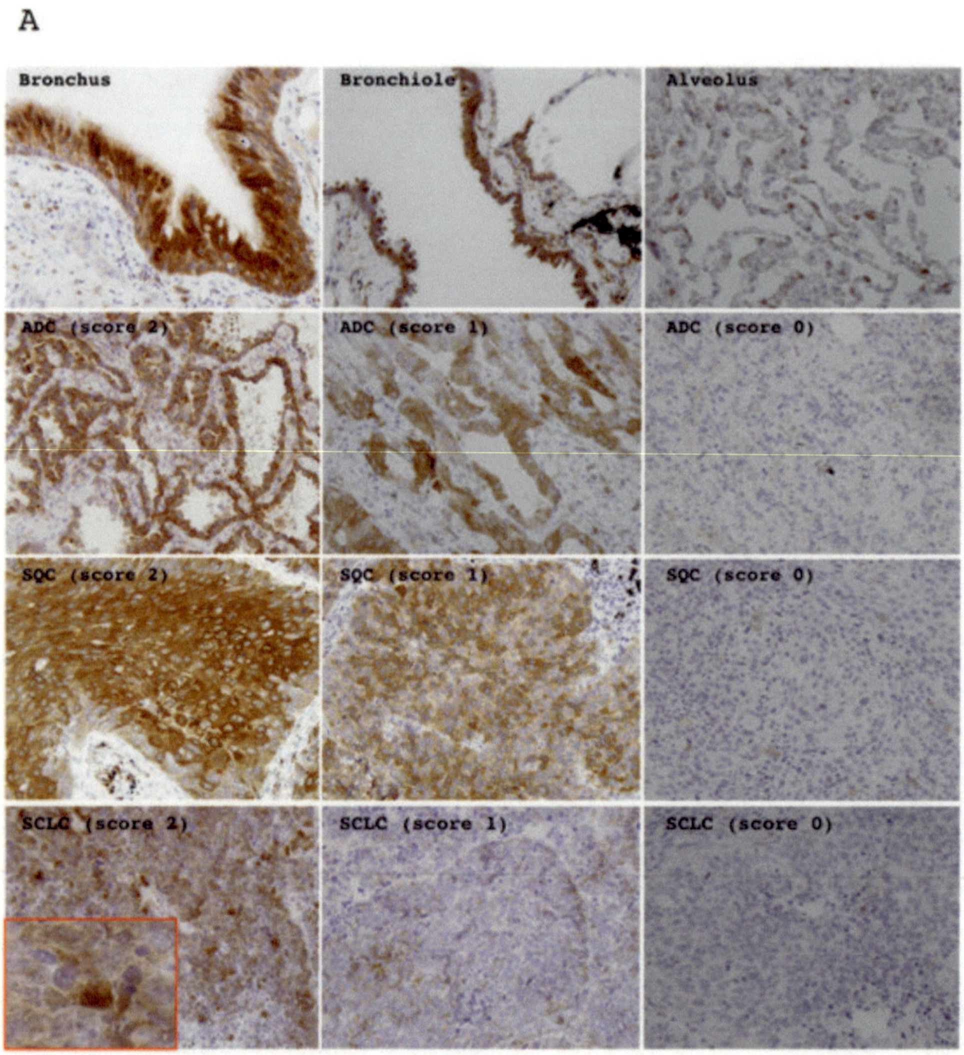
A
Bronchus
Bronchiole
Alveolus
ADC (score 2)
ADC (score 1)
ADC (score 0)
SQC (score 2)
SQC (score 1)
SQC (score 0)
SCLC (score 2)
SCLC (score 1)
SCLC (score 0)

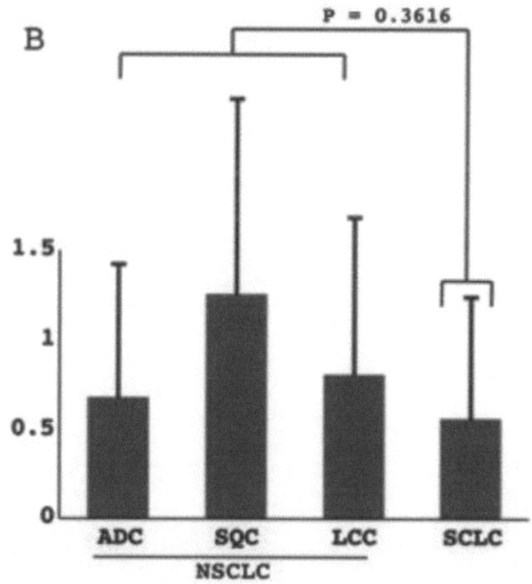

Fig. 7. Expression of ALDH1A1/ALDH2 (ALDH1/2) protein in non-cancerous airway epithelia and primary lung cancers. (A) Representative photographs of immunohistochemistry of surgical specimens of non-cancerous airway epithelia (top panels) and lung cancers (the other panels) are shown. Magnifications are ×200 in, non-cancerous airway epithelia (bronchus, bronchiole and alveolus), adenocarcinoma (ADC), squamous cell carcinoma (SQC) and small cell lung carcinoma (SCLC), and ×400 in the inset of SCLC. Levels of ALDH1/2 expression were evaluated according to a scoring system; negative (score 0), unequivocally strong (score 2), and positive but weaker than a score of 2 (score 1). (B) Seventy-nine tumors (49 ADCs, 16 SQCs, 5 large cell carcinomas, and 9 SCLCs) were examined. The mean and standard deviation (error bar) among each histological type are shown in graph. Differences were analyzed with Student's t-test, and P value is indicated. The experimental materials and methods are as follows. All cases examined were of lung cancer patients who underwent surgical resection at the Kanagawa Prefectural Cardiovascular and Respiratory Disease Center Hospital (Yokohama, Japan) between 2001 and 2008. Informed consent for research use was obtained from all the subjects providing materials. Tissue sections (4 μm thick), cut from the formalin-fixed and paraffin-embedded tissue block with largest tumor dimension, were deparaffinized and rehydrated, and incubated with 3% hydrogen peroxide to block endogenous peroxidase activities. The sections were incubated with 5% goat serum to block non-immunospecific protein binding. After antigen retrieval treatment, boiling in citrated buffer (0.01 M, pH6.0) to restore the masked epitope, the sections were incubated with a primary antibody, which non-selectively binds to both ALDH1A1 and ALDH2 (clone 44, BD Transduction). Immunoreactivity was visualized with an Envision detection system (DAKOcytomation, Carpinteria, CA), and the nuclei were counterstained with hematoxylin.

Category	Molecule	SCLC	NSCLC
Cell surface marker	CD133	1. Eramo A, *et al.* [42] Cancer cells isolated from surgical specimens 2. Jiang T, *et al.* [52] H1688 cell line 3. Meng X, *et al.* [48] *H446 cell line	1. Eramo A, *et al.* [42] Cancer cells isolated from surgical specimens 2. Jiang T, *et al.* [52] H460, H125, H322, and H358 cell lines 3. Levina V, *et al.* [50] H460 cell line 4. Chen YC, *et al.* [51] Cancer cells isolated from surgical specimens 5. Meng X, *et al.* [48] *A549 cell line
	PODXL-1	1. Koch LK, *et al.* [69] Immunohistochemical analysis in surgical specimen tissue sections	
	uPAR	1. Gutova M, *et al.* [54] H1417, H69AR, H211, H1688, H1882, and H250 cell lines	
Transporter	SP	1. Meng X, *et al.* [48] *H446 cell line	1. Ho MM, *et al.* [48] A549, H23, H460, HTB-58, H2170, and H441 cell lines 2. Meng X, *et al.* [48] *A549 cell line
	ABCG2		1. Sung JM, *et al.* [25] A549 cell line
Enzymatic activity	ALDH	1. Jiang T, *et al.* [52] Aldefluor assay in H1618 cell line 2. Moreb JS, *et al.* [93] RT-PCR, Western blotting, spectrophotometrical analysis and Aldefluor assay in SW210.5, H82, and SCLC-16HC cell lines	1. Ucar D, *et al.* [95] Spectrophotometrical analysis and Aldefluor assay in H522 cell line 2. Patel M, *et al.* [96]. Immunohistochemical analysis in surgical specimen tissue sections 3. Jiang F, *et al.* [49] Aldefluor assay in H460, H125, H322, and H358 cell lines 4. Moreb JS, *et al.* [93] RT-PCR, Western blotting, spectrophotometrical analysis and Aldefluor assay in A549, H522, H322, H157, H125, H460, H1299, LCLC-103H and ADLC-5M2H lung cancer cell lines, as well as Beas-2B non-cancerous airway cell line
Signaling pathway	Shh	1. Watkins DN, *et al.* [77] NCI-H1618, NCI-H60, NCI-H146, NCI-H209, NCI-H249, NCI-H82, and NCI-H417 cell lines 2. Yagui-Beltrán A, *et al.* [78] Review 3. Peacock CD, *et al.* [79] Review	1. Yagui-Beltrán A, *et al.* [78] Review 2. Peacock CD, *et al.* [79] Review
	Wnt/ β -catenin	1. Yagui-Beltrán A, *et al.* [78] Review 2. Peacock CD, *et al.* [79] Review	1. Yagui-Beltrán A, *et al.* [78] Review 2. Peacock CD, *et al.* [79] Review 3. Levina V, *et al.* [50] H460 cell line
Transcription factor	Bmi1	1. Koch LK, *et al.* [69] Immunohistochemical analysis in surgical specimen tissue sections	1. Dovey JS, *et al.* [85] Bronchioloalveolar carcinoma (mouse)
	4.Oct		1. Levina V, *et al.* [50] H460 cell line 2. Chen YC, *et al.* [51] Cancer cells isolated from surgical specimens

SCLC: small cell lung carcinoma; NSCLC: non-small cell lung carcinoma; PODXL-1: podocalyxin-like protein 1; uPAR: urokinase plasminogen activator receptor;

SP: side population; ABCG2: ATP binding cassette transporter superfamily member G2; ALDH: aldehyde dehydrogenase; Shh: Sonic hedgehog; Bmi1: B cell-specific Mo-MuLV integration site 1.
*These authors reported that both of CD133+ and CD133- cells and of SP cells and non-SP cells exhibited the cancer initiating activity.
The methods for analysis of ALDH activity and protein expression are specifically described, because the procedures employed may potentially lead to the differences in results.

Table 1. Cancer stem cell markers in small cell lung carcinoma amd non-small cell lung carcinoma

	NSCLC			SCLC
No. of cases analyzed	ADC [49]	SQC [16]	LCC [5]	[9]
Positive rate % [No.]	51.0% [25]	87.5% [14]	40.0% [2]	33.3% [3]

NSCLC, non-small cell lung carcinoma; SCLC, small cell lung carcinoma; ADC, adenocarcinoma;

SQC, squamous cell carcinoma; LCC, large cell carcinoma;

Chi-square test (among all, P = 0.0254; NSCLC versus SCLC, P = 0.154)

Immunohistochemical analysis was performed in formalin-fixed tumor sections using a primary antibody against

ALDH (BD transduction, Palo Alto, CA). Immunoreactivity was visualized with an Envision detection system (DAKO).

If 5% or more of neoplastic cells in a tumor showed immunohistochemical expression of ALDH, it was judged as positive.

Table 2. Positive rate of immunohistochemical ALDH1/2 expression among NSCLC and SCLC

Abbreviations

SCLC: small cell lung carcinoma; NSCLC: non-small cell lung carcinoma; SQC: squamous cell carcinoma; ADC: adenocarcinoma; LCC: large cell carcinoma; RB: retinoblastoma; TP53: tumor protein 53; EGFR: epidermal growth factor receptor; ASCL1: achaete-scute complex homolog 1; TTF-1: thyroid transcription factor-1; ALDH: aldehyde dehydrogenase; CSC: cancer stem cell; ABCG2, ATP binding cassette transporter superfamily member G2; CIC: cancer initiating cell; SP: side population; FACS: fluorescence activating cell sorting; UV: ultraviolet; uPAR: urokinase plasminogen activator receptor; uPA: urokinase plasminogen activator; Shh: Sonic hedgehog; BMP: bone morphogenetic protein; Bmi1: B cell-specific Mo-MuLV integration site 1; PODXL-1: podocalyxin-like protein 1; RT-PCR: reverse transcription polymerase chain reaction; mRNA, messenger ribonucleic acid: cDNA; complementary deoxyribonucleic acid; siRNA: small interfering RNA; PI: propidium iodide.

12. References

[1] Parkin, M., Tyczynski, JE., Boffetta, P., Samet, J., Shields, P., Caporaso, N. Lung cancer epidemiology and etiology. In: Travis, W.D., Brambilla, E., Muller-Hermelink, H.K., Harris, C.C. (eds). *Tumours of the lung. Tumours of the lung, pleura, thymus and heart. World Health Organization Classification of Tumours. Pathology & Genetics.* Lyon, IARC Press 2004; 12-15.

[2] Travis, W.D., Brambilla, E., Muller-Hermelink, H.K., Harris, C.C. (eds). IARC Press: Lyon, 2004; 9-124. Working group that convened for an editorial and consensus conference in Lyon, France, March 12-16, 2003. Tumours of the Lung. In: *World Health Organization Classification of Tumours. Pathology and Genetics of Tumours of the Lung, Pleura, Thymus and Heart.*

[3] Otto, W.R. (2002) Lung epithelial stem cells. *J Pathol, 197*, 527-535.

[4] Giangreco, A., Groot, K.R., Janes, S.M. (2007) Lung cancer and lung stem cells: strange bedfellows? *Am J Respir Crit Care Med, 175*, 547-553.

[5] Giangreco, A., Arwert, E.N., Rosewell, I.R., Snyder, J., Watt, F.M., Stripp, B.R. (2009) Stem cells are dispensable for lung homeostasis but restore airways after injury. *Proc Natl Acad Sci USA, 106,* 9286-9291.
[6] Blanpain, C., Horsley, V., Fuchs, E. Epithelial stem cells: turning over new leaves. (2007) *Cell, 128,* 445-458.
[7] Kitamura, H., Yazawa, T., Shimoyamada, H., Okudela, K., Sato, H. (2008) Molecular and genetic pathogenesis of lung cancer: differences between small-cell and non-small-cell carcinomas. *Open Pathol J, 2,* 106-114. Doi:10.2174/1874375700802010106
[8] Kitamura, H., Yazawa, T., Sato, H., Okudela, K., Shimoyamada, H. (2009) Small cell lung cancer: significance of RB alterations and TTF-1 expression in its carcinogenesis, phenotype, and biology. *Endcr Pathol, 20,* 101-107.
[9] Nuciforo, P., Fraggetta, F. (2004) Cancer stem cell theory: pathologists' considerations and ruminations about wasting time and wrong evaluations. *J Clin Patho1, 7,* 782-783.
[10] Clarke, M.F., Dick, J.E., Dirks, P.B., Eaves, C.J., Jamieson, C.H., Jones, D.L. (2006) Cancer stem cells--perspectives on current status and future directions: AACR Workshop on cancer stem cells. *Cancer Res, 66,* 9339-9344.
[11] Lobo, N.A., Shimono, Y., Qian, D., Clarke, M.F. (2007) The biology of cancer stem cells. *Annu Rev Cell Dev Biol, 23,* 675-699.
[12] Rapp, U.R., Ceteci, F., Schreck, R. (2008) Oncogene-induced plasticity and cancer stem cells. *Cell Cycle, 7,* 45-51.
[13] Kim, C.F., Dirks, P.B. (2008) Cancer and stem cell biology: how tightly intertwined? *Cell Stem Cell, 3,* 147-150.
[14] Yang, Y.M., Chang, J.W. (2008) Current status and issues in cancer stem cell study. *Cancer Invest, 26,* 741-755.
[15] Li, X., Lewis, M.T., Huang, J., Gutierrez, C., Osborne, C.K., Wu, M.F. (2008) Intrinsic resistance of tumorigenic breast cancer cells to chemotherapy. *J Natl Cancer Inst, 100,* 672-679.
[16] Li, L., Borodyansky, L., Yang, Y. (2009) Genomic instability en route to and from cancer stem cells. *Cell Cycle, 8,* 1000-1002.
[17] Hill, R.P. (2006) Identifying cancer stem cells in solid tumors: case not proven. *Cancer Res, 66,* 1883-1890.
[18] Kelly, P.N., Dakic, A., Adams, J.M., Nutt, S.L., Strasser, A. (2007) Tumor growth need not be driven by rare cancer stem cells. *Science, 317,* 337.
[19] Lewis, M.T. (2008) Faith, heresy and the cancer stem cell hypothesis. *Future Oncol, 4,* 585-589.
[20] Yoo, M.H., Hatfield, D.L. (2008) The cancer stem cell theory: is it correct? *Mol Cells, 26,* 514-516.
[21] Vezzoni, L., Parmiani, G. (2008) Limitations of the cancer stem cell theory. *Cytotechnology, 58,* 3-9.
[22] Rowan, K. (2009) Are cancer stem cells real? After four decades, debate still simmers. *J Natl Cancer Inst, 101,* 546-547.
[23] Sneddon, J.B., Werb, Z. (2007) Location, location, location: the cancer stem cell niche. *Cell Stem Cell, 1,* 607-611.

[24] Kitamura, H., Okudela, K., Yazawa, T., Sato, H., Shimoyamada, H. (2009) Cancer stem cell: implications in cancer biology and therapy with special reference to lung cancer. *Lung Cancer, 66,* 275-281.

[25] Sung, J.M., Cho, H.J., Yi, H., Lee, C.H., Kim, H.S., Kim, D.K. (2008) Characterization of a stem cell population in lung cancer A549 cells. *Biochem Biophys Res Commun, 371,* 163-167.

[26] Feldmann, G., Dhara, S., Fendrich, V., Bedja, D., Beaty, R., Mullendore, M., Karikari, C., Alvarez, H., Iacobuzio-Donahue, C., Jimeno, A., Gabrielson, K.L., Matsui, W., Maitra, A. (2007) Blockade of hedgehog signaling pancreatic cancer invasion and metastases: a new paradigm for combination therapy in solid cancers. *Cancer Res, 67,* 2187-96.

[27] Besson, A., Hwang, H.C., Cicero, S., Donovan, S.L., Gurian-West, M., Johnson, D. (2007) Discovery of an oncogenic activity in p27Kip1 that causes stem cell expansion and a multiple tumor phenotype. *Genes Dev, 21,* 1731-1746.

[28] Yin, A.H., Miraglia, S., Zanjani, E.D., Almeida-Porada, G., Ogawa, M., Leary, A.G., et *al.* (1997) AC133, a novel marker for human hematopoietic stem and progenitor cells. *Blood, 90,* 5002-5012.

[29] Wuchter, C., Ratei, R., Spahn, G., Schoch, C., Harbott, J., Schnittger, S., *et al.* (2001) Impact of CD133 (AC133) and CD90 expression analysis for acute leukemia immunophenotyping. *Haematologica, 86,* 154-161.

[30] Shmelkov, S.V., St. Clair, R., Lyden, D., Rafii, S. (2005) AC133/CD133/Prominin-1. *Int J Biochem Cell Biol, 37,* 715-719.

[31] Uchida, N., Buck, D.W., He, D., Reitsma, M.J., Masek, M., Phan, T.V., *et al.* (2000) Direct isolation of human central nervous system stem cells. *Proc Natl Acad Sci USA, 97,* 14720-14725.

[32] Pötgens, A.J., Bolte, M., Huppertz, B., Kaufmann, P., Frank, H.G. (2001) Human trophoblast contains an intracellular protein reactive with an antibody against CD133--a novel marker for trophoblast. *Placenta, 22,* 39-645.

[33] Salven, P., Mustjoki, S., Alitalo, R., Alitalo, K., Rafii, S. (2003) VEGFR-3 and CD133 identify a population of CD34+ lymphatic/vascular endothelial precursor cells. *Blood, 101,* 168-172.

[34] Richardson, G.D., Robson, C.N., Lang, S.H., Neal, D.E., Maitland, N.J., Collins, A.T. (2004) CD133, a novel marker for human prostatic epithelial stem cells. *Cell Science, 117 pt16,* 3539-3545.

[35] Piechaczek, C. (2001) CD133. *J Biol Regul Homeost Agents, 15,* 101-102.

[36] Yu, Y., Flint, A., Dvorin, E.L., Bischoff, J. (2002) AC133-2, a novel isoform of human AC133 stem cell antigen. *J Biol Chem, 277,* 20711-20716.

[37] Marzesco, A.M., Janich, P., Wilsch-Bräuninger, M., Dubreuil, V., Langenfeld, K., Corbeil, D., *et al.* Release of extracellular membrane particles carrying the stem cell marker prominin-1 (CD133) from neural progenitors and other epithelial cells *J Cell Science, 118 pt13,* 2849-2858.

[38] Taïeb, N., Maresca, M., Guo, X.J., Garmy, N., Fantini, J., Yahi, N. (2009) The first extracellular domain of the tumour stem cell marker CD133 contains an antigenic ganglioside-binding motif. *Cancer Lett, 278,* 164-173.

[39] Choi, D., Lee, H.W., Hur, K.Y., Kim, J.J., Park, G.S., Jang, S.H., et al. Cancer stem cell markers CD133 and CD24 correlate with invasiveness and differentiation in colorectal adenocarcinoma. *World J Gastroenterol, 15,* 2258-2264.

[40] Ahn, S.M., Goode, R.J., Simpson, R.J. (2008) Stem cell markers: insights from membrane proteomics? *Proteomics, 8,* 4946-4957.

[41] Klonisch, T., Wiechec, E., Hombach-Klonisch, S., Ande, S.R., Wesselborg, S., Schulze-Osthoff, K., *et al.* Cancer stem cell markers in common cancers - therapeutic implications. *Trends Mol Med, 14,* 450-460.

[42] Eramo, A., Lotti, F., Sette, G., Pilozzi, E., Biffoni, M., Di Virgilio. A., *et al.* (2008), Identification and expansion of the tumorigenic lung cancer stem cell population. *Cell Death Differ, 15,* 504-514.

[43] Wang, J., Sakariassen, P.Ø., Tsinkalovsky, O., Immervoll, H., Bøe, S.O., Svendsen, A., *et al.* (2008) CD133 negative glioma cells form tumors in nude rats and give rise to CD133 positive cells. *Int J Cancer, 122,* 761-768.

[44] Ogden, A.T., Waziri, A.E., Lochhead, R.A., Fusco, D., Lopez, K., Ellis, J.A., *et al.* (2008) Identification of A2B5+CD133- tumor-initiating cells in adult human gliomas. *Neurosurgery, 60,* 505-514.

[45] Shmelkov, S.V., Butler, J.M., Hooper, A.T., Hormigo, A., Kushner, J., Milde, T., *et al.* (2008) CD133 expression is not restricted to stem cells, and both CD133+ and CD133- metastatic colon cancer cells initiate tumors. *J Clin Invest, 188,* 2111-2120.

[46] Mizrak, D., Brittan, M., Alison, M.R. CD133: molecule of the moment. *J Pathol, 214,* 3-9.

[47] Bidlingmaier, S., Zhu, X., Liu, B. (2008) The utility and limitations of glycosylated human CD133 epitopes in defining cancer stem cells. *J Mol Med, 86,* 1025-1032.

[48] Meng, X., Wang, X., Wang, Y. (2009) More than 45% of A549 and H446 cells are cancer initiating cells: evidence from cloning and tumorigenic analyses. *Oncol Rep, 12,* 995-1000.

[49] Jiang, F., Qiu, Q., Khanna, A., Todd, N.W., Deepak, J., Xing, L, *et al.* (2009) Aldehyde dehydrogenase 1 is a tumor stem cell-associated marker in lung cancer. *Mol Cancer Res, 7,* 330-338

[50] Levina, V., Marrangoni, A.M., DeMarco, R., Gorelik, E., Lokshin, A.E. (2008) Drug-selected human lung cancer stem cells: cytokine network, tumorigenic and metastatic properties. *PLoS ONE, 2,* e3077.

[51] Chen, Y.C., Hsu, H.S., Chen, Y.W., Tsai, T.H., How, C.K., Wang, C.Y., *et al.* (2008) Oct-4 expression maintained cancer stem-like properties in lung cancer-derived CD133-positive cells. *PLoS ONE, 3,* e2637.

[52] Jiang, T., Collins, B.J., Jin, N., Watkins, D.N., Brock, M.V., Matsui, W., *et al.* (2009) Achaete-scute complex homologue 1 regulates tumor-initiating capacity in human small cell lung cancer. *Cancer Res, 69,* 845-854.

[53] Ito, T., Udaka, N., Okudela, K., Yazawa, T., Kitamura, H. (2003) Mechanisms of neuroendocrine differentiation in pulmonary neuroendocrine cells and small cell carcinoma. *Endocr Pathol, 14,* 133-139.

[54] Goodell, M.A., Brose, K., Paradis, G., Conner, A.S., Mulligan, R.C. (1996) Isolation and functional properties of murine hematopoietic stem cells that are replicating in vivo. *J Exp Med, 183,* 1797-1806.

[55] Wu, C., Alman, B.A. Side population cells in human cancers. *Cancer Lett, 268,* 1-9.

[56] Hirschmann-Jax, C., Foster, A.E., Wulf, G.G., Nuchtern, J.G., Jax, T.W., Gobel, U., *et al.* (2004) A distinct "side population" of cells with high drug efflux capacity in human tumor cells. *Proc Natl Acad Sci USA, 101,* 14228-14233.

[57] Hirschmann-Jax, C., Foster, A.E., Wulf, G.G., Goodell, M.A., Brenner, M.K. (2005) A distinct "side population" of cells in human tumor cells: implications for tumor biology and therapy. *Cell Cycle*, 4, 203-205

[58] Zhou, S., Schuetz, J.D., Bunting, K.D., Colapietro, A.M., Sampath, J., Morris, J.J., *et al.* (2001) The ATP binding cassette transporter Bcrp1/ABCG2 is expressed in a wide variety of stem cells and is a molecular determinant of the side-population phenotype. *Nat Med, 7,* 1028-1034.

[59] Telford, W.G., Bradford, J., Godfrey, W., Robey, R.W., Bates, S.E. (2007) Side population analysis using a violet-excited cell-permeable DNA dye. *Stem Cells, 25,* 1029-1036.

[60] Ho MM, Ng AV, Lam S, Hung JY. Side population in human lung cancer cell lines and tumors is enriched with stem-like cancer cells. *Cancer Res* 2007; 67:4827-4833.

[61] Sophos, N.A., Vasiliou, V. (2003) Aldehyde dehydrogenase gene superfamily: the 2009 update. *Chem Biol Interact, 143-144, 5-22.*

[62] Huang, E.H., Hynes, M.J., Zhang, T., Ginestier, C., Dontu, G., Appelman, H., *et al.* (2009) Aldehyde dehydrogenase 1 is a marker for normal and malignant human colonic stem cells (SC) and tracks SC overpopulation during colon tumorigenesis. *Cancer Res, 69,* 3382-3389.

[63] Jones, R.J., Barber, J.P., Vala, M.S., Collector, M.I., Kaufmann, S.H., Ludeman, S.M., *et al.* (1995) Assessment of aldehyde dehydrogenase in viable cells. *Blood, 85,* 2742-2746.

[64] Armstrong, L., Stojkovic, M., Dimmick, I., Ahmad, S., Stojkovic, P., Hole, N., *et al.* (2004) Phenotypic characterization of murine primitive hematopoietic progenitor cells isolated on basis of aldehyde dehydroganse activity. *Stem Cells, 22,* 1142-1151.

[65] Corti, S., Locatelli, F., Papadimitriou, D., Donadoni, C., Salani, S., Del Bo, R., *et al.* (2006) Identification of a primitive brain-derived neural stem cell population based on aldehyde dehydrogenase activity. *Stem Cells, 24,* 975-985.

[66] Ginestier, C., Hur, M.H., Charafe-Jauffret, E., Monville, F., Dutcher, J., Brown, M., et *al.* (2007) ALDH1 is a marker of normal and malignant human mammary stem cells and a predictor of poor clinical outcome. *Cell Stem Cell, 1,* 555-567.

[67] Dylla, S.J., Beviglia, L., Park, I.K., Chartier, C., Raval, J., Ngan, L., *et al.* (2008) Colorectal cancer stem cells are enriched in xenogeneic tumors following chemotherapy. *PLoS ONE, 3,* e2428.

[68] Storms, R.W., Trujillo, A.P., Springer, J.B., Shah, L., Colvin, O.M., Ludeman, S.M., *et al.* (1999) Isolation of primitive human hematopoietic progenitors on the basis of aldehyde dehydrogenase activity. *Proc Natl Acad Sci USA, 96,* 9118-9123.

[69] Koch, L.K., Zhou, H., Ellinger, J., Biermann, K., Höller, T., von Rücker, A., *et al.* (2008) Stem cell marker expression in small cell lung carcinoma and developing lung tissue. *Hum Pathol, 39,* 1597-1605.

[70] Lanza, F., Healy, L., Sutherland, D.R. Structural and functional features of the CD34 antigen: an update. *J Biol Regul Homeost Agents, 15,* 1-13.

[71] Nielsen, J.S., McNagny, K.M. (2008) Novel functions of the CD34 family. *J Cell Sci, 121pt22,* 3683-92.

[72] Doyonnas, R., Nielsen, J.S., Chelliah, S., Drew, E., Hara, T., Miyajima, A., McNagny, K.M. (2005) *Blood, 105,* 4170-4178.

[73] Gutova, M., Najbauer, J., Gevorgyan, A., Metz, M.Z., Weng, Y., Shih, C.C., *et al.* (2007) Identification of uPAR-positive chemoresistant cells in small cell lung cancer. *PLoS ONE, 2,* e243.

[74] Alfano, D., Franco, P., Vocca, I., Gambi, N., Pisa, V., Mancini, A., Caputi, M., Carriero, M.V., Iaccarino, I., Stoppelli, M.P. (2009) The urokinase plasminogen activator and its receptor: role in cell growth and apoptosis. *Thromb Haemost, 93,* 205-211.

[75] Van der Flier, L.G., Clevers, H. (2009) Stem cells, self-renewal, and differentiation in the intestinal epithelium. *Annu Rev Physiol, 71,* 5.1-5.20.

[76] Liao, X., Siu, M.K., Au, C.W., Chan, Q.K., Chan, H.Y., Wong, E.S., et al. (2009) Aberrant activation of hedgehog signaling pathway contributes to endometrial carcinogenesis through β-catenin. *Mod Pathol, 22,* 839-847.

[77] Watkins, D.N., Berman, D.M., Burkholder, S.G., Wang, B., Beachy, P.A., Baylin, S.B. (2003) Hedgehog signalling within airway epithelial progenitors and in small-cell lung cancer. *Nature, 422,* 313-317.

[78] Yagui-Beltrán, A., He, B., Jablons, D.M. (2008) The role of cancer stem cells in neoplasia of the lung: past, present and future. *Clin Transl Oncol, 10,* 719-725.

[79] Peacock, C.D., Watkins, D.N. (2008) Cancer stem cells and the ontogeny of lung cancer. *J Clin Oncol, 26,* 2883-2889.

[80] Lemjabbar-Alaoui, H., Dasari, V., Sidhu, S.S., Mengistab, A., Finkbeiner, W., Gallup, M., *et al.* (2006) Wnt and Hedgehog are critical mediators of cigarette smoke-induced lung cancer. *PLoS ONE, 1,* e93.

[81] Alison, M.R., Islam, S. (2009) Attributes of adult stem cells. *J Pathol, 217,* 144-160.

[82] Polakis, P. (2000) Wnt signaling and cancer. *Genes Dev, 14,* 1837-1851.

[83] Reya, T., Clevers, H. (2005) Wnt signalling in stem cells and cancer. *Nature, 434,* 843-850.

[84] Valk-Lingbeek, M.E., Bruggenman, S.W.M., van Lohuizen, M. (2004) Stem cell and cancer: poly-comb connection. *Cell, 118,* 409-418.

[85] Dovey, J.S., Zacharek, S.J., Kim, C.F., Lees, J.A. (2008) Bmi1 is critical for lung tumorigenesis and bronchioalveolar stem cell expansion. *Proc Natl Acad Sci USA. 105,* 11857-11862.

[86] Ovitt, C.E., Schöler, H.R. (1998) The molecular biology of Oct-4 in the early mouse embryo. *Mol Hum Reprod, 4,* 1021-1031.

[87] Basak, S.K., Veena, M.S., Oh, S., Huang, G., Srivatsan, E., Huang, M., Sharma, S., Batra, R.K. (2009) The malignant pleural effusion as a model to investigate intratumoral heterogeneity in lung cancer. *PLoS One, 4,* e5884.

[88] Collins, A.T., Berry, P.A., Hyde, C., Stower, M.J., Maitland, N.J. (2005) Prospective identification of tumorigenic prostate cancer stem cells. *Cancer Res, 65,* 10946-10951.

[89] Annabi, B., Lachambre, M.P., Plouffe, K., Sartelet, H., Béliveau, R. (2009) Modulation of invasive properties of CD133(+) glioblastoma stem cells: a role for MT1-MMP in bioactive lysophospholipid signaling. *Mol Carcinog, 48,* 910-919.

[90] Li, L., Neaves, W.B. (2006) Normal stem cells and cancer stem cells: the niche matters. *Cancer Res, 66,* 4553-4557.

[91] Hilbe, W., Dirnhofer, S., Oberwasserlechner, F., Schmid, T., Gunsilius, E., Hilbe, G., *et al.* (2004) CD133 positive endothelial progenitor cells contribute to the tumour vasculature in non-small cell lung cancer. *J Clin Pathol, 57,* 965-969.

[92] Moreb, J.S., Baker, H.V., Chang, L.J., Amaya, M., Lopez, M.C., Ostmark, B., Chou, W. (2008) ALDH isozymes downregulation affects cell growth, cell motility and gene expression in lung cancer cells. *Mol Cancer, 7,* 87.

[93] Moreb, J.S., Zucali, J.R., Ostmark, B., Benson, N.A. (2007) Heterogeneity of aldehyde dehydrogenase expression in lung cancer cell lines is revealed by Aldefluor flow cytometry-based assay. *Cytometry B Clin Cytom, 72,* 281-9.

[94] Moreb, J.S. (2008) Aldehyde dehydrogenase as a marker for stem cells. *Curr Stem Cell Res Ther, 3,* 237-46.

[95] Ucar, D., Cogle, C.R., Zucali, J.R., Ostmark, B., Scott, E.W., Zori, R., *et al.* (2009) Aldehyde dehydrogenase activity as a functional marker for lung cancer. *Chem Biol Interact, 178,* 48-55.

[96] Patel, M., Lu, L., Zander, D.S., Sreerama, L., Coco, D., Moreb, J.S. (2008) ALDH1A1 and ALDH3A1 expression in lung cancers: correlation with histologic type and potential precursors. *Lung Cancer, 59,* 340-349.

[97] Carpentino, J.E., Hynes, M.J., Appelman, H.D., Zheng, T., Steindler, D.A., Scott, E.W., Huang, E.H. (2008) Aldehyde dehydrogenase-expressing colon stem cells contribute to tumorigenesis in the transition from colitis to cancer. *Cancer Res, 69,* 8208-8215.

[98] Christ, O., Lucke, K., Imren, S., Leung, K., Hamilton, M., Eaves, A., Smith, C., Eaves, C. (2007) Improved purification of hematopoietic stem cells based on their elevated aldehyde dehydrogenase activity. *Haematologica, 92,* 1165-1172.

[99] Sisson, J.H. (2007) Alcohol and airways function in health and disease. *Alcohol, 41,* 293-307.

[100] Moriwaki, Y., Yamamoto, T., Higashino, K. (1997) Distribution and pathophysiologic role of molybdenum-containing enzymes. *Histol Histopathol, 12,* 513-524.

[101] Yin SJ. Alcohol dehydrogenase: enzymology and metabolism. Alcohol Alcohol Suppl. 1994;2:113-9.

[102] Cozens, A.L., Yezzi, M.J., Kunzelmann, K., Ohrui, T., Chin, L., Eng, K., Finkbeiner, W.E., Widdicombe, J.H., Gruenert, D.C. CFTR expression and chloride secretion in polarized immortal human bronchial epithelial cells. *Am J Respir Cell Mol Biol, 10,* 38-47.

[103] Masuda, A., Kondo, M., Saito, T., Yatabe, Y., Kobayashi, T., Okamoto, M., Suyama, M., Takahashi, T., Takahashi, T. (1997) Establishment of human peripheral lung epithelial cell lines (HPL1) retaining differentiated characteristics and responsiveness to epidermal growth factor, hepatocyte growth factor, and transforming growth factor β1. *Cancer Res, 57,* 4898-4904.

[104] Okudela, K., Hayashi, H., Ito, T., Yazawa, T., Suzuki, T., Nakane, Y., Sato, H., Ishi, H., KeQin, X., Masuda, A., Takahashi, T., Kitamura, H. (2004) K-ras gene mutation enhances motility of immortalized airway cells and lung adenocarcinoma cells via

Akt activation: possible contribution to non-invasive expansion of lung adenocarcinoma. *Am J Pathol, 164,* 91-100.

[105] Deshusses JM, Burgess JA, Scherl A, Wenger Y, Walter N, Converset V, Paesano S, Corthals GL, Hochstrasser DF, Sanchez JC. (2003) Exploitation of specific properties of trifluoroethanol for extraction and separation of membrane proteins. *Proteomics, 3,* 1418-1424.

[106] Zhan X, Desiderio DM. (2003) Spot volume vs. amount of protein loaded onto a gel: a detailed, statistical comparison of two gel electrophoresis systems. *Electrophoresis, 24,* 1818-1833.

8

Prostate and Colon Cancer Stem Cells as a Target for Anti-Cancer Drug Development

Galina Botchkina and Iwao Ojima
Stony Brook University, New York
USA

1. Introduction

With a worldwide cumulative incidence rate of 9.4%, colorectal cancer is the second leading cause of cancer deaths when both sexes are combined, and prostate cancer is the most commonly diagnosed malignancy and the second leading cause of cancer-related death in men (Jemal et al., 2009). Standard anti-cancer drugs often fail to provide a long-term cure of epithelial tumors, which represent about 90% of human cancers. Thus, response rates in phase I oncology trials were as low as 2.5% over the last decade (Roberts et al., 04; Kamb et al., 07). Such limited effectiveness of standard anti-cancer therapies has been recently attributed to the existence of relatively rare, highly drug resistant, quiescent or slow proliferating tumor-driving cells - cancer stem cells (CSCs). Tumor cells with a stem cell-like properties, such as self-renewal and ability to differentiate into multiple cell types characteristic for particular tumor have recently been identified in all major human tumors, including prostate and colon cancers (reviewed in Dalerba et al., 07a; Mimeault et al., 07). Accumulated knoweledge suggests that majority, if not all tumors possess a minor subpopulation of stem cells and a major (or bulk) mass of progenitors at different stages of their maturation. Malignant stem-like subpopulation within the tumors possesses exclusive tumor-initiating capacity *in vivo* (after serial transplantation to the immunodeficient mice) and high potential to induce 3D cancer spheroids *in vitro* (after serial passaging). Since CSCs are responsible for tumor initiation, development and metastasis, and are highly resistant to standard anti-cancer therapies, they are likely to be the most crucial target in the treatment of cancer. This new concept of carcinogenesis and new paradigm in anti-cancer therapy requires significant reconsideration of previously accepted criteria of the drug effectiveness and development of novel, physiologically and clinically more relevant experimental models. Although isolation and purification of the cancer-specific CSCs reamain to be problematic due to lack of the unique CSC surface markers and insufficient knowledge of the CSC biology, several methodological approaches allow for prospective isolation, purification and reasonable propagation of these cells. Applying these approaches, we and others previously have shown that prostate and colon tumor-initiating cells are functionally, genomically and morphologically different from their bulk tumor counterparts. In this chapter we will discuss novel criteria of the anti-cancer drug efficacy, and present our data on the CSC-targeted activities of a new-generation taxoids.

2. Prostate and colon CSC phenotypes

It is increasingly recognized now that, similarly to normal mammalilan tissues, tumors are organized hierarchically, comprising a minor population of the long-lived self-renewing stem cells, which also give rise to all the heterogeneous cell phenotypes due to ongoing differentiation. CSCs share some basic features and signal transduction pathways, such as Wnt, Shh, Notch, Bmi-1 and others with normal stem cells (Pardal et al., 2003; Reya & Clevers, 2005), and most of the CSC types have been identified and isolated using common cell surface markers. Although none of the currently available cell surface markers can be considered as universal or highly specific for CSCs, several markers were successfully used for prospective isolation of the tumor-initiating cells from diverse tumor types. Among them are the two most commonly used, CD133 (also known as AC133 and prominin-1) and CD44. Thus, several human cancer types, including brain tumors (Singh et al. 2003), kidney (Bussolati et al., 2005), prostate (Collins et al., 2005), hepatocellular (Suetsugu et al., 2006; Yin et al., 2007), colon (O'Brien etal., 2007; Ricci-Vitiani et al., 2007), and pancreatic (Hermann et al., 2007; Li et al., 2007) carcinomas have minor population of CD133-positive cells which have much higher tumorigenic and clonogenic potentials compared to their CD133-negative counterparts or unsorted cells. Other markers, including CD166, Musashi-1, CD29, CD24 (Vermeulen et al., 2008), and leucine-rich repeat-containing G-protein-coupled receptor 5 (Lgr5; Barker et al., 2007) were also suggested for isolation of CSCs.

CD133 is a cell-surface glycoprotein comprising five trans-membrane domains and two large glycosylated extracellular loops (Shmelkov et al., 2005). CD44 is also a multistructural and multifunctional cells surface adhesion molecule involved in cell-cell and cell-matrix interactions, stemness and tumour development, in part via β-catenin and Wnt signaling activation of the CD44 gene transcription (Ponta et al., 2003; Marhaba & Zoller, 2004). Although in many studies both CD44 and CD133 were used as a single cell surface markers and were reported as putative CSC markers, accumulated experimental data suggests that combination of several markers allows for better enrichment of cells with either exclusive or highly increased tumorigenicity in comparison to their bulk counterparts. Thus, the subfraction of prostate cancer cells with $CD44^{+}\alpha_2\beta_1^{hi}CD133^{+}$ phenotype was first described by Collins and colleagues (Collins et al., 2005) as possessing the highest *in vitro* proliferative potential, self-renewal, and the lack of androgen receptor expression. Of note, since normal prostate stem cells are also androgen independent (Isaaks, 1985; Collins et al., 2001; Richardson et al., 2004), it suggests they may be the cells of origin of prostate cancer. It remains to be established whether cancer-specific CSCs represent homogeneous or heterogeneous phenotypic populations. It is also unclear whether some commonly used markers, such as CD133 and CD44, are of equal functional importance. A recent study has demonstrated the unique role of CD133 in the normal and malignant colon, showing that $CD133^{+}$ normal stem cells at the base of crypts in the adult intestine (a stem cell niche) not only generate the entire intestinal epithelium, but give rise to all the neoplastic cells in mice colon tumors (Zhu et al., 2009a). However, another study has shown that only a knockdown of CD44, but not CD133, strongly prevented clonal formation and inhibited tumorigenicity in mice xenograft model (Du et al., 2008). Authors reported that $CD44^{+}$ did not colocalize with $CD133^{+}$ cells within colorectal cancer. Similar results reported by Horst and colleagues showed that the expression of CD133 correlates with that of CD166, while both do not correlate with CD44 (Horst et al., 2009). However, this data contradicts multiple reports showing not only the colocalization of the CD133 and CD44 in several types of human cancer (Collins et al., 2005; Dalerba et al., 2007b; Haraguchi et al., 2008; Zhu et al., 2009b), but also suggesting their combined expression as the best CSC marker (Haraguchi et al., 2008; Zhu et al., 2009b). Since clinical specimens of solid tumors are highly heterogeneous, and membrane expression of CD133 and CD44 undergo a complex post-translational regulation, it may significantly contribute to controversial interpretation of experimental data obtained by diverse experimental approaches.

Although the tumorigenic subset of colon cancer cells was initially identified as CD133-positive (O'Brien et al., 2007; Ricci-Vitiani et al., 2007), in several established cell lines and some clinical specimens both CD133 and CD44 are quite abundant and can not solely

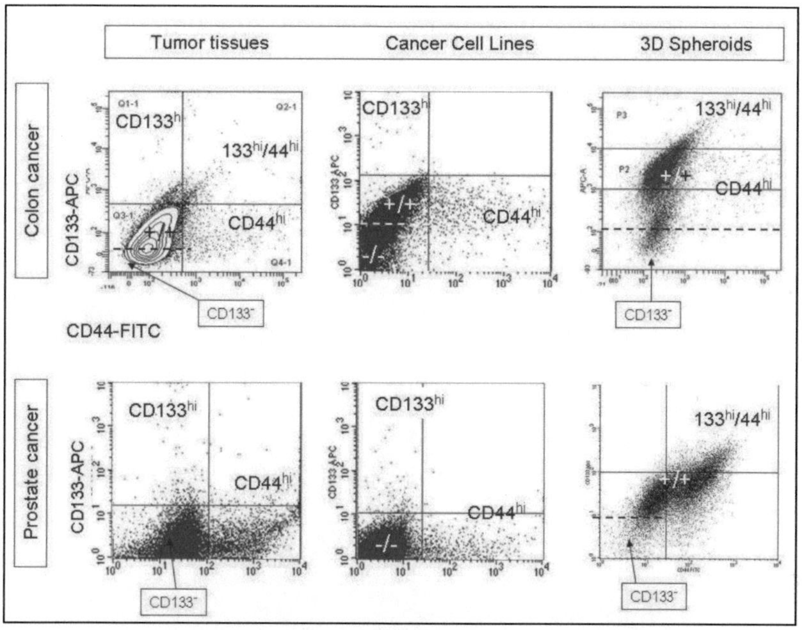

Fig. 1. Phenotypic analysis of colon and prostate cancer cells obtained from patient samples (left column), established cell lines (middle column) and 3D spheroids induced by $CD133^{hi}/CD44^{hi}$ subpopulations (right column). Majority of colon cancer cells of different origin are positive for CD133, CD44 (+/+). In contrast, bulk prostate cancer cells are negative for CD133, and negative or low positive for CD44. However, both cancer types possess minority subpopulations with high expression of each marker ($CD133^{hi}$; $CD44^{hi}$), or high combined expression ($CD133^{hi}/CD44^{hi}$). Both colon and prostate cancer spheroids induced by $CD133^{hi}/CD44^{hi}$ populations in general express much higher levels of these markers compared to parental cell lines, and much larger populations of cells with $CD133^{hi}/CD44^{hi}$.

demarcate the tumor-initiating cells. Clinical specimens often display highly variable levels of these markers, and in such cases combination of CD44 and CD166 with the epithelial-specific antigen (ESA; also known as the epithelial cell adhesion molecule, EpCAM) was suggested as more specific for colon CSCs (Dalerba et al., 2007b; Dylla et al., 2008). In addition, in some metastatic colon cancers and long-term maintained cell lines, such as HCT116, both $CD133^{+}$ and CD133-negative cell populations can induce tumors in NOD/SCID mice (Schmelkov et al., 2008; Botchkina et al., 2009). There is also some misinterpretation of the terminology concerning colon cancer cells, which may be *positive* for particular CSC markers, but only minority populations enriched with CSCs can express *high levels* of these markers. Thus, majority of cells in invasive long-term maintained HCT116 cell lines is *positive* for CD133, CD44 and CD166 (*Figure 1*; upper row; marked as +/+), which were considered as a good single markers for isolation of the minor subpopulation of tumorigenic cell in multiple cancer types and established cell lines. In contrast to the colon cancer cell lines, majority of the prostate PC-3 cells and their metastatic derivatives are negative for CD133, and only minor subpopulations express high levels of both CD133 and CD44 (*Figure 1*; lower row; *Figure 2*, upper row). However, only cells with *highest* levels of CD133 and CD44 (marked as $CD133^{hi}$ and $CD44^{hi}$) grown under stem cell-promoting conditions (type I collagen-coated surfaces, serum-free medium, low cell number and repeated cell sorting) allows for significant enrichemnt of prostate and colon CSCs and increase of their tumor-initiating and clonogenic capacities (Rowehl et al., 2008; Botchkina et

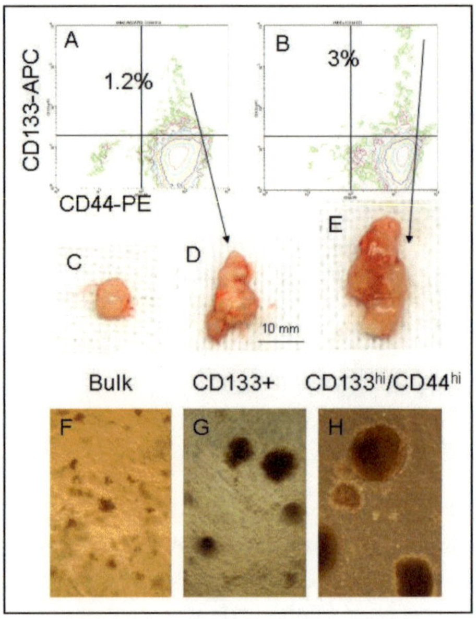

Fig. 2. Phenotypic (A, B), tumorigenic (C-E) and clonogenic (F-H) analyses of the prostate cancer cells. Subpopulation of $CD133^{hi}/CD44^{hi}$ cells is larger in repeatedly sorted cells (B; upper right). Mice tumor xenograrfts induced by $1x10^7$ of the unsorted (bulk) cancer cells (C), $1.5x10^3$ of one-time MACS sorted CD133+ cells (D), and by $1.5x10^3$ of repeatedly sorted and grown on type I collagen cells with higher ratio of $CD133^{hi}/CD44^{hi}$ phenotype (E). The FACS-sorted $CD133^{hi}/CD44^{hi}$ cells possess significantly higher sphere-forming capacity (H) in contrast to the unsorted (F) and MACS-sorted (G) cells.

al., 2009). Prostate and colon cancer spheroids induced by $CD133^{hi}/CD44^{hi}$ cell populations expressed much higher levels of these markers in general, and much more cells were highly positive for CD133 and CD44. Since cells with higher levels of expression of these cell surface markers (after repeated cell sorting and culturing under stemness-promoting conditions) possess significantly increased tumorigenic and clonogenic potentials (*Figure 2*; prostate cancer PC3MM2 cells are shown), it suggests that these cell populations are enriched with putative CSCs.

3. Cancer models

The relevance of the *in vivo* and *in vitro* cancer models to patient tumors remains to be a topic of controversy. Human cancers represent an extremely heterogeneous class of diseases, and each clinical case is unique pathologically and highly heterogeneous biologically in terms of gene expression patterns and levels, the tumor/host interactions, interecations between cells and the extracellular matrix, and many other. It is crucial to isolate tumorigenic cells from each cancer type and, ideally, from maximal possible number of clinico-pathologically different cases for their precise molecular characterization and designing of individual treatment strategies. In addition, cancer cells in general have high rates of genetic and epigenetic changes (Hill et al, 1984; Hill et al., 2006). It is established that long-term culturing can change a malignant phenotype of particular cell line, and same is true for *in vivo* passaging of human cancer xenografts as solid tumors in nonsyngenic host - immunodeficient mice. In this context, transplantation of the tumor cells directly derived from patients into immunodeficient mice (early passages without *in vitro* passaging) should recapitulate original tumors relatively closely. However, biopsy material is usually limited and contaminated with normal stem cells, therefore isolation of the rare putative CSCs is still problematic due to the lack of specific CSC markers. In contrast, established cancer cell lines do not have any normal stem cells, because they quickly loose their stemness and differentiate in standard culture condition. Therefore, cancer cell lines could be an attractive alternative source of cells for CSC research and drug development.

It is clear now that traditionally used monolayer of adherent cancer cells has a very limited relevance to the hierarchically organized *in vivo* tumors, because such cultures have unnatural cell-to-cell and cell-to-matrix contacts, which can significantly affect their phenotype, signal transduction pathways and drug response. Since monolayer cultures are directly exposed to medium content and are readily accessible to oxygen, which is an important signal for stem cell self-renewal, apoptosis, differentiation and migration (reviewed in Friedrich et al., 2009), biological and therapeutic studies on two-dimensional cancer cell cultures have limited clinical relevance and may lead to inaccurate conclusions. This model is even less suitable for stem cell-based studies, because even highly purified CSCs can undergo relatively fast differentiation after being placed in adherent culturing conditions. On the other hand, standard cancer cell lines represent virtually unlimited resource, therefore, it would be useful to have standardized experimental conditions for obtaining a highly tumorigenic and drug resistant CSCs in sufficient quantities, which is a prerequisite for preliminary screening/development of potentially effective CSC-targeted drugs, as well as for investigation of general properties of CSCs.

An alternative 3D model of free-floating cancer spheroids was established by Sutherland and colleagues long before the discovery of CSCs (Inch et al., 1970; Sutherland et al., 1971). This model is more closely related to original tumors with respect to cell morphology, metabolic and proliferative gradients, oxygen and drug penetration, cell-cell junctions, kinases activation and other parameters, compared to the cancer cell monolayers (Friedrich et al., 2009). Spheroid cells have an enhanced resistance to many of the commonly used anti-cancer drugs (Dessoize et al., 2000; Yoshida et al., 2008), showing dramatically lower cytotoxicity against 3D cancer spheroids compared to monolayer cultures, and exhibit chemoresistance which recapitulates this resistant phenotype *in vivo* (Dubessy et al., 2000; Durand et al., 2001; Friedrich et al., 2009). Increased resistance of spheroid cells to ionizing radiation was first demonstrated by Sutherland and colleagues (Inch et al., 1970; Sutherland et al., 1971). The floating cancer spheroids are organized hierarchically, similarly to the *in vivo* tumors, containing relatively small (although usually increased compared to the parental tumor) population of the tumorigenic cells and a large spectrum of their progenitors, the bulk tumor cells at different stages of differentiation. They can be passaged for many generations, suggesting that they contain a population of cells with extensive self-renewal capacity. Thus, the cancer spheroids induced by primary colon carcinoma cells select for cells that coexpress multiple CSC markers, including CD133, CD166, CD44, CD24, CD29 (Vermeulen et al., 2008) and Lgr5 (Barker et al., 2007). We found that both mice tumor xenografts and 3D spheroids induced by more purified phenotypic populations of cancer-specific tumorigenic cells ($CD133^{high}/CD44^{high}$ for prostate and colon cancer) have higher tumorigenic and clonogenic potentials, and much higher ratio of cells with original phenotype, even after several weeks in 3D culture (Rowehl et al., 2008; Botchkina et al., 2009). Striking correlation between ability to form compact 3D spheroids and invasive potential was recently demonstrated on ovarian cancer cells (Sodek et al., 2009). Although 3D cancer cell cultures were developed several decades ago, earlier studies focused on analyses of drug responses were usually limited to the relatively short-term gross evaluation of the inhibition of spheroid growth and apoptosis, but specific stem cell-related responses of spheroid cells were not studied. Recently, several mechanisms were suggested as a mediators of the CSC drug resistance, including replication quiescence, high expression of ABC transporters, active DNA repair, activation of anti-apoptotic pathways, down-regulation of the apoptotic machinery and others (Dean et al., 2005; Donnenberg et al., 2005; Mimeault et al., 2007).

Therefore, taking into account all of the above, early passage cancer floating spheroids induced by purified cancer-specific CSCs and early passage patient-derived mice tumor xenografts can be suggested as relatively suitable models for studying CSC-targeted drug efficacy. Both mice tumors and spheroids induced by purified CSCs contain higher ratios of cells with original transplanted phenotypes compared to parental sources. Since CSCs represent a dynamic population with dual potential, self-renewal versus generation of the committed progenitors, which eventually will differentiate into all mature cell phenotypes, isolated CSC phenotypes should be cultured, tested and treated under conditions designed to retain their "stemness" and preclude differentiation to the bulk tumor cells. The isolated cell phenotypes should be functionally tested for at lest major stem cell properties, including self-renewal capacity *in vivo* (ability of the particular cell phenotype to induce tumors in NOD/SCID mice after serial transplantations of the low cell number); self-renewal capacity *in vitro* (ability of the particular cell phenotype to induce 3D colonospheres during serial passaging under non-adherent, serum-free culture conditions), and plasticity (ability to produce all the differentiated cell phenotypes characteristic for particular tumor under standard culture conditions). In addition to standard methods of analysis of cytotoxicity, CSC-targeted drug activities should be also evaluated by functional analyses of stem cell-related properties, as well as by comparative genomic and molecular analyses.

4. Genomic characteristics of the prostate and colon CSCs

Genome-wide Gene Expression Profiling

We studied the genome-wide gene expression profiles of prostate and colon CSCs using high-density oligonucleotide microarrays (Affymetrix Gene Chip HG-U133 Set). To increase the discriminating power of the gene microarray assay, either repeatedly MACS-CD133 sorted and grown on type I collagen-coated surfaces at low density prostate PC3MM2 and colon HCT116 cells, or floating spheroids induced by $CD133^{high}/CD44^{high}$ phenotypes in serum-free MSCB medium were analyzed in comparison to their bulk adherent counterparts. In prostate tumorigenic cells, we have determined 213 genes with 10-100 fold increased activity out of 8994 differentially expressed ones, and 87 genes with 5-50 fold decreased activity (Rowehl et al., 2008). Among the most up-regulated genes were anti-apoptotic genes, including *BIRC5* (survivin), *CDC2, TOP2A, MYBL2, HELLS, ANGPTL* and others. Another largest population of genes was related to the cell cycle regulation and proliferation, including cyclin B, *CCNB1, CDC2, CDCA 2, 3, 5* and *8, BUB1, ANLN, ATM, FOXM1, TACC3, PLK4, SHCBP1, GTSE1* and others. Several "stemness" genes involved in developmental pathways, including *MYBL* and *SOX4* were also significantly upregulated. Of interest, the *ASPM* gene, which is responsible for accelerated human brain evolution and also is overexpressed in some human cancers (34) displayed 128-fold higher expression in prostate CSCs compared to the bulk tumor cells. Among significantly downregulated genes were those involved in regulation of apoptosis (*NUPR1, BCL2L1, TRIB3*); cell cycle/proliferation (*CDKN2B, TRIM13; SLC3A2*) and cell-cell and cell-matrix signaling (*S100A9, S100P, GDF15*).

In colon tumor-initiating cells, we have found that the microarray assay has much higher discriminating power in analysis of cells from floating spheres. Thus, we have determined more than 500 of significantly (3-120 fold) upregulated genes out of 4351 differentially expressed ones, and 436 genes which were downregulated by 3-1500 folds in colon CSCs grown as floating spheroids (Botchkina et al., 2009). For comparison, analysis of single-time MACS-$CD133^{+}$ cells versus unsorted cells has shown only 988 differentially expressed genes with 162 signifficantly up-regulated ones. It can be explained by constitutively high expression of CD133 by the majority of colon cancer HCT116 cells, which predominantly represent progenitor cells. We have determined that, similarly to the prostate CSCs, majority of the most upregulated genes were those related to anti-apoptosis (*APP*, Bcl3/NF*kappa* B2 complex, *BDNF, BIRC3, BIRC4, BTRC3, CBX4, CCAR1, CCPG1, CD74, DHCR24, FOXO3, HSPA1B, IGFBP3, IF16, NFKB1A, TBX3, TNFAIP3, TRIB3* and others); cell cycle/cell proliferation (*FOSB, IL-8, CCNG2, IGFBP3, TGFBP1, MXD1, INSIG1, EHF, CD74, CDC25A, HSMPP8*); and transcription factors (*ID2, ID2B, DENR, MXD1* and many others). Several stemness genes were also upregulated (NOTCH pathway; *APP, MIB1*; Wnt receptors *TGFB1I1, CSNK1D*). High number of genes regulating Ca^{2+} homeostatis and calmodulin binding also revealed significantly altered expression which is most likely connected with the altered induction and regulation of apoptosis in CSCs. The most significantly downregulated genes in HCT floating spheres were *HLI4* (1500-fold) which is responsible for heterophilic cell adhesion; apoptosis-related cytochrom *c, COX6A1* gene (300-fold), and *BCL2L1* which regulates the release of cytochrom *c* from mitochondria; *CXCL14* gene involved in cell-cell signaling (100-fold). Among other significantly downregulated genes were apoptosis-related *AP15, BAX, CASP2, CFL1, ENO1, FXR1, HSPD1, HSP90B1, FAS, Fas*-binding (*FBF1, NPM1), MVEGFA, RAD21, RHOB, SOCS2, VDAC1*, and many others; cell cycle/cell proliferation (ras *RHOB, CDV3, CDK8, NFYC*); genes involved in negative regulation of cell growth (*DCBLD2, POSTN, CDH11*); signal transduction (ATP binding: *SPARC, MAP3K2, HSP90AB1*); and heat shock protein genes (*HSP90B1, HSPD1*) which are required for antigen presentation. This data is in line with current knowledge that chemo- and radioresistance of CSCs is attributed to upregulation of anti-apoptotic genes, down-regulation of pro-apoptotic ones, active DNA repair, reactivation of some developmental signaling cascades, and other mechanisms (Dean et al., 2005; Mimeault et al., 2007).

Stem Cell-Related Gene Expression Profiling

We analyzed the floating spheroids induced by CD133^{high}/CD44^{high} cell populations derived from the three independent colon cancer cell lines, including HCT116, HT29 and DLD-1 with the stem cell pathway-specific PCR Array assay (*SA*Biosciences). Each array contains SYBR Green-based real-time PCR gene-specific assays for a set of 84 genes. Using filtering criteria of a 1.5 or greater fold-change in expression, we have analyzed differentially expressed genes in these three types of floating colonospheres compared to their bulk differentiated adherent counterparts (Botchkina et al., 2010). The most profound differences were observed in HCT116 spheroids grown from CD133^{high}/CD44^{high} cells (*Figure 4 A;* left histogram), which is in line with their higher sphere-forming and tumor-initiating capacities compared to cells of the same phenotype isolated from HT29 and DLD-1 lines. About one-fourth of the analyzed stem cell-related genes, including Wnt and Notch pathway genes responsible for self-renew and cell cycle regulation, were commonly up-regulated in all types of spheroids, with significantly higher levels of expression in HCT116 ones. Thus, 6 of 6 analyzed genes responsible for stem cell self-renewal (*SOX1, SOX2, MYST1, MYST2, NEUROG2* and *HSPA9*), and 3 of 5 genes regulating symmetrical/asymmetricasl cell division (*NOTCH1, NOTCH2* and *PARD6A*) were significantly up-regulated in the HCT116 CD133/CD44-high colonospheres compared to their bulk counterparts. The most significantly up-regulated genes in HT29 spheroids were *ACAN, ALPI, APC, ASCL2, CCND2, CD3D, CD4, CD8A, CD8B, COL2A1, COL9A1, DHH, DLL3, DTX1 FGF1, GJA1, S100B,SOX2, T, TERT* and *WNT1;* and in DLD-1 spheroids - *ALDH1A1, ASCL2, CCND2, CD4, COL1A1, DLL1, DTX1, FGF1, GJA1, IGF1, JAG1, MME, NCAM1,* and *NOTCH1.*

In metastatic prostate cancer PC3MM2 cell line, majority of the analyzed stemness genes were also dramatically up-regulated in spheroids induced by CD133^{high}/CD44^{high} cells compared to their bulk counterparts (*Fig.4 B;* left histogram), wich is in line with the Affymetrix microarray data. Multiple developmental genes, including *NOTCH1, NOTCH2, NUMB, DTX2, DLL3, JAG1, WNT1, MYC, SOX1, SOX2,* and genes involved in general regulation of stem cells self-renewal and maintenance, including *NEUROG2, MYST1, MYST2, HSPA9B, DLL1, PPARD, FRAT, CD44, COL2A1, DVL1, TERT, ASCL2, BTRC* and others were overactivated. The ABC transporters-related gene, *ABCG2* was also up-regulated in prostate spheroids compared to the corresponding adherent cell cultures, which together with the upregulated anti-apoptotic and down-regulated pro-apoptotic genes might explain dramatic increase in the resistance to drug treatment of 3D spheroids versus adherent cancer cell cultures.

Accumulated data suggest that recently discovered transcription factors essential for stem cells self-renewal and maintenance of pluripotency, including OCT4, SOX2, c-Myc and Klf4 (Takahashi et al., 2006; 2007), are closely related to cancer invasion, metastasis and CSC maintenance. Thus, expression of the SOX2 and OCT4 was associated with less differentiated phenotype, distant recurrence and poor prognosis for colorectal cancer (Tsukamoto et al., 2005; Saigusa et al., 2009). It was shown that some prostate cancers overexpress several genes typically associated with stem cells, including *Bcl-2, OCT3/4, BMI1, β-CATENIN, SMOOTHENED* and others, which indicates that these tissues may contained some significant ratios of the CSCs (reviewed in Mimeault & Batra, 2006). We have found that floating cancer spheroids contain a minority cell populations (about 3-4%of the spheroid cells) with high levels of expression of several transcription factors, including c-Myc, Oct4, Sox2 and NANOG. The flow cytometry data were confirmd with western blot analysis shown the presence of these proteins in total lysates of the spheroid cells, as well as in repeatedly sorted cells with CD133^{high}/CD44^{high} phenotype.

5. CSC-targeted activities of the new-generation taxoids

It is largely accepted now that effective anti-cancer drugs should be targeted toward the cancer-specific tumor-initiating cells, not only the bulk tumor cells. For advanced prostate cancer, androgen deprivation therapy remains the most widely used treatment modality. However, although it induces remission in about 90% of patients, in ~18 months all patients relapse with a hormone-refractory drug resistant disease, which is invariably fatal (overall median survival is 23-37 months). Such resistance to hormonal therapy was associated with the lack of androgen receptors on the putative prostate CSCs (Isaaks, 1999; Taplin & Balk, 2004; Maitland & Collins, 2008). Colon cancer is inherently drug-resistant due to multiple mechanisms that are still poorly characterized, so both CSCs and the progenitor cells can potentially contribute to chemotherapy tolerance.

Numerous studies have demonstrated that both CD133- and CD44-positive fractions in many cancer types are exceptionally resistant to standard anti-cancer therapies (Frank et al., 2003; Frank et al., 2005; Bao et al., 2006; Liu et al., 2006; Hong et al., 09; Vlashi et al., 09). Moreover, there is growing evidence that conventional therapeutic modalities focused on the tumor debulking may actually *promote* cancer progression by stimulating quiescent CSCs to divide symmetrically (self-renewal) and repopulate the tumor mass with undifferrentiated cells (Bao et al, 2006; Dirks, 2006 ; Eramo et al., 2006; Woodward et al., 2007; Todaro et al, 2007; Bleau et al., 2009). Multiple evidence indicate that the ratio of CD133^{+} cells correlates with tumor aggressiveness, histologic grade and clinical outcome (Al-Hajj et al, 2003; Liu et al., 2006; Zeppernick et al., 2008; Maeda et al., 2008; Horst et al., 2008; Wang et al., 2009). In colorecral cancer, elevated levels of CD133 expression were associated with distant recurrence (Yasuda et al., 2009) and resistance to chemo- and radiotherapy (Saigusa et al., 2010). The proportion of CD133^{+} cells in colon cancer metastases is higher than in primary tumors (Puglisi et al., 2009). Similar data were reported for CD44-positive cells (Hong et al, 09). There is also growing data that CSCs, in particular CD133-positive cells, express several pluripotency markers (Chen et al., 2008), which was linked to their chemo- and radioresistant properties. The expression of CD133, Sox2 and Oct4, was increased after treatment with chemo- (Levina et al., 2008) and radiation therapy (Saigusa et al., 2009), and was also associated with an unfavorable clinical outcome (Wang et al., 2009). Taken together, it can explain the well known fact that metastatic lesions are more resistant to treatment compared to primary tumors. Since CSCs, similarly to other types of stem cells, have almost unlimited ability to self-renew, treatment strategies can be focused either to direct elimination of tumor-initiating cells, abrogation of their stemness, or promotion of their differentiation. This new paradigm of cancer treatment requires development of novel drug molecules and additional, stem cell-relevant criteria to assess CSC drug responses.

Paclitaxel (Taxol®, Bristol-Myers Squibb) and its semisynthetic analog Docetaxel (Taxotere®, Aventis) are the most commonly used anti-cancer drugs and standard chemotherapy of colon and hormone-resistant prostate cancers. These taxanes bind to the β-tubulin subunit, accelerate the polymerization of tubulin, thereby stabilizing the microtubules and inhibiting their depolymerization, which results in the arrest of the cell division cycle and consequent apoptosis. Although both paclitaxel and docetaxel possess potent antitumor (debulking) activity, most treated patients ultimately manifest resistance to the drugs and recurrence of the disease, which is known to be associated with a more malignant phenotype and high mortality rates (Mimeault et al., 2007). Thus, two large phase III trials (TAX 327 and SWOG 9916; Southwest Oncology Group) have demonstrated that these drugs increased an overall survival in patients with hormone-refractory metastatic prostate cancer from 16-17 months to only 17.5-18.9 months (Roberts et al., 2004). To develop new taxane anticancer agents with fewer side effects, superior pharmacological properties, and improved activity against drug-resistant human cancers, extensive structure-activity relationship studies on taxol and its congeners have been performed in different laboratories. Several novel second- and third-generation taxoids with systematic modifications at the C2, C10, and C3′N positions were synthesized in Dr. Ojima's group (reviewed in Ojima & Das, 2009). It was determined that (i) the C3′-phenyl group was not an essential component for their potent activity and (ii) the modifications of the C10 position with certain acyl groups as well as the replacement of the phenyl group with an alkenyl or alkyl group at the C3′ position made compounds 1–2 orders of magnitude more potent than the parent drugs (paclitaxel and docetaxel) against drug resistant human breast cancer cell lines. These highly potent taxoids were termed "second-generation taxoids". Furthermore, we found that introduction of a substituent (e.g., MeO, N_3, Cl, F, etc.) to the *meta* position of the C2-benzoyl group of the second-generation taxoids, enhanced the activities 2–3 orders of magnitude higher than the parent drugs against different types of the drug-resistant cancer cells (Ojima & Das, 2009).

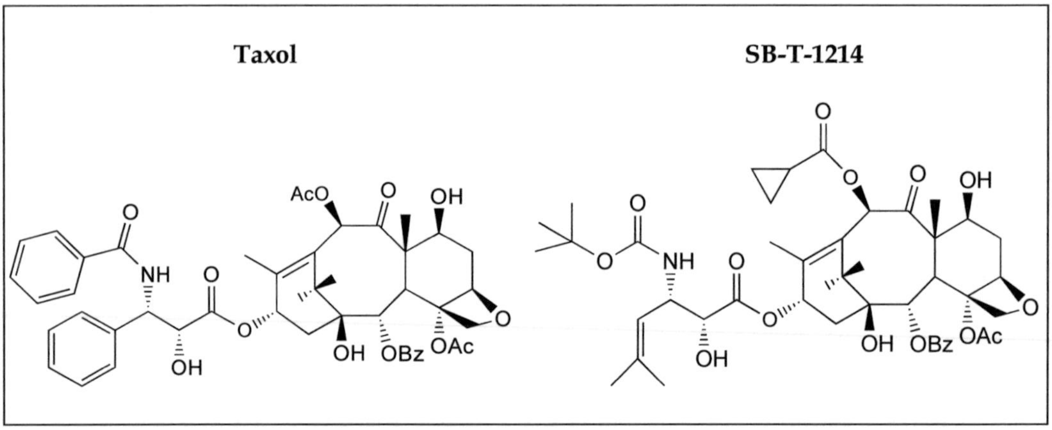

Fig. 3. Chemical structure of taxol (A) and new-generation taxoid, SB-T-1214 (B).

The antitumor activity of SB-T-1214 (*Figure 3*), one of the leading candidates among the new generation taxoids studied in our laboratory, was assayed *in vivo* against a Pgp+ DLD-1 human colon tumor xenograft in SCID mice, as well as against highly drug-resistant CFPAC-1 pancreatic tumor xenografts. The drug was administered intravenously in three doses 3 times using a 3-day regimen, starting from day 5 after DLD-1 subcutaneous tumor implantation. As anticipated, paclitaxel was ineffective against this highly drug-resistant (Pgp+) tumor at its optimal dose (60 mg/kg total dose). In contrast, SB-T-1214 has shown profound antitumor activity, with the best result at 60 mg/kg total dose, 20mg/kg x 3, wherein complete regression of the DLD-1 tumor was achieved in five of five mice (tumor growth delay was >201 days). Systemic toxicity profile has shown that there was only a 3-5% weight loss during the period of day 15 to day 20, and the drug was well tolerated by animals (Kuznetsova et al., 2006). Histopathological analysis of the hematoxylin and eosin stained tissue sections of the tumor xenografts recovered from the control (vehicle treated) mice revealed a large tumor areas with densely packed tumor cells (Botchkina et al., 2010), which uniformly expressed membrane-bounded immunoreactivity for human epithelial cell adhesion molecule, *h*EpCAM. Several small clusters of cells with high levels of CD133 expression were found predominantly within the outer areas of the tumors corresponding to the tumor invasive front, whereas scattered CD133+ cells were detected across the entire tumor areas. Flow cytometry analysis of the dissociated and immunomagnetically (MACS-*h*EpCAM) sorted mice tumor xenografts confirmed the presence of a minor population (about 4%) of human cancer cells with high combined expression of the CD133 and CD44. After three consequent treatments with the SB-T-1214, we observed a complete reduction in tumor volume. Residual tissues showed multiple inflammatory infiltrates and fibrosis, and were negative for human EpCAM and CD133. Since tumor growth delay was comparable with the lifespan of SCID mice, we hypothesized that this compound could affect timorigenic cell populations by modulation of some stemness genes and signaling pathways. To test this hypothesis, the CSC-specific effects of SB-T-1214 were studied on previously characterized three independent invasive colon cancer cell lines (HCT116, HT29 and DLD-1), as well as on highly metastatic derivative of the prostate PC-3 cell line, PC3MM2, which was kindly provided by M. D. Anderson Cancer Center (USA). The tumor-initiating cells were first isolated and enriched with a fluorescence activated cell sorting (FACS) based on highest combined expression of the CD133 and CD44. We have found that majority of cells in all selected colon cancer cell lines grown at standard adherent conditions expressed moderate levels of CD133, CD44 and CD166. However, all three cell lines possessed minority cell populations with highest expression of CD133, which coincided with high expression of CD44 ($CD133^{high}/CD44^{high}$). Then selected cell subpopulations were subjected to further purification and propagation using several approaches, which include repeated cell sorting, short-term culturing at low cell density on type I collagen-coated surfaces, growing cells in serum-free stem cell medium and others. To confirm that selected cell phenotypes posess the stem cell-related characteristics, they were subjected to functional and genomic analyses as we previously described (Rowehl et al., 2008; Botchkina et al., 2009). We have determined that even without additional purification, the acutely isolated $CD133^{high}/CD44^{high}$ cells derived from all three colon cancer cell lines possessed relatively high efficiency in forming dense floating multicellular spheroids in non-adherent cultures with serum-free medium in contrast to their corresponding bulk counterparts, which produced a few loose flat colonies. Dissociated spheroid cells retained an original cell phenotype and expressed all the studied commonly used stem cell surface markers, including CD133, CD44, CD166, *h*EpCAM, CD49b, and CD117. Immunohistochemical analysis of spheroid cells revealed a minority cell population expressing high levels of nuclear β–catenin.

In our previous studies we have found that short-term culturing of repeatedly sorted cells on type I collagen-coated surfaces in serum-free stem cell medium led not only to the retaining, but to significant increase of the ratios of the tumor-initiating cell phenotypes. This data is in line with a recent study showing that human colorectal carcinoma cells grown on type I collagen in serum-free medium undergo an epithelial-mesenchymal-like transition and downregulation of E-cadherin and β-catenin at cell-cell junctions (Kirkland et al., 2009). Authors have found that collagen type I inhibited cell differentiation, increased clonogenicity and promoted expression of CD133 and Bmi1, indicating that it promoted expression of a stem cell-like phenotype in colon cancer cells. Therefore, the CSC-targeted effects of the SB-T-1214 were tested under two experimental conditions: a) using purified CSCs grown adherent to the type I collagen, which promote stemness and retain selected cell phenotypes in undifferentiated state; and b) using 3D spheroid cultures induced by the purified CSCs, which also allow for enrichment of CSCs and retaining of the undifferentiated phenotype in major cell population. As we mentioned above, spheroid cells are highly resistant to standard treatment modalities, possess high tumorigenic and clonigenic potentials, and express many markers of stemness, including CD133, CD166, CD44, CD24, CD29 (Rowehl et al., 2008; Vermeulen et al., 2008; Botchkina et al., 2009) and Lgr5 (Barker et al., 2007). As discussed above, these features are characteristic for the most aggressive clinical cases with poor prognosis and, therefore, selected approach seems clinically relevant and adequate for search of drugs with the potential to eradicate cancer.

Administration of 0.1-1μM SB-T-1214 for 48 hours induced a loss of integrity of the floating spheroids and apoptosis in about 90% of the sphere cells (Botchkina et al., 2010), with higher rates of cell death in adherent type I collagen cultures. Although about 11% of cells survived this treatment regimen, such cells displayed multiple abnormalities, including a greatly enlarged size, multiple nuclei, a significant increase in the number of long and knobby projections, and severe vacuolization. Many cells displayed a clear sign of the mitotic catastrophe. Most importantly, viable cells which survived this treatment regimen significantly lost the ability to form secondary spheroids, which indicates that colon CSC population was critically affected. Thus, 1000 of untreated HCT116 primary spheroid cells induced 125±6 secondary spheroids, HT29 - 75±7, and DLD-1 gave rise to 93±6 secondary spheroids, whereas the SB-T-1214-treated dissociated spheroid cells produced only 1.5±0.3, 4±0.6, and 3±0.4 secondary spheroids, correspondently ($P<0.01$). After placement on type I collagen surfaces, cells that survived drug treatment, displayed profound morphological abnormalities similar to those described above.

The CD133^{high}/CD44^{high}-induced colon and prostate cancer spheroids were further tested for the expression of stem cell-related genes before and after treatment with SB-T-1214 using PCR array assay (*SA*Biosciences). Each array contains SYBR Green-based real-time PCR gene-specific assays for a set of 84 genes. Using filtering criteria of a 1.5 or greater fold-change in expression, we have analyzed differentially expressed genes in three types of floating colonospheres compared to their bulk differentiated adherent counterparts, as well as before and after treatment with SB-T-1214. The most profound differences were observed in HCT116 spheroids grown from CD133^{high}/CD44^{high} cells (*Figure 4; left panel*), which is in line with their higher sphere-forming and tumor-initiating capacities. About one-fourth of the analyzed stem cell-related genes, including Wnt and Notch pathway genes responsible for self-renew and cell cycle regulation, were commonly up-regulated in all types of spheroids, with significantly higher levels of expression in HCT116 ones. Thus, 6 of 6 analyzed genes responsible for stem cell self-renewal (*SOX1, SOX2, MYST1, MYST2, NEUROG2* and *HSPA9*), and 3 of 5 genes regulating symmetrical/asymmetricasl cell division (*NOTCH1, NOTCH2* and *PARD6A*) were significantly up-regulated in the HCT116 CD133/CD44-high colonospheres compared to their bulk counterparts. The most significantly up-regulated genes in HT29 spheroids were *ACAN, ALPI, APC, ASCL2, CCND2, CD3D, CD4, CD8A, CD8B, COL2A1, COL9A1, DHH, DLL3, DTX1 FGF1, GJA1, S100B,SOX2, T, TERT* and *WNT1;* and in DLD-1 spheroids - *ALDH1A1, ASCL2, CCND2, CD4, COL1A1, DLL1, DTX1, FGF1, GJA1, IGF1, JAG1, MME, NCAM1,* and *NOTCH1.*

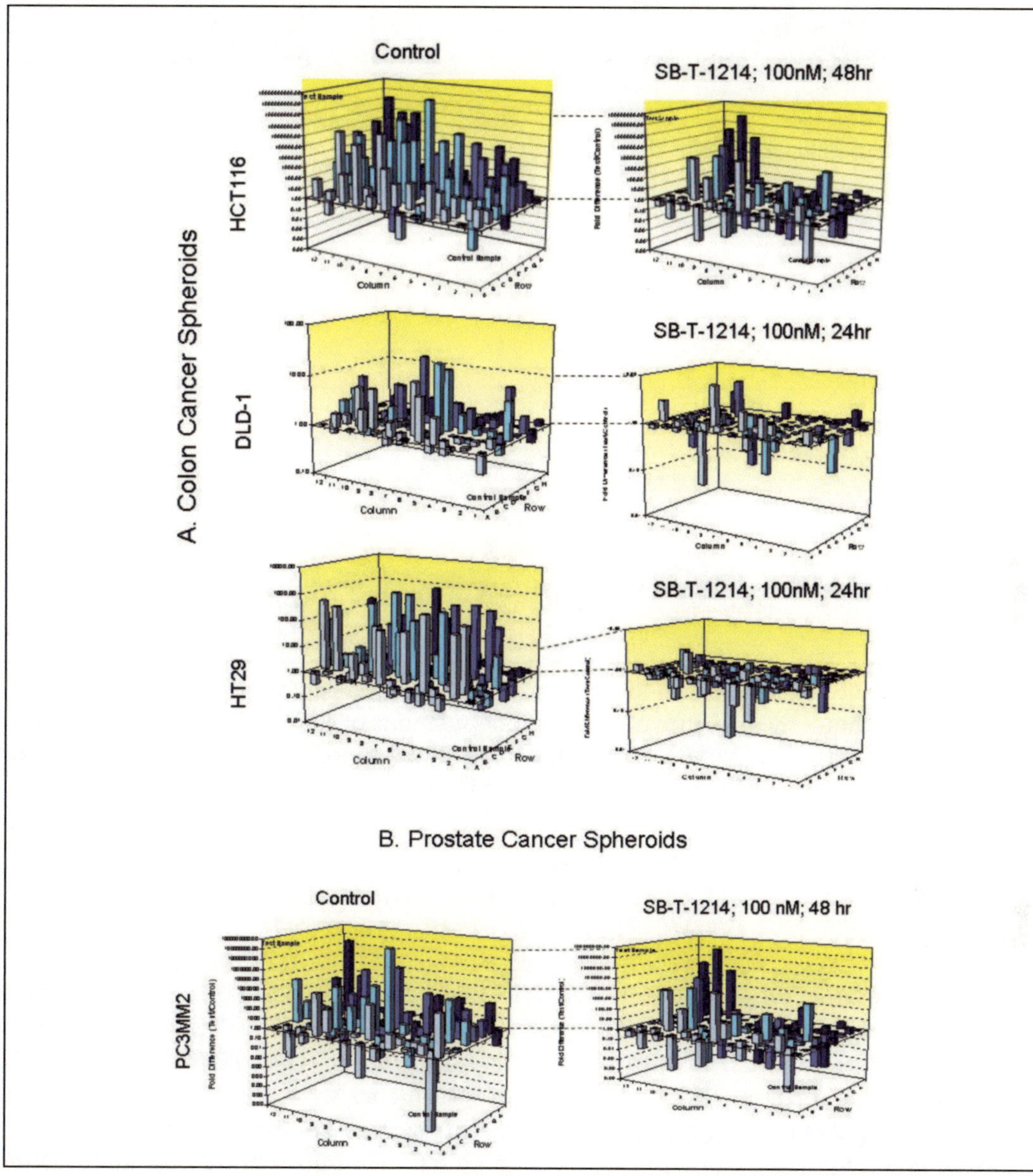

Fig. 4. Drug-induced alteration in the stem cell-related gene expression profiles (PCR Array assay) in colon and prostate cancer spheroids induced by CD133^{high}/CD44^{high} cell populations. A majority of the stemness genes were up-regulated in floating spheroids grown from CD133^{high}/CD44^{high} cells (upper half of each histogram) derived from colon HCT116, HT29and DLD-1 (A), as well as from PC3MM2 (B) cell lines in comparison with their corresponding bulk counterparts (lower half of each histogram). Treatment with 100nM SB-T-1214 for 24 or 48 hr induced down-regulation of a majority of the stem cell-related genes (right column). Importantly, relatively low concentrations of SB-T-1214 (100nM-1μM for 24 or 48 hr) induced dramatic down-regulation of the majority of stem cell-related genes in all three types of colonospheres, as well as in the prostate PC3MM2

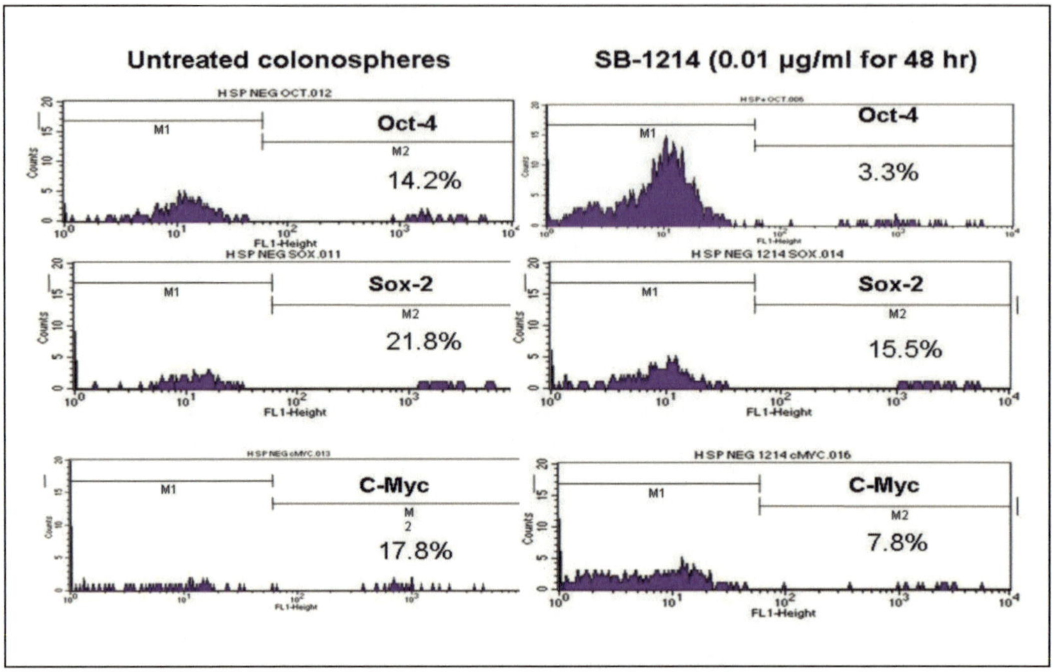

Fig. 5. Drug-induced alterations in the expression of the markers of pluripotency.
FACS analysis shows the presence of minor subpopulations of colon cancer cells within the 3D spheroids (left column), which express the three key pluripotency genes (Sox2, Oct4, and c-Myc). After treatment with SB-T-1214 percent of these cells was decreased (right column).

spheroids (*Figure 4, right panel*). The most significant drug-induced down-regulation of gene expression was detected: 1) in HCT116 colonospheres for *SOX1, RPL13A, BMP3, NEUROG2, GJB1, GJA1, ASCL2, CTNNA1, GDF2, ALPI, S100B, CD8B1, ACTB, CCND1, FGF1, PARD6A, DVL1, GDF3, ISL1, CD3D, MME, FGFR1, RB1, BMP1, AIN1, ALDH1A1, CD8A, PPARD, FZD1, NUMB, ABCG2*; 2) in HT29 colonospheres for *ACAN, ALPI, BMP3, CD3D, CD4, CD8A, CD8B, CDH2,COL2A1, COL9A1, DHH, DLL1, DLL3, DTX1, FGF1, FGF3, FZD1, GDF2, IGF1, MME, MYOD, NCAM1, NEUROG2, S100B, SOX2,* and *TERT*; 3) in DLD-1 colonospheres for *CD4, CDH2, COL1A1, DLL1, DTX1, IGF1, FGF3, FZD1, JAG1, KRT15, MSX1, NCAM1* and *NOTCH1*. Of note, many of these genes were related to the stem cells self-renewal, regulation of symmetric/asymmetric division and pluripotency.

We have found that the colonospheres induced by HCT116 cells with $CD133^{high}/CD44^{high}$ phenotype contained minority cell populations with high levels of expression of several markers, which are essential for pluripotency and self-renewal of embryonic stem cells (iPS-related genes) including c-MYC, SOX2, OCT3/4, LIN28, and NANOG (Botchkina et al., 2010). To analyze possible drug-induced alterations in the expression of these stem cell-specific transcription factors, which are low in abundance and present in a minority of colon cancer cell populations, we treated floating spheroids with 100nM of SB-T-1214 for 24 hours to induce such alterations, but avoid profound cell death. Importantly, both FACS and western blot analyses have shown that the expression of Oct-4, Sox-2, Nanog, Lin-28 and c-Myc was inhibited after a single treatment with relatively low drug concentration (*Figure 5*; FACS analysis is shown). These data are promising in light of a recent clinical study, which has demonstrated that expression of several iPS-related genes, in particular, LIN28 and SOX2 is significantly associated with lymph node metastasis (Saiki et al., 2009). It was recently demonstrated that treatment with 5-FU and oxaliplatin, a standard therapy for metastatic colon cancer, induced up to 30-fold enrichment of CD133+ and up to 2-fold enrichment of CD44+ cells in HT29 cell line (Dallas et al., 2009). These data are in line with our observation that after a single treatment with 100μM Paclitaxel for 24 hours, the clonogenic potential of the dissociated HT29 and DLD-1 spheres cells was significantly increased, so we can assume that post-treatment spheroids contained a higher proportion of putative colon CSCs compared to untreated spheroids.

Therefore, SB-T-1214 efficiently suppressed the majority of stem cell-related genes, including Wnt and Notch, and in particular, several essential markers of pluripotent embryionic stem cells, including *SOX-2, Oct-4 and c-Myc,* on both transcriptional and protein levels. Importantly, WNT activity is known to regulate the self-renewal of prostate cancer cells with stem cell characteristics independently of androgen receptor activity (Bisson & Prowse, 2009); while c-*myc* gene (c-Myc is a Wnt target) amplification has been associated with the appearance of hormone-independent prostate cancer (Nupponen et al., 1998; Bernard et al., 2003), and a significant increase of c-*myc* amplification has been observed as a consequence of anti-androgen treatment (Kaltz-Wittmer et al., 2000). Of note, c-Myc is not essential for normal stem cells (Oskarsson et al., 2006), which makes it an even more attractive target for therapeutic intervention. Therefore, inhibition of WNT and NOTCH signaling by SB-T-1214 can reduce the self-renewal of prostate cancer stem cells and improve therapeutic outcomes. Since we have studied the SB-T-1214 induced alterations in the stemness gene expression profiles using total cell lysates (equal amounts of the total RNA for PCR arrays and total protein for western blot analyses), the significant inhibition of the stem cell-related genes induced by SB-T-1214 is promising.

6. Conclusions

Taken together, our data strongly support the suggestion that prostate and colon cancers cells with high combined expression of CD133 and CD44 represent stem-like cells with high tumorigenic and sphere-forming potentials, and significantly up-regulated multiple developmental pathways characteristic for pluripotent stem cells. Several mechanisms, including up-regulation of the anti-apoptotic and down-regulation of pro-apoptotic pathways, as well as high levels of expression of ABC transporters, active DNA repair and others, can contribute to the resistance of CSCs to standard treatment. Our findings provide first evidence that a new-generation taxoid, SB-T-1214, possesses significant activity against 3D colon and prostate cancer spheroids induced by, and enriched with, drug resistant tumorigenic $CD133^{high}/CD44^{high}$ cell populations, and efficiently inhibits the expression of a majority of stem cell-related genes, including several key regulators of pluripotency and self-renewal of embryonic stem cells. Therefore, our data indicate that the long-term efficacy of SB-T-1214 against drug resistant tumors *in vivo* (Kuznetsova et al., 2006; Ojima &Das, 2009) may be explained by down-regulation of multiple stem cell-related genes in tumorigenic cell populations, in addition to known efficacy of taxoids as a mitotic poisons due to their binding to microtubules (Jordan & Wilson, 2004) in the proliferating pool of cancer cells. These findings should be further tested across a large series of clinical specimens of primary and metastatic lesions of prostate and colon cancers.

7. References

Al-Hajj M, Wicha MS, Benito-Hernandez A, Morrison SJ, and Clarke MF (2003) Prospective identification of tumorigenic breast cancer cells. Proc Natl Acad Sci USA 100:3983-3988.

Zeppernick F, Ahmadi R, Campos B, Dictus C, Helmke BM, Becker N, Lichter P, Unterberg A, Radlwimmer B and Herold-Mende CC. (2008) Stem Cell Marker CD133 Affects Clinical Outcome in Glioma Patients. Clinical Cancer Research *14*:123-129.

Bao, S.; Wu, Q.; McLendon, R.; Hao, Y.; Shi, Q.; Hjelmelad, A.; Dewhirst, M.; Bigner, D. & Rich, J. (2006) Glioma stem cells promote radioresistance by preferential activation of the DNA damage response, *Nature* 444:756–760.

Barker N, van Es JH, Kuipers J, Kujala P, van den Born M, Cozijnsen M, Haegebarth A, Korving J, Begthel H, Peters PJ, Clevers H. Identification of stem cells in small intestine and colon by marker gene Lgr5. *Nature* 449: 1003–1007, 2007.

Bisson, I. & Prowse, D. (2009) WNT signaling regulates self-renewal and differentiation of prostate cancer cells with stem cell characteristics. *Cell Research* 19:683–697.

Bernard, D.; Pourtier-Manzanedo, A.; Gil, J.& Beach, D. (2003) Myc confers androgen-independent prostate cancer cell growth. *J. Clin. Invest.* 112(11): 1724-1731.

Bleau AM, Hambardzumyan D, Ozawa T, Fomchenko EI, Huse JT, Brennan CW, Holland EC. (2009) PTEN/PI3K/Akt pathway regulates the side population phenotype and ABCG2 activity in glioma tumor stem-like cells. Cell Stem Cell. 4(3):226-35.

Botchkina, I.; Rowehl, R.; Rivadeneira, D.; Karpeh, M.; Crawford, H.; Dufour, A.; Ju, J.; Weng, Y.; Leyfman, Y.; & Botchkina, G.I. (2009). Phenotypic Subpopulations of Metastatic Colon Cancer Stem Cells: Genomic Analysis. *Cancer Genomics and Proteomics*, 6(1), 19-30.

Botchkina, G.; Wang, Y.; Savitt, A.; Rowehl, R.; Leyfman, Y.; Wang, H.; Zhu, S.; Ju, J.; Zuniga, E.; Das, M.; & Ojima, I. New-generation taxoid SB-T-1214 inhibits stem cell-related gene expression in three-dimensional cancer spheroids induced by two phenotypic subpopulations of colon tumor-initiating cells. *Molecular Cancer* 9:192, 2010.

Bussolati B, Bruno S, Grange C, Buttiglieri S, Deregibus MC, Cantino D and Camussi G (2005) Isolation of renal progenitor cells from adult human kidney. Am J Pathol 166:545-555.

Chen YC, Hsu HS, Chen YW, Tsai TH, How CK, Wang CY, Hung SC, Chang YL, Tsai ML, Lee YY, Ku HH, Chiou SH: Oct-4 expression maintained cancer stem-like properties in lung cancer-derived CD133-positive cells. PLoS One 2008, 3(7):e2637.

Csete M: Oxygen in the cultivation of stem cells. Stem cell biology: Development and plasticity, Ann NY Acad 2005, 1049:1-8.

Dalerba P, Cho RW, and Clarke MF: Cancer Stem Cells: Models and Concepts. Annual Rev Med 2007a,58:267-284.

Dalerba P, Dylla SJ, Park IK, Liu R, Wang X, Cho RW, Hoey T, Gurney A, Huang EH, Simeone DM, Shelton AA, Parmiani G, Castelli C, and Clarke MF: Phenotypic characterization of human colorectal cancer stem cells. PNAS USA 2007b, 104:10158-63.

Dallas NA, Xia L, Fan F, Gray MJ, Gaur P, van Buren G 2nd, Samuel S, Kim MP, Lim SJ, Ellis LM: Chemoresistant colorectal cancer cells, the cancer stem cell phenotype, and increased sensitivity to insulin-like growth factor-I receptor inhibition. Cancer Res 2009, 69(5):1951-7.

Dean, M.; Fojo, T., & Bates, S. (2005). Tumor stem cell and drug resistance. Nat Rev Cancer 2005, 5:275-284.

Desoize, B. & Jardillier, J. Multicellular resistance: a paradigm for clinical resistance? Crit. Rev. Oncol. Hematol. 36, 193–207 (2000).

Dirks PB (2006) Cancer: Stem cells and brain tumours. *Nature* 444, 687-688.

Donnenberg VS, Donnenberg AD. Multiple drug resistance in cancer revisited: the cancer stem cell hypothesis. J. Clin. Pharmacol 2005, 45:872–877.

Du L, Wang H, He L, Zhang J, Ni B, Wang X, Jin H, Cahuzac N, Mehrpour M, Lu Y, Chen Q: CD44 is of Functional Importance for Colorectal Cancer Stem Cells. Clin Cancer Res 2008, 14: 6751-6760.

Dubessy C, Merlin JM, Marchal C & Guillemin F: Spheroids in radiobiology and photodynamic therapy. Crit Rev Oncol Hematol 2000, 36, 179–192.

Durand RE & Olive PL: Resistance of tumor cells to chemo- and radiotherapy modulated by the three-dimensional architecture of solid tumors and spheroids. Methods Cell Biol 2001, 64, 211–233 (2001)

Eramo A, Ricci-Vitiani L, Zeuner A, Pallini R, Lotti F, Sette G, Pilozzi E, Larocca LM, Peschle C and De Maria R. (2006) Chemotherapy resistance of glioblastoma stem cells *Cell Death and Differentiation*13, 1238–1241.

Frank NY, Pendse SS, Lapchak PH, Margaryan A, Shlain D, Doeing C, Sayegh MH and Frank MH (2003) Regulation of progenitor cell fusion by ABCB5 P-glycoprotein, a novel human ATP-binding cassette transporter, J Biol Chem 278:47156–47165.

Frank NY, Margaryan A, Huang Y, Schatton T, Waaga-Gasser AM, Gasser M, Sayegh MH, Sadee W and Frank MH (2005) ABCB5-mediated doxorubicin transport and chemoresistance in human malignant melanoma. Cancer Res 65:4320–4333.

FriedrichJ, Siedel C, Ebner R, Kunz-Schughart LA (2009) Spheroid-based drug screening: considerations and practical approach. Nature Protocols 4:309-324.

Hamilton G: Multicellular spheroids as an in vitro tumor model. Cancer Lett 1998, 131:29-34.

Haraguchi M, Ohkuma M, Sakashita H, Matsuzaki S, Tanaka F, Mimori K, Kamohara Y, Inoue H and Mori M: $CD133^{+}CD44^{+}$ Population Efficiently Enriches Colon Cancer Initiating Cells. Ann Surgical Oncol 2008, 15:2927-2933.

Hermann PC, Huber SL, Herrler T, Aicher A, Ellwart JW, Guba M, Bruns CJ, and Heeschen C (2007) Distinct Populations of Cancer Stem Cells Determine Tumor Growth and Metastatic Activity in Human Pancreatic Cancer. Cell Stem Cell 1:313-323.

Hill RP, Chambers AF, Ling V, and Harris JF (1984) Dynamic heterogeneity: rapid generation of metastatic variants in mouse B16 melanoma cells. Science 224:998-1001.

Hill RP (2006) Identifying Cancer Stem Cells in Solid Tumors: Case Not Proven. Cancer Research 66:1891-1896.

Hong SP, Wen J, Bang S , Park S , Song SY : CD44-positive cells are responsible for gemcitabine resistance in pancreatic cancer cells. Internatiionl J Cancer 2009, 125(10):2323-31.

Horst D, Kriegl L, Engel J, et al. CD133 expression is an independent prognostic marker for low survival in colorectal cancer. Br J Cancer. 2008;99(8):1285–9.

Horst D, Kriegl L, Engel J, Kirchner T, Jung A: Prognostic Significance of the Cancer Stem Cell Markers CD133, CD44, and CD166 in Colorectal Cancer. Cancer Investigation 2009, 27: 844 - 850.

Inch WR, McCredie JA and Sutherland RM: Growth of nodular carcinomas in rodents compared with multi-cell spheroids in tissue culture. Growth 1970, 34;271–282.

Isaaks JT. The biology of hormone refractory prostate cancer. Why does it develop? (1999) Urol. Clin. North. Am. 26(2): 263-273.

Jemal A, Siegel R, Ward E, Hao Y, Xu J, Thun MJ: Cancer statistics. CA Cancer J Clin 2009, 59:225-249.

Jordan MA and Wilson L: Microtubules as a target for anticancer drugs. Nat Rev Cancer 2004, 4(4):253-65.

Kaltz-Wittmer, C, et al. (2000) FISH analysis of gene aberrations (MYC, CCND1, ERBB2, RB, and AR) in advanced prostatic carcinomas before and after androgen deprivation therapy. Lab. Invest. 80:1455-1464.

Kamb A, Wee S, Lengauer C: Why is cancer drug discovery so difficult? Nature Rev Drug Discovery 2007, 6: 115-120.

Kirkland SC. (2009) Type I collagen inhibits differentiation and promotes a stem cell-like phenotype in human colorectal carcinoma cells. *Br J Cancer.* 101(2):320-326.

Kondo T. Stem cell-like cancer cells in cancer cell lines. Cancer Biomark. 2007;3(4-5):245-50.

Kuznetsova L, Chen J, L. Sun X, Wu A, Pepe JM, Veith P, Pera RJ, Bernacki and Ojima I: Syntheses and Evaluation of Novel Fatty Acid-2nd-generation Taxoid Conjugates as Promising Anticancer Agents. Bioorg Med Chem Let, 2006, 16:974-977.

Levina V, Marrangoni AM, DeMarco R, Gorelik E, Lokshin AE. Drug-selected human lung cancer stem cells: cytokine network, tumorigenic and metastatic properties. PLoS ONE 2008; 3(8):e3077.

Li C, Heidt DG, Dalerba P, Burant CF, Zhang L, Adsay V, Wicha M, Clarke MF, and Simeone DM (2007) Identification of pancreatic cancer stem cells. Cancer Res 67:1030-7.

Lin EH, Hassan M, Li Y, et al. Elevated circulating endothelial progenitor marker CD133 messenger RNA levels predict colon cancer recurrence. Cancer. 2007;110(3):534–42.

Liu G, Yuan X, Zeng Z, Tunici P, Ng H, Abdulkadir IR, Lu L, Irvin D, Black KL and Yu JS (2006) Analysis of gene expression and chemoresistance of CD133+ cancer stem cells in glioblastoma. Mol. Cancer 5:67.

Maeda S, H Shinchi H, Kurahara H, Y Mataki Y, Maemura K, Sato M, Natsugoe S, Aikou T and S Takao S (2008) CD133 expression is correlated with lymph node metastasis and vascular endothelial growth factor-C expression in pancreatic cancer. British J Cancer 98:1389-1397.

Marhaba R, Zöller M. (2004) CD44 in cancer progression: adhesion, migration and growth regulation. J Mol Histol. 35(3):211-31.

Maitland NJ and Collins AT (2008) Prostate cancer stem cells: a new target for therapy. J. Clinical Oncology 26 (17): 2862-2870.

Mehra N, Penning M, Maas J, et al. Progenitor marker CD133 mRNA is elevated in peripheral blood of cancer patients with bone metastases. Clin Cancer Res. 2006;12(16):4859–66.

Mimeault M and Batra SK (2006) Recent advances on multiple tumorigenic cascades involved in prostatic cancer progression and therapies. *Carcinogenesis* 27(1): 1-22.

Mimeault M, Hauke R, Mehra PP, Batra SK. (2007) Recent advances in cancer stem/progenitor cell research: therapeutic implications for overcoming resistance to the most aggressive cancers. J. Cell. Mol. Med. 11:981-1011.

Mueller-Klieser W: Three-dimensional cell cultures: from molecular mechanisms to clinical applications. Am J Physiol 1997, 273, C1109–C1123.

Naor D, Sionov RV, Ish-Shalom D. CD44: structure, function, and association with the malignant process. Adv Cancer Res. 1997;71:241-319.

Nupponen, NN, Kakkola, L, Koivisto, P, Visakorpi, T. (1998) Genetic alterations in hormone-refractory recurrent prostate carcinomas. Am. J. Pathol. 153:141-148.

O'Brien CA, Pollett A, Gallinger S, Dick J (2007) A human colon cancer cell capable of initiating timor growth in immunodeficient mice. Nature 445:106-110.

Ojima I and Das M: Recent Advances in the Chemistry and Biology of New Generation Taxoids. J Nat Prod 2009, 72(3):554-65.

Oskarsson T, Essers MA, Dubois N, Offner S, Dubey C, Roger C, Metzger D, Chambon P, Hummler E, Beard P and Trumpp A. (2006) Skin epidermis lacking the c-myc gene is resistant to Ras-driven tumorigenesis but can reacquire sensitivity upon additional loss of the p21Cip1 gene, Genes Dev 20, 2024-9.

Pardal R, Clarke MF, and Morrison SJ (2003) Applying the principles of stem cell biology to cancer. *Nat Rev Cancer* 3:895-902.

Ponta H, Sherman L, Herrlich PA: CD44: From adhesion molecules to signalling regulators. Nat Rev Mol Cell Biol 2003, 4(1):33-45.

Puglisi MA, Sgambato A, Saulnier N, Rafanelli F, Barba M, Boninsegna A, Piscaglia AC, Lauritano C, Novi ML, Barbaro F, Rinninella E, Campanale C, Giuliante F, Nuzzo G, Alfieri S, Doglietto GB, Cittadini A, Gasbarrini A: Isolation and characterization of CD133+ cell population within human primary and metastatic colon cancer. Eur Rev Med Pharmacol Sci 2009, Suppl 1:55-62.

Reya T and Clevers H (2005) Wnt signaling in stem cells and cancer. *Nature* 434:843-850.

Ricci-Vitiani L, Lombardi DG, Pilozzi E, Biffoni M, Todaro M, Peschle C, De Maria R (2007) Identification and expansion of human colon-cancer-initiating cells. Nature 445:111-115.

Roberts TG, Goulart BH, Squitieri L, Stallings SC, Halpern EF, Chabner BA, Gazelle GC, Finkelstein SN, Clark JW. (2004) Trends in the risks and benefits to patients with cancer participating in phase 1 clinical trials. JAMA 292: 2130-2140.

Rowehl RH, Crawford H, Dufour A, Leyfman Y, J. Ju, and Botchkina GI (2008) Genomic Analysis of Prostate Cancer Stem Cells Isolated from Highly Metastatic Cell Line. Cancer Genomics and Proteomics, 5(6), 301-309.

Saigusa S, Tanaka K, Toiyama Y, Yokoe T, Okugawa Y, Ioue Y, Miki C, Kusunoki M. Correlation of CD133, OCT4, and SOX2 in rectal cancer and their association with distant recurrence after chemoradiotherapy. Ann Surg Oncol. 2009 Dec;16(12):3488-98.

Saigusa S, Tanaka K, Toiyama Y, Yokoe T, Okugawa Y, Kawamoto A, Yasuda H, Morimoto Y, Fujikawa H, Inoue Y, Miki C, Kusunoki M. Immunohistochemical features of CD133 expression: Association with resistance to chemoradiotherapy in rectal cancer. Oncol Rep. 2010 Aug;24(2):345-50.

Saiki Y, Ishimaru S, Mimori K, Takatsuno Y, Nagahara M, Ishii H, Yamada K, Mori M. Comprehensive analysis of the clinical significance of inducing pluripotent stemness-related gene expression in colorectal cancer cells. Ann Surg Oncol. 2009 Sep;16(9):2638-44.

Santini MT & Rainaldi G: Three-dimensional spheroid model in tumor biology. Pathobiology 1999, 67, 148–157.

Shmelkov SV, Clair R, Lyden D, Rafii S (2005) AC133/CD133/Prominin-1. Int J Biochem Cell Biol 37:715-719.

Shmelkov SV, Butler JM, Hooper AT, Hormigo A, Kushner J, et al. (2008) CD133 expression is not restricted to stem cells, and both CD133 and CD133 metastatic colon cancer cells initiate tumors. *J Clin Invest* 118:2111-2120.

Singh SK, Clarke ID, Terasaki M, Bonn VE, Hawkins C, Squire J, Dirks PB (2003) Identification of a cancer stem cell in human brain tumors. Cancer Res 63:5821–5828.

Sodek KL Ringuette MJ, Brown, TJ (2009) Compact spheroid formation by ovarian cancer cells is associated with contractile behavior and an invasive phenotype. *Int. J. Cancer*, 124 (9) : 2060-2070.

Sutherland RM, McCredie JA and Inch WR. Growth of multicellular spheroids in tissue culture as a model of nodular carcinomas. J Nat Cancer Inst 1971, 46:113–120.

Suetsugu A, Nagaki M, Aoki H, Motohashi T, Kunisada T, Moriwaki H (2006) Characterization of CD133+ hepatocellular carcinoma cells as cancer stem/progenitor cells. Biochem and Biophys Res Comm 351:820-824

Takahashi, K; Yamanaka, S (2006) Induction of pluripotent stem cells from mouse embryonic and adult fibroblast cultures by defined factors. *Cell* 126:663–676.

Takahashi, K., Tanabe, K., Ohnuki, M., Narita, M., Ichisaka, T., Tomoda, K. and Yamanaka, S. (2007) Induction of pluripotent stem cells from adult human fibroblasts by defined factors. *Cell* 131, 861–872.

Taplin ME, Balk SP (2004) Androgen receptor: a key molecule in the progression of prostate cancer to hormone independence. J. Cell. Biochem. 91:483–490.

Thorne, R.; Legg J.; & Isacke C. (2004). The role of the CD44 transmembrane and cytoplasmic domains in co-ordinating adhesive and signalling events. Journal of Cell Science 117, 373-380.

Todaro M, Alea MP, Stefano AB, Cammareri P, Vermeulen L, Iovino F, Tripodo C, Russo A, Gulotta G, Medema JP, Stassi G. (2007) Colon cancer stem cells dictate tumor growth and resist cell death by production of interleukin-4. *Cell Stem Cell* 1:389-402.

Tsukamoto T, Mizoshita T, Mihara M, et al. Sox2 expression in human stomach adenocarcinomas with gastric and gastric-and-intestinal-mixed phenotypes. Histopathology. 2005;46(6):649–58.

Vermeulen L, Todaro M, de Sousa Mello F, Sprick MR, Kemper K, Perez Alea M, Richel DJ, Stassi G, Medema JP. Single-cell cloning of colon cancer stem cells reveals a multi-lineage differentiation capacity. Proc Natl Acad Sci U S A. 2008 Sep 9;105(36):13427-32.

Vlashi E, McBride WH, Pajonk F. Radiation responses of cancer stem cells. J Cell Biochem 2009

Wang Q, He W, Lu C, Wang Z, Wang J, Giercksky KE, Nesland JM, Suo Z: Oct3/4 and Sox2 are significantly associated with an unfavorable clinical outcome in human esophageal squamous cell carcinoma. Anticancer Res 2009, 29(4):1233-41.

Woodward, W.A., Chen, M.S., Behbod, F., Alfaro, M.P., Buchholz, T.A., and Rosen, J.M. (2007). Proc. Natl. Acad. Sci. USA 104, 618-623.

Yasuda H, Tanaka K, Saigusa S, Toiyama Y, Koike Y, Okugawa Y, Yokoe T, Kawamoto A, Inoue Y, Miki C, Kusunoki M. Elevated CD133, but not VEGF or EGFR, as a predictive marker of distant recurrence after preoperative chemoradiotherapy in rectal cancer. Oncol Rep. 2009 Oct;22(4):709-17.

Yin S, Li J, Hu C, Chen X, Yao M et al. (2007) CD133 positive hepatocellular carcinoma cells posess high capacity for tumorigenicity. Int J Cancer 120:1444-1450.

Zeppernick F, Ahmadi R, Campos B, Dictus C, Helmke BM, Becker N, Lichter P, Unterberg A, Radlwimmer B and Herold-Mende CC. (2008) Stem Cell Marker CD133 Affects Clinical Outcome in Glioma Patients. Clinical Cancer Research *14*:123-129.

Zhu L, Gibson P, Currle DS, Tong Y, Richardson RJ, Bayazitov IT, Poppleton H, Zakharenko S, Ellison DW, Gilbertson RJ. (2009a) Prominin 1 marks intestinal stem cells that are susceptible to neoplastic transformation. Nature, 457(7229):603-607.

Zhu Z, Hao X, Yan M, Yao M, Ge C, Gu J, Li J. (2009) Cancer stem/progenitor cells are highly enriched in CD133(+)CD44(+) population in hepatocellular carcinoma. Int J Cancer, Aug 26 (e-pub)

Part 3

Niches and Vascularization

9

Importance of Stromal Stem Cells in Prostate Carcinogenesis Process

Farrokh Asadi[1,2], Gwendal Lazennec[2] and Christian Jorgensen[2]
[1]City Colleges of Chicago and the University of Illinois at Chicago,
[2]Cellules souches mesenchymateuses, environnement articulaire et immunotherapies de la Polyarthrite rhumatoide INSERM: U844, IFR3, Universite Montpellier I,
[1]USA
[2]France

1. Introduction

Prostate cancer is a significant health concern for men throughout the world, responsible for the highest rate of morbidity after lung cancer, and its etiology still remains unclear (Siegel et al, 2007). Death from prostate cancer occurs largely in patients with the aggressive androgen-insensitive metastatic disease. Conventional therapies for prostate cancer, especially in its androgen-insensitive form, may result in the survival of small population of resistant cancer stem cells with tumor-initiating potential that are believed to be responsible for cancer relapse. Prostate stem cells may represent a major target for mutations leading to cancer as their longevity assures continued presence during the long latency between exposure and cancer development (Pierce & Wallace, 1971; Reya et al, 2001). The existence of stem cells in the prostate is probably best illustrated by animal studies investigating the effect of androgen on the prostate. Castration leads to rapid involution of the prostate, but once androgen levels are restored; the gland completely regenerates due to, possibly, existence of a long-lived prostate stem cell population (Isaacs etal, 1987). It is generally believed that cancer relapse in patients may be due to this small population of cancer stem cells within the tumor mass which are resistant to conventional therapies.

To date, prostate cancer stem cell researchers are facing many obscurities: 1) the amount of knowledge about prostate stem cells is limited due in part, to the small amounts of primary tumor samples available for investigation; 2) complexity in distinguishing between normal and malignant prostate cells based on surface markers alone; 3) problems due to confirmational analysis of data resulted from cell line experiments with those obtained from primary tumor counterparts; 4) although some investigators are strong supporter of xenograft propagation of human tumors, but the mouse stromal environment is very different from the human prostate stromal niche; and 5) exploitation of the prostate orthotropic xenograft, are also difficult to establish, and there are high rates of mortality. However, the combinatorial use of primary samples, xenografts and cell lines will likely provide the tools for the most rigorous prostate cancer scientists who are studying the complexity of cross-talking between prostatic epithelial cells and stromal stem cells (Marian & Shay, 2009).

This chapter briefly describes what is currently known about this emerging field of prostate cancer- stromal stem cell biology, which is bringing new knowledge to a global disease and may hopefully reveal new ideas and targets to assist in early detection, prognosis, and monitoring of prostate cancer.

2. Anatomy of the prostate

The normal human prostate gland is an organ consisting of a glandular part and a stromal part which can also be divided further on the basis of zones and lobes. The outermost part is called peripheral zone (PZ) and it consists of 70% part of the normal prostate gland in an adult man. It is in the peripheral part that most of prostate cancers occur. The central zone (CZ) is nearly 25% of the normal prostate gland. The central zone surrounds the ejaculatory ducts and the prostate cancers in this region are more serious and in many cases they may even affect the seminal vesicles. The third zone or the transition zone accounts for 5% of prostate volume and this region is responsible for the prostate enlargement problems. The last zone known as anterior fibro-muscular zone or stroma doesn't contain any glandular parts but consists of a variety of cells including fibroblasts, nerves, infiltrating lymphocytes, macrophages, endothelial cells, and smooth muscle cells (Figure 1).

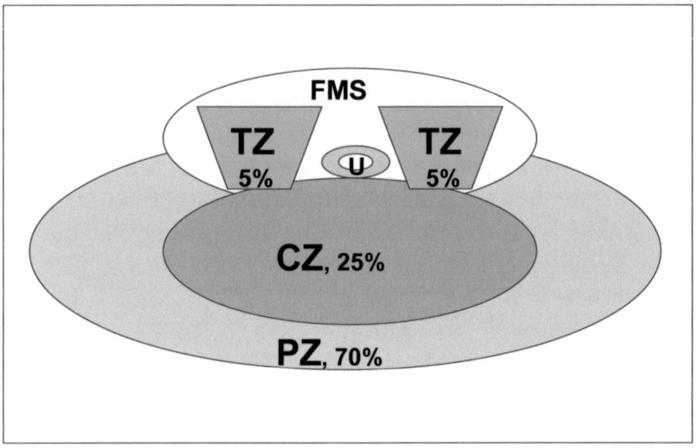

Fig. 1. **Prostate zones.** PZ, peripheral zone; CZ, central zone; TZ, transitional zone; U, urethra

3. Cellular characteristics of the prostate

Glandular part comprised of three anatomically distinct epithelial cell populations that can be distinguished by their morphological characteristics, functional significance, and relevance for carcinogenesis (Abate-Shen & Shen, 2000). **Prostatic proliferative basal cells** form a layer along the basement membrane of each prostatic duct, and **luminal secretory cells** form a layer above the basal cells. The basal cell express K5/14, CD44 (Liu etal, 1997), and BCL-2 markers (McDonnell et al, 1992). The luminal cells express prostate specific antigen (PSA), prostate acid phosphotase (PAP), androgen receptor (AR), and keratins K8/18 markers (Liu etal, 1997). More recently, an **intermediate phenotype** expressing a mixture of basal and luminal markers, with either co-expression of K5 and K18 in the absence of K14 or of K5 together with PSA, have been described (Verhagen et al, 1992; Bankhoff et al, 1994; Xue et al, 1998). **Neuroendocrine cells** are minor population scattered throughout the basal layer and are identified by the expression of neuroendocrine markers such as synaptophysin and chromogranin A. The prostate also contains several types of **stromal cells** including fibroblasts, myofibroblasts, and smooth muscle cells (Figure 2).

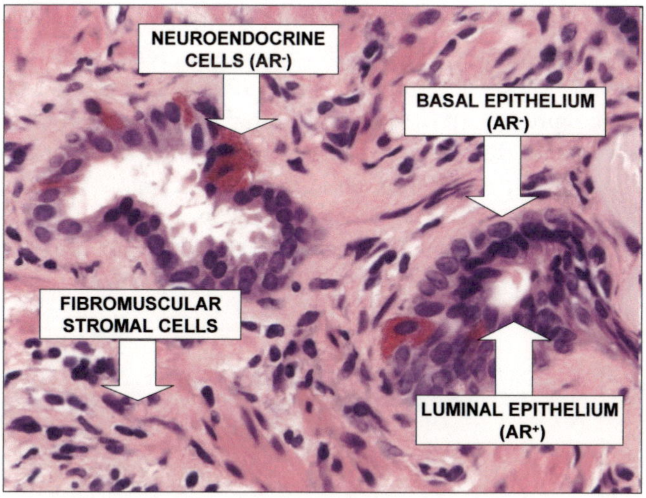

Fig. 2. Hematoxylin-Eosin staining of human prostate tissue, showing both glandular and stromal parts.

A classical androgen cycling experiments suggested that the prostate epithelium contain a stem cell population (English et al, 1987). When rodents are deprived of androgens, the prostate atrophies due to the apoptosis of terminally differentiated luminal cells that are dependent on androgen for growth and proliferation (English et al, 1987). When androgen is replaced, the prostate regenerates and resumes normal secretory function. It was shown that this experiment could be repeated for many sequential cycles and that a stem cell population must exist within the prostate (Isaacs, 1985). These findings have led to the traditionally held hypothesis that prostate stem cells (PSCs) reside within the basal layer of the gland (English et al, 1987). This was supported by findings that mice null for the basal cell marker *p63* were born without the prostate (Mills et al, 1999; Mills et al, 2002; Yang et al, 1999; Signoretti et al, 2000). It was also found that human basal cells express BCL-2, an anti-apoptotic protein that is commonly expressed by tissue stem cells (Verhagen,A.P., etal. 1992). Moreover, it was reported that BCL-2 lies downstream of parathyroid hormone-related peptide (PTHrP), an anti-apoptotic and osteoclastogenic growth factor, in a pathway that controls cellular proliferation and differentiation (Amling, M. et al. 1997).

4. Prostate epithelium differentiation model

The traditional model for prostate epithelial differentiation proposes that the epithelium is composed of multiple stem cell units (Isaacs & Coffey, 1989; Bonkhoff et al, 1994; Bankhoff & Remberger, 1996; Qiu et al, 1998; van Leenders et al, 2000; Hudson et al, 2000) where the prostate stem cells (PSCs) that has unlimited self-renewal capacity but only rarely proliferates residing in the basal cell layer. When PSCs proliferate, they provide progeny that differentiate into transit-amplifying cells (TACs). The TACs subsequently differentiate into either the luminal secretory cells or basal cells which can be easily distinguished by light microscopy (Litvinov,I.V., et al, 2006; Bonkhoff et al, 1994; Bankhoff & Remberger, 1996) (Figure 3). Neuroendocrine cells are not distinguishable under the light microscope but can be identified by electron microscopy or immunohistochemical staining with antibodies against neuroendocrine markers. Number of neuroendocrine cells are higher in the transition zone and peripheral zone than in the central zone, suggesting that they may be involved in disease processes associated with these areas, such as nodular prostatic hyperplasia and prostate cancer (Santamaria et al, 2002). This model is supported by the existence of TACs that express both basal- and luminal cell-specific cytokeratins in both fetal and adult stages of prostate development as well as identification of intermediate cells in invitro cultures of primary prostate epithelium (Wang et al. 2001; Xue et al, 1998; van Leenders et al, 2000; Uzgare, A.R. et al. 2004; Garraway, L.A., et al, 2003; Tokar, E.J. et al, 2005). Several other studies have also suggested basal cells can differentiate into luminal cells in vitro (Robinson et al, 1998; Tran, et al, 2002; Liu, et al, 1997).

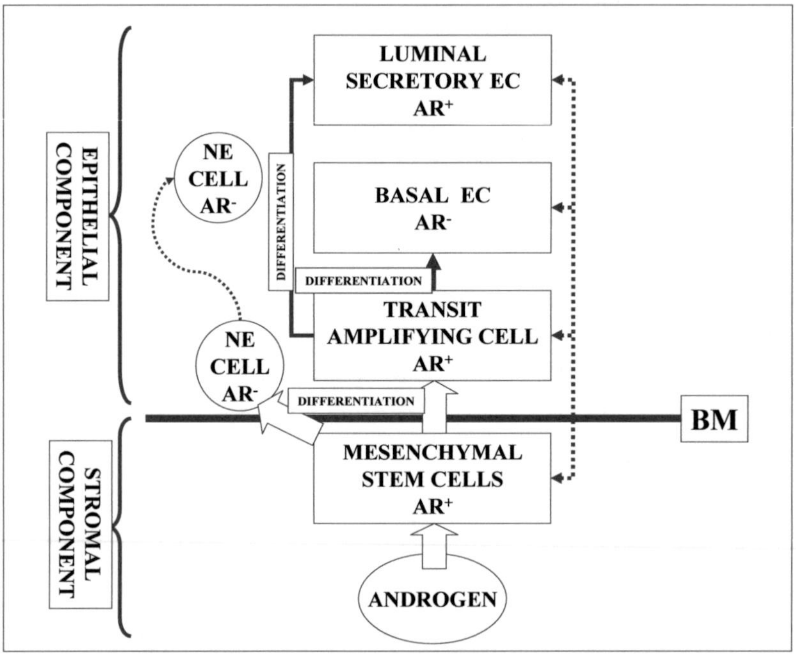

Fig. 3. **prostate developmental process.** Self-renewing prostate stem cells give rise to transit-amplifying cells of intermediate phenotype that may express both basal and luminal cell markers during their maturation. These cells theoretically possess transient self-renewal activity and produce large numbers of terminally differentiated secretory luminal cells. (*Adapted from Yin Sung et al, 2009*).

In human prostate adenocarcinoma, the majority of cancer cells express luminal cell-specific markers such as cytokeratin 8 (CK8), CK18, and prostate-specific antigen (PSA). Cells that solely express basal cell markers such as CK5, CK14, and p63 rarely observed (Okada, et al, 1992). This has led some investigators to suggest that prostate cancers are derived from luminal cell progenitor or mature luminal cell that has acquired self-renewal activity through mutations (Lawson & Witte, 2007). However, some reports have indicated that prostate cancer may originate in an intermediate or transit-amplifying epithelial cell that precedes luminal cell differentiation (Verhagen, etal, 1992; Tran etal, 2002; Reiter etal, 1998). Identification of intermediate cells that co-express both basal and luminal cell markers (Verhagen, etal, 1992), as well as prostate stem cell antigen (PSCA), a presumed marker of normal late-intermediate prostate cells which is often up-regulated in prostate cancers (Tran etal, 2002; Reiter etal, 1998) have been also reported.

5. Prostate adenocarcinoma

Most prostate tumors are adenocarcinomas, sharing numerous common features with other prevalent epithelial cancers, such as breast and colon cancer. A distinguishing feature of prostate cancer is its intimate association with aging, and clinically detectable prostate cancer is not generally manifest until age of 60 or 70 (Abate-Shen & Shen, 2000). To identify specific gene expression patterns of prostate tumor epithelial and adjacent stromal cells, in a most recent study, researchers utilized Laser Capture Microdissection (LCM) analysis and identified nearly 500 genes whose expression was significantly different between epithelial and stromal cells (Gregg et al, 2010). One important finding was the differential expression of *WT1* in prostate cancer epithelial cells that suggests a potential role for *WT1* in prostate cancer. Several reports have shown that the androgen-insensitive prostate cancer cells increase the expression of IGF-1 and IGF-1R compared with the androgen-sensitive cancer cells (Krueckl et al, 2004; Nickerson et al, 2001). A recent study suggests that local secretion of IGF-1 in the prostate stroma mediates tumor-stromal cell interactions of prostate cancer to accelerate tumor growth (Kawada et al, 2006).

Although prostate cancers are phenotypically and behaviorly similar in many respect to luminal secretory cells, recent studies suggest that prostate cancer may arise from a more immature cell types located within the basal or luminal cell layer (Vehagen etal, 1992; Nagle etal, 1987; De Marzo etal, 1998; Bui etal, 1998). In addition, it is hypothesized that prostate cancer, like other epithelial and nonepithelial cancers, must arise from stem or progenitor cells rather than from a terminally differentiated cell type (De Marzo et al, 1998). In the prostate, p63, the p53 homologue, is expressed only in basal cells and most importantly p63 (-/-) mice do not develop the prostate (Signoretti, etal, 2000). This finding suggest that p63 is required for prostate development and support the hypothesis that basal cells represent and/or include prostate stem cells. Furthermore, the presence of surface integrins on prostate stem cells suggests that these cells share common pathways with stem cells in other tissues (Collins, etal, 2001). Basal cells also express the anti-apoptotic protein BCL-2 and BCL-2 expression may help cells resist apoptotic stimuli such as high TGFβ production resulting from androgen depletion (Kelly & Yin, 2008). Most recently, Howard Hughes Medical Institute (HHMI) scientists Owen N. Witte and his colleagues at the University of California, Los Angeles (UCLA) found that basal cells from primary benign human prostate tissue can initiate prostate cancer in immunodeficient mice (Goldstein etal, 2010). Moreover, it was shown that the cooperative effects of transcriptional factors and androgen receptor in basal cells results in loss of basal cells and expansion of luminal cells expressing prostate-specific antigen and alpha-methylacyl-CoA racemase. As a result, they concluded that histological characterization of cancers does not necessarily correlate with the cellular origins of the disease. It may be years before investigators will know whether the experimental model developed by Witte and his colleagues might have a similar impact on prostate cancer. However, scientists can at least now begin to use the model to test suspected prostate cancer oncogenes systematically and in a more efficient manner with the goal of finding new targets for drug development. This chapter aims to outline recent concepts of stem cells role during the carcinogenesis process and bone metastses in prostate cancer.

6. Importance of androgens in prostate cancer initiation and progression

Prostate cancer development and growth is dependent on androgens and can be suppressed by androgen ablation monotherapy. However, due to the emergence of androgen-independent prostate tumor growth, prostate cancer recurs as androgen-insensitive and highly metastatic (Wang et al, 2007). There are two natural potent androgens in the mammal including humans. Although testosterone is the major androgen secreted from the testes, dihydrotestosterone (DHT) is the main androgen in the prostate to mediate the androgen action via the AR. Only one AR has been identifies so far, a member of the steroid/nuclear receptor superfamily, which is a ligand-dependent transcription factor. When androgens bind to the AR, this results in a conformational change within the AR, leading to the recruitment of co-regulators and transcription factors which mediate androgen-target gene expression. Although it is well known that androgens are important for prostate development and for the pathogenesis of prostate cancer, the precise mechanism as to how androgens control these processes are not yet fully understood. Furthermore, evidence for the direct modulation of androgen-AR actions by other hormones within the prostate cells emerging. For example, androgen actions in the prostate can be modulated by estrogens via estrogen receptors (ER). There are two known isoforms of the ER, ER_{α} and ER_{β} , which are both co-expressed with AR in the normal as well as tumors of the prostate (Zhu, 2005). Androgen-induced prostate epithelial cell proliferation is also regulated by an indirect pathway involving paracrine mediators produced by stromal cells, such as insulin-like growth factor (IGF), fibroblast growth factor (FGF), and epidermal growth factor (FGF) (Cunha & Donjacour, 1989; Byrne et al, 1996). In prostate epithelial cells, the androgenic signal engages secreted many cytokines which affects the prostate tumor microenvironment by inducing angiogenesis and stromal cell growth and differentiation (Zhu & Kyprianou, 2008).

Progressive prostate cancer is treated with androgen deprivation therapy, which causes an initial regression due to the androgen-sensitive nature of the vast majority of prostate cancer cells (Webster et al, 2005). However, a major problem in human prostate cancer is evolution of tumor cell populations toward androgen-insensitivity as well as resistance to apoptosis-inducing therapies and their tendency to metastasize. Prostate cancer preferentially metastasizes to the bone marrow stroma of the axial skeleton in up to 90% of patients and this is the principal cause of prostate cancer morbidity and mortality. This tendency arises from complexed molecular pathways that together lead to local invasion, extravassation and distal migration from the primary site followed by endothelial attachment, transmigration and site-specific metastasis. Androgen-induced prostate epithelial cell proliferation and differentiation is regulated by pathways involving paracrine mediators produced by stromal cells and this suggests that androgens are not sufficient to promote carcinogenesis. A key component of the search for new treatment strategies is an improved understanding of the differences between apoptosis-sensitive and apoptosis-resistant prostate cancer cells. Therefore, more effective therapies that can not only eradicate localized tumors but also prevent their metastasis are needed.

As is the case with normal prostate development, the growth of prostatic neoplasms is generally dependent on androgens, especially on 5a-dihydrotestosterone (DHT). Men castrated when young or men with inherited deficiency of 5a-reductase do not develop prostate cancer. Since the first observation (Hugginc & Hodges,1941), hormonal therapy remains the critical therapeutic option for advanced forms of prostate cancer. Multiple strategies have been used to reduce serum levels of androgens or interfere with their function via the androgen receptor (AR). However, the appropriate choice/timing and actual benefits of hormonal therapy in various situations still remain controversial (Figure 4).

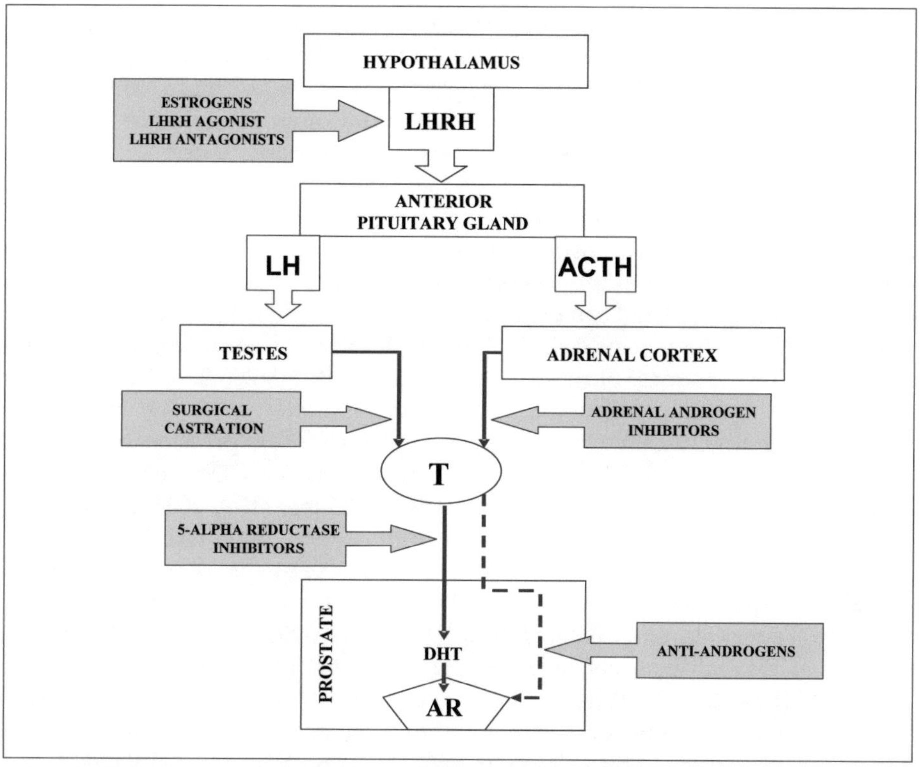

Fig. 4. **Current strategies for prostate cancer hormonal therapy.** LH-RH, luteinizing hormone releasing hormone; LH, luteinizing hormone; ACTH, adrenocorticotropic hormone; T, testosterone; 5α-R, 5α-reductase; DHT, dihydrotestosterone; AR, androgen receptor (*Adapted from Hiroshi et al (2004), THE prostate).*

7. Prostate cancer stem cells (PSCa)

In general, cancer stem cells can be defined as cells in the tumor with a tumor initiating potential. Normal stem cells are characterized by three properties: 1) capability of self-renewal; 2) strict control on stem cell numbers; 3) ability to divide and differentiate to generate all functional elements of that particular tissue (Bixby et al, 2002). Compared to normal stem cells, the cancer stem cells are believed to have no control on the cell number. Cancer stem cells form very small numbers in whole tumor and they are said to be responsible for the growth of the tumor cells (Sagar et al, 2007).

The cancer stem cell hypothesis was described more than 150 years ago (Virchow, 1860), but the new ideas came with the studies done in leukemia, where it was shown that a single cell with the CD34+/CD38- phenotype had the capacity of inducing the disease in NOD-SCID mice (Bonnet & Dick, 1997). More recently, cancer stem cells have been identified from solid tumors (Al-Hajj et al, 2003; Singh et al, 2003). There are several strategies to isolate prostate cancer initiating cells. The most common strategy used is identification of surface markers that share the same immunological profile with normal prostate stem cells. One of these markers is CD44, an adhesion molecule with multiple functions that appears to be important in tumor dissemination and metastasis (Draffin et al,2004; Naor etal, 2008; Ponta etal,2003). The CD44 cells also show properties of progenitor cells, and while these cells are AR^- they have the capacity to differentiate into AR^+ cells (Patrawala et al, 2006). Subsequent study has shown that $CD44^{high}/\alpha_{2\beta1}$ $integrin^{high}$ cells were more tumorigenic than $CD44^{low}/\alpha_2\beta_1$ $integrin^{low}$ cells when injected in immunocompromised mice (Patrawala etal, 2007).Putative prostate cancer stem cells have significant levels of telomerase, a ribonucleoprotein enzyme responsible for telomere elongation, indicating that they are an excellent target for telomerase inhibition therapy (Marian & Shay, 2009).
The progression to androgen-insensitive prostate cancer during androgen ablation therapy has led to speculation that prostate tumors may contain a small population of androgen-insensitive cells that survive and can expand in the absent of androgen (Litvinov et al, 2003). Since normal adult prostate stem cells (PSCs) are androgen-insensitive, it is reasonable to suspect they may be the source of these cells (Lawson & Witte, 2007). It has been described that the primary human prostate cancer cell subpopulation with the highest in vitro proliferative potential is negative for androgen receptor (AR) expression, and is suspected for normal PSCs (Collins etal, 2005). These cells also possess a $CD44^+\alpha_2\beta_1{}^{hi}CD133^+$ marker profile that is characteristic of normal human PSCs (Collins, et al, 2005; Richardson, et al, 2004). Utilizing several human prostate xenograft tumors and cell lines, it has been demonstrated that the $CD44^+$ cells, including PTHrP over-expressing PC3 cells, display enhanced proliferative activity in vitro and increased tumor-initiating and metastatic activity in vivo (Pacrawala, etal, 2006). These $CD44^+$cells are likewise AR^- and express higher mRNA levels of several stem cell markers including OCT3/4, BM11, β-CATENIN, and SMOOTHEND (Lawson & Witte, 2007). Human telomerase reverse transcriptase-imortalized primary human prostate cancer cell line has been shown to regenerate prostate tumors in mice that resembled the original patient tumor with respect to histopathology and Gleason score (Gu, etal, 2007). Regenerated tumors also contained basal, luminal, and neuroendocrine-like cancer cells, suggesting the clone of origin of the lines had multilineage differentiation capacity.
Common anticancer treatments such as radiation and chemotherapy do not eradicate the majority of cancer stem cells (Guzman et al, 2002; Jones etal, 2004). Cancer stem cells resistance to these therapeutics may be mediated by several stem cell-related mechanisms, including replication quiescence, activation of antiapoptotic pathways, and multi-drug transporter expression (Lawson & Witte, 2007). Androgen ablation therapies for invasive and metastatic prostate cancers may also spare prostate cancer stem cells (Litvinov etal, 2003). Research should therefore be aimed at developing therapeutics that can selectively target the prostate stem cell population rather than more differentiated prostate cancer cells. Clinical trials should likewise be designed to measure drug efficacy by examining their ability to eradicate prostate cancer stem cells rather than to measure bulk tumor regression (Lawson & Witte, 2007).

8. Multipotent stromal stem cells (MSCs) and their roles in the prostate cancer

Stem cells can be divided into three main categories: embryonic, germinal, and somatic. Embryonic stem cells originate from the inner cell mass of the blastcyst and are omnipotent, having indefinite replicative life span due to their telomerase expression (Soltysova, etal, 2005). Germinal stem cells are derived from primary germinal layers of embryo, and they differentiate into progenitor cells to produce specific organ cells (Sagar et al, 2007). Somatic/adult stem cells are progenitor cells as they are less totipotent i.e. less replicative life span than embryonic stem cells. They exist in mature tissues such as haematopoietic, neural, gastrointestinal and mesenchymal tissues (Sagar et al, 2007). The most commonly used adult stem cells are derived from bone marrow named haematopoietic stem cells, mesenchymal stem cells, and multipotent stromal stem cells (Kim et al, 2005).

Multipotent stromal stem cells (MSCs), or nonhematopoietic mesenchymal stem cell, were identified about 40 years ago (Friedenstein et al, 1974) in the bone marrow and were described as spindle shaped that proliferate to form colonies. These cells attach to plastic and are able to differentiate under defined *in vitro* conditions into multiple cell types present in many different tissues. The interaction between epithelial and stroma-forming non-hematopoietic bone marrow stem cells or multipotent mesenchymal stem cells (MSCs), such as fibroblasts, play a critical role in the development of both organs and tumors (Nelson & Bissell, 2006). This cross-talk is bidirectional and usually paracrine in nature. Multipotent MSCs have a fibroblast-like appearance that not only colonize numerous organs, but also are attracted to wounds and solid tumors especially. MSCs features include their ability to differentiate into cells of mesodermal lineage, such as bone, cartilage, and fat cells (Dominici et al, 2006). In addition, MSCs may transdifferentiate into cells of ecto- or endodermal lineages such as nerve, muscle, and epithelial cells (Ucelli et al, 2008). The plasticity of these cells, combined with their migratory potential and their preference for injured tissue, makes MSCs an ideal tool for therapeutic histogenesis (Brook et al, 2007). MSCs also enter tumors because cancer cells secrete chemokines that attract MSCs, and increase their migratory activity (Dwyer et al, 2007; Lin et al, 2008). In tumors, MSCs may alter the behavior of the cancer cells and may also differentiate to carcinoma-associated fibroblasts (CAF), which are known to be involved in cancer progression (Mishra et al, 2008). A recent report suggest that hMSCs enhance migratory potential of cancer cells by activating E-cadherin, a protease that down-regulates cell-cell adhesion and promoting cancer progression (Dittmer et al, 2009). Interestingly, MSCs have little effect on the migration of more aggressive breast cancer cells that already had lost E-cadherin. Instead, these highly aggressive cancer cells benefit from the interaction with hMSCs in a different way in that they aquire an increased potential to metastasize (Ditter et al, 2009; Karnoub et al, 2007). Yet, currently too little is known about hMSCs to get a clear picture of what the functions of hMSCs are in cancer progression. Among the many questions that remain are whether hMSCs act primarily on cancer cells as stem cells or as differentiated cells such as CAFs, and whether, under certain conditions, hMSCs may actually heal "cancerous wounds", which would explain why, in some cases, hMSCs suppress cancer growth (Dittmer, 2010).

9. Characteristics of multipotent stromal stem cells

MSCs and MSC-like cells have been identified to exist in and can be isolated from a large number of adult tissues, including the prostate, where they are postulated to carry out the function of replacing and regenerating local cells that are lost to normal tissue turnover, injury, or aging (Chen & Tuan, 2008). There is no uniformly accepted clear and specific definitive phenotype or surface markers for the prospective isolation of MSCs. The minimal requirement for a population of cells to qualify as MSCs, as suggested by the International Society for Cytotherapy includes: (a) they must be plastic adherent under standard culture conditions, (b) they should express CD105, CD73, and CD90 and lack of expression of CD45, CD34, CD14, or CD11b, CD79α or CD19, and HLA-DR surface molecules, and (c) they should possess tripotential mesodermal differentiation capability into osteoblasts, chondrocytes, and adipocytes (Dominici et al, 2006).

Growth factors that have regulatory effects on MSCs include members of the transforming growth factor- beta (TGF-β) superfamily, the insulin-like growth factors, the fibroblast growth factors, the platelet-derived growth factor, and Wnts. Among these growth factors, TGF-βs, including TGF-β_1, TGF-β_2, and TGF-β_3, as well as bone morphogenetic protein (BMPs) are the most potent inducers to promote chondrogenesis of MSCs (Chen & Tuan, 2008). For hMSCs, TGF-β_2 and TGF-β_3 were shown to be more active than TGF-β_1 in promoting chondrogenesis (Barry et al, 2001). PTHrP also plays a regulatory role in MSC terminal differentiation. When human bone marrow MSCs from osteo arthritis patients were cultured in a 3-D polyglycolic acid scaffold in the presence of TGF-β_3, upregulated expression of collagen X was significantly suppressed by the presence of PTHrP whereas expression of other cartilage-specific matrix proteins was not affected (Kafienah et al, 2007).

MSCs are a source of soluble pro-angiogenic factors that act synergistically on endothelial cells to promote vasculogenesis and angiogenesis. These include: angiopoietin-1 (Ang1), vascular endothelial growth factor (VEGF), and growth factors such as platelet-derived growth factor (PDGF), fibroblast growth factor-2 & 7 (FGF-2/7), cytokines interleukin-6 (IL-6) and tumor necrosis factor alpha (TNF-α) as well as plasminogen activator (Honczarenko et al, 2006; Kinnaird et al, 2004). In addition, MSCs secrete chemokines such as IL-8, which is involved in the recruitment of endothelial progenitors (Honczarenko et al, 2006).

The ability of MSCs to migrate to tumor sites has encouraged investigation into the possibility of using these cells as gene delivery mechanisms (Studeny et al, 2004; Studeny et al, 2002). Naïve MSCs have been shown to inhibit tumor growth, prompting the use of these cells as tumor inhibitory cells in vivo (Khakoo et al, 2003).

The importance of cross-talk between cancer cells and other components of the microenvironment has been increasingly recognized. In vitro and co implantation models combining prostate tumor cells and hMSCs hold great promise as a system in which the interaction between tumor and stroma can be manipulated and studied. A better understanding of the interplay between hMSCs and the tumor cells will be important in developing strategies for improved treatment that take into account the influence of the microenvironment on tumor survival and growth.

10. Epithelial-stromal interactions in the prostate cancer

As with many other tissues, prostate formation is initiated as a consequence of interactions between epithelial and mesenchymal tissues. Chemokines, produced by tumor cell as well as by the stromal environment, and their Cognate receptors have been shown to regulate multiple steps during the prostate carcinogenesis (Vindrieux, et al, 2009). Because neoplastic foci arise in the epithelial compartment, the role of the stromal compartment in carcinogenesis has been relatively neglected. The role of epithelial-mesenchymal interactions in prostate formation has been defined through elegant tissue recombination studies performed by Cunha and colleagues (Cunha et al, 1987; Cunha 1996). Their studies have led to the following principal conclusions:

1. Prostatic differentiation requires both epithelial and mesenchymal components.
2. Specificity for the mesenchymal component is relatively stringent.
3. Specificity for the epithelial component is relatively broad.
4. During prostate development, androgens initially act on the mesenchyme, and prostate does not form when urogenital mesenchyme is defective in androgen receptor.
5. Human epithelium and rodent mesenchyme (and vice versa) can be recombined to form prostate, supporting the validity of rodent prostate as a model for the human gland.

The interaction between epithelial and stroma-forming cells plays a fundamental role in the development of both normal organs and tumors (Nelson & Bissel, 2006). Recent studies suggest that cell of the microenvironment of solid tumors constitutes a permissive milieu for the induction, selection and expansion of cancer cells (Liotta & Kohn, 2001; Bhowmick et al, 2004; Maffini et al, 2004). Conversely, neoplastic cells may modify the microenvironment through cell communication proteins, in particular growth factors. Genetic profiling of solid tumors has shown abnormal gene expression in both cancer cells and cells from the microenvironment (Allinen et al, 2004). Elucidating the role of the microenvironment is a major concern in finding ways to disrupt this vicious circle and induce cancer cell apoptosis. Because interactions between the epithelial and stromal components are essential for all stages of normal prostate growth and development, it is likely that aberrant interactions play a significant role in prostate carcinogenesis (Abate-Shen & Shen, 2000).

Decreased E-cadherin expression is correlated with various indices of prostate cancer progression including grade, local invasiveness, dissemination into the blood, and tumor relapse after radiotherapy (Loric et al, 2001; Mason et al, 2002; Ray et al, 2006). In contrast, markers of a mesenchymal phenotype including N-cadherin, osteoblast-cadherin, and WAP-type four disulfide core/ps20 proteins (WFDC-1) are all up regulated by prostate cancer cells (Tomita et al, 2000; McAlhany et al, 2004; Jaggi et al, 2006). Increased levels of the extracellular domain of N-cadherin have also detected in the serum of prostate cancer patients (Derycke et al, 2006). The functional importance of decreased E-cadherin levels has also been demonstrated in prostate cancer cells with its inverse correlation with cellular motility and protease expression (Chunthapong et al, 2004). These changes in epithelial and mesenchymal markers and the loss of prostatic glandular architecture are consistent with the general differentiated phenotype of aggressive prostate cancer cells, although decisive evidence for EMT remains elusive (Hugo et al, 2007). The proof of principal for EMT in prostate cancer has emerged from studies using *in vitro* and *in vivo* models of prostate cancer progression. EGF can induce EMT in Du145 cells due to caveolae-dependent endocytosis of E-cadherin followed by transcriptional down regulation by Snail (Lu et al, 2003), and inhibition of EGF signaling restores E-cadherin levels (Yates et al, 2007). In contrast, loss of the epithelium-specific transcription factor prostate-derived ETS factor (PDEF), which is down regulated by TGFβ, induces EMT in PC3 cells (Gu et al, 2007). In addition, over-expression of PSA and kallikerin-related peptidase (KLK4), both potential activators of pro-EGF and latent TGFβ2, results in EMT in PC3 cells (Whitbread et al, 2006). While PSA and KLK4 are part of normal prostatic secretions, they leak into the tumor microenvironment due to the disruption of glandular architecture during cancer progression, suggesting a link between tissue architecture and EMT (Hugo et al, 2007). The cadherin profile and invasiveness of prostate cancer cells correlates with androgen-insensitivity (Jennbacken et al, 2006), and the androgen receptor is also absent or lowly expressed in PC3 and Du145 cells. Therefore, it is likely that perturbation of the androgen receptor axis has a permissive effect on EMT as aggressive prostate cancer cells exhibit increased plasticity and loose their luminal epithelial phenotype, including androgen receptor expression during tumor progression (Hugo, et al, 2007). Cancer cells may also modify the microenvironment through cell communication proteins, such as cytokines, and MET has been recognized in a number of mesenchymal tumors. In prostate cancer, co-culture of DU145 prostate cancer cells with hepatocytes resulted in re-expression of E-cadherin (Yates et al, 2007). This is consistent with findings in clinical material, in which membranous E-cadherin was detected in hepatic metastasis using immunohistochemistry, and vimentin was absent in the tumor cells. In the Dunning prostate cancer model, mapping of FGF receptor-2(IIIb) in primary tumors, typically where the tumor cells were in contact with the stroma (Oltean et al, 2006).

11. Role of multipotent stromal stem cells in metastatic prostate cancer in the bone

The ability of prostate cancer cells to penetrate the basement membrane and then invade the interstitial stroma to initiate the metastatic process is largely mediated by proteolysis. It has been shown that CXCL12-CXCR4 interactions may play a role in the metastasis of prostate cancer to bone (Tiachman, et al, 2002), and the expression of CXCR4 and its interaction with CXCL12 may aid in facilitating the migration, invasion and matrix metalloproteinases (MMPs) expression by prostate tumor cells (Singh et al, 2004) .
Prostate and breast cancers show a high propenicity to metastasize to bone. Whereas breast cancer triggers preferentially an osteoclast reaction with bone resorption and consequent osteolytic lesions, prostate cancer elicits predominantly an osteoblast response resulting in osteosclerotic lesions, and preferentially metastasizes to the bone marrow stroma of the axial skeleton.(Mundy, 1997). Tumor-microenvironment interactions are crucial in bone metastases and genetic studies using laser captured microdissection and gene expression profiling of clinical specimens confirmed gene expression changes in prostate cancer cells and adjacent stroma (Gregg, et al, 2010). Co-culture of bone multipotent stromal cells with human prostate cancer cell line, LNCaP, induced permanent genetic, morphologic, and behavioral changes in LNCaP cells (Rhee et al, 2001). A recent study supports the concept of permanent genetic and behavioral changes of prostate cancer epithelial cells after being either co-cultured with prostate or bone multipotent stromal cells as three-dimensional prostate organoids or grown as tumor xenografts in mice (Sung et al, 2008).

1. **osteoblastic metastasis in prostate cancer**: Osteogenesis is achieved by differentiation of multipotent stromal stem cells into chondrocytes followed by endochondral ossification. Many stimulating factors have been identified with respect to osteogenesis in prostate cancer. There are three types of endothelin (ET-1, -2 and -3), which acts through the endothelin receptors Eta and ETb. They are synthesized in vascular endothelial cells and are involved in processes such as regulation of vascular endothelial tones and bone formation, amongst others (Clarke et al, 2009). It was shown that exogenous ET-1 induces prostate cancer proliferation and enhances the mitogenic effects of insulin-like growth factor and epidermal growth factor (Nelson, 2003). ET-1 production is a major factor in osteoblast overstimulation and osteogenesis (Guise &

Yin, 2003). Prostate epithelial cells produce ET-1 and its receptor, Eta is present throughout the prostate gland (Nelson et al, 1999). Experiments using an osteoblast mouse model (Guise & Yin, 2003) showed that tumors producing ET-1 act via Eta receptors on osteoblasts to stimulate accelerated osteogenesis. This abnormal activity is blocked by the ET-1 inhibitors (Nelson, 2003). Other osteoblastogenic factors include up-regulation of the Wnt pathways and production of cytokines such as bone morphogenetic protein, TGF-β, IGF, vascular endothelial growth factor, platelet-derived growth factor and MDA-BF (Logothetis & Lin, 2005). A further interesting aspect of the cytokine balance in prostate cancer metastasis relates to PTHrP, which is produced in prostate cancer bone metastases (Boyden et al, 2002). The prostate specific antigen (PSA) cleaves PTHrP and possibly shifts the prostate bone metastasis from osteolytic to osteogenesis (Cramer et al, 1996; Iwamura et al, 1996). In addition, PTHrP is known as an important local factor for osteogenesis by regulating chondrogenesis in a manner that attenuates chondrocyte hypertrophy (Amizuka et al, 2000). PSA can also cleave insulin-like growth factor binding protein (IGFBP-3), which in turn increases the level of IGF-1. This too would have the effect of shifting the axis of stimulation by the metastatic prostate cancer cells towards increased osteoblast activity (Cohen et al, 1994) (Figure 5).

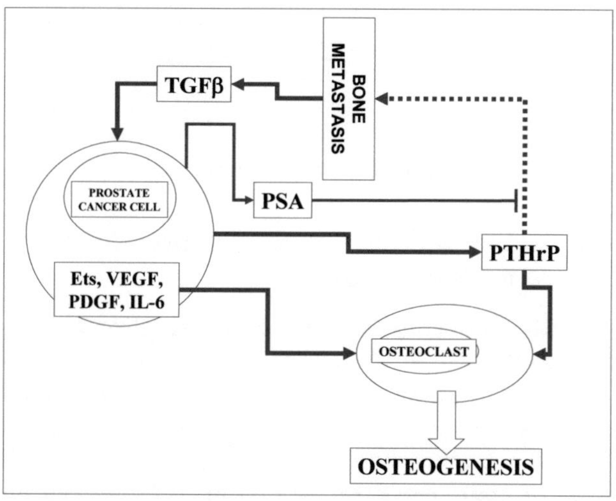

Fig. 5. Model of osteoblastic bone metastasis in prostate cancer.

2. **osteoclastic metastasis in prostate cancer**: It has been demonstrated that osteoblastic metastasis also involves considerable osteolysis (Reddi et al, 2003; Oades et al, 2002). Both the osteolysis itself and the factors released from bone matrix during bone resorption contribute to the vicious cycle of osteoblastic lesions (Clarke et al, 2009). Osteoclast recruitment, differentiation and activation by tumors are related to the osteoblast stimulation that results from osteoblastic over-expression of NF-κB (RANK ligand) and the production of osteoprotegerin (Jung et al, 2004). When PTHrP is present, osteoclasts differentiate in the absence of other stimulatory agents, suggesting that PTHrP plays a facilitating role (Clarke et al, 2009). On the other hand, androgen ablation increases osteoclastic bone resorption and bone loss (Smith et al, 2005; Krupski et al, 2004). The increased bone resorption due to androgen deprivation may result in a

more fertile environment for the development of bone metastasis. Furthermore, PSA is thought to contribute to prostate cancer metastasis through its protease activity and its ability to induce epithelial-mesenchymal transition and cell migration (Whitbread et al, 2006). Taken together, both osteoblasts and osteoclasts cooperate to actuate the settlement and growth of prostate cancer in bone (Ye et al, 2007) (Figure 6).

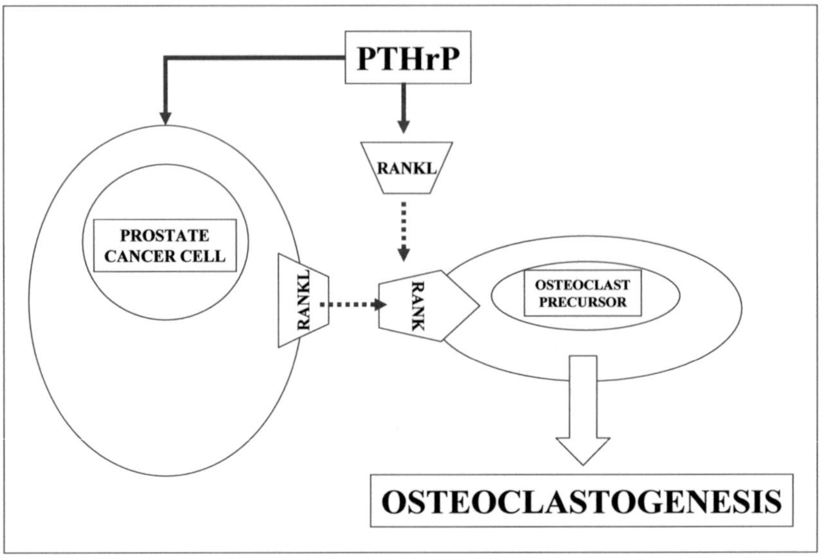

Fig. 6. Model of osteoclastic bone metastasis in prostate cancer.

12. Importance of parathyroid hormone-related protein in prostate carcinogenesis and bone metastases

PTHrP is produced by neuroendocrine, luminal, and basal stromal cells of the prostate and has been immunohistochemically identified in primary prostate cancer tissues (Iwamura ET AL, 1993.) as well as in higher levels in more advanced prostate carcinoma (Asadi et al, 1996). Additionally, it has been shown that expression of nuclear-targeted PTHrP can protect mesenchymal stem cells and chondrocytes (Figure 8) from apoptosis (Henderson et al, 1995). Other studies of androgen-sensitive LNCaP prostate cell lines *in vitro* provide interesting insights into potential mechanisms of PTHrP action. This cell line provides a good model for assessing the effects of PTHrP expression because the parental cell line produces no detectable PTHrP. Expression of full-length PTHrP in this cell line was protective against phorbol 12-myristate 13-acetate (PMA)-induced apoptosis, whereas the expression of NLS-deleted PTHrP in the same cells had no effect on apoptosis (Dougherty et al, 1999). This experiment confirms a previous study (Henderson et al, 1995) that PTHrP acts as an inhibitor of apoptosis.

In addition to anti-apoptotic role, PTHrP is produced by more than 90% of bone metastases (Powel et al, 1990), leading to the concept that local PTHrP production by cancer cells that reach bone promotes the bone resorption process, thus favoring tumor establishment and expansion. The experimental model that has provided the most support for this is one in which PTHrP-producing human breast cancer cells have established themselves and grown as lytic deposits in bone after injection into the arterial circulation of immune-deficient mice (Yoneda et al, 1997; Guise et al, 1996).

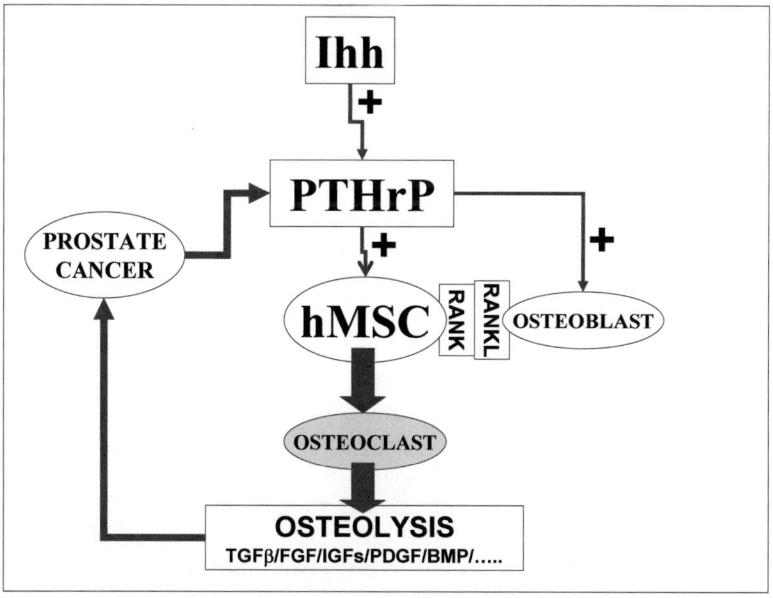

Fig. 8. Tumor cells produce PTHrP that stimulates hMSCs differentiation and osteoclast formation. Stimulated osteoclasts produce potent osteolytic factors that enhancing the effect of PTHrP.

PTHrP was originally discovered as a systemic humoral factor that is released by tumor cells and causes humoral hypocalcaemia of malignancy (HHM) (Suva et al, 1987; Wysolmerski and Broadus, 1994; Rankin et al, 1997; Grill et al, 1998). The hypercalcemic activity of PTHrP is based on its partial homology to parathyroid hormone (PTH) and by being able to bind to the parathyroid hormone 1 receptor (PTH1R) with equal affinity as PTH (Horiuchi et al, 1987; kemp et al, 1987; Juppner et al, 1991). Although PTHrP mediates its calcemic effects through PTH1R, there is evidence for a separate PTHrP receptor (Pearce et al, 1995). This is indicated by the observations that fragments not containing the N-terminal domain are present outside of cells, and that those fragments are able to interfere with cellular function when added exogenously (Soifer et al, 1992; Wu et al, 1996; Massfelder et al, 1997; Luparello et al, 2001). In particular, the mid-regional PTHrP (67-86) peptide, devoid of a functional NLS, has been shown to mobilize calcium through a phospholipase c-dependent pathway in squamous carcinoma cells (Orloff et al, 1996). This PTHrP domain is known to interact with an uncharacterized receptor, but different from the PTH1R in osteoblasts (Valin et al., 1997, 2001; Alonso et al., 2008). It has been previously demonstrated that PTHrP (107-139) can rapidly increase VEGF expression in human osteoblastic cells (Esbrit et al., 2000).
PTHrP is also expressed by non-transformed cells in almost all tissues (dePapp and Stewart, 1993) where it serves specific functions as an autocrine or paracrine factor (Moseley and Gillespie, 1995; Philbrick et al, 1996; Strewler, 2000). In embryogenesis, PTHrP plays an essential role in mammary gland and bone development (Vortkamp et al, 1996; Wysolmerski et al 1998). Disruption of the PTHrP gene in mice leads to fatal skeletal dysplasia (Karaplis et al, 1994; Karaplis and Deckelbaum, 1998). In the developing bone,

PTHrP secreted from periarticular perichondrium activates PTH1R on chondrocytes, therby preventing premature ossification (Vortkamp et al, 1996). The widespread expression of PTHrP in normal tissue was the first evidence that the protein had a role in normal physiology. Normal subjects do not have detectable circulating levels of PTHrP, suggesting that in normal physiology PTHrP acts as a local regulator or cytokine in the tissue where it is produced.

Recent evidence suggests the importance of parathyroid hormone-related protein (PTHrP) in tumor progression, androgen-insensitive and resistance of prostate cancer cells to apoptosis (Asadi et al, 1996; Asadi and Kukreja, 2005; Asadi et al, 2010; Wu et al, 1998; Gujral et al, 2001; Tovar and Falzon, 2002). PTHrP is a mediator of cellular growth and differentiation and is involved in mesenchymal-epithelial interactions in several tissues (Hardy, 1992; Van de Stolpe etal, 1993, Wysolmerski etal, 1994). It has been shown that PTHrP and the PTH/PTHrP receptor are expressed in cells of the adipocytic lineage and that PTHrP signaling by the cAMP-dependent PKA enhances MAPK activity, leading to phosphorylation of PPARγ, the master regulator of adipocyte differentiation, and thereby repression of the adipogenic differentiation program (Chan et al, 2001). Immunohistochemical studies have also identified PTHrP in a subpopulation of stromal cells located in the red pulp of the spleen, primarily in a subcapsular distribution (Funk et al, 1995). A most recent study has pointed out that in oral squamous cell carcinoma a suitable microenvironment has been provided for osteoclast formation not only by producing IL-6 and PTHrP but also by stimulating stromal cells to synthesize these proteins (Kayamori et al, 2010). Interestingly, BCL-2, an anti-apoptotic gene, lies downstream of PTHrP in a signaling pathway that regulates osteogenesis during development (Amling et al, 1997). It has been suggested that BCL-2 serves to regulate apoptotic cell death during embryonic development. In adult, BCL-2 expression is limited to renewing stem cell populations such as those found in prostatic glandular epithelia (Hockenbery et al, 1991). Osteoclastogenesis is a stromal-cell dependent process that is also mediated by PTHrP through receptor activator of nuclear factor κB (RANK)/RANK ligand and osteoprotegerin system (Clines & Guise, 2005). Tumor cells produce PTHrP, an osteoclastogenic factor, that stringers stromal stem cells to express receptor activator of NF-κB ligand (RANKL) which in turn binds to and activates osteoclast precursors and causing them to mature.

Since PTHrP over-expression correlates inversely with androgen sensitivity and results in resistance to apoptotic injuries in prostate cancer cells, it is important to control the level of PTHrP expression in these cells. Recent studies indicate that adenovirus E1A oncogene has strong tumor suppression activities that involve conversion of apoptosis-resistant cells to apoptosis-sensitive cells (Shisler et al, ; Cook et al, ; Yageta et al,; Breckenridge et al,; Shao,). Most recently, it has been shown that expression of the adenoviral E1A protein expression in apoptosis-resistant PC-3 cells sensitized these prostate cancer cells to TNF-α-induced apoptotic cell death. Furthermore, it was shown that the effect of E1A on PTHrP expression was through repression of the transcriptional activity of the PTHrP P3 promoter (Asadi et al, 2010).

PTHrP transcripts are translated into three different isoforms, PTHrP (-36/139), PTHrP (-36/141), and PTHrP (-36/173). They all contain the N-terminal signal sequence for entrance into the endoplasmic reticulum and the coding regions between residues 1 and 139 (Martin et al, 1991; Philbrick et al, 1996; Strewler, 2000). The isoforms PTHrP (-36/141) and the human-specific PTHrP (-36/173) products feature extended C-terminus (Dittmer, 2004) (Figure 7). The PTHrP protein is post-translationally cleaved at a number of dibasic sites leading to the removal of the pre-pro sequence between -36 and +1 and to a limited fragmentation of the protein (Diefenbach-Jagger et al, 1995; Dittmer et al, 1996; Wu et al, 1996). These fragments contain one or more of the three functional domains which are the N- terminal (PTHrP 1-36), the mid region (PTHrP 38-94) and the C-terminal domain (PTHrP 107-139) (Dittmer, 2004). The mid-region domain is able to enter the nucleus. It contains a nuclear localization sequence (NLS) which allows PTHrP to accumulate in the nucleus and to bind to RNA (Massfelder et al, 1997; Henderson et al, 1995; Aarts et al, 1999). Nuclear targeting can be further achieved by residues 66-94 which is recognized by importin β (Lam et al, 1999a; Cingolani et al 2002). The mid-region sequence also holds a CDK 1(cdc2)/CDK2 phosphorylation site. Following its phosphorylation, PTHrP is retained in the cytoplasm suggesting that the activity of nuclear PTHrP is regulated by the cell cycle (Lam et al, 1999b; Dittmer, 2004). The C-terminal domain, also called osteostatin, is able to inhibit bone resorption and, thereby, antagonizes the action of the N-terminal domain of PTHrP (Fenton et al, 1994; Cornish et al, 1997). The C-terminal domain also harbors four potential targets for kinases at residues 119, 130, 132, and 138 whose mutation from a serine or threonine to an alanine blocked the mitogenic activity of PTHrP in vascular smooth muscle cells (Fiaschi-Taesch et al, 2004). The sequence between residues 140 and 173 has been shown to interfere with the nuclear localization of PTHrP and to raise the cAMP level (Goomer et al, 2000; Hastings et al, 2004). Previous studies have reported that the half-life of all three transcripts of PTHrP mRNA ranges from 30 min to more than 3h, depending on the cell type (Heath etal, 1995; Werkmeister etal, 1998, Benitez-Verguizas etal, 1999).

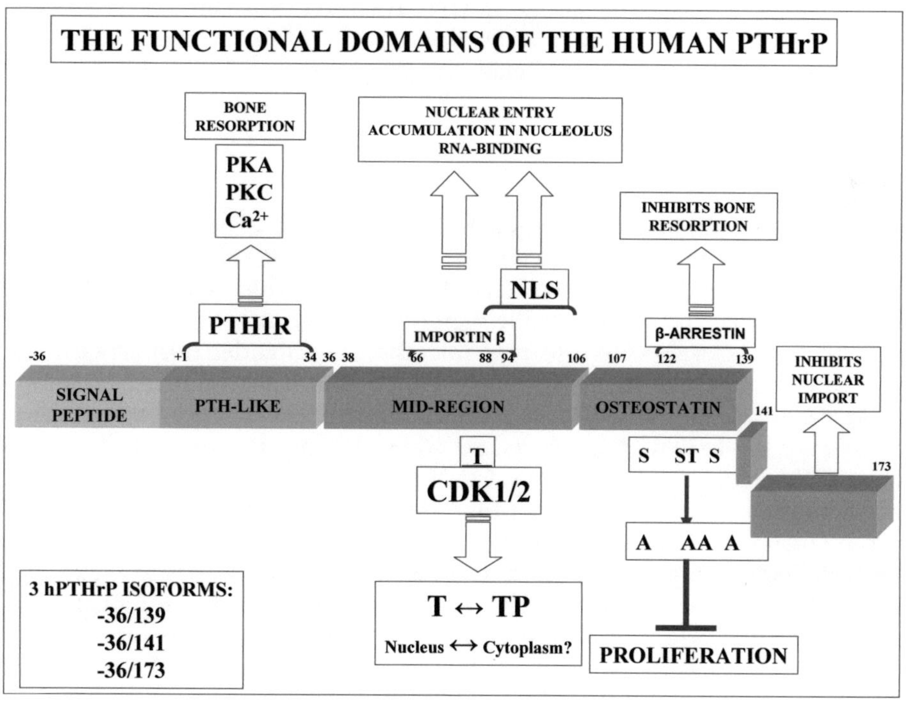

Fig. 7. **The functional domains of the human PTHrP protein.** T, Thr; TP, phosphorylation of Thr ; SSTS, residues :Ser^{119}, Ser^{130}, Thr^{132}, Ser^{138} ; AAAA, alanines; CDK, cyclin-dependent kinase; GPCR, G-protein coupled receptor (*Adapted from Dittmer, 2004*).

13. Therapeutic applications of multipotent stem cells (MSCs)

Despite significance advances in the field of gene therapy for cancer, two major obstacles remain that continue to limit the clinical potential of this approach: lack of tumor tropism of vectors; and stimulation of an immune response (Dwyer, et al, 2010). The fact that MSCs have a natural tropism for tumors and their metastases, can be differentiated into several different cell types in vitro, their relative ease of expansion in culture, and their immunologic characteristics clearly make MSCs and MSC-like cells a promising source of stem cells for tissue regeneration an cancer gene therapy (Lazennec & Jorgensen, 2008). Applications of MSCs in cancer treatment has gained considerable attention, with studies reporting engineered MSCs specifically targeting multiple tumor types followes by local secretion of therapeutic proteins. In a number of tumor models, MSCs expressing IFNβ has been shown to result in decreased tumor burden and increased animal survival (Studeny, et al, 2002; Nakamizo, et al, 2005;Kidd, et al, 2010). MSCs engineered to secrete IL-12 and embedded in a matrix adjacent to tumors were also reported to have a significant therapeutic effect (Eliopoulos, et al, 2008). MSCs expressing the hepatocyte growth factor antagonist NK4 in vivo were also found to prolong animal survival by inhibiting tumor-associated angiogenesis, lymphoangiogenesis and induction of cancer cell apoptosis (Kanehira, et al, 2007). Further, MSCs secreting IL-2 (Nakamura, et al, 2004; Stagg, et al, 2004), IL-12 (Eliopoulos, et al, 2008; Chen, et al, 2008) were shown to elicit an immunological reaction, and to stimulate inflammatory cell infiltration of the tumor tissue. Because MSCs are resistant to TRAIL-induced apoptosis, MSCs secreting TRAIL have been used in models of lung,breast,cervical and brain cancers in vivo, resulting in significant anti-tumor effects (Grisendi, et al, 2010; Loebinger et al, 2009; Mohr, et al, 2008; Kim, et al, 2008;Sasportas, et al,2009). The potential for MSC-mediated tumor promotion, however, is a significant concern and must be addressed.

14. Future research

At present, the cancer treatment is targeted at its proliferation potential and its ability to metastasize, and hence the majority of treatments are targeted at rapidly dividing cells and at molecular targets that represent the bulk of the tumor. This may explain the failure of treatments to eradicate the disease or the recurrence of the cancer (Reya et al, 2001). For tumors in which the cancer stem cells play role, three possibilities exist (Sagar et al, 2007): first, the mutation of normal stem cells or progenitor cells into cancer stem cells can lead to the development of the primary tumor. Second, during chemotherapy, most of the primary tumor cells may be destroyed but if cancer stem cells are not eradicated, they become refractory cancer stem cells and may lead to recurrence of tumor. Third, the cancer stem cells may immigrate to distal sites from the primary tumor and cause metastasis. Cancer stem cells are relatively quiescent compared to other cancer cells and do not appear to have the hyper-proliferation signals activated such as tyrosine kinase. These make the cancer stem cells resistant to the toxicity of the anti-cancer drugs, which traditionally target the rapidly dividing cells (Sagar et al, 2007). In addition, the tumor suppressor gene PTEN, polycomb gene *Bmi1* and the signal transduction pathways such as the Sonic Hedgehog (Shh), Notch and Wnt that are crucial for normal stem cell regulation, have been shown to be deregulated in the process of carcinogenesis (Galderisi et al, 2006; Groszer et al, 2001; Park et al, 2003). One approach to target the cancer stem cells may be the identification of the markers that are specific for the cancer stem cells compared to normal stem cells.

It has been suggested (Cunha et al, 1987) that during the embryogenesis of the prostate androgens do not initiate this regulation directly within the prostate epithelial cells. Instead, androgen ligand/AR interactions occur in embryonic prostatic stromal cells inducing these cells to synthesize and release soluble procrine factors in which their functions are to regulate the growth and development of prostatic epithelial cells (Cunha et al, 1987). Human adipose tissue-derived MSCs (hAT-MSCs) have been recently engineered, by retrovirus transduction, to express the suicide gene cytosine deaminase::uracil phosphoribosyltransferase (CD::UPRT). The ability of yeast cytosine deaminase expressing AT-MSCs (CD_y-AT-MSC) to convert the relatively nontoxic 5-fluorocytosine (5-FU) along with their ability to target tumor sites and micrometastases and to have a low immunogenic potential, makes thes cells a unique tool to convert prodrug to cytotoxic drugs directly within the tumor mass (Altaner, 2008). Previous results from *in vivo* experiments showed that CD_y-AT-MSCs, administered subcutaneously as a mixture with tumor cells, or intravenously significantly inhibited the growth of human colon adenocarcinoma (Kucerova et al, 2007) and human melanoma xenografts in nude mice treated with 5-FC (Kucerova, 2008). In a most recent study, the feasibility and efficacy of CD_y-AT-MSCs as cellular vehicle of the therapeutic gene CD::UPRT in the treatment of human prostate cancer has been tested (Cavarretta et al, 2010). It was demonstrated that AT-MSCs expressing fusion yeast CD::UPRT gene, when systematically administered in combination with the pro-drug 5-FC to human prostate tumor-bearing mice, were able to inhibit the prostate tumor growth (Cavarretta et al, 2010).

One possible therapeutic molecule for prostate cancer is interferon-β, which suppresses tumor cell growth by induction of differentiation, S-phase accumulation, and apoptosis (Dong et al, 1999; Qin et al, 1997). A most recent study describes the potential of genetically modified MSCs, constitutively expressing IFN-β in reducing tumor growth in a therapy model of prostate cancer lung metastasis (Ren et al, 2009). Targeted homing of MSC producing IFN-β, at tumor sites in the lungs was found to mediate anti-tumor effects by multiple mechanisms including induction of apoptosis, anti-angiogenesis and by increasing natural killer cell activity (Ren et al, 2009).

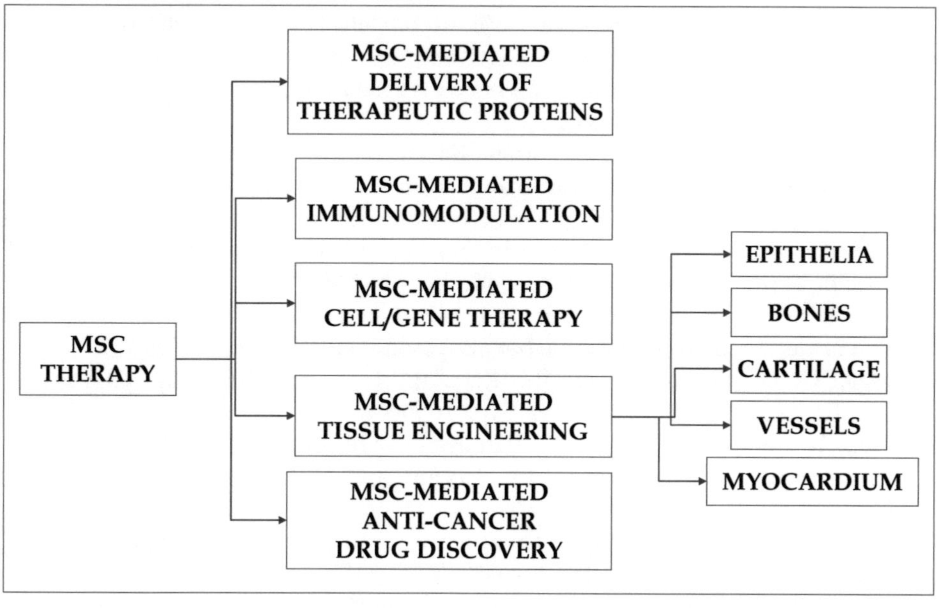

15. References

Abate-Shen,C., & Shen,MM., (2010). Molecular genetics of prostate cancer. Genes & Development, 14:2410-2434.

Abate-Shen, C., and Shen, M.M. (2000). Molecular genetics of prostate cancer. Genes Dev: 14:2410-2434.

Al-Hajj,M., Wicha,MS., Benito-Hernandez,A., Morrison,SJ., Clarke,MF. ((2003). Prospective identification of tumorigenic breast cancer cells. Proc.Natl.Acad.Sci.USA. 100:3983-3988.

Altaner,C. (2008). Prodrug cancer gene therapy. Cancer Lett. 270:191-201.

Amizuka,NH.,Warshawsky,JE., Henderso,D., Karap,AC., (1994). PTHrP-depleted mice show abnormal epiphyseal cartilage development and altered endochondral bone formation. J.CellBiol.,126:1611-1623.

Amling M.,Neff,N.,Tanaka,S.,Inoue,D., Baron,R., (1997). BCL-2 lies downstream of PTHrP in a signaling pathway that regulates chondrocyte maturation during skeletal development. J. Cell Biol. 136(1):205-213.

Asadi, F, SC Kukreja, B Boyer, AM Vales, and J. Cook. E1A Expression Inhibits PTHrP P3 Promoter Activity and Sensitizes Human Prostate Cancer Cells to TNF-induced Apoptosis. *International Urology & Nephrology*. DOI: 10.1007/s11255-009-9699-6, 2010. Paginated issue under print.

Asadi,F., & Kukreja,S. (2005). PTHrP expression in prostate cancer. Review: Crit. Rev. Euk.Gene Exp. 15(1): 28-42.

Asadi,F., Farraj,M., Sharifi,R., Malakouti,S., Antar,S., Kukreja,S. (1996). Enhanced expression of PTHrP in prostate cancer as compared with benign prostatic hyperplasia. Hum.Pathol, 27: 1319-1323.

Barry,F.,Boynton,RE.,Liu,B.,Murphy,JM. (2001). Chondrogenic differentiation of mesenchymal stem cells from bone marrow:differentiation-dependent gene expression of matrix components. Exp.Cell Res. 268:189-200.

Benitez-Verguizas J.,Loarte,D.,Esbrit,P., (1999). Effects of transforming growth factor beta on cell growth and PTHrP in Walker 256 tumor cells. Life Sci. 65:1807-1816.

Bixby,S., Kruger,CM., Morrison,SJ., (2002). Cell-intrinsic differences between stem cells from different regions of the peripheral nervous system regulate the generation of neural diversity. Neuron, 35:643-656.

Bonkhoff,H. & Remberger,K., (1996). Differentiation pathways and histogenetic aspects of normal and abnormal prostatic growth: a stem cell model. Prostate, 28:98-106.

Bonkhoff H.,Stein,U., Remberger,K. (1994). Multidirectional differentiation in the normal, hyperplastic and neoplastic human prostate: simultaneous demonstration of cell-specific epithelial markers. Hum. Pathol. 25:98-106.

Bonnet,D., & Dick,JE.,(1997). Human acute myeloid leukemia is organized as a hierarchy that originates from a primitive hematopoietic cell. Nat.Med. 3:730-737.

Breckenridge,DG. & Shore,GC. (2000). Regulation of apoptosis by E1A and Myc oncoproteins, Crit.Rev.Euk.Gene Exp., 10:273-280.

Broadus,AE., & Stewart,AF., (1994). Parathyroid hormone related protein. In the Parathyroids. J.P. Bilezikian, M.A. Levine, and R. Marcus, editors. Raven Press, Ltd., New York, 259-294.

Brook,G.,Cook,M.,Atkinson,K. (2007). Therapeutic applications of mesenchymal stromal cells. Semin.Cell Dev.Biol. 18:846-858.

Bubendorf,L.,Schopfer,A.,Wagner,U., (2000). Metastatic patterns of prostate cancer: an autopsy study of 1589 patients. Hum.Pathol., 31:578-583.

Bui, M., & Reiter,RE., (1998). Stem cell genes in androgen-independent prostate cancer. Cancer metastasis Rev. 17:391-399.

Byrne R.L., Leung,H., Neal,DE., (1996). Peptide growth factors in the prostate as mediators of stromal epithelial interaction. British J Urol. 77:627-633.

Chen,X.,Lin,X.,Zhao,J.,Zhao,X., (2008). A tumor-selective biotherapy with prolonged impact on established metastases based on cytokine gene-engineered MSCs. Mol.Ther., 16:749-756.

Chanthapong,J. Seftor,EA., Hendrix,MJC. (2004). Dual roles of E-cadherin in prostate cancer invasion. J.Cell Biochem. 91:649-661.

Clines G.A. & Guise T.A. (2005). Hypercalcemia of malignancy and basic research on mechanisms responsible for osteolytic and osteoblastic metastasis to bone. Endocrine-related Cancer. 12:549-583.

Collins,AT., Habib,FK, Maitland,NJ, Neal,DE., (2001). Identification and isolation of human prostate epithelial stem cells based on $\alpha_2\beta_1$-integrin expression. J.Cell Sci. 114:3865-3872.

Collins, A.T., etal (2005). Prospective identification of tumorigenic prostate cancer stem cells. Cancer Res. 65:10946-10951.

Cook,JL., Routes,BA.,Walker,TA>,Colvin,KL.,Routes,JM. (1999). E1A induction of cellular susceptibility to killing by cytolytic lymphocytes through target cell sensitization to apoptotic injury. Exp. Cell Res. 251:414-423.

Cunha G.R. & Donjacour A.A. (1989). Mesenchymal-epithelial interactions in the growth and development of the prostate. Cancer Treatment Res. 46:159-175.

De Marzo, A.M., Nelson,WG., Meeker,AK., Coffey,DS., (1998). Stem cell features of benign and malignant prostate epithelial cells. J.Urol. 160:2381-2392.

Derycke,L.,De Wever,O.,Bracke,M. (2006). Soluble N-cadherin in human biological fluids. Int.J.Cancer. 119:2895-2900.

Di Sant'Agnese,PA., de Mesy Jensen,KL., Agarwal,MM., (1985). Human prostatic endocrine-paracrine cells. Distributional analysis with a comparison of serotonin and neuro-specific enolase immunoreactivity and silver stains. Arch.Pathol.Lab.Med., 109:607-612.

Dittmer,J. (2010). Mesenchymal stem cells: "repair cells" that serve wounds and cancer? The Scientific World J.10:1234-1238.

Dittmer,A.,Hohlfeld,K.,Dittmer,J. (2009). Human mesenchymal stem cells induce E-cadherin degradation in breast carcinoma spheroids by activating ADAM10. Cell Mol.Life Sci. 66:3053-3065.

Dittmer,J., (2004). The importance of PTHrP for cancer development. Gene Thr.Mol.Biol.,8:451-464.

Dominici,M., Le Blanc,K. Mueller,I.,Horwitz,E. (2006). Minimal criteria for defining multipotent mesenchymal stromal cells. The International Society for Cellular Therapy Position Statement. Cytotherapy. 8:315-317.

Draffin,JE., McFarlane,S., Hill,A., Johnston,PG., Waugh, DJ., (2004). CD$$ potentiates the adherence of metastatic prostate and breast cancer cells to bone marrow endothelial cells, Cancer Res. 64:5702-5711.

Dwyer,RM.,Khan,S,Barry,FP.,O'Brien,T,Kerin,MJ., (2010). Advances in mesenchymal stem cell-mediated gene therapy for cancer. Stem Cell Res. Ther. 1:25-32.

Dwyer,RM.,Potter-Beirne, Kerin,MJ. (2007). Monocyte chemotactic protein-1 secreted by primary breast tumors stimulates migration of mesenchymal stem cells. Clin.Cancer Res.13:5020-5027.

Eliopoulos,N.,Francois,M.,Galipeau,J., (2008). Neo-organoid of marrow mesenchymal stromal cells secreting IL-12 for breast cancer therapy., Cancer Res. 68:4810-4818.

English, H.F., Santen, R.J., and Isaacs, J.T., (1987). Response of glandular versus basal rat ventral orostatic epithelial cells to androgen withdrawal and replacement. Orostate. 11: 229-242.

Foster C.S. (2000). Pathology of benign prostatic hyperplasia. Prostate. 9(supple):4-14.

Friedenstein,AJ,Deriglasova,UF,Luria,EA. (1974). Precursors for fibroblasts in different populations of heamatopoietic cells as detected by the in vitro colony assay method. Exp.Hematol. 2:83-92.

Funk JL, Lausier J, Moser AH, Shigenaga JK, Huling S, Nissenson RA, Strewler GJ, Grunfeld C, Feingold KR. (1995).Endotoxin induces parathyroid hormone-related protein gene expression in splenic stromal and smooth muscle cells, not in splenic lymphocytes. Endocrinology. 136(8):3412-21.

Galderisi,U., Cipollaro,M.,Giordano,A., (2006). Stem cells and brain cancer. Cell Death Differ., 13:5-11.

Gao,J., Arnold,JT., Isaacs, JT. (2001). Conversion from a paracrine to an autocrine mechanism of androgen-stimulated growth during malignant transformation of orostatic epithelial cells. Cancer Res. 61:5038-5044.

Garraway,L.A., et al (2003). Intermediate basal cells of the prostate: invitro and in vivo characterization. Prostate.55:206-218.

George K. Chan, Ron A. Deckelbaum, Isabel Bolivar, David Goltzman and Andrew C. Karaplis (2001).PTHrP Inhibits Adipocyte Differentiation by Down-Regulating PPARγ Activity via a MAPK-Dependent Pathway. Endocrinology Vol. 142, No. 11 4900-4909

Goldstein A.S., etal, (2010). Identification of a cell origin for human prostate cancer. Science. 329(5991):568-571.

Golomb E.,Kruglikova,A., Dvir,D., Parnes,N.,Abramovici,A, (1998). Induction of atypical prostatic hyperplasia in rats by sympathomimetic stimulation. Prostate. 34:214-221.

Goltzman,D., Hendy,GN., Banville,D., (1989). PTHrP: molecular characterization and biological properties. Trends Endocrinol.Metab., 1:39-44.

Goto,K., et al., (2006). Proximal prostatic stem cells are programmed to regenerate a proximal-distal ductal axis. Stem Cells, 24:1859-1868.

Gregg,JL., Brown,KE., Mintz,EM., Piontkivska,H., Fraizer,GC. (2010) Analysis of gene expression in prostate cancer epithelial and interstitial stroma cells using laser capture microdissection. BMC Cancer, 10:165.

Grisendi,G.,Bussolari,R.,Cafarelli,L.,Dominici,M.,(2010).Adipose-derived mesenchymal stem cells as stable source of tumor necrosis factor-related apoptosis-inducing ligand delivery for cancer therapy., Cancer Res. 70:3718-3729.

Grozer,M., Erickson,R.,Wu,H., (2001). Negative regulation of neural stem/progenitor cell proliferation by the PTEN tumor suppressor gene in vivo.Science,294:2186-2189.

Gu,G., etal.(2007). Prostate cancer cells with stem cell characteristics reconstitute the original human tumor in vivo. Cancer Res. 67:4807-4815.

Gu,X.,Zerbini,LF.,Yang,Q.,Libermann,TA. (2007). Reduced PDEF expression increases invasion and expression of mesenchymal genes in prostate cancer cells. Cancer Res. 67:4219-4226.

Guzman,M.L. etal (2002). Preferential induction of apoptosis for primary human leukemic stem cells. Proc.Natl.Acad.Sci.USA. 99:16220-16225.

Hall,JA., Maitland,NJ., Stower,M., Lang,SH., (2002). Primary prostate stromal cells modulate the morphology and migration of primary prostate epithelial cells in type 1 collagen gels. Cancer Res. 62:58-62.

Hardy M.H. (1992). The secret life of the hair follicles. Trends Genet. 8:55-61.

Heath,J.K.,Southby,J.,Fukumoto,S.,Gillespie,MT., (1995). EGF-stimulated PTHrP expression involves increased gene transcription and mRNA stability. Biochemical J. 307:159-167.

Henderson,JE., Amizuka,N., Goltzman,D.,Karaplis,AC. (1995). Nuclear localization of PTHrP enhances survival of chondrocytes under conditions that promote apoptotic cell death. Mol.cell Biol. 15:4064-4075.

Hockenbery,D.M.,Zutter,M.,Hickey,W.,Nahm,M.,Korsmeyer,SJ.,(1991).BCL-2 protein is topographically restricted in tissues characterized by the apoptotic cell death. Proc.Natl.Acad.Sci.USA. 88:6961-6965.

Hudson,DL., O'Hare,M., Watt,FM, Masters,JR., (2000). Proliferative heterogeneity in the human prostate: evidence for epithelial stem cells. Lab.Invest., 80:1243-1250.

Hugginc C, Hodges CV. Studies on prostatic cancer. Cancer Res, (1941); 1:293-297

Isaacs, J.T., (1985). Control of cell proliferation and cell death in the normal and neoplastic prostate: a stem cell model in benign prostatic hyperplasia. C.H. Rodgers et al., editors. Department of Health and Human Services. Washington DC, USA. NIH. Bethesda, Maryland, USA. 85-94.

Isaccs,JT. & Coffey,DS., (1989). Etiology and disease process of benign prostatic hyperplasia. Prostate Suppl. 2:33-50.

Jaggi,M.,Nazemi,T.,Abrahams,NA.,Balaji,KC. (2006). N-cadherin switching occurs in high Gleason grade prostate cancer. Prostate. 66:193-199.

Jemal A, Siegel R, Ward E, Murray T, Xu J, Thun MJ, (2007). Cancer statistics. CA Cancer J Clin; 57: 43–66

Jones,R.J., etal. (2004). Cancer stem cells: are we missing the target? Natl. Cancer Inst. 96:583-585.

Juppner,H., Abou-Samra,AB., Kronenberg,HM., (1991). A G protein-linked receptor for PTHrP. Science(Wash. DC). 254:1024-1026.

Kafienah,W.,Mistry,S.,Hollander,AP. (2007). Three-dimensional cartilage tissue engineering using adult stem cells from osteoarthritis patients. Arthritis Rheum. 56:177-187.

Kanehira,M.,Xin,H.,Hoshino,K.,Saijo,Y., (2007). Targeted delivery of NK4 to multiple lung tumors by bone marrow-derived mesenchymal stem cells. Cancer Gene Ther.,14:894-903.

Karaplis,AC.,Luz,A.,Mulligan,RC., (1994). Lethal skeletal dysplasia from targeted disruption of the PTHrP gene. Genes Dev.8:277-289.

Kartsogiannis,V., (1997). Temporal expression of PTHrP during endochondral bone formation in mouse and intramembranous bone formation in an in vivo rabbit model. Bone,1:385-391.

Karnoub,AE.,Dash,AB.,Vo,AP., Weinberg,RA. (2007). Mesenchymal stem cells within tumor stroma promote breast cancer metastasis. Nature. 449:557-563.

Kelly K. & Yin J.J. (2008). Prostate cancer and metastasis initiating stem cells. Cell Res. 18:528-537.

Khakoo,AY.,Pati,S.Anderson,S. (2003). Human mesenchymal stem exert potent antitumorigenic effects in a model of kaposi's sarcoma. J.Exp.Med. 203:1235-1247.

Kidd,S.,Caldwell,L.,Marini,FC., (2010). Mesenchymal stem cells alone or expressing interferon-beta suppress pancreatic tumors in vivo, an effect countered by anti-inflammatory treatment. Cytotherapy (Epub ahead of print).

Kim,CF.,Jackson,EL.,Woolfenden,AE.,Jacks,T.,(2005).Identificationof bronchioalveolar stem cells in normal lung and lung cancer. Cell, 121:823-835.

Kim,SM.,Lim,JY.,Park,SI.,Jeun,SS., (2008). Gene therapy using TRAIL-secreting human umbillical cord blood-derived mesenchymal stem cells against intracranial glioma. Cancer Res., 68:9614-9623.

Kou Kayamori, Kei Sakamoto, Tomoki Nakashima, Hiroshi Takayanagi, Kei-ichi Morita, Ken Omura, Su Tien Nguyen, Yoshio Miki l, Tadahiro Iimura, Akiko Himeno, Takumi Akashi, Hisafumi Yamada-Okabe, Etsuro Ogata and Akira Yamaguchi (2010). Roles of Interleukin-6 and Parathyroid Hormone-Related Peptide in Osteoclast Formation Associated with Oral Cancers, American Journal of Pathology. *176:968-980*

Krueckl,SL., Sikes,RA, Edlund,NM., et al. (2004). Increased insulin-like growth factor I receptor expression and signaling are components of androgen-independent progression in a lineage-derived prostate cancer progression model. Cancer Res. 64: 8620-9.

Krupsi,TL., Lee,WC., Litwin,MS., (2004). Natural history of bone complications in men with prostate carcinoma initiating androgen deprivation therapy. Cancer., 101:541-549.

Kucerova,L.,Matuskova,M.,Bohovic,R. (2008). Cytosine deaminase expressing human mesenchymal stem cells mediated tumor regression in melanoma bearing mice. J.Gene Med. 10:1071-1082.

Kucerova,L., Altanerova,V. Altaner,C. (2007). Adipose tissue-derived human mesenchymal stem cells mediated prodrug cancer gene therapy. Cancer Res. 67:6304-6313.

Lanske,B., Karaplis,AC.,Lee,K.,Mulligan,RC., (1996). PTH/PTHrP receptor in early development and Indian hedgehog-regulated bone growth., Science 273, 663-666.

Lawson D.A. and Witte O.N. (2007). Stem cells in prostate cancer initiation and progression. J Clin Invest. 117(8):2044-2050.

Lazennec?G. & Jorgensen,C. (2008). Concise review: Adult multipotent stromal cells and cancer: Risk or benefit?, Stem Cells, 26:1387-1394.

Lin,SY.,Yang,J,Gold,J. (2008). The isolation of novel mesenchymal stromal cell chemotactic factors from the conditioned medium of tumor cells. Exp.Cell Res. 314:3107-3117.

Litvinov, I.V. et al. (2003). Is the Achilles' heel for prostate cancer therapy a gain of function in androgen receptor signaling? J. Clin. Endocrinol.Metab. 88:2972-2982.

Litvinov, I.V., et al. (2006). Low-calcium serum-free defined medium selects for growth of normal prostatic epithelial stem cells. Cancer Res. 66: 8598-8607.

Liu,A.Y., et al.(1997). Cell-cell interaction in prostate gene regulation and cytodifferentiation. Proc. Natl. Acad. Sci.USA. 94:10705-10710.

Loebinger,MR.,Edaouddi,A.,Davis,D.,Janes,SM., (2009). Mesenchymal stem cell delivery of TRAIL can eliminate metastatic cancer. Cancer Res.,69:4134-4142.

Logothetis,CJ.,&Lin,SH., (2005). Osteoblasts in prostate cancer metastasis to bone. Nat.Rev.Cancer, 5:21-28.

Loric,S.,Paradis,V.,Gala,JL,Eschweg,P. (2001). Abnormal E-cadherin expression and prostate cell blood dissemination as markers of biological recurrence in cancer. Eur.J.Cancer. 37:1475-1481.

Lu,Z.,Ghosh,S.Wang,Z,Hunter,T. (2003). Downregulation of caveolin-1 function by EGF leads to the loss of E-cadherin, increased transcriptional activity of beta-catenin, and enhanced tumor cell invasion. Cancer Cell. 4:499-515.

Mangin,M.,Webb,AC.,Barton,DE., (1988). Identification of a cDNA encoding a PTHrP from human tumor associated with HHM. Proc.Natl.Acad.Sci.USA.,85:597-601.

Marian,CO., and Shay,JW. (2009). Prostate tumor initiating cells: A new target for telomerase inhibition therapy? Biochimica et Biophysica Acta, 289-296.

Mason,MD.,Davies,G.,Jiang,WG. (2002). Cell adhesion molecules and adhesion abnormalities in prostate cancer. Crit.Rev.Oncol.Hematol. 41:11-28.

McAlhany,SJ.,Ayala,GE.,Rowley,DR. (2004). Decreased stromal expression and increased epithelial expression of WFDCI/ps20 in prostate cancer is associated with reduced recurrence-free survival. Prostate. 61:182-191.

McDonnell T.J. (1992). Expression of the protooncogene BCL-2 in the prostate and its association with emergence of androgen-independent prostate cancer. Cancer Res. 52:6940-6944.

Mills, A.A., et al (1999). p63 is a p53 homologue required for limb and epidermal morphogenesis. Nature. 398:708-713.

Mills, A.A., Qi Y., and Bradly, A. (2002). Conditional inactivation of p63 bu Cre-mediated excision. Genesis. 32: 138-141.

Mishra,PJ., Humeneniuk,R., Banerjee,D. (2008). Carcinoma-associated fibroblast-like differentiation of human mesenchymal stem cells. Cancer Res. 68:4331-4339.

Mohr,A.,Lyons,M.,Deedigan,L.,Zwacka,R., (2008). Mesenchymal stem cells expressing TRAIL lead to tumor growth inhibition in an experimental lung cancer model. J;Cell Mol.Med.,12:2628-2643.

Moseley,JM., (1991). Immunohistochemical detection of PTHrP in human fetal epithelia. J;Clin.endocrinol.Metab. 73:478-484.

Nagle R.B., Ahmann,FR., McDanniel,KM., Celniker,A., (1987). Cytokeratin characterization of human prostatic carcinoma and its derived cell lines. Cancer Res. 47:281-286.

Nakamizo,A.,Marini,F.,Studeny,M.,Andreeff,M.,Lang,FF. (2005). Human bone marrow-derived mesenchymal stem cells in the treatment of gliomas., Cancer Res., 65:3307-3318.

Nakamura,K.,Ito,Y.,Kawano,Y.,Hamada,H.; (2004). Antitumor effect of genetically engineered mesenchymal stem cells in a rat glioma model. Gene Ther.,11:1155-1164.

Naor,D., Wallach-Dayan,SB., Zahalka,MA., Sionov,RV., (2008). Involvement of CD44, a molecule with a thusand faces, in cancer dissemination, Semin.Cancer Biol, 18:260-267.

Nickerson,T., Chang,F., Lorimer,D., Smeekens, SP., et al. (2001). In vitro progression of LAPC-9 and LNCaP prostate cancer models to androgen independence is associated with increased expression of insulin-like growth factor I receptor. Cancer Res. 61:6276-80.

Nowell,PC., and Hungerford,DA. (1960). Chromosome studies on normal and leukemic human leukocytes. J.Natl.Cancer Inst., 25:85-109.

Oades,GM.,Coxon,J,Colston,KW., (2002). The potential role of bisphosphonates in prostate cancer. Prostate Cancer Prostatic Dis., 5:264-272.

Okada,H., etal (1992). Keratin profiles in normal/hyperplastic prostates and prostate carcinoma. Virchows Arch.A Pathol.Anat.Histopathol. 421:157-161.

Oltean, S.,Sorg,BS.,Garcia-Blanco,MA. (2006). Alternative inclusion of fibroblast growth factor receptor 2 exon IIIc in dunning prostate tumors reveals unexpected epithelial mesenchymal plasticity. Pro.Natl.Acad.Sci.USA. 103:14116-14121.

Pacrawala,L.,etal (2006). Highly purified CD44+ prostate cancer cells from xenograft human tumors are enriched in tumorigenic and metastatic progenitor cells. Oncogene. 25:1696-1708.

Park,IK.,Qian,D., Clarke,MF., (2003). Bmi-1 is required for maintenance of adult self-renewing haematopoietic stem cells. Nature, 423:302-305.

Parrawala,L., Calhoun,T., Schneider-Broussard,R., Li,H., Bahatia,B.,Tang,S., et al (2006). Highly purified CD44+ prostate cancer cells from xenograft human tumors are enriched in tumorigenic and metastatic progenitor cells, Oncogene, 25:1696-1708.

Patrawala,L., Calhoun,T., Schneider-Broussard,R.,Tang,DG., et al (2007). Hierarchial organization of prostate cancer cells in xenograft tumors: the CD44+alpha2beta1+ cell population is enriched in tumor-initiating cells. Cancer Res., 67:6796-6805.

Peehl,D.M. (1996). Cellular biology of prostatic growth factors. Prostate. 6(Suppl):74-78.

Pierce,G.B. & Wallace,C. (1971). Differentiation of malignant to benign cells. Cancer Res. 31:127-134.

Ponta,H., Sherman,L., Herrlich,PA. (2003). CD44: from adhesion molecules to signaling regulators, Nat.Rev.Mol.Cell Biol. 4:33-45.

Qui,Y., Robinson,D., Pretlow,TG., Kung,HG., (1998). Etk/Bmx, a tyrosine kinase with a pleckstrin-homology domain, is an effector of phosphotidylinositol 3′-kinase and is involved in interleukin 6-induced neuroendocrine differentiation of prostate cancer cells. Proc.Natl.Acad.Sci.USA.,95:3644-3649.

Ray,ME.,Mehra,R.,Shah,RB. (2006). E-cadherin protein expression predicts prostate cancer salvage radiotherapy outcomes. J.Urol. 176:1409-1414.

Reya,T. Morrison,SJ., Clarke,MF., Weissman,IL., (2001). Steme cells, cancer and cancer stem cells. Nature. 414:105-111.

Reddi,AH., Moha,S., (2003). Mechanisms of tumor metastasis to the bone:challenges and opportunities. J.BoneMiner Res.,5:264-272.

Reiter, R.E., etal. (1998). Prostate stem cell antigen: a cell surface marker overexpressed in prostate cancer. Proc.Natl.Acad.Sci.USA. 95:1735-1740.

Richardson,G.D., Robson,CN., Lang,SH., Neal,DE., Collins,TA. . (2004). CD133, a novel marker for human prostatic epithelial stem cells. J.CellSci.117:3539-3545.

Robinson, E.J. et al (1998). Basal cells are progenitors of luminal cells in primary cultures of differentiating human prostatic epithelium. Prostate. 37:149-160.

Roudier,MP.,True,LD.,Higano,CS., (2003). Phenotypic heterogeneity of end-stage prostate carcinoma metastatic to bone. Hum.Pathol.,34:646-653.

Salm,SN., et al. (2005). TGF-beta maintains dormancy of prostatic stem cells in the proximal region of ducts. J.Cell Biol.170:81-90.

Santamaria,L., Martin,R., Martin,JJ., Alonso,L., (2002). Stereologic estimation of the number of neuroendocrine cells in normal human prostate detected by immunohistochemistry. Appl.Immunohistochem.Mol.Morphol., 10:275-281.

Saspotas ?LS.,Kasmieh,R.,Wakimoto,H.,Shah,K., (2009). Assessment of therapeutic efficacy and fate of engineered human mesenchymal stem cells for cancer therapy. Proc.Natl?Acad.Sci.USA., 106:4822-4827.

Sellers,RS.,Luchin,AI.,Richard,V.,Rosol,TJ., (2004). Alternative splicing of PTHrP mRNA : expression and stability. J.Mol.Endocrinol., 33:227-241.
Shah,RB.,Mehra,R.,Chinnaiyan,AM., (2004). Androgen-independent prostate cancer is heterogenous group of diseases: lessons from a rapid autopsy program. Cancer Res., 64:9209-9216.
Shao,R.,Tsi,EM., Hung,MC. (2001). E1A inhibition of radiation-induced NF-kappaB activity through suppression of IKK activity and I-kappaB degradation independent of Akt activation. Cancer Res. 61:7413-7416.
Signoretti, S.,Waltregny,D., Dilks,J;, Isaac,B., Loda,M. (2000). p63 is a prostate basal cell marker and is required for prostate development. Proc. Am.J.Pathol. 157:1769-1775.
Signoretti, S., et al. (2005). p63 regulates commitment to the prostate cell lineage. Proc. Natl.Acad.Sci.USA. 102:11355-11360.
Singh,SK., Clarke,ID., Terasaki,M., Bonn,VE., Hawkins,C., Dricks,PB. (2003). Identification of a cancer stem cell in human brain tumors. Cancer Res. 63: 5821-5828.
Shisler,J., Duerksen-Hughs,P., Gooding,LR. (1996). Induction of susceptibility to TNF by E1A is dependent on binding to either p300 or p105-Rb and induction of DNA synthesis. J.Virol., 70:68-77.
Smith,MR., Lee,WC.,Pashos,CL., (2005). Gonadotropin-releasing hormone agonists and fracture risks;a claims-based cohort study of men with nonmetastatic prostate cancer. J.Clin.Oncol.,23:7897-7903.
Soltysova,A.,Altanerova,V., Altaner,C., (2005). Cancer stem cells. Neoplasma, 52:435-440.
Stagg,J.,Lejeune,L.,Paquin,A., Galipeau,J. , (2004). Marrow stromal cells for IL-2 delivery in cancer immunotherapy. Hum.Gene Ther. 15:597-608.
Strewler, GJ., (2000). The physiology of PTHrP. N.Engl.J.Med., 342:177-185.
Strewler,GJ.,Stern,PH.,Jacobs,JW, Nissenson,RA., (1987). PTHrP from human renal carcinoma cells. Structural and functional homology with PTH. J.Clin.Invest., 80:1803-1807.
Studeney,M., Marini,FC.,Dembinski,JK. (2004). Mesenchymal stem cells: potential precursors for tumorstroma and targeted-delivery vehicles for anticancer agents. J.Natl.Cancer Inst. 96:1593-1603.
Studeney,M.,Marini,FC.,Zompetta,C.,Andreeff,M., (2002). Bone marrow-derived mesenchymal stem cells as vehicle for interferon-beta delivery into tumors.,Cancer Res.,62:3603-3608.
Suda,N., (1996). Expression of PTHrP in cells of osteoblast lineage. J.Cell Physiol.166:94-104.
Suva,LJ., Winslow,REH.,Wettenhall,RG.,Chen,EY., (1987). A PTHrP implicated in malignant hypercalcemia: cloning and expression. Science (Wash.DC)., 237:893-896.
Tiachman,RS., Cooper,C.,Keller,ET., (2002). Use of stromal cell-derived factor-1/CXCR4 pathway in prostate cancer metastasis to bone. Cancer Res., 62:1832-1837.
Tokar,EJ., Ancrile,BB., Cunha,GR., Webber,MM. (2005). Stem/progenitor and intermediate cell types and the origin of human prostate cancer. Differentiation, 73:463-473.
Tomita,K.,vanBokhoven,A.,Schalken,JA. (2000). Cadherin switching in human prostate cancer progression. Cancer Res. 60:3650-3654.
Tran,C.P.,Lin,C., Yamashiro,J., Reiter,RE.,(2002). Prostate stem cell antigen is a marker of late intermediate prostate epithelial cells. Mol. Cancer Res.1:113-121.
Tsujimura,A., et al. (2002). Proximal location of mouse prostate epithelial stem cells: a model of prostatic homeostasis. J.cell Biol., 157:1257-1265.

Uzagare, A.R. et al.(2004) In vitro culturing and characteristics of transit amplyfying epithelial cells from human prostate tissue. J. Cell. Biochem. 91:196-205.
Van de Stolpe,A.,Karperien,M., Bruckner,P., (1993). PTHrP as an endogenous inducer of parietal endoderm differentiation. J.Cell Biol.120:235-243.
Van Leenders,G., Dijkman, H., Ruiter,D., Schalken, J.,(2000). Demonstration of intermediate cells during human prostate epithelial differentiation in situ and in vitro using triple staining confocal scanning microscopy. Lab.Invest. 80:1251-1258.
Verhagen,A.P.,Ramaker,FCS., Aalders,TW., Schalken,JA., (1992). colonization of basal and luminal cell-type cytokeratins in human prostate cancer, Cancer Res. 52:6182-6187
Vindrieux,D., Escobar,P.,Lazennec,G., (2009). Emerging roles of chemokines in prostate cancer. Endocrine-related Cancer,16:663-673.
Virchow,R. (1860). Cellular pathology, R.M. De Witt, London.
Wang X,Yin,L., Rao,P.,Stein,R., Heston,WD., (2007). Targeted treatment of prostate cancer. J Cellular Biochem. 102: 571-579.
Wang, Y., Hayward,S., Cao,M., Cunha,G. (2001). Cell differentiation lineage in the prostate. Differentiation. 68:270-279.
Webster WS, Small EJ, Rini BI, Kwon ED, (2005). Prostate cancer immunology: biology, therapeutics, and challenges. J Clin Oncol; 23: 8262–8269
Werkmeister J.R.,Blomme,EA.,Weckmann,MT.,Rosol,TJ., (1998). Effect if TGFβ on PTHrP secretion and mRNA expression by normal human keratinocytes. In vitro Endocrine. 8:291-299.
Whitbread,AK.,Nicole,DL.,Clements,JA., (2006). The role of kallikrein-related peptidases in prostate cancer: potential involvement in an epithelial to mesenchymal transition. Biol.Chem.,387:707-714.
Wysolmerski,JJ.,Stewart,AF.,Martin,TJ., (2001). Physiological actions of PTH and PTHrP . V. Epidermal, mammary, reproductive and pancreatic tissue. In the parathyroids. 2nd edition. JP; Bilezikian,RL. Marcus and MA. Levine, editors. Academic press Inc. San Diego, California, USA/London, United Kingdom. 275-291.
Wu,G.,Iwamura,M., Greshagen,S. (1998). Characterization of the cell-specific expression of PTHrP in normal and neoplastic prostate tissues. Urology, 51: 110-120.
Wysolmerski J.J.,Broadus,AE.,Zhou,J.,Fuchs,E.,Philbrick,WM.,(1994). Overexpression of PTHrP in the skin of transgenic mice interferes with hair follicle development. Proc.Natl.Acad.Sci.USA. 91:1133-1137.
Xue,Y., Smedts,F., Debruyne,FM., Schalken, JA, (1998). Identification of intermediate cell types by keratin expression in the developing human prostate. Prostate. 34:292-301.
Yageta,M., Tsunoda,H., Oda,K. (1999). The adenovirus E1A domains required for induction of DNA replication in G2/M arrested cell coincide with those required for apoptosis. Oncogene. 18:4767-4776.
Yang, A. et al, (1999). p63 is essential for regenerative proliferation in limb, craniofacial and epithelial development. Nature. 398:714-718.
Yates,CC.,Shepard CR.,Wells,A. (2007). Co-culturing human prostate carcinoma cells with hepatocytes leads to increased expression of E-cadherin. Br.J.Cancer.96:1246-1252.
Yuan-Shan Zhu (2005). Molecular basis of steroid action in the prostate. Cell Sci. 4:
Zhu M.L. & Kyprianou N. (2008). Androgen receptor and growth factor signaling cross-talk in prostate cancer cells. Endocrine-related Cancer. 15: 841-849.

10

Cancer Stem Cells and Their Niche

Guadalupe Aparicio Gallego[1], Vanessa Medina Villaamil[1],
Silvia Díaz Prado[1,3] and Luis Miguel Antón Aparicio[2,3]
[1]*INIBIC, A Coruña University Hospital, A Coruña*
[2]*Medical Oncology Service, A Coruña University Hospital, A Coruña*
[3]*Medicine Department, University of A Coruña, A Coruña*
Spain

1. Introduction

Stem cells within many tissues are thought to reside within a niche formed by a group of surrounding cells and their extracellular matrices, which provide an optimal microenvironment for the stem cells to function. In general, the niche is thought to consist of a highly organized microenvironment in which various factors, such as signals coming from secreted cytokines, extracellular matrix interactions, and intercellular adhesion, are thought to work cooperatively to maintain the undifferentiated stem cell phenotype. Among stem cells, adult stem cells are often localized into specific niches where they utilize many, but not necessarily all, of the external and intrinsic factors used by the embryonic counterparts in selecting a specific fate. Within the niche, stem cells are able to maintain their ability for self-renewal as well as their potential so that, consequently, detachment from the niche compartment induces stem cell differentiation and loss of self-renewal. Thus, when a stem cell begins to divide, it is thought that one daughter cell remains into niche to replace the original stem cell whereas other daughter cell is expelled out of niche and starts its process of differentiation. In this process, a cell retains self-renewal and differentiation inhibitory factors, so that keep being stem cell, whereas another daughter cell is destined to proliferate during a certain number of divisions for finally differentiate along a particular lineage. This latter daughter cell will receive too few stemness factors to maintain as stem cell, and/or inherit proliferation and/or differentiation factors that can overcome its stem cell phenotype. To maintain tissue homeostasis and correct functioning of organism, the number of daughter cells that retain stem cell identity must be strictly controlled such that differentiated cells can be generated in response to any injury. Likewise, the rate of division of stem cells into niche must be tightly controlled since an overproduction of daughter cells destined to be differentiated may be harmful because may result in cancer generation. In the present chapter, we speculate cancer stem cell niche for as well as the mechanisms that influence on the generation of daughter cells.

2. General concept

The concept of a stem cell niche was first proposed in 1978 by Schofield (Schofield, 2004), as a specific microenvironment in which adult stems cells reside in their tissue of origin.

Within the niche, stem cells are able to maintain their ability for self-renewal, as well as their multipotentially, and consequently, detachment from the niche compartment induces stem cell differentiation and loss of self-renewal.

The ability of stem cells to reside within niches is an evolutionarily conserved phenomenon. Adult stem cells are often localized to specific niches where they utilize many, but not necessarily all, of the external and intrinsic cues used by the embryonic counterparts in selecting a specific fate.

The regulation of the stem cell niche can therefore directly dictate the characteristic of an organ, and it is common that the regulation of the stem cell niche has a major influence on the function and morphology of an organ. This flexible regulation of the stem cell niche could have been a relatively easy way to acquire radically different stem cells types during evolution.

Stem cells within many tissues are thought to reside within a niche formed by a group of surrounding cells and their extracellular matrices, which provide an optimal microenvironment for the stem cells to function. In general, the niche is thought to consist of a highly organized microenvironment in which various factors, such as secreted cytokines, extracellular matrix interactions, and intercellular adhesion, are thought to work cooperatively to maintain the undifferentiated stem cell phenotype (Conti et al., 2005).

The identification of a niche within any tissue involves knowledge of the location of the stem cells. According to literature reported, to prove that a niche is present, the stem cell must be removed and subsequently replaced while the niche persists, providing support to the remaining exogenous cells (Sprandling et al., 2001).

Conceptually, a stem cell niche is a recess in a supporting medium that provides protection and nourishment to an individual, yet exclusion from molecules that may cause differentiation or mutation. Then, where the niche is well defined, the stem cells are virtually enveloped by differentiated cells, specialized to house and interact with the stem cells (Tulina & Matrevis, 2001; Morrison et al., 1997). The protective niches are composed not only of stem cells but also a diverse gathering of neighbouring differentiated cell types which secrete and organize a rich milieu of extracellular matrix and other factors that allow stem cells to manifest their unique intrinsic properties, including the ability to self renew, while keeping their pack-set of differentiation programs on hold. It is the combination of the intrinsic characteristics of stem cells and their microenvironment that shapes their properties and defines their potential.

Various lines of evidence suggest that once a stem cell niche is formed in a tissue, stem cells take up long-term residence there. Inside the niche, stem cells are often quiescent; outside the niche, stem cells must either possess sufficient intrinsic factors to overcome differentiation or succumb too much of fate. Direct physical interactions between stem cells and their non stem cell neighbours in the niche are critical in keeping stem cells in this specialized compartment and in maintaining stem cell character.

The niche is critical in maintaining the intrinsic self-renewing; undifferentiated character of the resident stem cells and the niche's microenvironments is both proliferation- and differentiation-inhibitory. The normal microenvironment, established by signals from the various other cells (stroma) that normally surround the niche seen to be important in maintaining the slow-cycling properties of labelled-retaining cells (LRCs) and keeping them in reserve. When stem cells cannot be identified or isolated in a particular organ, their existence may be inferred from kinetics studies of 5´-bromo-2´-deoxyuridine (BrdU) incorporation. Because stem cells are believed to be slowly dividing, the presence of labelled-retaining cells can identify the anatomical location of a stem cell niche.

Niche function

The protective niches are composed not only of stem cells but also a diverse gathering of neighbouring differentiated cells types which secrete and organize a rich milieu of extracellular matrix and other factors that allow stem cells to manifest their unique intrinsic properties, including the ability to self renew, while keeping their repertoire of differentiation programs on hold.

Without the appropriate microenvironment of specific intracellular interactions and cellular organization, the stem cell can become an undesirable beast; it is the combination of the intrinsic characteristics of stem cells and their microenvironment that shapes their properties and defines their potential. Direct physical interactions between stem cells and their non stem cell neighbours in the niche are critical in keeping stem cells in this specialized compartment and in maintaining stem cell character.

Regulating stem cell self-renewal is an essential feature of the niche. In the niche, regulating the balance between symmetric and asymmetric stem cell divisions becomes critical in maintaining proper stem cell number within the niche and in meeting the demand for differentiated cells within its surrounding tissue.

For a daughter to be a stem cell, it must retain self-renewal ad differentiation inhibitory factors. For a daughter destined to proliferate and differentiate along a particular lineage, this progeny cell must either receive too few stemness factors to maintain this state, and/or inherit proliferation and/or differentiation factors that can overcome this state.

To maintain tissue homeostasis, the number of daughter cells that retain stem cell identity must be strictly controlled such that differentiated cells can be generated in response to, for example wounding while the stem cell pool is simultaneously replenished but not expanded. The stem cells physically attach to the niche and, when they divide, orient their mitotic spindles with respect to the niche, so that one daughter inherits the attachment and stays in the niche, whereas the other daughter is displaced away from the niche and activates expression of genes that launch this cell along the differentiation pathway (Chen & McKearin, 2003; Kiger et al., 2000; Xie & Spradling, 2000; Yamashita et al., 2003).

The regulatory mechanisms of stem cell division within the niche to produce, on average, one stem cell and one cell committed to differentiate is as yet unknown, although there is no shortage of potential models (Loeffler & Roeder, 2002). When a stem cell divides, the possible outcomes are that two stem cells (A) are produced, that two daughter cells destined

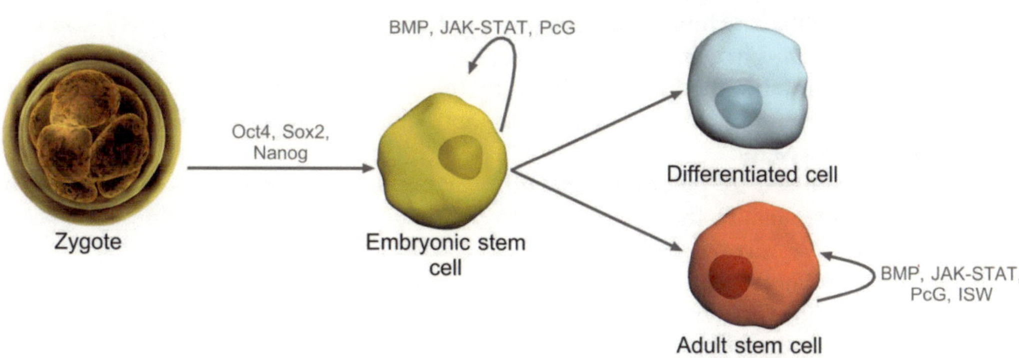

Fig. 1. Stem cell division.

to differentiate (B) cells are produced, or that there could be an asymmetric division resulting in one A and one B cell.

The process by which stem cells give rise to terminally differentiated cells occurs through a variety of committed progenitor cells (or transient amplifying cells), often overlapping in their differentiation capacity. During commitment, stem cells can undergo extensive proliferation and sequential differentiation, accompanied by a decrease in self-renewal capability to produce mature cells. The primary function of this transit population is to increase the number of mature cells produced by each stem cell division.

3. Structural architecture of the niche

Known niches are turning out to contain a high level of structural and regulatory complexity both in number and diversity cells. The association of stem cells with niches is also dynamic, and the same type of stem cell can use different niches at different times or under different physiological conditions.

The nature of the niche in terms of its composition and in the aspects of stem cell microenvironment is still not understood. The environment of the stem cells, the stem cell niche, defines the properties of the stem cell as much as the stem cell itself. The niche can be identified as the environment that sustains the stem cell population and is instructive in the differentiation and proliferation of the progeny.

Emerging evidence indicates that a specialized microenvironment, the stem cell niche, is one of the factors regulating normal stem cell maintenance and self-renewal. The stem cell niche controls stem cell maintenance and the crucial choice between self-renewal and the initiation of differentiation (Sprandling et al., 2001). Thus stem cells appear to require paracrine signals from the cellular niche in which they reside to maintain their identity and self-renewal capacity. As a result, the number of stem cells within a particular tissue can be regulated by controlling the number or size of available niches.

There is ample evidence that the maintenance of a functional tissue (i.e. epithelium) results from extensive regulation by and interaction with components of the extracellular matrix (ECM). Retention and loss of stem cells from the niche may be best achieved by regulating their adhesion to the ECM. No unequivocal molecular determinant of the stem cell niche has yet been identified, but there is an enormous potential for cross-talk between niche stem cells and the ECM. Mesenchymal matrix, subepithelial fibroblast, and myofibroblast may play a crucial role in defining the stem cell niche.

The molecular glue that anchors stem cells (SCs) to their niches is at least in part E-cadherin, which along with its partner, β-catenin in vertebrates, concentrates at stem cell niche borders. Cadherins and catenins participate in the formation of specialized intercellular junctions, called adherent junctions, which can be remodelled by virtue of their association with the actin cytoskeleton.

N-cadherin is expressed by putative stem/progenitor cells in the epithelial stem cell niche. N-cadherin is a member of the classic cadherin family that mediates cell-to-cell adhesion (Takeichi, 1991). N-cadherin may be a critical cell-to-cell adhesion molecule between epithelial stem/progenitor cells and their corresponding niche cells in the epithelium.

Other putative players in establishing stem cell relation are the integrins, which mediate adhesion of cells to a basal lamina composed of extracellular matrix (ECM). Elevated levels of integrins are often characteristic of stem cells, and loss function studies (in mice) reveal that both integrins and adherent functions play a critical roles in maintaining the location,

adhesiveness , and proliferative status of epithelial cells within tissues (Watt & Hohar, 2000). β_1-integrins, specially ($\alpha_4\beta 1$, $\alpha_5\beta_1$) have been reported to play a vital role in the early interaction of hematopoietic progenitor cells (HPCs) with the bone marrow (BM) niche (Voura et al., 1997; Papayannopoulou et al., 2001).
Adhesion between SCs and the surrounding support cells is important for holding stem cells within the niche, close to self-renewal signals and away from differentiation cues. Clusters of adherent junction are observed between stem cells and adjacent cells.
Gap junction intercellular communication via transfer of small molecules may also be involved in the survival and differentiation of early stem cells. The presence of *gap junctions* between SCs and adjacent support cells, coupled with the eventual loss of SCs, suggest that signaling via *gap junctions* may play a role in stem cell maintenance or may help physically maintain SCs in their niche.
Niche is in essence different, although there might be similarities in their structural architecture.

Microenvironment

The development of the most organs in vertebrates depends on a complex set of inductive interactions between epithelium and mesenchyme. These sequential and reciprocal interactions lead to the determination of stem cell fate and the organization of cells into tissues and organs. In the development, changes in gene expression patterns of several growths factors, transition factors, cell surface molecules, and structural molecules of the extracellular matrix have been implicated during the progressive determination of epithelial and mesenchymal cells. Similarly, in stem cell biology the niche describes the specialized microenvironment that supports stem cell maintenance and actively regulates cell function and proliferation (Li & Neaves, 2006; Yin & Li, 2006; Zhang & Li, 2008). A similar model has been suggested to delineate the interactions of malignant cells with their microenvironment at the primary tumor and at metastatic sites (Scadden, 2006; Sneddon & Werb, 2007; Psaila et al., 2006).
This microenvironment comprises supportive (non-malignant) stromal cells, soluble factors, vascular networks, nutrients and metabolic components, and the structural extracellular matrix (ECM) architecture (Folkman, 2002; Weigelt & Bissell, 2008; Joyce & Hanahan, 2004). A tumor-permissive immunological of inflammatory microenvironment is also required (Mantovani et al., 2008). Similar to stem cells, cancer cells seem to reside within highly distinct microenvironments, supported by uniquely specialized carcinoma-associated fibroblasts (Kalluri & Zeisberg , 2006). Epithelial-mesenchymal transition requires loss of cell-cell contacts and gain of cell motility.

Stroma

The stromal cells are the most important constituent of the niche structure, and they play important roles in both structural and functional maintenance and promotion for subsequent development as a matter of basic physiological need. The shaping of the niche structure is under continuous dynamics, most possibly due to regeneration oriented need of the constituent factors within the niche entity. Indeed as early as in 1978 (Schofield, 1978) has discussed about the stem cell niche where it was proposed that adult stem cells reside within a complex microenvironment of different cell types and extra-cellular matrix molecules that dictate stem cell self-renewal and progeny production in vivo (Schofield, 1978; Owen, 1998). Subsequent to the these first works it was propounded that the stromal cells should be the following criteria: they are found in the extravascular compartment, they participate in providing physical and functional support for the stem cells, they are not of stem cell lineage, and they are numbers of stromal system (Scadden, 2006; Deans & Moseley, 2000; Blau et al., 2001).

The stromal cells are now known to constitute a group of cells that act as the supportive "mattress" on which the maturing precursor stem and the progenitor cells rest directly (Bianco & Riminucci, 1998). The stromal cells exert their effect on stem cell via direct cell-cell interaction as well as by releasing soluble factors (Ryan et al., 1991; Dittel et al., 1993; Watt, 2000). It is also presumed that normal cells in turn also might receive signals provided stem cells. Stromal cells provide extrinsic signals that maintain the stem cell niche and regulate the repopulation of stem cells. However, very little is known about the structural microcompartments as well as the factors that govern the growth, maintenance and localization of stromal cells. The formulation of stromal structure engraved in the form of a matrix and their role in constituting microenvironment nest the niche (Law & Chaudhuri, 2007), but the crosstalk between stromal cells for the generation of healthy stem cells are yet to explore (Rattis et al., 2004).

The presence nearly the niche of cell types termed the stromal cells, including fibroblast, macrophages, the reticular cells and adipocytes are all known to exhibit phagocytic activity under the event of emergency. They can act as the scavenger cells to clear up the niche structure and provide potential protective machinery against the foreign invasion.

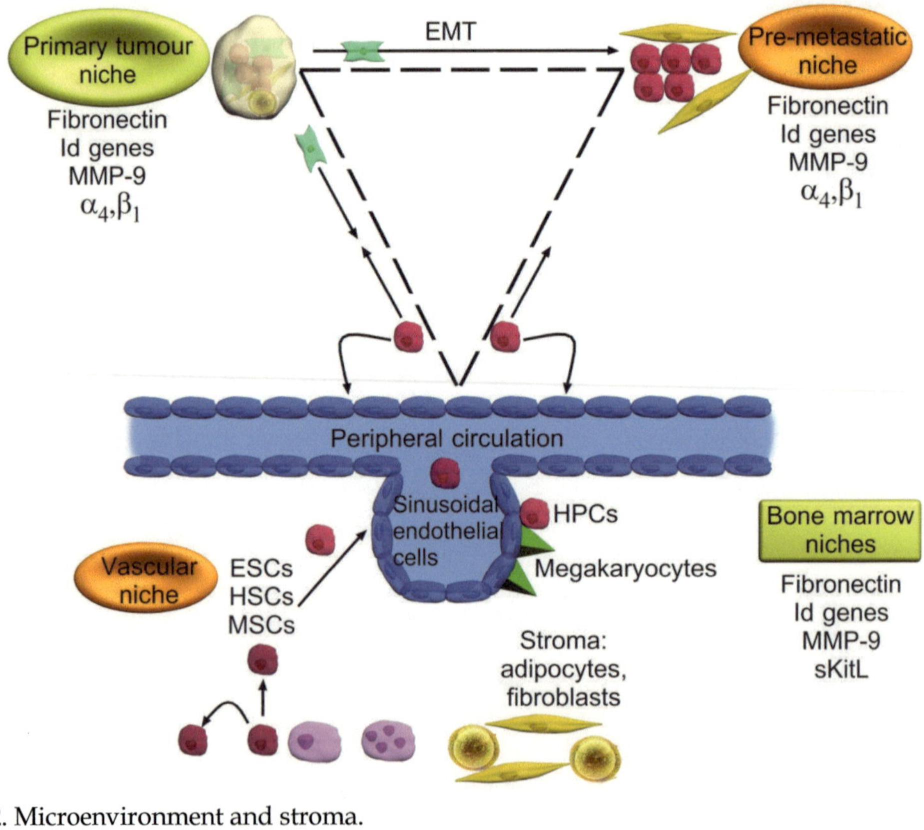

Fig. 2. Microenvironment and stroma.

Presumably, they form an immunological barrier surrounding the in vivo niche (Scadden, 2006). Stromal cell exhibit cytotoxic and phagocytic activity, and constitute the machinery of antigen presenting cell (APC) along with the stromal cell association as is found with the macrophages and the dendritic cells (Sujata & Chauduri, 2008).

Cancer cells and their associated stromal cells secrete a multitude of chemokines that direct the migration, proliferation, and differentiation of the vascular cell network to support the primary tumor and metastatic environment. A growing body of evidence recognizes the multiple signal transduction pathways, the details of the epithelial-to-mesenchymal transition, and the contribution of cell-to-cell and cell-to-matrix interaction as essential elements of the complex multistep process of metastasis. Molecular cross-talk between tumor-stromal as well as stromal-stromal components may enable synergy in the promotion of tumor progression (Burger & Kipps, 2006; Orimo et al., 2005). Also there are demonstrated that SDF-1 gradients mediate HSC retention within bone marrow niches, and growing evidence suggests that CXCR4-expressing cancer cells home to bone is a similar fashion, where they may lodge in the pre-existing supportive stromal microenvironment (Muller et al., 2001; Kaifi et al., 200). Stromal derived factor (SDF)-1, as is the case in bone marrow stroma, was highly expressed mediating recruitment and adherence of $CSCR4^{+}$ expressing tumor cells (Kucia et al., 2005).

Inflammatory cells

The intriguing association between tumor and inflammation has long been a subject of research (Cousens & Werb, 2002). To date, little is known about the pro-inflammatory secreted factors that mediate the crosstalk inside the niche. Recently there are demonstrated that primary tumor cells secrete TGFβ, and TNFα, inducing the expression of the

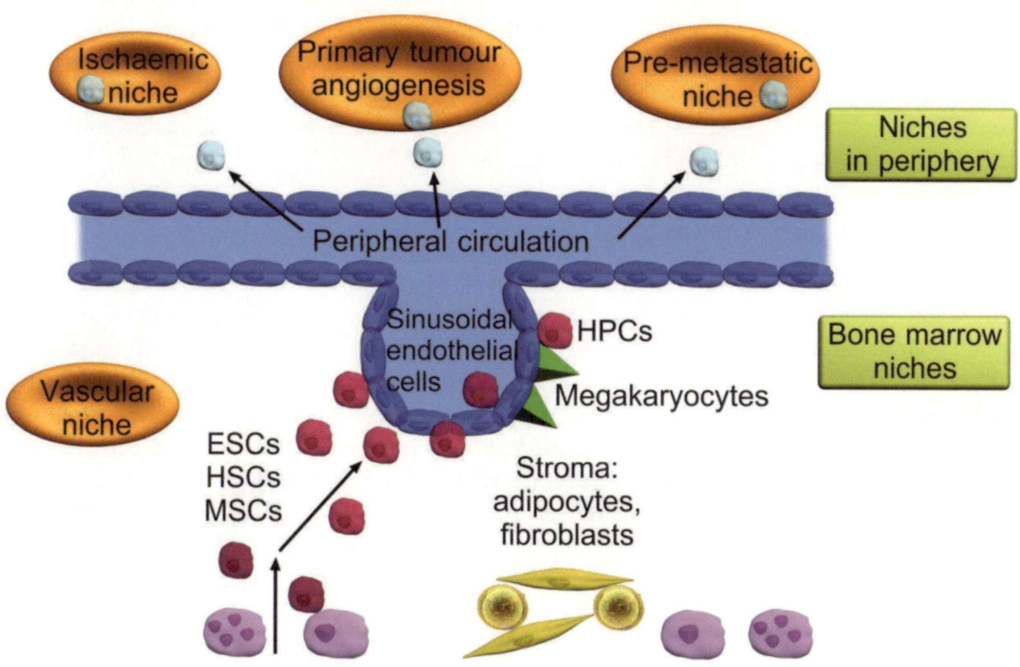

Fig. 3. Representative image of microenvironment.

proinflammatory chemokines S100A8 and S100A9, in the premetastatic microenvironment (Kucia et al., 2005). These chemoattractants increase the homing and engraftment of macrophage antigen 1 (Mac1)-expressing myeloid cells to the premetastatic niches. Activation of NF-kB signaling in macrophages in a serum amyloid A3 (SAA3) dependent fashion was also demonstrated (Hiratsuka et al., 2008). SAA3, a protein implicated in phagocyte chemoattraction, is up regulated in premetastatic niche by the inflammatory chemoattractant S100A8 and S100A9 (Hiratsuka et al., 2008). This finding raises the hypothesis that NF-kB in the premetastatic niche could be working to prepare a metastatic-like environment for primary tumor cells (Peinado et al., 2008). Nuclear factor kappa B (NF-kB) is a transcription factor that plays a pivotal role in connecting inflammation and cancer (Naugler & Karin, 2008).

Cell adhesion molecules

Individual cells in their particular environment adhere to the extracellular matrix (ECM) and their neighbours via integrin-containing and cadherin-containing complexes, respectively. Integrin-mediated adhesion to the ECM and cadherin-mediated adhesion between cells within developmental and physiological compartments are dynamically regulated.

A basic function of the niche is to anchor stem cells in the appropriate microenvironment. This function is mediated by adhesion molecules, including and adherent complex composed of cadherin and catenin. It has been reported that different forms of β-catenin interact with different protein complex. That is, the heterodimeric form of β-catenin/α-catenin interacts with membrane-bound cadherin, and the monomer form interacts with Tcf in nuclei (Gottardi & Gumbioner, 2004). It is, therefore, reasonable to proposed that β-catenin is a key molecule bridging two states of stem cells (Fuchs et al., 2004): the arrested state when stem cells are attached to the niche through the cadherin-β-catenin adhesion interaction (Zhang et al., 2003; Song & Xie, 2002) and the activated state in which β-catenin is nuclearly localized (Lowry et al., 2005; He et al., 2004).

A complex interplay of cytokines, chemokines, proteolytic enzymes and adhesion molecules maintain SC anchorage to the niche infrastructure.

4. Stem cell division and cancer

The processes which make possible that a cell gives rise to two daughter cells are defined as cell division cycle. These processes involve specific regulatory networks that impinge so that is strictly controlled both in time and space. Progression through the cell division cycle requires duplication of the genetic material and the delivery of the newly duplicated genomes to the two daughter cells during mitosis which represent one of the key processes in living organisms. This genetic duplication occurs in coordination with an increase in cellular components and changes in cell architecture. Balance between stem cell division and differentiation implies a fine coupling of cell division control, cell cycle arrest and reactivation, replication and differentiation.

In principle, stem cells can rely either completely on symmetric divisions or on a combination of symmetric and asymmetric divisions. The evidence for symmetric stem-cell divisions is strong, but the idea are that most stem cells can divide by either symmetric or asymmetric modes of division according to the fates of its daughter cells and the balance between these two modes is controlled by developmental and environmental signals.

Normally, SC divide asymmetrically (Cleevers, 2005) as a result of the asymmetric localization of cortical cell polarity determinants, such as Partner of Inscuteable (PINS) and atypical protein kinase C (aPKC), and cell fate determinants i.e Numb and Prospero, and regulated alignment of the mitotic spindle. For example when the machinery that regulates asymmetric divisions is disrupted, neuroblasts begin dividing symmetrically and form tumors (Lee et al., 2006; Albertson& Doe, 2003; Caussinus & Gonzalez, 2005). Cell clones lacking PINS are tumorigenic (Lee et al., 2006; Caussinus & Gonzalez, 2005), and cell clones lacking the cell fate determinants Numb or Prospero are also tumorigenic (Caussinus & Gonzalez, 2005). On the other hand it's known that the machinery that promotes asymmetric cell divisions has an evolutionary conserved role in tumor suppression (Cleevers, 2005).
Most stem cells have the ability to switch between asymmetric and symmetric modes of division, and that the balance between these two modes of division is defective in cancer disease. The adenomatous polyposis coli (APC) gene that regulates asymmetric division by stem cells in the intestinal epithelium is an important tumor suppressor in the mammalian colonic mucosa (Joslyn et al., 1991; Groden et al., 1991; Kinzler et al., 1991). Consistent with this tumorigenic potential, aPKC has been also identified as an oncogene in human lung cancers (Regala et al., 2005a; Regala et al., 2005b), and loss of Numb may be involved in the hyperactivation of Notch pathway signaling observed in breast cancers (Pece et al., 2004; Stylianou et al., 2006). In summary it is speculated that asymmetric division may suppress carcinogenesis, in addition to its role in maintaining a balance between stem cells and differentiated progeny.

Symmetric versus asymmetric division

Cell split in two at the end step of each division cycle. This division normally bisects through the middle of the cell and generates two equal daughters. When stem cells (SC) divide, their daughters either maintain SC identity or initiate differentiation. Conceptually, there are only three potential outcomes for SC after division: 1) a symmetrical division leading to net expansion of SC; 2) a symmetrical division that leads to the production of differentiated cells; and 3) an asymmetrical division leading to the maintenance of the SC population (Morrison & Kimble, 2006; Knoblich, 2008; Gonczy & DiNardo, 1996).
One SC can divide asymmetrically, producing one differentiating cell to maintain the tissue in a homeostatic state, or symmetrically, producing other SC; some mammalian SC populations may undergo both asymmetric and symmetric divisions depending on their circumstances (Chenn & McConnell, 1995). In summary, two main types of mechanism govern asymmetric cell division: the first, named intrinsic, relies on the asymmetric partitioning of cell components that determine cell fate; and the second, known as extrinsic, involves the asymmetric placement of daughter cells relative to external cues (Morrison & Kimble, 2006).
The relative proportion of symmetric divisions depending on their circumstances (Takahashi et al., 1996); the relative proportion of symmetric divisions appears to change over time, with symmetric divisions predominating at early time points when the SC pool would be expected to be expanding (Chenn & McConnell, 1995; Horvitz & Herskowitz, 1992). Whether this indicates that a single cell can switch from a symmetric to an asymmetric mode of cell division is not clear.
Asymmetry can manifest itself in two ways, namely by the unequal partitioning of cell-fate determinants and by the generation of daughter cells of different sizes. The mitotic spindle

is a key regulator of both of these events. First, its orientation controls the axis of cell division and can determine whether localized cell-fate determinants are segregated symmetrically or asymmetrically (Rappaport, 1996; Strome, 1993). Second, the position of the spindle within the dividing cell is thought to determine the relative size of two daughter cells (Rappaport, 1986; Albertson, 1984). The asymmetric segregation of cell-fate determinants and the generation of daughter cells of different sizes rely on the correct orientation and position of the mitotic spindle. The simple switch between symmetric and asymmetric segregation is achieved by changing the orientation of cell division: in vivo labelling mitotic spindles images reveals that the asymmetric spindle is formed in the same plane as symmetric spindle, but rotates before cell division. The direction of rotation usually correlates with the position of the centrosome at interphase: the spindle rotates in an anticlockwise direction when the centrosome is basal and clockwise when it is apical. Second, the cleavage furrow is not positioned equidistant between the spindle poles. As apical microtubules elongate and basal microtubules shorten, the midbody moves basally until it is positioned asymmetrically between the two spindle poles, at the site of the cleavage furrow, and the consequence are the generation of daughter cells of different sizes. The dogma indicates that the cleavage furrow always forms and generated two daughter cells of identical sizes equidistant from the spindle pole.

We have known that the asymmetric stem cell division is dictated by the spindle itself becoming asymmetric at anaphase. Microtubules on the apical side of the cell elongate, while those on the basal side become shorter. As the astral microtubules become longer, and seemingly more abundant, the apical aster enlarges, and the basal aster is concomitantly reduced in size (Kaltschmidt et al., 2000). Astral microtubules have been proposed to be involved in specifying the site of the cleavage furrow at cytokinesis (Rappaport, 1990; Oegema K & Mitchison, 1997).

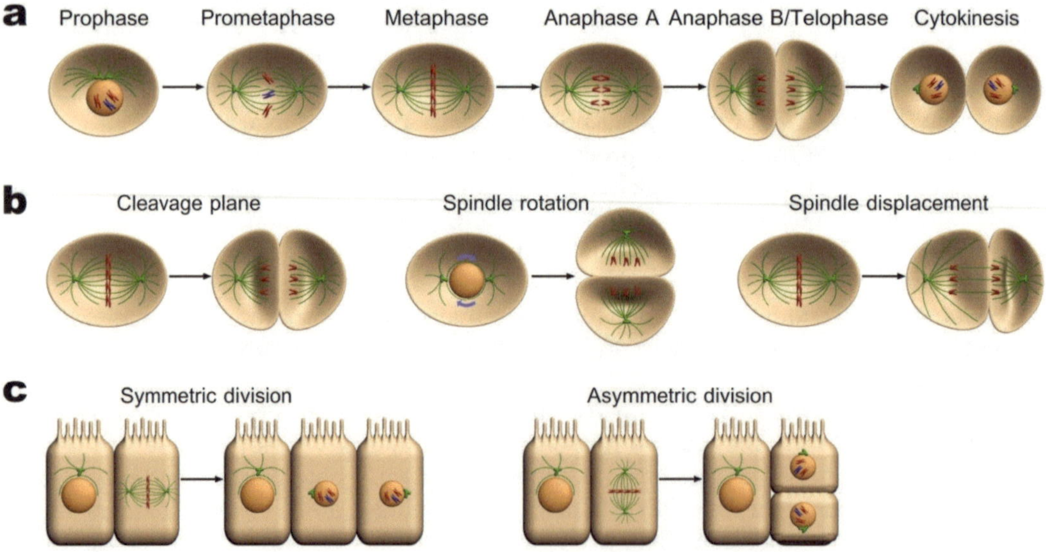

Fig. 4. A, B- Different phases of cell division and spindle rotation. C- Symmetric versus asymmetric stem cell division.

The stem cell niche functions to house regulate symmetric and asymmetric mitosis of stem cells; this regulation is affected through the action of various signalling pathways such as Wnt, Hh, Notch, Bmp, and probably others. Niche-forming cells are stimulated by growth factors and in turn, produce ligands (i.e. Delta), that act on stem cell receptors (i.e. Notch) to initiate stem cells mitosis or specify differentiation. Niche cells, the microenvironment they create, including the space between them, are features of a niche that allow it to maintain the stem cells, while preventing its differentiation and directing tissue growth and renewal through its daughters (Kiger et al., 2001).

5. Cell cycle in normal and tumor stem cells

Adult stem cells are often relatively slow-cycling cells able to respond to specific environmental signals and generate new stem cells or select a particular differentiation.
Exactly when and how most somatic stem cell niches develop is still a mystery, and in the world of stem cell niches, there are considerable variations in niche design. Some stem cells of adult mammals don't seem to have a specified niche within their respective tissue (i.e. skeletal muscle). In other cases, however, a stem cell compartment is established within a developing tissue, and cells within this niche are then activated in response to specific environment cues (i.e. skin, hair follicles, epidermis, mammary gland, lung, brain).
Stem cell repopulation is hierarchically organized and is intrinsically controlled by the intracellular cell cycle machinery. Their function appears to be highly associated with the differentiation stage in stem/progenitor pools. The negative regulation is important for maintaining homeostasis, especially at the stem cell level under physiological cues or pathological insults. By contrary disruption of cell cycle inhibition may contribute to the formation of the so-called cancer stem cells (CSCs) that are currently hypothesized to be partially responsible for tumorigenesis and recurrence of cancer. While a complex array of extracellular signals and intracellular transduction pathways certainly participate in the distinct response, the cell cycle machinery, as a final step, must communicate with the specific regulatory cues (Steinman & Nussenzweig, 2002) and cell cycle regulators must play key roles in this process.
The slow cycling feature seems to be a common behaviour in most adult stem cell types if not al, and their relative quiescence of stem cells may prevent their premature exhaustion lifespan, but it has been considered to be one of the hurdles in the context of the cancer recurrence and metastases propagation.
Stem cell (SC) quiescence is maintained by the balance between positive and negative proliferative factors: A variety of cell-cycle regulatory proteins, transcription factors, and cell-signaling molecules have been shown to regulate the quiescence of primitive stem/progenitor cells. The slow cycling feature seems to be a common feature in most adult stem cell types if not all (Potten, 1997; Bonfanti et al., 2001; Palmer TD et al., 2001). The relative quiescence of stem cells may prevent their premature exhaustation in vivo, but it has been considered to be one of the hurdles in the context of the in vivo cancer recurrence and/or metastasis.
The molecular principles of cell cycle regulation have been defined largely, and a number of surveillance checkpoints monitor the cell cycle and halt its progression. In mammalian cells, the cell cycle machinery that determines whether cells will continue proliferating or will cease dividing and differentiate appears to operate mainly in the G1 phase. Cell cycle progression is regulated by the sequential activation and inactivation of CDKs (Sherr, 1994;

Sherr & Roberts, 1995). In somatic cells, movement through Gi and into the S phase is driven by the active form of the cyclin D1, 2, 3/CDK4, 6 complex and the subsequent phosphorylation retinoblastoma (Rb) protein (Classon & Harlow, 2002). In parallel, the c-Myc pathway also directly contributes to the G1/S transition by elevating the transcription for cyclin E and cdc25A (Bartek & Lukas, 2001).

Several cell-cycle regulators have been shown to play critical roles in SC and/or progenitor cells proliferation, including p21, p27, p57, p16, p18 , and also the D-type cyclins (cyclin D1, D2, and D3) and their catalytic partners Cdk4 and Cdk6 . SC cell fate decisions are also regulated by several transcription factors (gfi-1, Pbx-1, MEF/ELF4, c-myc). Interestingly, many studies indicate that tumor-suppressor genes, including PTEN, p53, retinoblastoma (Rb), PML, APC, and FBw7, may play critical roles in maintaining SCs in a quiescent state. p18, a strong inhibitor for stem cell self-renewal has been suggested to be involved in the symmetric division of precursor cells in developing mouse brain (Tschan et al., 1999) and HSC self-renewal (Cheng et al., 2000; Yuan et al., 2004). The absence of p18 causes enhanced stem cell renewal, leading to an increased stem cell pool. The regulation for p18 gene and protein in stem cells is unclear at this moment. Given the striking outcome of p18 absence on stem cell renewal, it would be of great appeal to specifically look for the link of p18 with the several major signaling pathways controlling stem cell self-renewal.

p21, a gatekeeper for quiescent stem cells, is reduced in progenitor populations while is abundant in quiescent human HSCs (Stier et al., 2003; Dcos et al., 2000). Therefore, p21

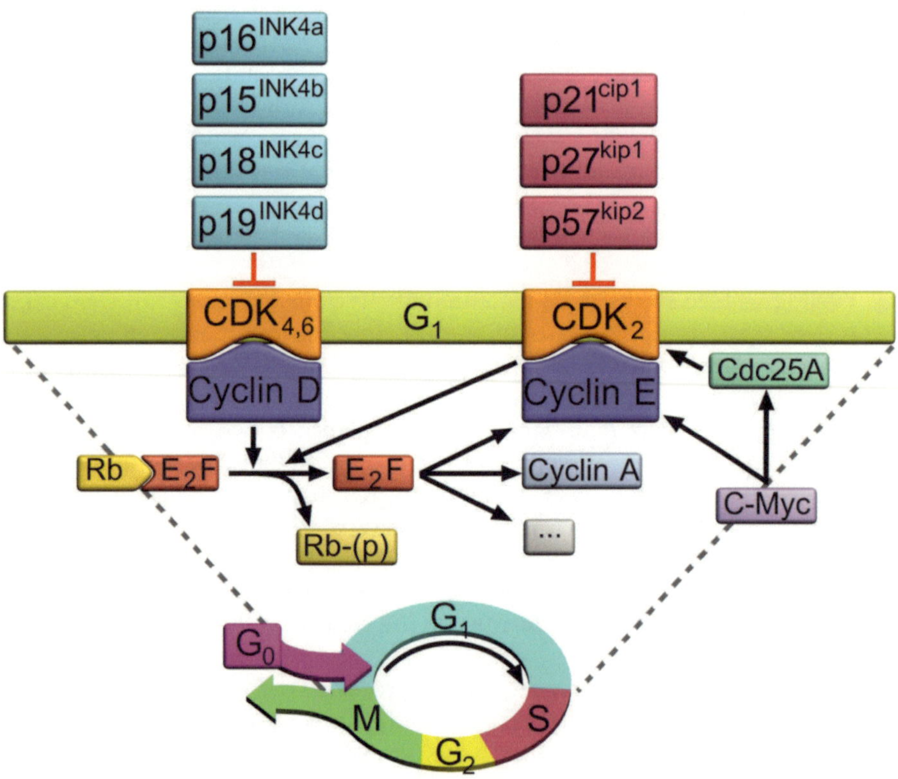

Fig. 5. Cell cycle regulators.

governs cell cycle entry of stem cells, and its absence leads to increased proliferation of the primitive cells (Cheng et al., 2000) , suggesting that restricted cell cycling is crucial to prevent premature stem cell depletion and death under conditions of stress.

p27, a progenitor-specific inhibitor to the repopulation efficiency, appears to accumulate at points in which signals for mitosis affect cell cycle regulators, and it has been shown to serve as an important regulator at a restriction point of mitogenic signals in many cell types (Coast et al., 1996). As progenitor cells are highly responsive to growth factors, though in a tissue-specific fashion, p27 must be a critical cell cycle mediator of many cytokines in progenitor cells (Polyak et al., 1995; Cashman et al., 1999). Thus, modulating p27 expression in a small number of stem cells without necessarily expanding the cells may translate into effects on the majority of mature cells.

The p16-Rb, of the family of "pocket proteins" that also includes p107 and p130, plays an important role in regulating the G1 checkpoint, cellular differentiation, apoptotic cell death, permanent cell-cycle arrest, and chromosomal stability (Sherr & Roberts, 1995; Classon & Harlow, 2002). pRb is likely to participate in the regulation of quiescence because its acute somatic inactivation is sufficient for Go-arrested cells to re-enter the cell cycle. Similarly, formation of p130/E2F4 complexes is thought to be a characteristic of Go and during the transition of cells from G1 to Go, p130 undergoes a specific phosphorylation event leading to its association with E2F4 (Sherr & Roberts, 1995).

6. Signaling from a support cell niche

One of the critical questions in the adult stem cell field concerns the mechanisms that regulate the decision between self-renewal and differentiation. Adult stem cells have two fundamental properties: a long-term capacity to divide and the ability to produce daughter cells that either retain stem cell identity or initiate differentiation along the appropriate lineage(s). The balance between self-renewal and initiation of differentiation is crucial. If too many daughter cells initiate differentiation, the stem cell population may be depleted. Conversely, if too many daughter cells maintain stem cell identity, the stem cell population may expand out of proportion, providing a pool of proliferative, incompletely differentiated cells that could mutate and became tumorigenic.

Physical attachment to the niche may be a feature of many adult stem cell systems, with the kind of functional complex depending on the nature of the niche; stem cells attach directly to somatic niche by adherent junctions. A general picture of how the stem cells niche mechanisms might work to control stem cell number and maintain the correct balance between self-renewal and differentiation is emerging. This process involves complex crosstalk between intercellular and intracellular mechanisms. First, the size, or number of stem cell niches defines the correct number of stem cells by sending short-range signal(s) for self-renewal or maintenance to the neighbouring stem cells. Second, cell-cell adhesion between supporting niche cells and stem cells enables stem cells to remain tightly associated with the niche. Third, stem cells are polarized with respect to the niche. Finally, stem cells polarized through contact with the niche can orient their mitotic spindles to ensure the normally asymmetric outcome of stem cell divisions by reliable placing one daughter cell firmly within the niche.

Within their niche apical-basal location determines stem cell self-renewal and/or differentiation. Theoretically, sister cells can either be in a planar orientation where both cells remain in direct contact with the basal lamina and host cells, or in an apical-basal orientation where one daughter cell is pushed toward the basal lamina and the other cell apically toward the host cell. Taken together, this behaviour demonstrates that niche plays an important role in the maintenance of stem cell identity of newly divided daughter cells. The daughter cell attached to the basal lamina remains pluripotential, whereas the daughter that loses contact with the basal lamina up-regulates stem cell marker of differentiation and becomes a committed adult cell.

Stem cells are usually located adjacent to support cells that secrete factors, required for maintaining stem cell identity. Cell-cell adhesion between stem cells and niche cells is required for stem cell maintenance, physically maintaining stem cells within the niche and ensuring that stem cells are held close to self-renewal signals emanating from the microenvironment. Recent advances have provided important insights into the role played by the microenvironment in regulating stem cell identity and the asymmetric generation of committed daughter cells (Fuchs et al., 2004; Knoblich, 2001; Moore KA & Lemischka, 2006). Within the stem cell niche, signaling pathways such as Notch, Wnt, BMP/TGFβ, and STAT and proteins such as Num, PRA, PKCζ, LGL, and NUMA have implicated in the regulation of asymmetric cell division (Fuchs et al., 2004; Knoblich, 2001; Moore KA & Lemischka, 2006, Betschinger & Knoblich, 2004; Knoblich et al., 1995; Rhyu et al., 1995).

Hypoxia support the niche

Hypoxic microenvironments also occur during embryogenesis and in the adult, where one consequence may be the creation of niches that maintain pluripotential cells.

Stem cells reside in tissue regions, the niche that are low in vasculature and that are thought to provide a low-oxygen environment (Cipolleschi et al., 1993; Suda et al., 2005; Nilsson et al., 2001). Stem cells are harboured in vivo in a low-oxygen environment, and with the consequent hypothesis that self-renewal potential of stem cells is strictly linked to the capacity of these cells to survey in a hypoxic environment. The control of stem cell survival and the regulation of hypoxia response are intimately coupled and they share common control gene/pathways (Sansone et al., 2005). Recent data indicate that the stem cell regulatory Notch pathway share in an interplay with the hypoxia response modulator HIF-1α to promote the onset of a stem/undifferentiated phenotype (Gustafson et al., 2005).

There is evidence that hypoxia affects stem cell function and survival (Cejudo-Martin & Johnson, 2005; Covello et al., 2006). In vitro, hypoxia actively maintains a stem cell immature phenotype, induces a loss of differentiation markers, and blocks differentiation. In vivo, stem cells express higher levels of hypoxia-regulated genes than do the more mature progeny, as well as high levels of glycolitic enzymes.

In hematopoietic stem cells niche, Notch signalling induces/regulates diverse cell fate decisions during development (Singh et al., 2000). Also, as an intracellular second messenger, nitric oxide (NO) is implicated in the trafficking of hematopoietic progenitors (Zhang et al., 2007) and in the recruitment of stem/progenitor cells (Aicher et al., 2003; Ihle et al., 1998).

Many works has revealed that active niche that supports self-renewal of stem cells via activation of the Janus-kinase (JAK)-signal transducer and activator of transcription (STAT) pathway within the adjacent stem cells. JAKs are non-receptor tyrosine kinases that mediate signaling downstream of many mammalian cytokines and growth factors receptors, in part by phosphorylation and activation of STAT (Ihle et al., 1998). The signal for stem cell self-renewal is transduced from the activated JAL via STAT.

Some of the effects of hypoxia on stem cells correlate with the effects of Notch signaling on these cells. Notch is able to both maintain the pluripotential state of some cells and induce specific cell fates. Notch also influences proliferation and survival.

Hypoxia is a pathophysiological component of many disorders, including cancer (Semenza, 2001). Hypoxia controls many important aspects of cellular life, and a recently discovered function of hypoxia is to regulate differentiation in stem/precursor cells. In addition to their influences on proliferation and differentiation of various stem/progenitor cells populations, hypoxia altering cellular energy metabolism and angiogenesis. Recent studies suggest the existence of an intimate and functionally important interaction between Notch and hypoxia-inducible factor (HIF)-1α, a transcription factor that regulates many genes involved in the response to hypoxia, including factors that promote angiogenesis (Gordan & Simon, 2007).

Hypoxia activates Notch-responsive promoters and increases of Notch direct downstream genes. The Notch intracellular domain interacts with HIF-1α, a global regulator of oxygen homeostasis, and HIF-1α is recruited to Notch-responsive promoters upon Notch activation under hypoxic conditions.

The link between Notch signaling and hypoxia represents a novel facet of the hypoxic response. In the canonical hypoxic response, hypoxia acts by altering the stability and activity of HIF-1α leading to binding of HIF-1α to HRE-containing regulatory elements in specific target genes and activation of such genes e.g. VEGF, PGK, EPO, PDGF, and GLUT1. The difference between the canonical hypoxic response and the transfer of hypoxic information into the Notch signaling pathway results in the activation Notch response genes.

Regulatory pathways

Genetic studies of stem cell regulation have indeed revealed the operation of multiple regulatory circuits in many stem cell niches. Now, there are to consider two types of regulatory pathways in stem cells: those that active intrinsically with stem cells themselves (Oct4, Sox2, Nanog); and those that mediate interactions with their neighbours (Notch, Hh, Wnt, BMP, JAK/STAT).

1-Notch signaling

Notch encodes a transmembrane receptor that is cleaved to release an intracellular domain (Nicd) that is directly involved in transcriptional control and many components of the Notch pathway are expressed in the precursor cell compartment of the developing vertebrate (Artavanis- Tsakonas, 2002; Andromtsellis-Theotokis et al., 2006).

Notch receptor activation induces the expression of the specific target genes and enhancer of split 3 (Hes3) and Sonic Hedgehog (SHh) through rapid activation of cytoplasm signals, including the serine/threonine kinase Akt, the transcription factor STAT3 and mammalian target of rapamycin, and thereby promotes the survival of somatic stem cells.

The rapid effect of Delta4 (Dll4) on stem cells survival suggested that cytoplasm survival signals were induced in addition to slower transcriptional responses traditionally attributed to Notch activation.

Downstream of Akt, mammalian target of rapamycin (mTOR) is a key regulator of cell growth. Jag1 caused transit phosphorylation of mTOR. Like DAPT, the mTOR inhibitor rapamycin blocked the survival effect of Dll4. Jag1 induced phosphorylation of MSK1 and LKB1 kinases, which have been intensively studied as drug targets in diabetes and cancer (Alessi et al., 1998). The PDK1 and p70 ribosomal S6 kinase components of the insulin signaling pathways are known to limit mTOR activation.

The p38 mitogen-activated protein kinase is also a potential inhibitor of survival because it acts downstream of JAK and antagonizes growth of many cell types by activating MSK (Deak et al., 1998; Lavoie et al., 1996). JAK and p39 inhibitors increased survival in stem cells. Combined JAK abd p38 inhibition neither did nor substantially improves survival, further indicating that JAK may act through p38 to antagonize the survival pathway in stem cell niche. These data suggest that Notch acting through STAT3 promotes, and that p38 antagonizes, survival.

2- JAK/STAT

Although the surrounding microenvironment or niche influences stem cell fate decisions, few signals that emanate from the niche specify stem cells self-renewal.
A number of search have revealed that active niche supports self-renewal of stem cells (SCs) via activation of the Janus-Kinase (JAK)-signal transducer and activator of transcription (STAT) pathway within the adjacent SCs (Tulina & Matrevis, 2001; Kiger et al., 2000). JAKs are non-receptor tyrosine kinases that mediate signaling downstream of many cytokine and growth factor receptors of mammalians, in part by phosphorylation and activation of STAT (Ihle et al., 1998).
JAKs mediate signaling downstream of many mammalian cytokine and growth factor receptors, often by phosphorylation and activation of STAT proteins; STAT was required autonomously for stem cell maintenance.
Mutations on the JAK-STAT pathway resulted in stem cell loss, whereas JAK-STAT activation by cell loss ectopic expression caused unrestricted stem cell self-renewal. The signal transducers and activators of transcription (STAT) (Jove, 2000) family consist of seven members that are genetically localized to three chromosomal regions (Copeland et al., 1995).

3-NO

The capacity to generate new cells from stem cells niche is preserved along span life. Quiescent SC of the adult niches become activated and generates rapidly dividing transit-amplifying (TA) fells.
Nitric oxide (NO) an intercellular messenger, exerts antiproliferative effects on several cells and facilitate cell differentiation. However it is not clear if the actions are due to direct cytostatic action of NO on the stem cell niche precursors or whether they are an indirect consequence of changes in niche blood flow or cell-to-cell contact activity produced by NOS inhibition. The mechanism involved in the NO stemness action is also unknown at present. Based on previous finding that NO decreases stem cell proliferation in the subventricular zone (SVZ) we hypothesized that NO may participate in the control of stem cell niche proliferation and differentiation.
NO, is a physiological inhibitor of stem cell proliferation/differentiation in adult stem cell niches that exert a direct, 6-GMP-independent antiproliferative effect on stem cell progenitor without affecting cell survival. NO prevent the EGF-induced transphosphorylation of AKT, which are required for multipotent progenitor self-renewal, and NOS inhibition enhanced stem cell niche phosphor-AKT and reduced nuclear $p27^{Kip}$. It was demonstrated that AKT phosphorylates the CDK inhibitor $p27^{Kip1}$ and prevents its translocation to the nucleus thus allowing cell cycle progression. Given that $p27^{Kip1}$ has been identified as a key regulator of the cell cycle specifically in transit-amplifying C cells this is probably that the mechanism by which NO-induced inhibition of AKT results in decreased multipotent precursor's proliferation. It is interesting to note a probably dissimilar distribution of $p27^{Kip1}$ in stem cell

niche, with a scared patron in the highly proliferative stem cell niche zone and abundant in the peripheral zone, where precursor that migrates arrest proliferation and differentiate.

Soluble factors

Under steady-state conditions, most stem cells are in contact with basal membrane and stromal cells, and are maintained in G0 phase of cell cycle (Cheng et al., 2000), while a small fraction is in S or G2/M phase of the cell cycle. The equilibrium between these two compartments is dictated by the bioavailability of stem cell-active cytokines, which are bound to the extracellular matrix or tethered to the membrane of stromal cells.

Local secretion of proteases may alter the stem cell-stromal cell interaction. The proteolytic cleavage of vascular cell adhesion molecule-1, expressed by stromal cells will be an essential step contributing to the mobilization of stem/progenitor cells. On the other way matrix metalloproteinase (MMPs) promote the release of extracellular matrix-bound or cell-surface-bound cytokines (Vu & Werb, 2000), such as vascular endothelial growth factor (VEGF), and can contribute to the release of stem cell-active cytokines following stress that shifts stem/progenitor cells from a quiescent to a proliferative niche.

7. miRNAs and stem cell

MicroRNAs (miRNAs) are a covered family of small regulatory molecules that function by modulating protein production. Each miRNA may regulate hundreds of different protein-coding genes. Each miRNA gene encodes a mature miRNA between 21-25 nucleotide (nt) long (Kim & Nam, 2006), non-coding RNAs that inhibit gene expression at the post-transcriptional level. They are transcribed as parts of longer molecules, up to several kilobases in length (pri-miRNA), that are processed in the nucleus into hairpin RNAs of 70-100 nt by the double-stranded RNA-specific ribonuclease, Drosha (Cullen, 2004; He & Hannon, 2004; Nakahara & Carthew, 2004; Bartel & Bartel, 2003; Ambros, 2001).The hairpin pre-miRNA are then transported to the cytoplasm by exportin 5 where they undergo final processing by a second, double-strand specific ribonuclease, known as Dicer. In animals, single-stranded miRNAs are incorporated into RNA induced silencing complexes (RISC) that bind primarily to specific messenger RNA (mRNA) at specific sequence motifs within the 3´untranslated region (3´UTR) of the transcript, which are significantly, although not completely, complementary to the miRNA.

Most characterized miRNAs from animals repress gene expression by blocking the translation of complementary messenger RNAs into protein; they interact with their targets by imperfect base-pairing, to mRNA sequences within the 3´UTR (He & Hannon, 2004).

Experimental evidence has suggested that small RNAs regulate stem cell character in animals (Bernstein E, et al., 2003; Carmell et al., 2002), and moreover, some miRNAs are differentially expressed in stem cells, suggesting a specialized role in stem cell regulation (Suh et al., 2004; Houbaviy et al., 2003).

Recently, the stem cell and miRNA fields have converged with the identification of stem-cell-specific miRNAs (Houbaviy et al., 2003). In addition to canonical miRNAs, mirtrons and shRNA-derived miRNAs have also been identified in mouse embryonic stem (ES) cells. It is now clear that miRNAs provide a new dimension to the regulation of stem cell functions. Based on their function in translational attenuation, miRNAs seem to regulate stem cell fate and behaviour by fine-tuning the protein levels of various factors that are required for stem cell or niche cell functions. One important function of miRNAs in ES cells is to regulate cell cycle progression during stem cell differentiation.

The overall function of the miRNA pathway in EC cell has been evaluated in humans and mice by analysing the phenotypes of two proteins that have crucial roles in the production of mature miRNAs: DGCR8 and Dicer mutants (Bernstein et al., 2003).

Stem cells have distinct miRNA signatures, and their assessment have been done by cloning sequencing of miRNA from stem cells. Deep sequencing of miRNAs from stem cells has revealed the identity of the specific miRNAs that are expressed in stem cells and might function in self-renewal and differentiation of stem cells.

In addition, different molecules may regulate postnatal stem cell niches (Palma et al., 2005; Shi et al., 2005). Dicer-1 (Dcr-1) is essential for processing miRNAs, whereas Dicer-2 (Dcr-2) is required for siRNAs; loss of Dcr-1 completely disrupts the miRNA pathway and only has a weak effect on the siRNA pathway. Thus Dcr-1 is required for cell autonomously in the stem cell niche for cell divisions that developing more differentiated cells.

Regulatory role of miRNAs

Transcription factors are essentials players in stem cell self-renewal and differentiation (Pevny & Placzek, 2005; Ross et al., 2003). However, post-transcriptional gene regulation is emerging as another essential and, until recently, unexpected regulator of development. Many different classes of small non-coding RNAs are present in stem cells, with diverse roles including RNA modification and chromatin remodelling (Mattick & Makunin, 2005).

Recently there are identified a large family of small non-coding miRNAs, which are likely key post-transcriptional players in stem cells and their differentiated progeny (Bartel, 2004). The cloning and sequencing of small RNAs using conventional methods revealed that the miR-290-295 cluster and miR-296 are specific to stem cells and that their levels decreases as the stem cells differentiate. Simply the miR-290-295 cluster has specific role in maintaining pluripotency (Singh et al., 2008): the real role of miR-290-295 is to induce differentiation. In contrast miR-21 and miR-22 increase substancially follow the induction of differentiation: these miRNAs might have important roles in stem cell differentiation (Kim & Nam, 2006; Singh et al., 2008).

miRNAs are especially attractive candidates for regulation stem cell self-renewal and cell fate decisions, as their ability to simultaneously regulate many targets provides a means for coordinated control of concerted gene action.

miRNAs are 21-25 nt, non-coding RNAs that are expressed in a tissue-specific and developmentally regulated manner and comprise approximately 1% of the total genes in the animal genome (Bartel, 2004). Although direct evidence for a functional role of miRNAs in stem cell biology is just emerging, hints regarding their involvement based on expression patterns, predicted targets, and over-expression studies suggest that they will be key regulators.

miRNA are likely important regulators for stem cell self-renewal: distinct sets of miRNAs are specifically expressed in pluripotent ES cells but not in differentiated embryonic bodies or in adult tissues, suggesting a role for miRNAs in stem cell self-renewal (Kim & Nam, 2006). Loss of Dicer1 causes embryonic lethality and loss of stem cell populations (Nakahara & Carthew, 2004; Wienholds et al., 2003), and in the other way, Argonaute family members are required for maintaining germline stem cells in differentiated organisms (Carmell et al., 2002).

As stem cells differentiate, they down-regulate stem cell maintenance genes and activate lineage-specific genes. These transitions require a rapid switch in gene expression profiles.

Although the transcription factor pool is replaced, remaining transcripts that were highly expressed in the previous stage need to be silenced. miRNAs are uniquely poised to rapidly effect such changes through simultaneous repression of many targets of any remaining transcripts. This would predict that miRNAs are also transcriptional regulated in different cell types such that there is extensive crosstalk between transcription and post-transcriptional regulation and that distinct miRNAs are active in particular lineages (Kanellopoulou et al., 2005; He & Hannon, 2004).
Since then, miRNAs have been implicated in a wide variety of developmental and metabolic pathways in both invertebrates and vertebrates, including cell differentiation, proliferation, programmed cell death, the number of functional miRNAs target pairs identified to date is minimal (He & Hannon, 2004).

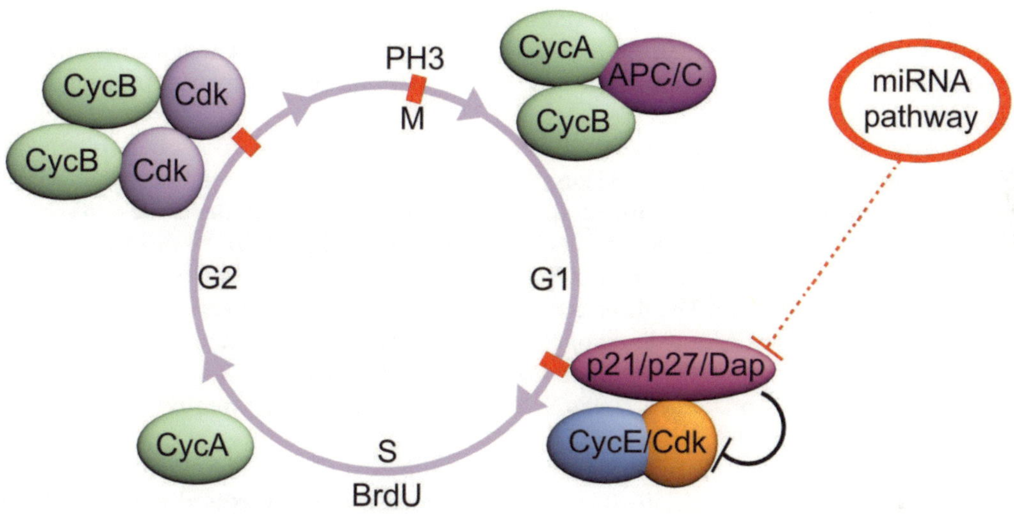

Fig. 6. miRNA pathway and stem cells cell cycle.

miRNA function in embryonic and adult stem cells

The functions of miRNAs in somatic tissue stem cells have also been identified, and their mechanisms of action are to regulate adult stem cell proliferation and differentiation. Evidence for this activity comes from experiments demonstrating that ES cells that were deficient in miRNA processing enzymes exhibited defects in their capacity for differentiation and self-renewal (Murchison et al., 2005; Wang et al., 2007). In addition, Dicer deficiency is embryonic lethal, and Dicer deficient embryos exhibit greatly reduced expression of Oct4 suggesting a stem cell defect (Kloosterman & Plasterk, 2006). The pluripotent property of ES cells is subject to regulation by the homeobox transcription factors, Oct4 and Nanog, which are essential regulators of early development and ES identity (Chambers et al., 2003; Mitsui et al., 2003; Nichols et al., 1998): it has been suggested that Oct4 initiates pluripotency state whereas Nanog maintains it (Chambers et al., 2007).
Little is known with respect to mechanisms by which miRNA function in controlling the developmental potential of ES cells, and it is largely unknown how ES cell-specific transcription factors and miRNA work together. The three stem factors (Oct4, Sox2, and Nanog) were found to occupy the promoters on many transcription factors and of 14 miRNAs (Boyer et al., 2005).

The actions of miRNA have been shown to regulate several developmental and physiological processes including stem cell differentiation, haematopoiesis, cardiac and skeletal muscle development, neurogenesis, etc... (Tay et al., 2008).

8. Tumor stem cell concentric niche model

Current investigations on primary cultures of solid tumors are generally conducted on random portions (i.e regionally undetermined) of surgically resected tumor or metastatic samples. It has been reported the existence of two types of cancer stem cells (CSCs) primary cancer stem cells (pCSCs) and/or metastatic cancer stem cells (mCSCs). But at intratumoral areas it can demonstrated the existence of two types of cancer stem cells (CSCs) within different regions of the same human tumor in relation to the pO2 gradient: the tumor mass characterized by a phenotypically immature anoxic core surrounded by a proliferating hypoxic layer, the more vascularised and more oxygenated peripheral area characterized by the presence of more differentiated cell types, with cells expressing pro-angiogenic signaling.

This model describes intratumoral areas in order to define potential phenotypic heterogeneity and differential expression of molecular signaling pathways in correlation to the oxygen tension gradient within the tumor mass. Thus there are identified three layers: the internal core, the intermediate, and the peripheral layers, based on the distance from the anoxic central core, to define their molecular and phenotypic features in correlation to the hypoxic concentric gradient. The three concentric layers bear quite diverse cell phenotypes.

The inner, highly hypoxic/anoxic core, characterized by stem cells with low proliferation index, and intermediate, mildly hypoxic layer, lining the anoxic core, with immature and proliferating tumor precursor cells, and the peripheral, more predominantly committed/differentiated cells.

Immunohistological analyses revealed that both the core and the intermediate layer were characterized by high level of HIF-1α expression which is over-expressed with VEGF. The expression of both Glut1 and CAIX was higher in the core, progressively undetectable at the periphery of the tumor.

Analysis of cell cycle marker Ki67 indicated that the inner core and, particularly, the intermediate-hypoxic area had the highest proliferation rate, whereas in the peripheral area, Ki67 expression was very low.

The intermediate portion is a thin transition area between the partially necrotic core and the peripheral area, which is defined by the presence of tumor angiogenesis. Nevertheless, VEGF highly expressing cells, characterized by poor HIF-1α expression, were found in the peripheral and more vascularised layer of the tumor mass. The expression of CD34, antigen constitutively expressed on endothelial cells, is found at the peripheral layer, the area highly enriched in CD34+ vessels.

Tumor cells derived from the intermediate area tended to form spheroids in vitro and displayed the highest proliferation rate, confirmed also by Ki67 expression, compared with cells from the core and from the peripheral area. Conversely, cells from the peripheral areas appeared more morphologically differentiated.

Moreover, cells recovered from the intermediate layer resulted to form the highest number of big size spheroids, whereas cells from the inner core formed small size spheroids; oppositely, cells derived from the peripheral area did not generate spheroids but rapidly differentiated. These behaviour support the assumption that stem cells, which are found to

be mainly located within the inner core, are characterized by a lower proliferation rate compared with committed precursors.
It has been shown that malignant tumors are characterized by a hypoxic microenvironment, which correlates with tumor aggressiveness (Azuma et al., 2003; Helczynska et al., 2003; Jogi et al., 2002), and over-activity of hypoxia inducible factor-1α (HIF-1α), the best described low oxygen sensor, is implicated in tumor progression (Smith et al., 2005). Recent data suggest that HIF-1α and multiple HIF-regulated genes are preferentially expressed in cancer stem cells in comparison with non-stem tumor cells and normal cell progenitors.
Importantly, hypoxia is also implicated in the regulation of several developmental critical signaling pathways, such as Notch (Gustafson et al., 2005), and, as were reported, bone morphogenic proteins (BMPs) (Pistollato et al., 2009) and Akt/mTOR pathways (170). Also HIF-2α has been described as a proto-oncogene.
Moreover, we speculate that the hypoxic signature is crucial in determining the epigenetic activation (HIF-1α, Glut1, and CAIX) and/or inhibition (BMP, Akt/mTOR/Stat3) of signaling pathways involved in the maintenance of the stem cell pool.

9. The pre-metastatic niche

Metastasis is know as a cascade of molecular/cellular events involving tumor cell intravasation, transport and immune evasion within the circulatory systems, arrest a secondary site, extravasations and finally colonization and growth (Chambers et al., 2002). Dissemination of tumor cells is a prerequisite for metastasis, but the two processes are not synonymous. Less than 1% of cancer cells entering the blood circulation successfully generate metastatic foci (Fidler, 1970; Fidler et al., 1977; Liotta et al., 1978; Varani et al., 1980; Mehlen & Puisieux, 2006).
Certain characteristics distinguish those cells able to colonize secondary tissues from other circulating tumor cells. The genetic and phenotypic make-up of a tumor is a major determinant of metastatic efficiency, but a receptive microenvironment is a requisite for establishing primary/secondary tumor growth. Gene-expression *signatures* that correlate with overall tumor metastatic efficiency (van der Vijver et al., 2002), and also those that can predict metastasis to a random organ have been described (Chang et al., 2004). The poor prognosis *signatures* encode not only genes important for intrinsic tumor cell cycle regulation, but also cell surface receptors and proteins expressed by the tissue stroma, such as matrix metalloproteinases, highlighting the importance of tumor cell-stroma interaction (Chang et al., 2008). Additionally, a transcriptional *signature* of fibroblast serum response has been shown to predict cancer progression (Kang et al., 2003). However, the factors underlying metastatic *dormancy*, and the dichotomy between tumor dissemination and metastatic establishement, remain enigmatic.
Bone marrow-derived hematopoietic progenitors cells (HPCs) recently emerged as key in initiating the early changes in metastatic cascade, creating a receptive microenvironment at designated sites for distant tumor growth and establishing the *pre-metastatic niche* (Kaplan et al., 2005).
Seminal research works demonstrated a key role for bone marrow-derived HPCs in *priming* distant tissues for tumor cell implantation and proliferation. BM-derived VEGFR-1$^+$ cells preceded the arrival of tumor cells and VEGFR-2$^+$ endothelial progenitor cells (EPCs), which migrate to established VEGFR-1$^+$ clusters. The pre-metastatic niches may function as physiological niches, and allow the VEGFR-1$^+$ cells to maintain expression of primitive cell

surface markers. It is possible that VEGFR1 activation, which leads to increased activity of epithelial-to-mesenchymal transition-associated transcription factors Snail, Twist, and Slug in the primary tumors, may also regulate VEGFR-1+ HPCs in the *pre-metastatic niche* (Yang et al., 2006).

Proangiogenic cytokines such VEGF induce homing of endothelial progenitor cells (EPCs), expressing VEGFR-2, to the tumor site, along with HPCs expressing VEGFR1.

These VEGFR-1+ HPCs are essential for stability and growth of the neovasculature (Lyden et al., 2001; Raffi et al., 2002; Okamoto et al., 2005; Carmeliet et al., 2001; Li et al., 2006). A tumors´s chemokine profile can greatly influence the contribution of the stromal microenvironment, such that those tumors co-expressing both VEGF and its family member placental growth factor (PIG), which exclusively signals through VEGFR-1, have a more aggressive metastatic phenotype (Marcellini et al., 2006).

10. References

Aicher, A; Heeschen, C; Mildner-Rihm, C; et al. (2003) Essential role of endothelial nitric oxide synthase for mobilization of stem and progenitor cells. *Nat Med.* 9: 1370-1376.

Aicher, A.; Heeschen, C.; & Dimmeler, S. (2004) The role of NOS3 in stem cell mobilization. *Trends Mol Med.* 10: 421-425.

Albertson D. (1984) Formation of the first cleavage spindle in nematode embryos. *Dev Biol.* 101:61-72.

Albertson R. & Doe CQ. (2003) Dlg, Scrib and Lgl regulate neuroblast cell size and mitotic spindle asymmetry. *Nature Cells Biol.* 5:166-170.

Alessi DR.; Kozlowski M.T.; Weng Q.P.; et al. (1998) 3-Phsphoinositide-dependent protein kinase 1 (PDK1) phosphorylates and activates the p70 S6 kinase in vivo and in vitro. *Curr Biol* 8:69-81.

Ambros V. (2001) microRNAs: tiny regulators with great potential. *Cell* 107: 823-826.

Androutsellis-Theotokis A.; Leker R.R.; Soldner F.; et al. (2006) Notch signaling regulates stem cell numbers in vitro and in vivo. *Nature* 442:823-826.

Artavanis- Tsakonas S.; Rand M.D., & Lake R.J. (2003) Notch signaling: cell fate control and signal integration in development. *Science* 296: 1655-1657.

Azuma Y.; Chou S.C.; Lininger R.A. et al. (2003) Hypoxia and differentiation in squamous cell carcinomas of the uterine cervix: Pimonidazole and involucrin. Clin *Cancer Res* 9:4944-4952.

Bartek J. & Lukas J. (2001) Pathways governing Gl-S transition and their response to DNA damage *FEBS Lett* 490:117-122.

Bartel B. & Bartel D.P. (2003) MicroRNAs: at the root of plant development? *Plant Physiol* 132:709-717.

Bartel DP. (2004) MicroRNAs: genomics, biogenesis, mechanism, and function *Cell;* 116: 281-297

Bernstein E.; Kim S.Y.; Carmell M.A. et al. (2003) Dicer is essential for mouse development. *Nature Genet* 35: 215-217.

Betschinger J.; Knoblich J.A. (2004) Dare to be different: asymmetric cell division in Drosophila, C. Elegans and vertebrates. *Curr Biol* 14: 674-R685

Betschinger J.; Mechtler K. & Knoblich J.A. (2003) The Par complex directs asymmetric cell division by phosphorylating the cytosesqueletal Lgl, *Nature* 422: 326-330.

Bianco P. & Riminucci M. (1998) The bone marrow stroma in vivo: ontogeny, structure, cellular composition and changes in disease. In: *Marrow stromal cell culture.* Beresford JN eds .United Kingdom: Cambridge University Press; 10-25.

Blau H.M.; Brazelton T.R. & Weiman J.M. (2001) The evolving concept of a stem cell: Entity or Function? *Cell* 105:829-841.

Bonfanti L.G.A.; Galli R. & Vescovi A.L. (2001) In: *Stem Cells and CNS Development.* Rao MS (ed). Humana Press: Totowa, NJ 31-48.

Boyer L.A.; Lee T.I.; Cole M.F.; et al. (2005) Core transcriptional regulatory circuitry in human embryonic stem cells. *Cell* 122:947-956.

Burger J.A. & Kipps T.J. (2006) CXCR4: a key receptor in the crosstalk between tumor cells and their microenvironment. *Blood* 107:1761-1767.

Carmeliet P. ; Moons L. ; Luttun A., et al. (2001) Synergism, between vascular endothelial growth factor and placental growth factor contributes to angiogenesis and plasma extravasations in pathological conditions. *Nat Med* 7:575-583

Carmell M.A., Xuan Z., Zhang M.Q. et al. (2002) The Argonaute family: tentacles that reach into RNAi, developmental control, stem cell maintenance, and tumorigenesis *Genes Dev* 16: 2733-2742.

Cashman J.D.;Clark-Lewis I.; Eaves A.C.; et al. (1999) Stromal-derived factor 1 inhibits the cycling of very primitive human hematopoietic cells in vitro and in NOD/SCID mice *Blood* 94:3722-3729.

Caussinus E. & Gonzalez C. (2005) Induction of tumor growth by altered stem-cell asymmetric division in Drosophila melanogaster. *Nature Genet* 37:1125-1129.

Cejudo-Martin P. & Johnson R.S. (2005) A new Notch in the HIF belt: How hypoxia impacts differentiation. *Dev Cell* 9: 575-576.

Chambers A.F.; Groom A.C. & McDonald I.C. (2002) Dissemination and growth of cancer cells in metastatic sites. *Nature Rev Cancer* 2:563-572.

Chambers I.; Colby D.; Robertson M. et al. (2003) Functional expression cloning of Nanog, a pluripotency sustaining factor in embryonic stem cells. *Cell* 113:643-655.

Chambers I.; Silva J.; Colby D. et al. (2007) Nanong safeguards pluripotency and mediates germline development. *Nature* 450:1230-1234.

Chang H.J.; Sneddon J.B.; Alizadeh A.A et al. (2004) Gene expression signature of fibroblast serum response predicts human cancer progression: similarities between tumors and wounds. *PLoS Biology* 2, E7.

Chen, D & McKearin, D. (2003) Dpp signaling silences bam transcription directly to establish asymmetric divisions of germline stem cells. *Curr Biol.* 13, 1786-1791.

Cheng T.; Rodrigues N.; Dombkowski D.; et al. (2000) Stem cell repopulation efficiency but not pool size is governed by p27 (kip1). *Nat Med* 6:1235-1240.

Cheng T.; Rodrigues N.; Shen H.;et al. (2000) Hematopoietic stem cell quiescence maintained by p21cip1/waf1. *Science* 287:1804-1808.

Chenn A. & McConnell S.K. (1995) Cleavage orientation and the asymmetric inheritance of Notch1 immunoreactivity in mammalian neurogenesis. *Cell* 82:631-641

Cipolleschi M.G.; Dello Sbarba P. & Olivotto M. (1993) The role of hypoxia in the maintenance of hematopoietic stem cells. *Blood* 82: 2031-2037.

Classon M. & Harlow E. (2002) The retinoblastoma tumour suppressor in development and *cancer Nat rev Cancer* 2:910-917.

Cleevers H. (2005) Stem cells, asymmetric division and cancer. *Nature Genet* 37:1027-1028.

Coast S.; Flanagan W.M.; Nourse J. et al. (1996) Accommodating haploinsufficient tumour suppressor genes in Knudson's model *Science* 272:877-880.

Conti L.; Pollard S.M.; Gorba T.; et al. (2005) Niche-independent symmetrical self-renewal of a mammalian tissue stem cell. *PLos Biol.* 3, E283.

Copeland N.G.; Gilbert D.J.; Schindler C., et al. (1995) Distribution of the mammalian Stat gene family in mouse chromosomes. *Genomics* 29:225-228.

Cousens L.M. & Werb Z. (2002) Inflammation and cancer. *Nature* 420:860-867.

Covello K.L.; Kehler J.; Yu H.; et al. (2006) HIF-2 alpha regulates Oct-4: Effects of hypoxia on stem cell function, embryonic development, and tumor growth. *Genes Dev* 20:557-570.

Cullen BR. (2004) Transcription and processing of human microRNAs precursors. *Mol Cell* 16:861-865.

Deak M.; Clifton A.D.; Lucocp L.M. et al. (1998) Mitogen-and stress-activated protein jinase-1 (MSK1) is directly activated my MAPK and SAPK2 (p38, and may mediate activation of *CREB. EMBO J* 17:4426-441.

Deans R.J. & Moseley A.B. (2000) Mesenchymal stem cells: Biology and potential clinical uses. Exp Haematol 28:875-884.

Dittel B.N.; Mc Carthy J.B., Wayner E.A., et al. (1993) Regulation of human B-cell precursor adhesion to bone marrow stromal cells by cytokines that exert opposing effects on the expression of vascular cell adhesion molecule-1 (VCAM-1) *Blood* 81:2272-2282.

Ducos K.; Panterne B.; Fortunel N. et al. (2000) p21(cip1) mRNA is controlled by endogenous transforming growth factor-beta1 in quiescent human hematopoietic stem/progenitor cells. *J Cell Physiol* 184:80-85.

Fidler I.J. & Nicolson C.L. (1977) Fate of recirculating B16 melanoma metastatic variant cells in parabiotic syngeneic recipients. *J Nat Can Inst* 58:1867-1877

Fidler I.J. (1970) Metastasis: Quantitative analysis of distribution and fate of tumor embolilabeled with 125 I-5-iodo-2´-deoxyuridine. *J Nat Cancer Inst* 45:773-782

Folkman J. (2002) Role of angiogenesis in tumor growth and metastases. *Semin Oncol* 29:15-18

Fuchs E.; Tumbar T. & Guasch G. (2004) Socializing with the neighbors : stem cells and their niche. *Cell* 116:769-778

Gonczy P. & DiNardo S. (1996) The germ line regulates somatic cyst cell proliferation and fate during Drosophila spermatogenesis. Development 122:2437-2447

Gordan J.D. & Simon M.C. (2007) Hypoxia-inducible factors: central regulators of the tumor phenotype. *Curr Opin Gene Dev* 17(1):71-7.

Gottardi C.J.; Gumbioner B.M. (2004) Distionct molecular forms of beta-catenin are targeted to adhesive or transcriptional complexes. *J Cell Biol* 167:339-349.

Groden J, et al. (1991) Identification and characterization of the familial adenomatous polyposis coli gene. *Cell* 66:589-600.

Gustafson M.V.; Zheng X.; Pereira T, et al. (2005) Hypoxia requires notch signaling to maintain the undifferentiated cell state. *Dev Cell* 9:617-628

He L. & Hannon G.J. (2004) MicroRNAs: small RNAs with a big role in gene regulation. *Nature Rev Genet* 5:522-531

He X.C.; Zhang J.; Tong W.G., et al. (2004) BMP signaling inhibits intestinal stem cell self-renewal through suppression of Wnt-beta-catenin signaling. *Nat Genet* 36:1117-1121.

Helczynska K.; Kronblad A.; Jogi A; et al. (2003) Hypoxia promotes a dedifferentiated phenotype in ductal breast carcinoma in situ. *Cancer Res* 63:1441-1444

Hiratsuka S.; Watanabe A.; Sakurai Y. et al. (2008) The S100A8-serum amyloid A3-TLR4 paracrine cascade establishes a pre-metastatic phase. *Nat Cell Biol* 10(11):1349-55.

Horvitz H.R. & Herskowitz I. (1992) Mechanisms in asymmetric cell division: two Bs or not two Bs,that is the question. *Cell* 68:237-255

Houbaviy H.B.; Murray M.F. & Sharp P.A. (2003) Embryonic stem cell-specific microRNAs. *Dev Cell* 5:351-358.

Ihle J.N.; Stravapodis D.; Parganas E. et al (1998) The roles of Jaks and Stats in cytokine signaling. *Cancer J Sci Am* 4(suppl):84-91.

Jogi A.; Ora I.; Nilsson H. et al. (2002) Hypoxia alters gene expression in human neuroblastoma cells toward an immature and neural crest-like phenotype. *Proc Natl Acad Sci USA* 99:7021-7026.

Joslyn G., et al. (1991) Identification of deletion mutations and three new genes at the famlial polyposis locus. *Cell* 66:601-613.

Jove R. (2000) STAT signaling. *Oncogene* 19:2445-2465.

Joyce J.A. & Hanahan D. (2004) Multiple roles for cysteine cathepsins in cancer. *Cell Cycle* 3:1516-1619.

Kaifi J.T.; Yekebas E.F.; Schurr P. t al. (2005) Tumor-cell homing to lymph nodes and bone marrow and CXCR4 expression in esophageal cancer. *J Natl can Inst* 97:1840-1847.

Kalluri R. & Zeisberg M. (2006) Fibroblasts in cancer. *Nat Rev Cancer* 6:392-401.

Kaltschmidt J.A.; Davidson C.; Brown N.H. et al. (2000) Rotation and asymmetric of the mitotic spindle direct asymmetric cell division in the developing central nervous system.*Nat. Cell Biol* 2:7-12.

Kanellopoulou C.; Muljo S.A.; Kung A.L. et al. (2005) Dicer-deficient mouse embryonic stem cells are defective in differentiation and centromeric silencing. Genes Dev 19:489-501

Kang Y.; Siegel P.M.; Shu W. et al. (2003) A multigenetic program mediating breast cancer metastasis to bone. *Cancer Cell* 3:537-549

Kaplan R.N.; Riba R.D.; Zacharoulis S. et al. (2005) VEGFR1-positive haematopoietic bone marrow progenitors initiate the premetastatic niche. *Nature* 438:820-827

Kiger A.A.; White-Cooper H. & Fuller M.T. (2000) Somatic support cells restrict germline stem cell self-renewal and promote differentiation. Nature 407:750-754

Kiger A.A.; Jones D.L.; Schulz C. et al. (2001) Stem cell self-renewal specified by JAK-STAT activation in respond to a support cell cue. *Science* 294, 2542-2545.

Kim V.N. & Nam J.W. (2006) Genomics of microRNA. *Trends Gent* 22:165-173.

Kinzler K.W. et al. (1991) Identification of FAP locus genes from chromosome 5q21. *Science* 253:661-665.

Kloosterman W.P. & Plasterk R.H. (2006) The diverse functions of microRNAs in animal development and disease. *Dev Cell* 11:441-450

Knoblich J.A.; Jan L.Y. & Jan Y.N. (1995) Asymmetric segregation of Numb and Prospero during cell division. *Nature* 377:624-627

Knoblich J.A. (2001) The Drosophila nervous system as a model for asymmetric cell division. *Symp Soc Exp Biol* 53:75-89

Knoblich J.A. (2008) Mechanisms of asymmetric stem cell division. *Cell* 132:583-597

Kucia M.; Reca R.; Miekus K., et al. (2005) Trafficking of normal stem cells and metastasis of cancer stem cells involve similar mechanisms: Pivotal role of the SDF-1-CXCR4 axis. *Stem Cells* 23:879-894.

Lavoie J.N.; Lállemain G.; Brunet A. et al. (1996) Muller R, Pouyssegur J. Cyclcin D1 expression is regulated positively by the p42/p44MAPK and negatively by the p38/HOGMAPK pathway. *J Biol Chem* 271: 20608-20616.

Law S. & Chaudhuri S. (2007) Niche theory, stem-stromal imbalance and aplastic anaemia. *J Stem Cells* 2:1-10

Lee C.Y.; Robinson K.J. & Doe CQ. (2006) Lgl, Pins and aPKC regulate neuroblasts self-renewal versus differentiation. *Nature* 439:594:598.

Li B.; Sharpe E.E.; Maupin A.B., et al. (2006) VEGF and PIGF promote adult vasculogenesis by enhancing EPC recruitment and vessel formation at the site of tumor neovascularisation. *Faseb J* 20:1495-1497.

Li L. & Neaves W.B. (2006) Normal stem cells and cancer stem cells: the niche matters. *Cancer Res* 66:4553-4557.

Liotta L.A.; Wembu D.; Saini R.K. et al. (1978) In vivo monitoring of the death rate of artificial murine pulmonary micrometastaes. *Cancer Res* 38:1231-1236.

Loeffler M. & Roeder I. (2002) Tissue stem cells: definition, plasticity, heterogeneity, self-organization, and models a conceptual approach. *Cells Tiss Organs* 171, 8-26.

Lowry W.E.; Blanpain C.; Nowak JA, et al. (2005) Defining the impact of β-catenin/Tcf transactivation of epithelial stem cells. *Genes Dev* 19:1596-1611

Lyden D.; Hattori K.; Dias S. et al. (2001) Impaired recruitment of bone-marrow-derived endothelial and hematopoietic precursor cells blocks tumor angiogenesis and growth. *Nat Med* 7:1194-1201.

Mantovani A.; Allavena P.; Sica A. et al (2008) Cancer- related inflammatinon. *Nature* 454:426-444

Marcellini M.; De Luca N.; Riccioni T. et al (2006 Increased melanoma growth and metastasis spreading in mice overexpressing placenta growth factor. *Am J Pathol* 169:643-654

Mattick J.S. & Makunin IV. (2005) Small regulatory RNAs in mammals. *Hum Mol Genet* 14:R121-R132

Mehlen P. & Puisieux A. (2006) Metastasis: a question of life or death. *Nature Rev Cancer* 6:449-458.

Mitsui K.; Tokuzawa Y.; Itoh H. et al (2003) The homeo-protein Nanog is required for maintenance of pluripotency in mouse epiblast and ES cells. *Cell* 113:631-642.

Moore K.A. & Lemischka I.R. (2006) Stem cells and their niches. *Science* 311:1880-1885.

Morrison, S.J.; Shah N.M. & Anderson DJ. (1997) Regulatory mechanisms in stem cell biology. *Cell* 88: 287-298.

Morrison S.D.J & Kimble J. (2006) Asymmetric stem-cell divisions in development and cancer. *Nature* 441:1068-1074.

Muller A.; Homey B.; Soto H. et al (2001) Involvement of chemokine receptors in breast cancer metastasis. *Nature* 410:50-56.

Murchison E.P.; Partridge J.F.; Tam O.H., et al (2005) Characterization of Dicer-deficient murine embryonic stem cells. *Proc Natl Acad Sci USA* 102:12135-12140.

Nakahara K. & Carthew R.W. (2004) Expanding roles for miRNAs and siRNAs in cell regulation. *Curr Opin Cell Biol* 16:127-133

Naugler W.E. & Karin M. (2008) NF-kappaB and cancer-identifying targets and mechanisms.*Curr Opin Genet Dev* 18:19-26

Nichols J.; Zevnik B.; Anastassiadis K., et al. (1998) Niwa H, Klewe-Nebenius D, Chambers I, et al. Formation of pluripotent stem cells in the mammalian embryo depends on the POU transcription factor Oct4. *Cell* 95:379-391.

Nilsson S.K.; Johnston H.M. & Coverdale J.A. (2001) Spatial localization of transplanted hemopoietic stem cells: Interferences for the localization of stem cell niches. *Blood* 97, 2293-2299.

Oegema K. & Mitchison T.J. (1997) Rappaport rules: cleavage furrow induction in animal cells. *Proc Natl Acad Sci USA* 94:4817-4820.

Okamoto R.; Ueno M.; Yamada Y. et al. (2005) Hematopoietic cells regulate the angiogenic switch during tumorigenesis. *Blood* 105:2757-2783.

Orimo A.; Gupta P.B.; Sgroi D.C. et al. (2005) Stromal fibroblasts present in invasive human breast carcinomas promote tumor growth and angiogenesis through elevated SDF-1/CXCL12 secretion. *Cell* 121:335-348.

Owen M.E. (1998) The marrow stromal cell system. In:Beresford JN eds. *Marrow stromal cell culture.* United Kingdom: Cambridge University Press. ; pp 1-9

Palma V.; Lim D.A.; Dahmane N. et al. (2005) Sonic hedgehog controls stem cell behavior in the postnatal and adult brain. *Development* 132:335-344

Palmer T.D.; Schwartz P.H.; Taupin P. et al. (2001). Cell culture. Progenitor cells from human brain after death. *Nature* 411:42-43.

Papayannopoulou T.; Priestley G.V.; Nakamoto B.; et al. (2001) Molecular pathways in bone marrow homing: Dominant role of $\alpha_4\beta_1$ over β_2-integrins and selectins. *Blood* 98: 2403-2411.

Pece S, et al. (2004) Loss of negative regulation Numb over Notch is relevant to human breast carcinogenesis. *J Cell Biol* 167:215-221.

Peinado H.; Raffi S. & Lyden D. (2008) Inflammation joins the "niche". *Cancer cell* 14:347-349

Pevny L. & Placzek M. (2005) SOX genes and neural progenitor identity. *Curr Opin Neurobiol* 15:7-13.

Pistollato F.; Rampazzo E.; Abbadi S. et al. (2009) Molecular mechanisms of HIF-1alpha modulation induced by oxygen tension and BMP2 in glioblastoma derived cells. *Plos One* 4:e6206

Pistollato F.; Chen H.L.; Rood B.R. et al. (2009) Hypoxia and HIF1alpha repress the differentiate effects of BMPs in high-grade glioma. *Stem cell* 27:7-17

Polyak K.; Lee M.H.; Erdjument-Bromage H. et al. (1994) Cloning of p27Kip1, a cyclin-dependent kinase inhibitor and a potential mediator of extracellular antimitogenic signals.*Cell* 78:59-66

Potten MLAC (ed). (1997) *Stem Cells and Cellular Pedigrees- A Conceptual Introduction.* Academic Press: London

Psaila B.; Kaplan R.N.; Port E.R. et al. (2006) Lyden D. Priming the "soil" for breast cancer metastasis: the premetastatic niche. *Breast Dis* 26:65-74

Rafii S.; Lyden D.; Benezra R. et al (2002) Vascular and haematopoietic stem cells: novel targets for anti-angiogenesis therapy. *Nature* 2 : 826-835

Rappaport R. (1996) *Cytokinesis in Animal Cells* (Cambridge Univ Press, Cambridge, 1996)

Rappaport R. (1986) Establishment of the mechanism of cytokinesis in animal cells. *Int Rev Cytol* 105:245-281

Rappaport R. (1990) *Role of mitotic apparatus in furrow initiation.* Ann NY, Academic Sci.

Rattis F.M.; Voermans C. & Reya T. (2004) Wnt signaling in the stem cell niche. *Curr Opin Haematol* 11:88-94

Regala R.P., et al. (2005) Atypical protein kinase Ciota is an oncogene in human non-small cell lung cancer. *Cancer Res* 65:8905-8911

Regala R.P., et al. (2005) Atypical protein kinase Ciota plays a critical role in human lung cancer cell growth and tumorigenicity. *J Biol Chem* 280:31109-31115.

Rhyu M.S.; Jan L.Y. & Jan YN. (1994) Asymmetric distribution of numb protein during division of the sensory organ precursor cell confers distinct fates to daughter cells. *Cell* 76:477-491

Ross S.E., Greenberg M.E. & Stiles C.D. (2003) Basic helix-loop-helix factors in cortical development. Neuron 39:13-25

Ryan D.H.; Nuccie B.L.; Abboud C.N. et al. (1991)Vascular cell adhesion molecule-1 and the integrin VLA-4 mediate adhesion of human B cell precursors to cultured bone marrow adherent cells. *J Clin Invest* 88:995-1004.

Sansone P.; Storci G.; Giovannini C. et al (2007) p66Shc/Notch-3 interplay controls self-renewal and hypoxia survival in human stem/progenitor cells in mammary gland expanded in vitro as mammospheres. *Stem Cells* 25: 807-815.

Scadden D.T. (2006) The stem-cell niche as an entity of action. *Nature* 441:1075-1079

Schofield R. (1978) The relationship between the spleen colony forming cell and the haematopoietic stem cell. *Blood Cells* 4:7-25

Semenza G.L. (2001) Hypoxia-inducible factor 1: oxygen homeostasis and disease pathophysiology. *Trends Mol Med* 7:345-350

Sherr C.J. (1994) G1 phase progression: cycling on cue. *Cell* 79:551-555

Sherr C.J. & Roberts J.M. (1995) Inhibitors of mammalian G1 cyclin-dependent kinases. *Genes Dev* 9:1149-1163.

Shi Y.; Chichung Lie D.; Taupin P. et al. (2004) *Nature* 427:78-83.

Singh S.K.; Kagalwala M.N.; Parker- Thornburg J. et al. (2008). REST maintains self-renewal and pluripotency of embryonic stem cells. *Nature* 453:223-227.

Singh N.; Phillips R.A.; Iscove N.N.; et al. (2000) Expression of notch receptors, notch ligands, and fringe genes in hematopoiesis. *Exp Hematol* 28: 527-534.

Smith K.; Gunaratnam L.; Morley M. et al. (2005) Silencing of epidermal growth factor receptor suppresses hypoxia-inducible factor-2-driven VHL-/- renal cancer. *Cancer Res* 65:5221-5230

Sneddon J.B. & Werb Z. (2007) Location, location, location: the cancer stem cell niche. *Cell Stem Cell* 1:607-611

Song X.; Xie T. D. (2002) E-cadherin-mediated cell adhesion in the Drosophila ovary. *Proc Natl Acad Sci USA* 99:14813-14018.

Sprandling A.; Drummond-Barbosa D. & Kai T. (2001) Stem cells find their niche. *Nature* 414: 98-104.

Steinman R.M. & Nussenzweig M.C. (2002) *Proc Natl Acad Sci USA* 99:351-358.

Stier S.; Cheng T.; Forhert R. et al. (2003) Ex vivo targeting of p21Cip1/Waf1 permits relative expansion of human hematopoietic stem cells. *Blood* 102:1260-1266.

Strome S. (1993) Determination of cleavage planes. *Cell* 72:3-6.

Stylianou S.; Clarke R.B. & Brennan K. (2006) Aberrant activation of notch signaling in human breast cancer. *Cancer Res* 66:1517-1525.

Suda T.; Raia F. & Hirao A. (2005) Hematopoietic stem cells and their niche. *Trends Immunol.* 26:426-433.

Suh M.R. et al. (2004) Human embryonic stem cells express a unique set of microRNAs. *Dev Biol* 270:488-498.

Suh M.R.; Lee Y.; Kim J.Y. et al. (2004) Human embryonic stem cells express a unique set of microRNAs.*Dev Biol* 270:488-498

Sujata L. & Chaudhuri S. (2008) Stem cell niche, the microenvironment and immunological crosstalk. *Cell Mol Immunol* 5:107-112.

Takashahi T.; Nowakowski R.S. & Caviness VS. (1996) The leaving or Q fraction of the murine cerebral proliferative epithelium; a general model of neocortical neurogenesis. *J Neurosci* 16:6183-6196.

Takeichi M. (1991) Cadherin cell adhesion receptors as a morphogenetic regulator. *Science* 251:1451-1455.

Tay Y.; Zhang J.; Thomson A.M. et al. (2008) MicroRNAs to Nanog, Oct4 and Sox2 coding regions modulate embryonic stem cell differentiation. Nature 455(7216):1124-8.

Tschan M.P.; Peters U.R.; Cajot J.F. et al. (1999) The cyclin-dependent kinase inhibitors p18INK4c and p19INK4d are highly expressed in CD34+ progenitor and acute myeloid leukaemic cells but not in normal differentiated myeloid cells.*Br J Haematol* 106:644-651

Tulina N. & Matrevis E. (2001) Control of stem cell self-renewal in Drosophila spermatogenesis by JAK-STAT signalling. *Science* 294:2546-2549.

van der Vijver M.J.; He Y.D., van´t Veer L.J. et al. (2002) Gene-expression signature as a predictor of survival in breast cancer. *N Engl J Med* 347:1999-2002.

Varani J.; Lowett E.J.; Elgebay S. et al. (1980) In vitro and in vivo adherence of tumor cells variants correlated with tumor formation. *Am J Pathol* 101:345-352.

Voura E.B.; Billia F.; Iscove N.N. et al. (1997) Expression mapping of adhesion receptor genes during differentiation of individual hematopoietic progenitors. *Exp Hematol* 25: 1172-1179.

Vu T.H. & Werb Z. (2000) Matrix metalloproteinases:effectors of development and normal physiology. *Genes Dev* 14:2123-2133.

Wang Y.; Mevid R.; Melton C. et al. (2007) DGCR8 is essential for microRNA biogenesis and silencing on embryonic stem cell self-renewal. *Nat Genet* 39:380-385.

Watt F.M. & Hogan BLM. (2000) Out of Eden: Stem cells and their niches. *Science* 287:1427-1430.

Weigelt B. & Bissell M.J. (2008) Unraveling the microenvironmental influences on the normal mammary gland and breast cancer. *Semin Cancer Biol* 18:311-321

Wienholds W.E.; Koudijs M.J.; van Eeden F.J. et al. (2003) The microRNA-producing enzyme Dicer1 is essential for zebrafish development. *Nat Genet* 35:217-218.

Xie T.; Spradling A.C. (2000) A niche maintaining germ line stem cells in the Drosophila ovary. *Science* 290: 328-330.

Yamashita Y.M.; Jones D.L.; Fuller M.T. (2003) Orientation of asymmetric stem cell division by the APC tumor suppressor and centrosome. *Science* 301:1547-1550.

Yang AD, Camp ER, fan F, et al. (2006) Vascular endothelial growth factor receptor-1 activation mediates epithelial to mesenchymal transition in human pancreatic carcinoma cells. *Cancer Res* 66:46-55.

Yin T. & Li L. (2006) The stem cell niches in bone. *J Clin Invest* 116:1195-1201.

Yuan Y.; Shen H.; Franklin D.S. et al. (2004) In vivo self-renewing divisions of haematopoietic stem cells are increased in the absence of the early G1-phase inhibitor, p18INK4C. *Nat Cell Biol* 6:436-442.

Zhang J. & Li L. (2008) Stem cell niche: microenvironment and beyond. *J Biol Chem* 283:9499-9503.

Zhang J.; Niu C.; Ye L. et al. (2003) Identification of the haematopoietic stem cell niche and control of the niche size. *Nature* 425:836-841

Zhang Y.; Wittner M.; Bouamar H. et al. (2007) Identification of CXCR4 as a new nitric oxide-regulated gene in human CD34+ cells. *Stem Cells* 25:211-219.

11

The Stem Cell Niche: The Black Master of Cancer

Maguer-Satta Véronique
Inserm U590, University Claude Bernard Lyon I, Lyon
France

1. Introduction

Different populations of cancer cells co-exist within the same tumor; some have properties that closely resemble those of normal stem cells, which gave rise to the concept of cancer stem cells. Interestingly, these particular cancer cells express the same surface markers as normal stem cells, suggesting that cancer can sometimes arise from the malignant transformation of stem cells, such as established for some leukemias. The cancer stem cell model predicts that, even if "conventional" cancer cells can be killed, only the destruction of cancer stem cells allows full recovery. This demonstrates the importance of treatments targeting cancer stem cells for patient outcome. Therapeutic innovations will emerge from a better understanding of the biology and environment of cancer stem cells. Indeed, the tumor environment can create a niche favoring the survival and proliferation of cancer stem cells. It also contributes to resistance against therapy-induced apoptosis by providing both physical and physiological protection. Clinically, it is crucial to get rid of these treatment-resistant quiescent cells and to adapt the therapeutic strategy to reach the cancer stem cells sheltered in niches. In fact, most cancers likely recur because cancer stem cells escape treatment, survive and regenerate the tumor. Current hypotheses under evaluation suggest that this resistance may be due to the preservation of normal stem cell protective mechanisms such as their location in a niche, deregulation of drug efflux/influx transporter expression or alterations in apoptotic, cell cycle and DNA repair mechanisms. In this context, one of the key issues is that cancer stem cell self-renewal is dependent on close interactions with the stem cell niche which regulate the different developmental signaling pathways and are often found deregulated in cancer. However, investigations of the role of the microenvironment in adult stem cell transformation and resistance, especially in solid tissues, have started only recently, likely because of the major technical difficulties involved. Despite this delay, and thanks in part to studies in the hematopoietic system, a gold standard model for stem cell biology, great advances have been made in understanding the importance of the stem cell-microenvironment crosstalk in both normal and cancer tissues. We have now reached the point where conventional anti-cancer strategies can give way to more innovative combined therapy to target these interactions and "re-access" cancer stem cell regulation controls. Targeting these mechanisms by taking advantage of potential differences in the biology of normal and cancer stem cells, such as differences in surface phenotype, self renewal/quiescence and stem cell-niche interactions, might allow successful cancer stem cell targeting and improve cancer treatment outcome. This chapter focuses on the main issues to be considered for efficient and specific targeting of cancer stem cells within their niche. First we will present the different kinds of adult somatic stem cell niches, their characteristics and functions in normal tissues, which have been particularly well described and studied in the hematopoietic system. We will review recent data on the control by the niche of cell self-renewal, quiescence, differentiation and survival/apoptosis. Then we will discuss the involvement of the cancer stem cell microenvironment in cancer initiation, in the maintenance of residual disease and in treatment escape, a combination of mechanisms that likely drive cancer relapse in both hematopoietic and solid tumors. In conclusion, we will discuss the main therapeutic approaches currently under development and evaluation for targeting interactions of cancer stem cells with their neighboring partners. It is already foreseeable that combinations of conventional therapeutic approaches with specific cancer stem cell-targeting treatments might efficiently cure cancer.

2. Stem cell niches: a critical cell survival architect

More than 30 years ago, the existence of special spatially defined areas that were suspected to supply factors necessary to the survival and development of cells capable to regenerate tissues in adult organisms was postulated (Schofield, 1978). It was suggested that the local environment was critical to maintain cell survival through the delivery of special signals by the so-called "niche" that directs cell proliferation, differentiation and apoptosis. A number of studies have clearly demonstrated that the stem cell niche constitutes a key regulator of stem-cell fate by balancing self-renewal and differentiation (Blanpain et al., 2004; Fuchs et al., 2004; Zhang et al., 2003; Calvi et al., 2003). This concept was later extended to solid tissues and cancers (Moore and Lemischka, 2006; Li and Neaves, 2006). Over the last decades the existence, composition and functions of adult stem cell niches have begun to be elucidated, mainly in the hematopoietic system and, more recently, in solid tissues.

2.1 The hematopoietic model

The concept of stem cell niche was first described in the hematopoietic system. It was proposed that the bone marrow environment, where hematopoietic stem cells reside, is capable to regulate the maturation of hematopoietic stem cells by controlling the balance between two main mechanisms, stem cell quiescence/maintenance, and differentiation and production of mature blood components (Schofield, 1978). However, in order to allow for tissue turnover or injury repair, the stem cell niche must also permit stem cell activation and recruitment for proliferation/differentiation (Schofield, 1978). The normal bone marrow microenvironment (the hematopoietic "niche") regulates the dormancy, survival and non-differentiation of hematopoietic stem cells (Li and Li, 2006) in response to various external signals, therefore constituting a dynamic system. In addition, the niche interacts with stem cells; it does not only behave as an active regulator but also receives feedback from stem cells which actively contribute to the organization of their own niche (Fuchs et al., 2004). Adhesion to both matrix proteins and stromal cells and exposure to their soluble factors (cytokines, morphogens) controls the self-renewal and differentiation of hematopoietic stem cells (Ross and Li, 2006). In this regard, mesenchymal stem cells have been shown to play a central role in the stem cell niche in hematopoietic and other tissues (Docheva et al., 2007; Dazzi et al., 2006). They can differentiate into osteoblasts, the major regulators of hematopoiesis, and secrete many matrix proteins, morphogens, growth factors and cytokines (Calvi et al., 2003; Zhang et al., 2003). Interestingly, it has also been reported that infusion of *ex vivo*-expanded mesenchymal stem cells enhances hematopoietic stem cell engraftment, thus participating actively in stem cell homing (Dazzi et al., 2006). Immune cells are also an important component of the stem cell niche (Yang, 2007). Mesenchymal stem cells inhibit the immunological functions of antitumor lymphocytes such as natural killer cells (Sotiropoulou et al., 2006) and cytotoxic T lymphocytes (Djouad et al., 2003). Interactions between the different components appear to be important in controlling stem cell function, as illustrated by the impact of mesenchymal stem cells on immune cells (Benvenuto et al., 2007). Finally, inflammatory and oxidative stresses, associated with microenvironmental elements, constitute important regulators of hematopoietic stem cell functions (Ito et al., 2006). Recently, a step forward was made with the identification of different subsets of hematopoietic stem cells such as dormant or homeostatic stem cells. This discovery immediately implied the likely existence, within the bone marrow, of distinct hematopoietic niches supporting and controlling the different hematopoietic stem cell types. Two main types of niches are commonly distinguished according to their location, composition and function on hematopoietic stem cells: the osteoblastic/endosteal niche and the vascular niche. *In situ* experiments have located hematopoietic stem cells within the trabecular-bone area (Zhang et al., 2003). The niche that contains the most dormant stem cells is described as a hypoxic place close to the endosteum which contains osteoblasts, fibroblasts, osteoclasts, perivascular structures and sympathetic neurons (Burness and Sipkins, 2010; Trumpp et al., 2010). The control of the size and composition of the niche has been reported to involve a number of different factors such as Notch or the Bone Morphogenetic Proteins (Kiel and Morrison, 2008; Zhang et al., 2003). Interestingly, this family of proteins has also been known for several years to be a key factor in the control of hematopoietic stem cell fate (Sadlon et al., 2004; Maguer-Satta and Rimokh, 2004). In the bone marrow environment, hypoxia has been initially described to regulate hematopoietic differentiation, in particular toward the erythroid lineage, likely to counteract oxygen deprivation after an injury episode (Perry et al., 2007). Conversely, within the endosteal niche, the hypoxic environment appears to protect the long-lived, deeply dormant stem cells from the toxic effects of oxidative damage caused by reactive oxygen species that otherwise could conduct to the alteration of the stem cell pool. On the other hand, oxygenated perivascular niches represent a network of sinusoids composed of endothelial cells, reticular cells and megakaryocytes (Trumpp et al., 2010). Their function seems to promote hematopoietic stem cell proliferation and differentiation, in particular during blood recovery after an injury. Even if dormant cells could theoretically also locate in vascular niches, these niches remain the principal sites where bone marrow hematopoietic stem cells are mobilized to the peripheral circulation, together with differentiated hematopoietic cells (Burness and Sipkins, 2010). This mechanism is mainly regulated by the SDF-1/CXCR4 chemokine pathway that directs the passage of the cells from or toward the bone marrow. To maintain blood homeostasis, a flux of homeostatic hematopoietic stem cells migrates from endosteal niches through perivascular niches to the circulation. Therefore a continuous traffic of hematopoietic stem cells is observed from one niche to another and to the peripheral circulation, then back to the bone marrow and supposedly to dormancy.

2.2 Insight in solid tissue stem cell niches

As in the hematopoietic system, the niche in solid tissues is defined as the physiological microenvironment which keeps the stem cells quiescent until their self-renewal. The same applies to other stem cell niches present in various tissues and containing various partners

(Blanpain et al., 2004; Moore and Lemischka, 2006). Despite the technical difficulties of investigating the niche composition, location and function in solid mammalian tissues, some examples have been reported in the neural system and in the intestinal and various other epithelia (Burness and Sipkins, 2010). A number of elements common to solid tissue and hematopoietic stem cell niches have then been identified, including cell-cell and cell-extra cellular matrix interactions, as well as diffusible signaling factors mediating signal transduction in order to maintain stem cell survival and self-renewal. For example, in the nervous system the functional interactions of the vascular niche between neural stem cells and endothelial cells through junctional contacts are involved in the increased proliferation of neural stem cells. Similar to neurogenic niches in the hippocampus, neurovascular interaction has been observed in the sub-ventricular zone where numerous polarized stem cells establish connections with the endothelial cells of blood vessels through long basal processes. These stem cells also extend short apical processes to connect to ependymal cells that line the surface of lateral ventricles (Vazin and Schaffer, 2010). Recent data in intestine, brain, hair follicle or skin suggest that, like hematopoietic stem cells in the bone marrow, two main categories of stem cell niches might exist in solid tissues. Evidence in support of this theory comes in part from the observation that in tissues containing low cycling stem cells, participation in homeostasis and repair requires that cells rapidly switch from a quiescent to proliferative state. As in the hematopoietic system, two functional types of niches could be distinguished, one allowing rapid entry into proliferation, as required for tissue regeneration, and one that would maintain long-term growth and self-renewal (Greco and Guo, 2010). Interestingly, another bi-compartmentalization has been proposed for epithelial tissues based on cellular components of the niche. The two compartments would be the epithelial niche where stem cells are in direct contact with the basal lamina and the stromal niche where stem cells interact with another cell type in contact with basal lamina (Morrison and Spradling, 2008). Each type of epithelium has its own mechanism to regenerate from local stem cells. The different stem cell populations cooperatively regenerate all terminally differentiated cell types within the tissue. The microenvironment of epithelial stem cells is generally located near a basement membrane and the stem cells are part of the basal layer. Supportive cells present within the niche protect the stem cells from exogenous factors. Following differentiation, stem cell progenies migrate along the basement membrane and leave the niche (Verstappen et al., 2009). Epithelial niches might be limited by the presence of specific molecules within the extracellular matrix or on neighboring tissues. On the other hand, stromal niches appear to develop independently of the presence of stem cells and to maintain their morphology even after stem cell loss (Morrison and Spradling, 2008). Both types of niches depend on cell-cell junction molecules and stem cells are in contact with their progenies. In all cases and in any proposed classification, the role of niches in solid tissues is the same as in the hematopoietic system, namely to maintain and protect the stem cell pools which are crucial for tissue homeostasis. In all systems, this mechanism appears to be dependent on stem cell interactions with their close environment. A permanent dialogue through recurrent adhesion molecules such as cadherins or integrins is required to maintain stem cell architecture and shape, but this mechanism also constitutes a key regulator of asymmetrical division, and therefore self-renewal, as we will discuss now (Marthiens et al., 2010).

3. The guardian of key features of stem cells

The niche is critical to maintaining stem cell quiescence, the intrinsic self-renewal and undifferentiated character of resident stem cells, but it also regulates exogenous stem cells that tend to home back to that specific microenvironment.

3.1 Asymmetric cell division

Regulating the balance between symmetrical and asymmetrical divisions is critical to maintain the proper number of stem cells within the niche and meeting the demand for differentiated cells in surrounding tissues. Asymmetric cell division is one of the key features of stem cells that allows simultaneous self-renewal and differentiation. Asymmetric division is the process by which a single cell gives rise to two different daughter cells, a major strategy for the generation of cell diversity during the development or renewal of an organism/organ/tissue (Fuchs et al., 2004). However, it is also important to note that asymmetric division is not the only way to maintain stem cell self-renewal since two identical daughter cells are also specified entirely by their position and external signals derived from cells outside the niche (Conti et al., 2005). In particular, this process has been reported to occur in stem cell amplification during regeneration (Morrison and Kimble, 2006). Experiments in *Drosophila* and *Caenorhabditis elegans* have identified three major steps to achieve asymmetrical division: establishment of polarity, localization of fate determinant to one or the other cell pole, and subsequent regulation of the plane of cell cleavage. Upon division, the fate determinants will be asymmetrically distributed between the two daughter cells, one of them retaining stem cell features while the other one is driven toward a more differentiated stage (Marthiens et al., 2010). A number of genetic determinants have been shown to be involved in the intrinsic mechanism that dictates asymmetrical division (Faubert et al., 2004) but the exact pathways involved and their connection with extrinsic elements are still under investigation. However, thanks to studies in animal models like *Caenorhabditis elegans*, great progress has been made in understanding how the stem cell niches give instructive signals to drive asymmetric divisions in order to orchestrate the flow and cell fate of committed progenitors in a spacio-temporally controlled fashion. Asymmetry can be governed by the proximity to the cellular environment, such as the defined niches, that exerts extrinsic physical tension to achieve asymmetrical distribution of the mitotic spindles. Astral microtubules are physical structures that determine centrosome and spindle positioning. The aster traction to one pole of the cell results from a complex network of interactions between cell surface molecules, intra-cellular microtubules and intrinsic elements. Certain adhesion molecules such as APC, cadherins and integrins, have been shown to be involved in this process (Fuchs et al., 2004; Marthiens et al., 2010). For example, the role of cell-to-cell interactions mediated by β1-Integrins is crucial for the maintenance of stemness, especially in the hematopoietic stem cells that home back to the bone marrow (Gottschling et al., 2007). Authors have shown that β1-integrins play a significant role not only in the interaction between hematopoietic stem cells and mesenchymal stem cells but also in the regulation of the long-term fate of hematopoietic stem cells by favoring initial self-renewing divisions and the survival of primitive hematopoietic stem cells. This role of β1 integrin in asymmetrical division has also been demonstrated in solid tissue stem cells such as in the skin or the mammary gland (Marthiens et al., 2010). Therefore close interactions between stem cells and their neighbor cells within the stem cell niche allow adhesion molecules to control the angle of cell division by interacting with astral microtubules that regulate centrosome positioning. In cancer, the loss of this ability of asymmetrical division is thought to lead to the over amplification of a pool of cells that progressively drives to tumorigenesis.

3.2 Stem cell quiescence

The crucial point for the body to achieve homeostasis throughout life is to be able to preserve the stem cell pools from exhaustion and alteration. To that aim, the body employs a strategy involving specialized stem cell niches, such as the osteoblastic/endosteal niche in the hematopoietic system and the so-called epithelial niche for epithelium tissues that, by their defined composition, are capable to display quiescent signaling to the resident stem cells (Trumpp et al., 2010; Morrison and Spradling, 2008). In order to maintain stem cells through time, it is important that self-renewal divisions of dormant stem cells occur only transiently, for example in response to a physiological need or to injury. Niche components, such as extracellular matrix molecules (laminin, fibronectin, collagen, glycosaminoglycans), provide a physical framework and instructive signals that regulate stem cells, in particular by participating to the maintenance of cell quiescence. It has been described, for instance, that β-integrin regulates the maintenance of neural stem cells and directly induces the expression of other cell surface receptors that relay information to the neural stem cells. Extracellular-matrix molecules also serve to immobilize and locally increase the concentration of a number of soluble signaling molecules such as the Bone Morphogenetic Proteins, Sonic Hedgehog or Wingless proteins, involved in stem cell quiescence (Vazin and Schaffer, 2010). Several receptors have then been demonstrated to be involved in the specific signals that dictate stem cell quiescence, partly by preventing cell division and differentiation. These include the tyrosine kinase receptor Kit (i.e. CD117) that binds Stem Cell Factor (SCF), the receptor for angiopoietin 1 (ANG1) TIE2, the TromboPOietin (TPO) receptor (cytokine receptor MyeloProliferative Leukemia virus receptor, MPL) and the CXC-chemokine receptor 4 (CXCR4) that binds the Stromal Derived Factor 1 (SDF1). Signaling response to their respective ligands inhibits the division of cells, thus preserving their dormancy. In addition, dormant niches seem to be dependent upon low oxygen concentration environment to maintain stem cell dormancy mainly through HIF1α signaling (Guitart et al., 2010; Diabira and Morandi, 2008; Eliasson et al., 2010; Moreno-Manzano et al., 2010). In the hematopoietic system, it is now well known that hypoxia is one of the key factors of the endosteal niche that contribute to maintaining normal stem cells in a dormant stage (Trumpp et al., 2010). All these signals are actively coordinated and presented in a temporally and spatially regulated manner to ensure the balance between stem cell quiescence and activation (Trumpp et al., 2010).

3.3 Stem cell fate

To preserve the stem cell pool from exhaustion, self-renewal divisions of dormant hematopoietic stem cells seem to occur only transiently after injury or mobilization signals. In this particular situation which requires the release of stem cells from their dormant stage, both types of signals have been reported to induce a proteolytic environment that enzymatically cleaves physical hematopoietic-niche bonds. This allows stem cells to migrate from the endosteal niche to the vascular niche where they find proliferation/differentiation signals and eventually leave the bone marrow to be transported to the site of injury by the peripheral system (Trumpp et al., 2010). Therefore, the architectural design of a niche appears to be suited to particular needs of its resident stem cells and, conversely, stem cells may play an important role in organizing and specifying the niche as proposed in the context of breast by the dynamic reciprocity concept (Xu et al., 2009). One of the best described actors in self-renewal maintenance in different systems is the β1-Integrin. This protein belongs to the large family of heterodimeric receptors involved in cell-matrix and cell-cell adhesion. Integrins transduce both "Outside-In" and "Inside-Out" signals involved in cellular processes such as cell morphology, motility, proliferation, differentiation, inhibition of apoptosis and likely much more (Ho and Wagner, 2007; Docheva et al., 2007; Gottschling et al., 2007; Dylla et al., 2004). In some cases, like in the neural system (Hall et al., 2006) or breast (Shackleton et al., 2006; Stingl et al., 2006), some integrins are even considered as stem cell markers. Their key role in the hematopoietic system has been largely documented, mainly through their binding to fibronectin (main ligand of β1 integrin) or, to a lesser extent, to VCAM-1 (Levesque and Simmons, 1999), in diverse processes of hematopoietic stem cell regulation such as self-renewal, differentiation, mobility and apoptosis (Hurley et al., 1997; Hurley et al., 1995; Jiang et al., 2000a; Prosper and Verfaillie, 2001; Prosper et al., 1998; Priestley et al., 2006; Priestley et al., 2007; Scott et al., 2003). More recently their involvement in stem cell maintenance has been demonstrated in both murine (Taddei et al., 2008) and human (Bachelard-Cascales et al., 2010) breast and studies are currently investigating their role in the biology of stem cells in many other solid tissues. Understanding the fine-tuned regulation that switches stem cells from a deep dormant to a proliferating state is quite complex. As for quiescence maintenance, extracellular matrix-bound molecules such as the Bone Morphogenetic Proteins (Vazin and Schaffer, 2010) could also serve as main regulators to control stem cell self-renewal, proliferation or commitment, as described by us in the hematopoietic system (Jeanpierre et al., 2008; Maguer-Satta et al., 2006; Maguer-Satta and Rimokh, 2004; Maguer-Satta et al., 2003) or by others in the epithelial system (Blanpain and Fuchs, 2006), or for Notch and Sonic Hedgehog in the neural system (for review see (Fuchs et al., 2004; Morrison and Spradling, 2008)). Finally, stem cells respond differently to a two-dimensional substrate and a three-dimensional environment, thus activating different signaling pathways. Integrin signaling, for instance, is involved in extracellular matrix remodeling which controls the niche architecture and therefore impacts

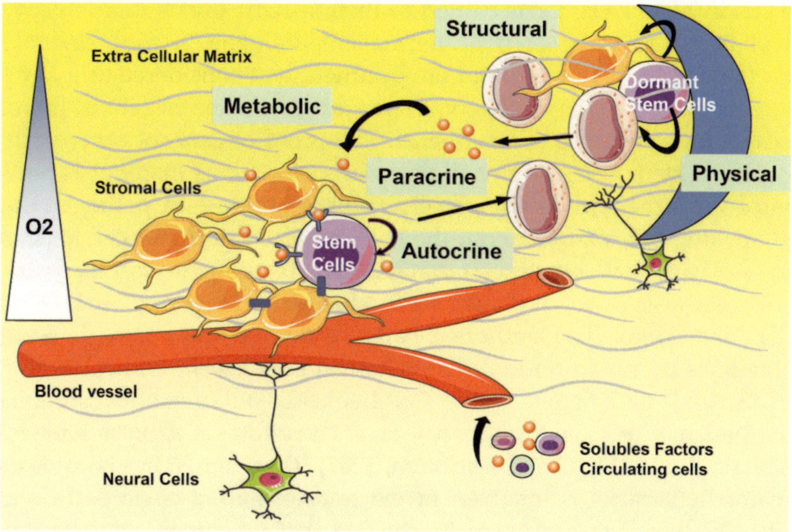

Fig. 1. Parameters of stem cells niches that drive stem cells behavior and/or the reverse, summary of the main parameters involved in stem cell behavior such as dormancy or inversely their commitment, migration. The same elements are involved in the permanent dialogue that exists between stem cells and their niche going from the stem cell toward its environment to modify or regulate its function. Each of these elements can be affected during cell transformation inducing cancer stem cell escape, resistance and persistence.

stem cell behavior and tumorigenesis (Larsen et al., 2006). This has been demonstrated in normal adult stem cells using variations of matrix elasticity to drive stem cell fate (Engler et al., 2006). Moreover, matrix remodeling, notably proteolytic breakdown of fibronectin giving rise to biologically active peptides or to domains of interaction with morphogens or TGFβ regulators, may be involved in the control of hematopoietic stem cell fate either by promoting cell proliferation or commitment toward specific lineages.
The different niche types defined share common features and activate common signal transduction pathways to achieve the slow-cycling, self-renewing, undifferentiated state of their residents (Fig. 1). For that, several different pathways display a number of crosstalks and multigene redundancies. Conversely, each niche is composed of different types of non stem cells and stem cells that constitute this environment and a same signaling pathway can control different cellular functions. Altogether this strongly suggests that the critical genes involved in stem cell fate are likely to vary with the different stem cell types and their location, even if the general mechanisms controlling their behavior remain the same.

4. The under-estimated initiator/actor of cancer

There is growing evidence that, although it has long been largely under-evaluated, the tumor microenvironment plays a very active role in tumor initiation and progression. More than twenty years ago, a few people went against the strong wave of genetic promoters as the only explanation for the etiology of cancer, and claimed that "mutations were not all" in oncogenesis. At that time some scientist argued that the tumor environment was also a major actor in cancer pathogenesis and that it should be taken into account in studies that pretend to understand and treat cancer (Ronnov-Jessen and Bissell, 2009). With the discovery of cancer stem cells, focus turned to their specific microenvironment and studies tried to elucidate the function of their permanent dialogue. It took several decades to actually reach the point where the tumor environment was considered as a key player at all stages of cancer. This led to major observations and gave some insight in its role in cancer initiation, escape and resistance to treatments. The proof of concept came once more from the hematopoietic system where a key clinical observation was made. It is now trivial that the bone marrow microenvironment plays an important role in pathogenesis. A review providing compelling information about the hematopoiesis of donor cell leukemia strongly supports this "seed and soil" hypothesis that has been hanging around for years in the field of solid tumor metastasis research (Paget, 1989; Mueller and Fusenig, 2004; Demicheli, 2001; Greig and Trainer, 1986). The authors clearly underline that, though seemingly rare, leukemia sometimes occurs in normal donor hematopoietic cells transplanted to leukemia patients. The disease is then named Donor Cell Leukemia and must be distinguished from a relapse of the patient's original malignancy as it constitutes a *de novo* leukemia affecting normal transplanted cells (Flynn and Kaufman, 2007). Therefore, it has become quite evident that the hematopoietic niche is involved in the transformation of normal donor cells into leukemia cells; this theory is supported by the fact that no cytogenetic abnormalities have been detected in donor cells. It is even suspected that, as the hematopoietic stem cells present in the graft are responsible for hematopoietic reconstitution in the recipient, Donor Cell Leukemia might arise from abnormal hematopoietic stem cell regulation by the patient's hematopoietic niche (Flynn and Kaufman, 2007). Therefore, the role of the tumor microenvironment in tumor initiation and progression through its different constituting elements (stromal and immune cells as well as extra cellular matrix molecules) is being increasingly acknowledged. Two main hypotheses could explain features of cancer stem cells: one proposes that transformed stem cell-like populations progressively evade their niche control while the other one considers that the niche itself could be altered during oncogenesis. Actual data document both aspects, indicating that tumors arise from complex combinations of alterations that trigger both the malignant cells and their environment.

4.1 Niche alteration: cause and consequence

A first step to identify and understand the role of niche alteration in cancer development has been the characterization of the cellular content of the niche. In established leukemia, several lines of evidence demonstrate that both cell and matrix components of the bone marrow microenvironment, such as integrins, are clearly modified (Ruoslahti, 1999). Mesenchymal stem cell alterations have then been investigated and several changes have been identified in their transcriptome, phenotype and functions from myeloma patients (Arnulf et al., 2007; Corre et al., 2007). In a number of myeloid or lymphoid leukemias, profound alterations of the bone marrow environment, such as myelofibrosis, are frequently reported. In myeloma, osteolytic lesions and differential expression of integrins and cytokines correlate with early oncogenic events (Hideshima et al., 2004). In Chronic Myelogenous Leukemia, bone marrow macrophages impair the mesenchymal cell support of hematopoiesis (Bhatia et al., 1995a), whereas in Acute Myeloid Leukemia, fibronectin and Wnt ligands are overexpressed (Simon et al., 2005). Alterations of the $\beta 1$ integrin, not in terms of membrane protein expression but rather as a defect in protein activation, has been shown to be involved in the loss of regulation of leukemic hematopoietic stem cells by the marrow stroma (Bhatia et al., 1995a; Bhatia et al., 1999; Jiang et al., 2000b; Jongen-Lavrencic et al., 2005; Lundell et al., 1997; Lundell et al., 1996). Original signaling pathways downstream of integrin ligation have been involved in normal and leukemic cell survival, proliferation and adhesion (Tabe et al., 2007; Dylla et al., 2004; Melikova et al., 2004). In solid tumors, integrins have also been involved at various levels in breast cancer biology, likely at the level of cancer stem cell (Bissell et al., 2005; Park et al., 2006; Faraldo et al., 2005; Faraldo et al., 2002; Faraldo et al., 2000; Taddei et al., 2003). In addition, a deregulated signal transduction in leukemic cells may allow them to escape microenvironmental control (Astier et al., 2003; Wilson et al., 2004; De Waele et al., 1999). Another example of niche alteration has been reported in solid tumors by pathologists who have described the frequent association of stromatogenesis and neoplasia. This stromatogenesis is an affection of the tumor-associated stroma characterized by many changes such as deregulated expression and organization of fibronectin and collagen, leading to modifications of the stroma-associated tumor that becomes more rigid. Other studies have shown that extracellular matrix stiffness perturbs the original epithelial morphogenesis by clustering integrins and inducing focal adhesion assembly to enhance specific signaling pathways (Paszek et al., 2005). Cells sense elevated extracellular matrix rigidity through their integrins and respond with modified signaling that in turn stimulate integrin expression or change their conformation to induce their activation. This response can be amplified by a signaling cascade involving different molecules (such as Rho, Rock, ERK) that drive surrounding cell proliferation and transformation and extracellular matrix rigidity (Larsen et al., 2006). As a consequence, the tumor microenvironment can send erroneous signals to niche cells, inducing accumulation of proteases and activation of soluble factors, all contributing to alter stem cell control. Altogether, these data indicate that most cancers are likely associated with modifications of the stem cell environment. One of the consequences possibly contributing to cancer initiation is the deregulation of asymmetric division control by the niche. When the asymmetric division machinery is perturbed tumor growth is observed (Caussinus and Gonzalez, 2005). In support of this hypothesis is also the fact that some gene products that induce asymmetric cell divisions function as tumor suppressor genes, such as reported for APC in colorectal cancer and melanoma. Conversely, gene products that favor symmetric cell divisions act as oncogenes in mammalian cells, such as PKC in lung cancer. Symmetric division then not only favors the expansion of stem cell numbers but might also increase the risk of aneuploidy and accumulation of secondary mutations by impaired mechanisms controlling the mitotic machinery (Morrison and Kimble, 2006). It then becomes important to understand the consequences of this matrix remodeling on normal and cancer stem cell behavior, in particular for drug resistance.

4.2 Cancer stem cells: natural reprogramming in "iPS" by the niche

Of particular interest in the context of cancer, niches have been demonstrated to be capable of reprogramming cells. An experimentally-vacated ovarian germline stem cell niche induced the division of foreign surrounding somatic stem cells which then have given rise to ovarian follicle cells and allowed the dedifferentiation of ectopic follicle progenitor cells at earlier stages of differentiation. These experiments have established the fact that a niche is a stable structure capable to direct cell fate even outside its initial intrinsic differentiation program (Kai and Spradling, 2003). These observations might be in part explained by the reprogramming power of physical constraint. A very elegant study has demonstrated that simple physical constraint can drive stem cells toward one lineage rather than another, indicating that both physical and cellular properties of niches are important in the control of stem cell behavior (Engler et al., 2006). In the past five years, stem cell research has made a major breakthrough by artificially inducing cell reprogramming. Yamanaka et al have developed a strategy that generates from mature differentiated cells a "stem cell-like" entity named iPS for "induced-Pluripotent Stem Cell". Reprogrammed cells display most of the properties of pluripotent stem cells, such as the ability to differentiate into functional mature cells, and present a number of epigenetic modifications (Boheler, 2009). It is intriguing that factors deregulated in the cancer niche, such as hypoxia, have recently been reported to significantly improve the iPS process (Yoshida et al., 2009). The origins of cancer stem cells are still debated and one can hypothesize that the transformation of a true stem cell, such as in Chronic Myelogenous Leukemia, is likely to be an infrequent event. Almost a decade ago, the option that cancer stem cells could arise from the reacquisition of stem cell characteristics emerged (Passegue et al., 2003). It is then tempting to suggest that one of the first steps in tumor initiation is the generation of cancer "iPS" induced by alterations occurring in the niche, such as a change in rigidity, extracellular matrix remodeling or oxygen concentration (Engler et al., 2006; Larsen et al., 2006; Heddleston et al., 2010). In support of this hypothesis is the fact that in cells classified as cancer stem cells the re-expression of embryonic genes or genes involved in self-renewal has often been described and shown to be involved in the cancer stem cell phenotype (Lessard and Sauvageau, 2003; Yin et al., 2010; Godmann et al., 2009). Finally, the niche could induce genetic or epigenetic changes in cancer stem cells (or vice versa) as observed using the iPS technology (Boheler, 2009). These changes provide a growth advantage and induce a differentiation blockade, causing their transformation into cancer stem cells (Issa, 2007; Wang and Dick, 2005).

4.3 Factors that control key surviving pathways

A large number of factors have been reported to favor cancer cell survival. Only a few particularly significant examples of the key role played by the niche in cancer stem cell behavior will be given here. The tumor microenvironment is often hypoxic, due essentially to chaotic vasculature, poor oxygen diffusion across the expanding tumor and irregular blood flow. The oxygenation status of tumor tissues cycles in both spatial and temporal manners. Several studies have shown that hypoxic conditions enhance the metastatic power of cancer cells likely through HIF-dependent pathways (Heddleston et al., 2010). During cancer initiation, a hypoxic environment might favor the transformation of the resident stem cells by potentiating the effect of genes associated with stemness like Notch. At the clinical level, there is a correlation between the presence of a hypoxic zone within the tumor and poor patient outcome, and this could be explained by an increased number of cancer stem cells (Heddleston et al., 2010). This might also explain the disappointing results obtained in some studies of single-agent vascular-targeted treatments aimed at depriving the tumor of oxygen by inhibiting its ability to generate a neo-vasculature in the hope to kill cancer cells. A side effect of this strategy might be a significant increase in the pool of drug-resistant cancer stem cells. However this does not preclude combining anti-angiogenic strategies with other specific anti-cancer stem cell therapies. As stated above, hypoxia has been reported to significantly improve the cell reprogramming by which mature differentiated cells give rise to iPS (Yoshida et al., 2009). The capacity of cancer stem cells to modulate the tumor environment has also been suspected. In solid tumors, several arguments suggest that cancer stem cells, as they are capable to survive in low oxygen concentration, stimulate angiogenesis in response to HIF-dependent signaling. This will help to increase the oxygen level within the growing tumor which otherwise conduct to necrosis of the under oxygenated tumor mass. With growing knowledge, hypoxia has become a critical microenvironment parameter. Indeed, HIF expression in cancer stem cells is now described to be responsible for cell proliferation and tumor survival (Heddleston et al., 2010). Later on during disease progression, continuous or increasing hypoxic conditions can lead to specific activation of local enzymes such as reported for lysyl oxidase, a well-known enzyme that crosslinks collagen. This enzymatic activity does not seem important for cancer initiation but appear essential for metastasis through activation of the protein FAK phosphorylation that stimulates cell migration and contributes to cancer spread (Larsen et al., 2006).

4.4 The perfect hide-out

Alteration of the permanent crosstalk between cancer stem cells and their microenvironment deregulates the balance between dormant and activated stem cells, contributing to tumor resistance (Besancon et al., 2009; White et al., 2006). A consequent literature has documented this aspect of cancer biology in both the hematopoietic context and solid tumors (Hall et al., 2007; Kleeff et al., 2007; Kaplan et al., 2006; Psaila et al., 2006; Tysnes and Bjerkvig, 2007; Lee and Herlyn, 2007b; Lee and Herlyn, 2007a; Mueller and Fusenig, 2004). The bone marrow microenvironment is largely involved in the pathogenesis and maintenance of malignant tumors of hematopoietic origin. In the microenvironment, leukemic stem cells represent a quiescent population of cells that are resistant to standard therapy and different from their normal counterparts. Moreover, mesenchymal stem cells, the second largest population of long-lived stem/progenitor cells in the bone marrow, could favor the growth of tumor cells and their survival by inducing anti-apoptotic signals and further resistance to chemotherapeutic agents, as reported in acute myeloid leukemia (Konopleva et al., 2009).

Integrins are known to be involved not only in regulating the proliferation of extracellular matrix (fibronectin) and stromal cells (osteoblasts, mesenchymal stem cells) but also in the chemoresistance of leukemic stem cells (Fernandez-Vidal et al., 2006; De Toni et al., 2006). Numerous studies indicate that cell-cell and cell-matrix adhesion molecules also protect tumors from treatments. Adhesive interactions between cells or between cells and the extracellular matrix can regulate apoptosis and cell survival in a wide variety of cell types. Several studies have demonstrated that drugs generate a stress-induced anti-apoptotic bcl-2 signaling pathway implicating β1 integrin and fibronectin interaction (Damiano, 2002). Interestingly, anti-β1 antibodies or antisense oligonucleotides enhance the apoptotic process (Hazlehurst et al., 2001). In small cell lung cancer, the emergence of resistance to chemotherapy has also been correlated to high expression of integrins in the extracellular matrix (Hodkinson et al., 2007). The authors have demonstrated that the extracellular matrix, via β1 integrin-mediated PI3-kinase activation, allows small cell lung cancer cells to escape treatment-induced cell cycle arrest, apoptosis and DNA damage. In the mammary system, it has also been demonstrated that β1-integrin plays a key role in treatment resistance (Park et al., 2008). Interestingly, we have demonstrated that β1-integin interaction with its ligand is required to maintain mammary stem cells in their niche at immature stage. Indeed, by using β1 blocking antibodies we have been able to induce further stem cell differentiation (Bachelard-Cascales et al., 2010). Altogether, these observations suggest that resistant breast cancer stem cells use β1-integrin to hide in the niche. In solid tumors, the microenvironment can protect stem cells from the oxygen deprivation due to rapid tumor cell proliferation and abnormal vessel formation (Keith and Simon, 2007). Therefore, the niche provides cancer stem cells with physical and physiological protection from anti-cancer drugs (Elrick et al., 2005).

5. A major target for cancer cure

Accumulated data clearly indicate that stem cell niches are key and active elements in cancer biology: they are involved in tumor initiation, progression and maintenance and therefore constitute an important target in anti-cancer therapy (Adams and Scadden, 2006; White et al., 2006). Observations indicate that the stem cell niche remains one of the key targets for future developments in cancer treatment. Two main strategies are currently developed based on the reciprocal dependence of the cancer stem cells and their niches. One is to attempt to awake quiescent cancer stem cells from dormancy and the other is to make them leave their protective niche. One should however keep in mind that selective anti-cancer stem cell treatments will not immediately eliminate differentiated cancer cells, and might therefore be prematurely dropped if their clinical activity is judged solely by the traditional response criteria of changes in the bulk of the tumor. This implies that re-examining both pre-clinical and clinical drug development paradigms in order to include the cancer stem cell concept might revolutionize the treatment of many cancers. Some drugs are already available that could act, at least in part, by killing cancer stem cells; however, no complete cure has been obtained to date, suggesting that further experimentation with cancer stem cell-targeted therapy is required (Besancon et al., 2009). The major problem for people developing these new drugs is to selectively target cancer stem cells whereas preserving normal stem cells. This question is indeed critical, since many studies have highlighted the extensive phenotypic and functional similarities between normal and cancer stem cells. A possible solution could be based on the fact that interactions between cancer stem cells and their environment are profoundly altered. The modified cell environment itself can even be considered a relevant treatment target, even if not malignant *per se*. Re-establishing a normal niche might also normalize its dialogue with cancer stem cells and some can imagine that this will help, in cooperation with more conventional therapy, to knock over cancer stem cells.

5.1 How to awake dormant stem cells

In this regard, the crucial role of adhesive interactions between tumor cells and the stroma in response to chemotherapy has been deciphered in various systems (Damiano, 2002; Haslam and Woodward, 2003). In chronic myelogenous leukemia, with the market release of anti-tyrosine kinase inhibitors specific for the fusion onco-protein BCR-ABL (imatinib) (Druker et al., 2001) and because of its toxicity, interferon α has been partially abandoned. But, interestingly, there is a re-emerging interest for interferon α in this indication. CD34+ leukemic samples from patients with BCR-ABL expression have been reported to contain quiescent leukemic stem cells that are particularly resistant to tyrosine kinase inhibitor treatments (Graham et al., 2002). These cells also have a defective integrin-cytoskeletal association that conducts *in vitro* to their restricted mobility (Bhatia et al., 1999). We may hypothesize that this favors chronic myelogenous leukemia stem cell quiescence, but *in vitro* treatment with interferon α restores the integrin-cytoskeletal association (Bhatia et al., 1999). A more recent study has shown that interferon α can also deplete the pool of chronic myelogenous leukemia stem cells and trigger their differentiation, whereas imatinib is only able to inhibit advanced differentiated chronic myelogenous leukemia progenitors (Angstreich et al., 2005). In T-cell leukemia, Kayo and coworkers have demonstrated the existence of side-population cells with stem-like properties, and shown that interferon α is able to trigger their differentiation and enhance their sensitivity to chemotherapy (Kayo et al., 2007). Consistent with these results, an advanced clinical phase 3 trial is currently exploring the efficacy of imatinib and interferon α combination therapy for the treatment of chronic myelogenous leukemia. In addition, several recent studies have reported that agents which can activate quiescent/dormant cells, such as cytokines (G-CSF (Holtz et al., 2007) and interferon α) or other compounds (arsenic trioxide-AS_2O_3), can be efficiently used to induce cancer stem cell cycling (for review see (Essers and Trumpp, 2010)). These examples indicate that it is possible to kill cancer stem cells by combining treatment approaches. It is necessary, first, to awake quiescent stem cells and direct them toward differentiation, likely associated with their release from tumor niches, thus rendering them more accessible to chemotherapy, and, second, to expose these stem cells to more conventional chemotherapeutic drugs (Konopleva et al., 2009). Finally, in glioma, evidence suggests that anti-angiogenic therapy might enhance the efficiency of chemotherapy by disrupting the vascular niche of stem cells (Folkins et al., 2007). The investigators propose that the loss of communication between stem cells and their niche elicits a reduction or loss of certain stem cell properties associated with drug resistance, including dormancy, high proliferation rate and DNA repair. These observations provide a rational explanation for the poor efficiency of anti-angiogenic therapies when used alone and suggest that their use in combination with chemotherapy might open new perspectives in cancer stem cell targeting. Indeed, the hypoxic tumor microenvironment favors cancer stem cell dormancy and survival, as we discussed earlier. Interestingly, HIF1α, in addition to its role on stem cell dormancy, has also been found to regulate stromal cell-derived factor 1 (SDF1/CXCL12) gene expression in endothelial cells that mediate the adhesion, migration and homing of CXCR4-expressing stem cells. This has been proposed to create a hypoxic microenvironment that facilitates the recruitment, retention and resting of cancer stem cells. This hypothesis is supported by recent data demonstrating the sensitivity of leukemic stem cells to anthracyclines, doxorubicin and daunorubicin, mediated in part by the inhibitory effect of the HIF1α pathway. Direct inhibitors of HIF1α are currently under clinical development and evaluation (for review see (Konopleva et al., 2009)). These data suggest that targeting the hypoxic pathway might then not only help to release cancer stem cells from their niche (as discussed below) but also contribute to shift them from quiescence/dormancy to active cycling, rendering them sensitive to conventional anti-mitotic chemotherapies.

5.2 How to release cancer stem cells from their niche

The niche favors the homing and retention of normal and cancer stem cells which remain in this safe environment, away from circulating cytotoxic drugs, during treatment. This protective role is mediated in part by the chemokine receptor 4 (CXCR4) and its ligand, the stromal cell-derived factor 1 (SDF1/CXCL12) (Larochelle et al., 2006; Papayannopoulou, 2004). Interestingly these molecules have been recently reported to be involved in stem cell dormancy (Trumpp et al., 2010). An antagonist of the CXCR4 receptor, AMD3100, has been investigated in several phase I to III clinical trials exploring hematopoietic stem cell mobilization in leukemic patients with the objective of proposing self-transplantation after cytotoxic chemotherapy (Larochelle et al., 2006). Also, disruption of the SDF1/CXCL12 axis during tumor progression has been shown to induce the migration of cancer stem cells and to make them re-accessible and therefore sensitive to cytotoxic drugs in various leukemia and solid tumors (Gazitt, 2004; Rubin et al., 2003; Yang et al., 2007; Burger and Burkle, 2007). AMD3100 is currently under clinical investigation in combination with a cocktail of mitoxantrone, etoposide and cytarabine (Burger and Burkle, 2007). The CXCR4/CXCL12 axis also constitutes a good anti-cancer stem cell target in at least two solid tumor models, breast and prostate cancers. Inhibition of the CXCR4/CXCL12 axis using another antagonist of the CXCR4 receptor, TN14003, has been explored in a mouse breast cancer metastasis model (Liang et al., 2004). Injection of human breast MDA-MB-231 cancer cells into the tail vein of mice induced several lung metastases. In mice treated with TN14003, metastases were dramatically reduced (Liang et al., 2004). Even if no clear causative link can be established with cancer stem cell depletion by the CXCR4 antagonist these data, combined with results obtained with AMD3100, tend to validate the CXCR4/CXCL12 axis, when expressed in the cancer stem cell subpopulation, as a good candidate for new treatment strategies. As this pathway is shared by both normal and cancer stem cells, concerns have been raised about the potential toxicity of targeting the CXCR4/CXCL12 axis. Normal stem cells would normally be protected from treatments by their microenvironment but, when mobilized, be suddenly exposed to cytotoxic drugs. One solution would be to combine the CXCR4 antagonists with monoclonal antibodies (see below) that would target specifically cancer (stem) cells while sparing their normal counterparts. Another possible approach for releasing cancer stem cells from their microenvironment would be to inhibit their physical attachment to the components of the niche. Obvious targets are the integrins which have been shown to be involved in cancer stem cell maintenance and resistance, as discussed earlier. Interestingly, only few treatments have demonstrated efficacy against this abnormality which is particularly important in the stem cell compartment, likely including leukemic stem cells. Indeed, in the hematopoietic system interferon α seems to be the most efficient, or at least the most documented, drug for restoring full normal functions of β1 integrin in chronic myelogenous leukemia cells (Bhatia et al., 1995a; Bhatia et al., 1995b). In chronic myelogenous leukemia, the role of the specific BCR-ABL fusion protein inhibitor imanitib on integrin correction is still debated as some studies report a partly restored integrin function in immature cells (Bhatia et al., 1998) while other indicate the inefficiency of the drug on integrin defects (Ramaraj et al., 2004; Wertheim et al., 2002). Novel therapeutic strategies must therefore be developed to inhibit integrin-mediated cell survival signals and likely improve response rates. This could be achieved by targeting the downstream signaling of the integrin pathway. It has been proposed that the integrin-linked kinase which interacts with the cytoplasmic domains of β1 and β3 integrins might constitute a good target. This kinase mediates a diversity of functions relating to its role in coupling integrins and growth factor receptors to downstream signaling pathways. Through its downstream targets protein kinase B/Akt and glycogen synthase kinase-3b, the integrin-linked kinase appears to be involved in several oncogenesis-related events, including suppression of apoptosis and promotion of cell survival, as well as cell migration and invasion. Furthermore, increased integrin-linked kinase expression and activity have been correlated with malignancy in several human tumor types, including breast, prostate, brain, and colon carcinomas (Yoganathan et al., 2002). For example, the role of β1-integrin in maintaining mammary stem cells (Bachelard-Cascales et al., 2010) and in the resistance of breast cancer cells (Park et al., 2008) make integrin-linked kinase an interesting target to prevent relapse and/or metastasis in breast or any other type of cancer.

5.3 Emerging strategies

Cell-based therapy has been evaluated for many years in different diseases including cancer. Infusion of *ex vivo*-expanded mesenchymal stem cells has been proposed to enhance hematopoietic stem cell engraftment, especially in the adjuvant setting to treat graft-versus-host disease in cancer therapy (Khakoo et al., 2006), on the basis of anti-tumor properties of mesenchymal stem cells (Elzaouk et al., 2006; Ramasamy et al., 2007). Interestingly and surprisingly, several studies have reported that normal neural stem cells are able to move toward and attach to cancer stem cells in the central nervous system, which makes them eligible tools for the specific delivery of cytotoxic drugs to cancer stem cells (Sakariassen et al., 2007). There is increasing evidence that cancer stem cells in different types of tumors and leukemia share a number of common features, in particular their need of a close interaction with their microenvironment. This suggests that diagnostic and therapeutic monoclonal antibodies and other molecules may be applicable across tumor types. Until recently, most antibody-based strategies targeted antigens expressed by mature differentiated or activated cells. Adhesion molecules, such as CD44 and members of the Integrin family, mainly mediate cell-cell interactions between normal and cancer stem cells and various components of the niche (Chan and Watt, 2001; Ghaffari et al., 1999; Dontu et al., 2005;Ruoslahti, 1999). Also the adhesion molecule CD44 has been demonstrated to be required in acute myeloid leukemia for the homing of leukemic stem cells to their microenvironment where they are maintained in an immature state (Jin et al., 2006). Therefore the use of CD44 as a specific anti-cancer stem cell target has been investigated. Experiments using H90, a specific anti-CD44 antibody, have shown that disturbance of CD44-mediated cell-cell or cell-extracellular matrix adhesion alters the homing and maintenance of acute myeloid leukemia stem cells. This causes their differentiation towards monocytic or granulocytic lineages and depletion of acute myeloid leukemia stem cells in the bone marrow. Moreover, H90-treated mice have shown a reduced homing capacity in secondary recipient organs such as spleen or the bone marrow of non-injected bones. Interestingly, H90 effects are specific for acute myeloid leukemia stem cells and no homing disturbance is observed when using normal cord blood stem cells. A study performed in serially transplanted mice has shown that H90-treated mice do not developed leukemia, contrary to non-treated mice (Jin et al., 2006). A study using the humanized anti-CD44 antibody ARH460-16-2, which binds to human acute myeloid leukemia $CD34^{+}CD38^{neg}$ cancer stem cells, has evidenced a convincing anti-tumor activity in an AML xenograft model (Abstract Number 3976, AACR2008). Moreover, because CD44 is also present and found effective in other cancer stem cells, such as in breast (Sheridan et al., 2006), prostate (Patrawala et al., 2007), colorectal (Dalerba et al., 2007), pancreatic (Li et al., 2007) and small cell lung (Gutova et al., 2007) cancers, the authors have demonstrated that this antibody also exerts broad effects in solid tumors (Abstract Number 3975, AACR2008). The ARH460-16-2 antibody has already completed Pre-Investigational New Drug evaluation by the FDA, which opens new promising perspectives for cancer treatment. The discovery of new markers of cancer stem cells from different tumor types has led to the development of many monoclonal antibodies in order not only to characterize and isolate the cancer stem cells but also to target them for treatment (for review see (Deonarain, 2008)). As therapeutic antibodies are about to enter large clinical trials, the next decade of translational research and development in this area should see marked improvement in cancer diagnosis, prevention and treatment.

6. Concluding remarks

It has been known that microenvironments that can impose normal tissue architecture can both suppress the malignant phenotype and instruct otherwise malignant multipotent cells to give origin to differentiated cells and engage in normal organ development. Aging, associated with an increase in the number of cell divisions in which the centrosome is not tightly associated with adherent junctions between cells, is suspected to decrease stem cell numbers within the niche. This indicates that the effect of aging on stem cells partly results from impaired niche regulation at different levels. In addition, there is accumulating evidence that continuous input from the microenvironment might also determine the risk and course of tumor development. The more insight we get into the stem cell niche, the more new questions and issues emerge. Among these could be the clarification of whether niches are transiently or permanently occupied, of how they maintain their activity and specialization through time, of how the organism controls the number, size and composition of these niches, and so much more. To complement the advancing knowledge of niche composition and characteristics before and after cancer development, the current challenge is to develop experimental models encompassing the complexity of three-dimensional tissue organization, multiple cell niches and extra-cellular-matrix composition and allowing to grasp the full significance of the microenvironment in normal and in cancer cells. This crucial step will achieve a full understanding of features and functions of the stem cell niches, a real "black master" involved in all phases of cancer development. These findings should translate into a double-barreled therapy targeting both the cancer stem cells and their tumor niche. This would allow elaborating treatments to target cancer stem cells within their niches and ensure access to deeply quiescent cancer stem cells, if such exist, in order to make cancer a curable disease. Complementary approaches, such as the recruitment of useful bystanders like immune cells, should help to kill cancer stem cells or destroy their supporting environment. Undoubtedly, a better understanding of cancer development will evolve into novel strategies of risk assessment, diagnosis, prognosis and therapy.

7. References

Adams,G.B. and Scadden,D.T. (2006). The hematopoietic stem cell in its place, *Nat. Immunol.* 7,4.,(333-337),

Angstreich,G.R., Matsui,W., Huff,C.A., Vala,M.S., Barber,J., Hawkins,A.L., Griffin,C.A., Smith,B.D., and Jones,R.J. (2005). Effects of imatinib and interferon on primitive chronic myeloid leukaemia progenitors, *Br. J. Haematol.* 130,3.,(373-381),

Arnulf,B., Lecourt,S., Soulier,J., Ternaux,B., Lacassagne,M.N., Crinquette,A., Dessoly,J., Sciaini,A.K., Benbunan,M., Chomienne,C., Fermand,J.P., Marolleau,J.P., and Larghero,J. (2007). Phenotypic and functional characterization of bone marrow mesenchymal stem cells derived from patients with multiple myeloma, *Leukemia* 21,1.,(158-163),

Astier,A.L., Xu,R., Svoboda,M., Hinds,E., Munoz,O., de Beaumont,R., Crean,C.D., Gabig,T., and Freedman,A.S. (2003). Temporal gene expression profile of human precursor B leukemia cells induced by adhesion receptor: identification of pathways regulating B-cell survival, *Blood.* 101,3.,(1118-1127),

Bachelard-Cascales,E., Chapellier,M., Delay,E., Pochon,G., Voeltzel,T., Puisieux,A., Caron,d.F., and Maguer-Satta,V. (2010). The CD10 enzyme is a key player to identify and regulate human mammary stem cells, *Stem Cells* 28,6.,(1081-1088),

Benvenuto,F., Ferrari,S., Gerdoni,E., Gualandi,F., Frassoni,F., Pistoia,V., Mancardi,G., and Uccelli,A. (2007). Human mesenchymal stem cells promote survival of T cells in a quiescent state, *Stem Cells* 25,7.,(1753-1760),

Besancon,R., Valsesia-Wittmann,S., Puisieux,A., de Fromentel,C.C., and Maguer-Satta,V. (2009). Cancer stem cells: the emerging challenge of drug targeting, *Curr. Med. Chem.* 16,4.,(394-416),

Bhatia,R., McGlave,P.B., Dewald,G.W., Blazar,B.R., and Verfaillie,C.M. (1995a). Abnormal function of the bone marrow microenvironment in chronic myelogenous leukemia: role of malignant stromal macrophages, *Blood* 85,12.,(3636-45),

Bhatia,R., McGlave,P.B., and Verfaillie,C.M. (1995b). Treatment of marrow stroma with interferon-alpha restores normal beta 1 integrin-dependent adhesion of chronic myelogenous leukemia hematopoietic progenitors. Role of MIP-1 alpha, *J Clin Invest* 96,2.,(931-9),

Bhatia,R., Munthe,H.A., and Verfaillie,C.M. (1998). Tyrphostin AG957, a tyrosine kinase inhibitor with anti-BCR/ABL tyrosine kinase activity restores beta1 integrin-mediated adhesion and inhibitory signaling in chronic myelogenous leukemia hematopoietic progenitors, *Leukemia* 12,11.,(1708-1717),

Bhatia,R., Munthe,H.A., and Verfaillie,C.M. (1999). Role of abnormal integrin-cytoskeletal interactions in impaired beta1 integrin function in chronic myelogenous leukemia hematopoietic progenitors, *Exp. Hematol.* 27,9.,(1384-1396),

Bissell,M.J., Kenny,P.A., and Radisky,D.C. (2005). Microenvironmental regulators of tissue structure and function also regulate tumor induction and progression: the role of extracellular matrix and its degrading enzymes, *Cold Spring Harb. Symp. Quant. Biol.* 70,(343-356),

Blanpain,C. and Fuchs,E. (2006). Epidermal stem cells of the skin, *Annu. Rev. Cell Dev. Biol.* 22,(339-373),

Blanpain,C., Lowry,W.E., Geoghegan,A., Polak,L., and Fuchs,E. (2004). Self-renewal, multipotency, and the existence of two cell populations within an epithelial stem cell niche, *Cell* 118,5.,(635-648),

Boheler,K.R. (2009). Stem cell pluripotency: a cellular trait that depends on transcription factors, chromatin state and a checkpoint deficient cell cycle, *J. Cell Physiol* 221,1.,(10-17),

Burger,J.A. and Burkle,A. (2007). The CXCR4 chemokine receptor in acute and chronic leukaemia: a marrow homing receptor and potential therapeutic target, *Br. J. Haematol.* 137,4.,(288-296),

Burness,M.L. and Sipkins,D.A. (2010). The stem cell niche in health and malignancy, *Semin. Cancer Biol.* 20,2.,(107-115),

Calvi,L.M., Adams,G.B., Weibrecht,K.W., Weber,J.M., Olson,D.P., Knight,M.C., Martin,R.P., Schipani,E., Divieti,P., Bringhurst,F.R., Milner,L.A., Kronenberg,H.M., and Scadden,D.T. (2003). Osteoblastic cells regulate the haematopoietic stem cell niche, *Nature* 425,6960.,(841-846),

Caussinus,E. and Gonzalez,C. (2005). Induction of tumor growth by altered stem-cell asymmetric division in Drosophila melanogaster, *Nat. Genet.* 37,10.,(1125-1129),

Chan,J.Y. and Watt,S.M. (2001). Adhesion receptors on haematopoietic progenitor cells, *Br. J. Haematol.* 112,3.,(541-557),

Conti,L., Pollard,S.M., Gorba,T., Reitano,E., Toselli,M., Biella,G., Sun,Y., Sanzone,S., Ying,Q.L., Cattaneo,E., and Smith,A. (2005). Niche-independent symmetrical self-renewal of a mammalian tissue stem cell, *PLoS. Biol.* 3,9.,(e283-

Corre,J., Mahtouk,K., Attal,M., Gadelorge,M., Huynh,A., Fleury-Cappellesso,S., Danho,C., Laharrague,P., Klein,B., Reme,T., and Bourin,P. (2007). Bone marrow mesenchymal stem cells are abnormal in multiple myeloma, *Leukemia* 21,5.,(1079-1088),

Dalerba,P., Dylla,S.J., Park,I.K., Liu,R., Wang,X., Cho,R.W., Hoey,T., Gurney,A., Huang,E.H., Simeone,D.M., Shelton,A.A., Parmiani,G., Castelli,C., and Clarke,M.F. (2007). Phenotypic characterization of human colorectal cancer stem cells, *Proc. Natl. Acad. Sci. U. S. A* 104,24.,(10158-10163),

Damiano,J.S. (2002). Integrins as novel drug targets for overcoming innate drug resistance, *Curr. Cancer Drug Targets.* 2,1.,(37-43),

Dazzi,F., Ramasamy,R., Glennie,S., Jones,S.P., and Roberts,I. (2006). The role of mesenchymal stem cells in haemopoiesis, *Blood Rev.* 20,3.,(161-171),

De Toni,F., Racaud-Sultan,C., Chicanne,G., Mas,V.M., Cariven,C., Mesange,F., Salles,J.P., Demur,C., Allouche,M., Payrastre,B., Manenti,S., and Ysebaert,L. (2006). A crosstalk between the Wnt and the adhesion-dependent signaling pathways governs the chemosensitivity of acute myeloid leukemia, *Oncogene* 25,22.,(3113-3122),

De Waele,M., Renmans,W., Jochmans,K., Schots,R., Lacor,P., Trullemans,F., Otten,J., Balduck,N., Vander,G.K., Van Camp,B., and Van,R., I (1999). Different expression of adhesion molecules on CD34+ cells in AML and B-lineage ALL and their normal bone marrow counterparts, *Eur. J. Haematol.* 63,3.,(192-201),

Demicheli,R. (2001). Tumour dormancy: findings and hypotheses from clinical research on breast cancer, *Semin. Cancer Biol.* 11,4.,(297-306),

Deonarain,M.P. (2008). Recombinant antibodies for cancer therapy, *Expert. Opin. Biol. Ther.* 8,8.,(1123-1141),

Diabira,S. and Morandi,X. (2008). Gliomagenesis and neural stem cells: Key role of hypoxia and concept of tumor "neo-niche", *Med. Hypotheses* 70,1.,(96-104),

Djouad,F., Plence,P., Bony,C., Tropel,P., Apparailly,F., Sany,J., Noel,D., and Jorgensen,C. (2003). Immunosuppressive effect of mesenchymal stem cells favors tumor growth in allogeneic animals, *Blood.* 102,10.,(3837-3844),

Docheva,D., Popov,C., Mutschler,W., and Schieker,M. (2007). Human mesenchymal stem cells in contact with their environment: surface characteristics and the integrin system, *J. Cell Mol. Med.* 11,1.,(21-38),

Dontu,G., Liu,S., and Wicha,M.S. (2005). Stem cells in mammary development and carcinogenesis: implications for prevention and treatment, *Stem Cell Rev.* 1,3.,(207-213),

Druker,B.J., Talpaz,M., Resta,D.J., Peng,B., Buchdunger,E., Ford,J.M., Lydon,N.B., Kantarjian,H., Capdeville,R., Ohno-Jones,S., and Sawyers,C.L. (2001). Efficacy and safety of a specific inhibitor of the BCR-ABL tyrosine kinase in chronic myeloid leukemia, *N. Engl. J. Med.* 344,14.,(1031-1037),

Dylla,S.J., Deyle,D.R., Theunissen,K., Padurean,A.M., and Verfaillie,C.M. (2004). Integrin engagement-induced inhibition of human myelopoiesis is mediated by proline-rich tyrosine kinase 2 gene products, *Exp. Hematol.* 32,4.,(365-374),

Eliasson,P., Rehn,M., Hammar,P., Larsson,P., Sirenko,O., Flippin,L.A., Cammenga,J., and Jonsson,J.I. (2010). Hypoxia mediates low cell-cycle activity and increases the proportion of long-term-reconstituting hematopoietic stem cells during in vitro culture, *Exp. Hematol.* 38,4.,(301-310),

Elrick,L.J., Jorgensen,H.G., Mountford,J.C., and Holyoake,T.L. (2005). Punish the parent not the progeny, *Blood* 105,5.,(1862-1866),

Elzaouk,L., Moelling,K., and Pavlovic,J. (2006). Anti-tumor activity of mesenchymal stem cells producing IL-12 in a mouse melanoma model, *Exp. Dermatol.* 15,11.,(865-874),

Engler,A.J., Sen,S., Sweeney,H.L., and Discher,D.E. (2006). Matrix elasticity directs stem cell lineage specification, *Cell* 126,4.,(677-689),

Essers,M.A. and Trumpp,A. (2010). Targeting leukemic stem cells by breaking their dormancy, *Mol. Oncol.*

Faraldo,M.M., Deugnier,M.A., Thiery,J.P., and Glukhova,M.A. (2000). Development of mammary gland requires normal beta 1-integrin function, *Adv. Exp. Med. Biol.* 480,(169-174),

Faraldo,M.M., Deugnier,M.A., Tlouzeau,S., Thiery,J.P., and Glukhova,M.A. (2002). Perturbation of beta1-integrin function in involuting mammary gland results in premature dedifferentiation of secretory epithelial cells, *Mol. Biol. Cell* 13,10.,(3521-3531),

Faraldo,M.M., Teuliere,J., Deugnier,M.A., Taddei-De La Hosseraye,I., Thiery,J.P., and Glukhova,M.A. (2005). Myoepithelial cells in the control of mammary development and tumorigenesis: data from genetically modified mice, *J. Mammary. Gland. Biol. Neoplasia.* 10,3.,(211-219),

Faubert,A., Lessard,J., and Sauvageau,G. (2004). Are genetic determinants of asymmetric stem cell division active in hematopoietic stem cells?, *Oncogene* 23,43.,(7247-7255),

Fernandez-Vidal,A., Ysebaert,L., Didier,C., Betous,R., De Toni,F., Prade-Houdellier,N., Demur,C., Contour-Galcera,M.O., Prevost,G.P., Ducommun,B., Payrastre,B., Racaud-Sultan,C., and Manenti,S. (2006). Cell adhesion regulates CDC25A expression and proliferation in acute myeloid leukemia, *Cancer Res.* 66,14.,(7128-7135),

Flynn,C.M. and Kaufman,D.S. (2007). Donor cell leukemia: insight into cancer stem cells and the stem cell niche, *Blood.* 109,7.,(2688-2692),

Folkins,C., Man,S., Xu,P., Shaked,Y., Hicklin,D.J., and Kerbel,R.S. (2007). Anticancer therapies combining antiangiogenic and tumor cell cytotoxic effects reduce the tumor stem-like cell fraction in glioma xenograft tumors, *Cancer Res.* 67,8.,(3560-3564),

Fuchs,E., Tumbar,T., and Guasch,G. (2004). Socializing with the neighbors: stem cells and their niche, *Cell* 116,6.,(769-778),

Gazitt,Y. (2004). Homing and mobilization of hematopoietic stem cells and hematopoietic cancer cells are mirror image processes, utilizing similar signaling pathways and occurring concurrently: circulating cancer cells constitute an ideal target for concurrent treatment with chemotherapy and antilineage-specific antibodies, *Leukemia* 18,1.,(1-10),

Ghaffari,S., Smadja-Joffe,F., Oostendorp,R., Levesque,J.P., Dougherty,G., Eaves,A., and Eaves,C. (1999). CD44 isoforms in normal and leukemic hematopoiesis, *Exp. Hematol.* 27,6.,(978-993),

Godmann,M., Gashaw,I., Katz,J.P., Nagy,A., Kaestner,K.H., and Behr,R. (2009). Kruppel-like factor 4, a "pluripotency transcription factor" highly expressed in male postmeiotic germ cells, is dispensable for spermatogenesis in the mouse, *Mech. Dev.* 126,8-9.,(650-664),

Gottschling,S., Saffrich,R., Seckinger,A., Krause,U., Horsch,K., Miesala,K., and Ho,A.D. (2007). Human mesenchymal stromal cells regulate initial self-renewing divisions of hematopoietic progenitor cells by a beta1-integrin-dependent mechanism, *Stem Cells* 25,3.,(798-806),

Graham,S.M., Jorgensen,H.G., Allan,E., Pearson,C., Alcorn,M.J., Richmond,L., and Holyoake,T.L. (2002). Primitive, quiescent, Philadelphia-positive stem cells from patients with chronic myeloid leukemia are insensitive to STI571 in vitro, *Blood* 99,1.,(319-325),

Greco,V. and Guo,S. (2010). Compartmentalized organization: a common and required feature of stem cell niches?, *Development* 137,10.,(1586-1594),

Greig,R.G. and Trainer,D.L. (1986). Shaping future strategies for the pharmacological control of tumor cell metastases, *Cancer Metastasis Rev.* 5,1.,(3-14),

Guitart,A., Hammoud,M., Dello,S.P., Ivanovic,Z., and Praloran,V. (2010). Slow-cycling/quiescence balance of hematopoietic stem cells is related to physiological gradient of oxygen, *Exp. Hematol.*

Gutova,M., Najbauer,J., Gevorgyan,A., Metz,M.Z., Weng,Y., Shih,C.C., and Aboody,K.S. (2007). Identification of uPAR-positive chemoresistant cells in small cell lung cancer, *PLoS. ONE.* 2,2.,(e243-

Hall,B., Andreeff,M., and Marini,F. (2007). The participation of mesenchymal stem cells in tumor stroma formation and their application as targeted-gene delivery vehicles, *Handb. Exp. Pharmacol.*180.,(263-283),

Hall,P.E., Lathia,J.D., Miller,N.G., Caldwell,M.A., and ffrench-Constant,C. (2006). Integrins are markers of human neural stem cells, *Stem Cells* 24,9.,(2078-2084),

Haslam,S.Z. and Woodward,T.L. (2003). Host microenvironment in breast cancer development: epithelial-cell-stromal-cell interactions and steroid hormone action in normal and cancerous mammary gland, *Breast Cancer Res.* 5,4.,(208-215),

Hazlehurst,L.A., Valkov,N., Wisner,L., Storey,J.A., Boulware,D., Sullivan,D.M., and Dalton,W.S. (2001). Reduction in drug-induced DNA double-strand breaks associated with beta1 integrin-mediated adhesion correlates with drug resistance in U937 cells, *Blood.* 98,6.,(1897-1903),

Heddleston,J.M., Li,Z., Lathia,J.D., Bao,S., Hjelmeland,A.B., and Rich,J.N. (2010). Hypoxia inducible factors in cancer stem cells, *Br. J. Cancer* 102,5.,(789-795),

Hideshima,T., Bergsagel,P.L., Kuehl,W.M., and Anderson,K.C. (2004). Advances in biology of multiple myeloma: clinical applications, *Blood.* 104,3.,(607-618),

Ho,A.D. and Wagner,W. (2007). The beauty of asymmetry: asymmetric divisions and self-renewal in the haematopoietic system, *Curr. Opin. Hematol.* 14,4.,(330-336),

Hodkinson,P.S., Mackinnon,A.C., and Sethi,T. (2007). Extracellular matrix regulation of drug resistance in small-cell lung cancer, *Int. J. Radiat. Biol.*(1-9),

Holtz,M., Forman,S.J., and Bhatia,R. (2007). Growth factor stimulation reduces residual quiescent chronic myelogenous leukemia progenitors remaining after imatinib treatment, *Cancer Res.* 67,3.,(1113-1120),

Hurley,R.W., McCarthy,J.B., and Verfaillie,C.M. (1995). Direct adhesion to bone marrow stroma via fibronectin receptors inhibits hematopoietic progenitor proliferation, *J. Clin. Invest* 96,1.,(511-519),

Hurley,R.W., McCarthy,J.B., Wayner,E.A., and Verfaillie,C.M. (1997). Monoclonal antibody crosslinking of the alpha 4 or beta 1 integrin inhibits committed clonogenic hematopoietic progenitor proliferation, *Exp. Hematol.* 25,4.,(321-328),

Issa,J.P. (2007). DNA methylation as a therapeutic target in cancer, *Clin. Cancer Res.* 13,6.,(1634-1637),

Ito,K., Hirao,A., Arai,F., Takubo,K., Matsuoka,S., Miyamoto,K., Ohmura,M., Naka,K., Hosokawa,K., Ikeda,Y., and Suda,T. (2006). Reactive oxygen species act through p38 MAPK to limit the lifespan of hematopoietic stem cells, *Nat. Med.* 12,4.,(446-451),

Jeanpierre,S., Nicolini,F.E., Kaniewski,B., Dumontet,C., Rimokh,R., Puisieux,A., and Maguer-Satta,V. (2008). BMP4 regulation of human megakaryocytic differentiation is involved in thrombopoietin signaling, *Blood.* 112,8.,(3154-3163),

Jiang,Y., Prosper,F., and Verfaillie,C.M. (2000a). Opposing effects of engagement of integrins and stimulation of cytokine receptors on cell cycle progression of normal human hematopoietic progenitors, *Blood.* 95,3.,(846-854),

Jiang,Y., Zhao,R.C., and Verfaillie,C.M. (2000b). Abnormal integrin-mediated regulation of chronic myelogenous leukemia CD34+ cell proliferation: BCR/ABL up-regulates the cyclin-dependent kinase inhibitor, p27Kip, which is relocated to the cell cytoplasm and incapable of regulating cdk2 activity, *Proc. Natl. Acad. Sci. U. S. A* 97,19.,(10538-10543),

Jin,L., Hope,K.J., Zhai,Q., Smadja-Joffe,F., and Dick,J.E. (2006). Targeting of CD44 eradicates human acute myeloid leukemic stem cells, *Nat. Med.* 12,10.,(1167-1174),

Jongen-Lavrencic,M., Salesse,S., Delwel,R., and Verfaillie,C.M. (2005). BCR/ABL-mediated downregulation of genes implicated in cell adhesion and motility leads to impaired migration toward CCR7 ligands CCL19 and CCL21 in primary BCR/ABL-positive cells, *Leukemia* 19,3.,(373-380),

Kai,T. and Spradling,A. (2003). An empty Drosophila stem cell niche reactivates the proliferation of ectopic cells, *Proc. Natl. Acad. Sci. U. S. A* 100,8.,(4633-4638),

Kaplan,R.N., Psaila,B., and Lyden,D. (2006). Bone marrow cells in the 'pre-metastatic niche': within bone and beyond, *Cancer Metastasis Rev.* 25,4.,(521-529),

Kayo,H., Yamazaki,H., Nishida,H., Dang,N.H., and Morimoto,C. (2007). Stem cell properties and the side population cells as a target for interferon-alpha in adult T-cell leukemia/lymphoma, *Biochem. Biophys. Res. Commun.* 364,4.,(808-814),

Keith,B. and Simon,M.C. (2007). Hypoxia-inducible factors, stem cells, and cancer, *Cell* 129,3.,(465-472),

Khakoo,A.Y., Pati,S., Anderson,S.A., Reid,W., Elshal,M.F., Rovira,I.I., Nguyen,A.T., Malide,D., Combs,C.A., Hall,G., Zhang,J., Raffeld,M., Rogers,T.B., Stetler-Stevenson,W., Frank,J.A., Reitz,M., and Finkel,T. (2006). Human mesenchymal stem cells exert potent antitumorigenic effects in a model of Kaposi's sarcoma, *J. Exp. Med.* 203,5.,(1235-1247),

Kiel,M.J. and Morrison,S.J. (2008). Uncertainty in the niches that maintain haematopoietic stem cells, *Nat. Rev. Immunol.* 8,4.,(290-301),

Kleeff,J., Beckhove,P., Esposito,I., Herzig,S., Huber,P.E., Lohr,J.M., and Friess,H. (2007). Pancreatic cancer microenvironment, *Int. J. Cancer* 121,4.,(699-705),

Konopleva,M., Tabe,Y., Zeng,Z., and Andreeff,M. (2009). Therapeutic targeting of microenvironmental interactions in leukemia: mechanisms and approaches, *Drug Resist. Updat.* 12,4-5.,(103-113),

Larochelle,A., Krouse,A., Metzger,M., Orlic,D., Donahue,R.E., Fricker,S., Bridger,G., Dunbar,C.E., and Hematti,P. (2006). AMD3100 mobilizes hematopoietic stem cells with long-term repopulating capacity in nonhuman primates, *Blood.* 107,9.,(3772-3778),

Larsen,M., Artym,V.V., Green,J.A., and Yamada,K.M. (2006). The matrix reorganized: extracellular matrix remodeling and integrin signaling, *Curr. Opin. Cell Biol.* 18,5.,(463-471),

Lee,J.T. and Herlyn,M. (2007a). Microenvironmental influences in melanoma progression, *J. Cell Biochem.* 101,4.,(862-872),

Lee,J.T. and Herlyn,M. (2007b). Old disease, new culprit: Tumor stem cells in cancer, *J. Cell Physiol* 213,3.,(603-609),

Lessard,J. and Sauvageau,G. (2003). Bmi-1 determines the proliferative capacity of normal and leukaemic stem cells, *Nature* 423,6937.,(255-260),

Levesque,J.P. and Simmons,P.J. (1999). Cytoskeleton and integrin-mediated adhesion signaling in human CD34+ hemopoietic progenitor cells, *Exp. Hematol.* 27,4.,(579-586),

Li,C., Heidt,D.G., Dalerba,P., Burant,C.F., Zhang,L., Adsay,V., Wicha,M., Clarke,M.F., and Simeone,D.M. (2007). Identification of pancreatic cancer stem cells, *Cancer Res.* 67,3.,(1030-1037),

Li,L. and Neaves,W.B. (2006). Normal stem cells and cancer stem cells: the niche matters, *Cancer Res.* 66,9.,(4553-4557),

Li,Z. and Li,L. (2006). Understanding hematopoietic stem-cell microenvironments, *Trends Biochem. Sci.* 31,10.,(589-595),

Liang,Z., Wu,T., Lou,H., Yu,X., Taichman,R.S., Lau,S.K., Nie,S., Umbreit,J., and Shim,H. (2004). Inhibition of breast cancer metastasis by selective synthetic polypeptide against CXCR4, *Cancer Res.* 64,12.,(4302-4308),

Lundell,B.I., McCarthy,J.B., Kovach,N.L., and Verfaillie,C.M. (1996). Activation-dependent alpha5beta1 integrin-mediated adhesion to fibronectin decreases proliferation of chronic myelogenous leukemia progenitors and K562 cells, *Blood.* 87,6.,(2450-2458),

Lundell,B.I., McCarthy,J.B., Kovach,N.L., and Verfaillie,C.M. (1997). Activation of beta1 integrins on CML progenitors reveals cooperation between beta1 integrins and CD44 in the regulation of adhesion and proliferation, *Leukemia* 11,6.,(822-829),

Maguer-Satta,V., Bartholin,L., Jeanpierre,S., Ffrench,M., Martel,S., Magaud,J.P., and Rimokh,R. (2003). Regulation of human erythropoiesis by activin A, BMP2, and BMP4, members of the TGFbeta family, *Exp. Cell Res.* 282,2.,(110-120),

Maguer-Satta,V., Forissier,S., Bartholin,L., Martel,S., Jeanpierre,S., Bachelard,E., and Rimokh,R. (2006). A novel role for fibronectin type I domain in the regulation of human hematopoietic cell adhesiveness through binding to follistatin domains of FLRG and follistatin, *Exp. Cell Res.* 312,4.,(434-442),

Maguer-Satta,V. and Rimokh,R. (2004). FLRG, member of the follistatin family, a new player in hematopoiesis, *Mol. Cell Endocrinol.* 225,1-2.,(109-118),

Marthiens,V., Kazanis,I., Moss,L., Long,K., and ffrench-Constant,C. (2010). Adhesion molecules in the stem cell niche--more than just staying in shape?, *J. Cell Sci.* 123,Pt 10.,(1613-1622),

Melikova,S., Dylla,S.J., and Verfaillie,C.M. (2004). Phosphatidylinositol-3-kinase activation mediates proline-rich tyrosine kinase 2 phosphorylation and recruitment to beta1-integrins in human CD34+ cells, *Exp. Hematol.* 32,11.,(1051-1056),

Moore,K.A. and Lemischka,I.R. (2006). Stem cells and their niches, *Science* 311,5769.,(1880-1885),

Moreno-Manzano,V., Rodriguez-Jimenez,F.J., Acena-Bonilla,J.L., Fustero-Lardies,S., Erceg,S., Dopazo,J., Montaner,D., Stojkovic,M., and Sanchez-Puelles,J.M. (2010). FM19G11, a new hypoxia-inducible factor (HIF) modulator, affects stem cell differentiation status, *J. Biol. Chem.* 285,2.,(1333-1342),

Morrison,S.J. and Kimble,J. (2006). Asymmetric and symmetric stem-cell divisions in development and cancer, *Nature* 441,7097.,(1068-1074),

Morrison,S.J. and Spradling,A.C. (2008). Stem cells and niches: mechanisms that promote stem cell maintenance throughout life, *Cell* 132,4.,(598-611),

Mueller,M.M. and Fusenig,N.E. (2004). Friends or foes - bipolar effects of the tumour stroma in cancer, *Nat. Rev. Cancer* 4,11.,(839-849),

Paget,S. (1989). The distribution of secondary growths in cancer of the breast. 1889, *Cancer Metastasis Rev.* 8,2.,(98-101),

Papayannopoulou,T. (2004). Current mechanistic scenarios in hematopoietic stem/progenitor cell mobilization, *Blood.* 103,5.,(1580-1585),

Park,C.C., Zhang,H., Pallavicini,M., Gray,J.W., Baehner,F., Park,C.J., and Bissell,M.J. (2006). Beta1 integrin inhibitory antibody induces apoptosis of breast cancer cells, inhibits growth, and distinguishes malignant from normal phenotype in three dimensional cultures and in vivo, *Cancer Res.* 66,3.,(1526-1535),

Park,C.C., Zhang,H.J., Yao,E.S., Park,C.J., and Bissell,M.J. (2008). Beta1 integrin inhibition dramatically enhances radiotherapy efficacy in human breast cancer xenografts, *Cancer Res.* 68,11.,(4398-4405),

Passegue,E., Jamieson,C.H., Ailles,L.E., and Weissman,I.L. (2003). Normal and leukemic hematopoiesis: are leukemias a stem cell disorder or a reacquisition of stem cell characteristics?, *Proc. Natl. Acad. Sci. U. S. A* 100 Suppl 1,(11842-11849),

Paszek,M.J., Zahir,N., Johnson,K.R., Lakins,J.N., Rozenberg,G.I., Gefen,A., Reinhart-King,C.A., Margulies,S.S., Dembo,M., Boettiger,D., Hammer,D.A., and Weaver,V.M. (2005). Tensional homeostasis and the malignant phenotype, *Cancer Cell* 8,3.,(241-254),

Patrawala,L., Calhoun-Davis,T., Schneider-Broussard,R., and Tang,D.G. (2007). Hierarchical organization of prostate cancer cells in xenograft tumors: the CD44+alpha2beta1+ cell population is enriched in tumor-initiating cells, *Cancer Res.* 67,14.,(6796-6805),

Perry,J.M., Harandi,O.F., and Paulson,R.F. (2007). BMP4, SCF, and hypoxia cooperatively regulate the expansion of murine stress erythroid progenitors, *Blood* 109,10.,(4494-4502),

Priestley,G.V., Scott,L.M., Ulyanova,T., and Papayannopoulou,T. (2006). Lack of alpha4 integrin expression in stem cells restricts competitive function and self-renewal activity, *Blood.* 107,7.,(2959-2967),

Priestley,G.V., Ulyanova,T., and Papayannopoulou,T. (2007). Sustained alterations in biodistribution of stem/progenitor cells in Tie2Cre+ alpha4(f/f) mice are hematopoietic cell autonomous, *Blood.* 109,1.,(109-111),

Prosper,F., Stroncek,D., McCarthy,J.B., and Verfaillie,C.M. (1998). Mobilization and homing of peripheral blood progenitors is related to reversible downregulation of alpha4 beta1 integrin expression and function, *J. Clin. Invest* 101,11.,(2456-2467),

Prosper,F. and Verfaillie,C.M. (2001). Regulation of hematopoiesis through adhesion receptors, *J Leukoc Biol* 69,3.,(307-16),

Psaila,B., Kaplan,R.N., Port,E.R., and Lyden,D. (2006). Priming the 'soil' for breast cancer metastasis: the pre-metastatic niche, *Breast Dis.* 26,(65-74),

Ramaraj,P., Singh,H., Niu,N., Chu,S., Holtz,M., Yee,J.K., and Bhatia,R. (2004). Effect of mutational inactivation of tyrosine kinase activity on BCR/ABL-induced abnormalities in cell growth and adhesion in human hematopoietic progenitors, *Cancer Res.* 64,15.,(5322-5331),

Ramasamy,R., Lam,E.W., Soeiro,I., Tisato,V., Bonnet,D., and Dazzi,F. (2007). Mesenchymal stem cells inhibit proliferation and apoptosis of tumor cells: impact on in vivo tumor growth, *Leukemia* 21,2.,(304-310),

Ronnov-Jessen,L. and Bissell,M.J. (2009). Breast cancer by proxy: can the microenvironment be both the cause and consequence?, *Trends Mol. Med.* 15,1.,(5-13),

Ross,J. and Li,L. (2006). Recent advances in understanding extrinsic control of hematopoietic stem cell fate, *Curr. Opin. Hematol.* 13,4.,(237-242),

Rubin,J.B., Kung,A.L., Klein,R.S., Chan,J.A., Sun,Y., Schmidt,K., Kieran,M.W., Luster,A.D., and Segal,R.A. (2003). A small-molecule antagonist of CXCR4 inhibits intracranial growth of primary brain tumors, *Proc. Natl. Acad. Sci. U. S. A* 100,23.,(13513-13518),

Ruoslahti,E. (1999). Fibronectin and its integrin receptors in cancer, *Adv Cancer Res* 76,(1-20),

Sadlon,T.J., Lewis,I.D., and D'Andrea,R.J. (2004). BMP4: its role in development of the hematopoietic system and potential as a hematopoietic growth factor, *Stem Cells* 22,4.,(457-474),

Sakariassen,P.O., Immervoll,H., and Chekenya,M. (2007). Cancer stem cells as mediators of treatment resistance in brain tumors: status and controversies, *Neoplasia.* 9,11.,(882-892),

Schofield,R. (1978). The relationship between the spleen colony-forming cell and the haemopoietic stem cell, *Blood Cells* 4,1-2.,(7-25),

Scott,L.M., Priestley,G.V., and Papayannopoulou,T. (2003). Deletion of alpha4 integrins from adult hematopoietic cells reveals roles in homeostasis, regeneration, and homing, *Mol. Cell Biol.* 23,24.,(9349-9360),

Shackleton,M., Vaillant,F., Simpson,K.J., Stingl,J., Smyth,G.K., Asselin-Labat,M.L., Wu,L., Lindeman,G.J., and Visvader,J.E. (2006). Generation of a functional mammary gland from a single stem cell, *Nature* 439,7072.,(84-88),

Sheridan,C., Kishimoto,H., Fuchs,R.K., Mehrotra,S., Bhat-Nakshatri,P., Turner,C.H., Goulet,R., Jr., Badve,S., and Nakshatri,H. (2006). CD44+/, *Breast Cancer Res.* 8,5.,(R59-

Simon,M., Grandage,V.L., Linch,D.C., and Khwaja,A. (2005). Constitutive activation of the Wnt/beta-catenin signalling pathway in acute myeloid leukaemia, *Oncogene* 24,14.,(2410-2420),

Sotiropoulou,P.A., Perez,S.A., Gritzapis,A.D., Baxevanis,C.N., and Papamichail,M. (2006). Interactions between human mesenchymal stem cells and natural killer cells, *Stem Cells* 24,1.,(74-85),

Stingl,J., Raouf,A., Eirew,P., and Eaves,C.J. (2006). Deciphering the mammary epithelial cell hierarchy, *Cell Cycle* 5,14.,(1519-1522),

Tabe,Y., Jin,L., Tsutsumi-Ishii,Y., Xu,Y., McQueen,T., Priebe,W., Mills,G.B., Ohsaka,A., Nagaoka,I., Andreeff,M., and Konopleva,M. (2007). Activation of integrin-linked kinase is a critical prosurvival pathway induced in leukemic cells by bone marrow-derived stromal cells, *Cancer Res.* 67,2.,(684-694),

Taddei,I., Deugnier,M.A., Faraldo,M.M., Petit,V., Bouvard,D., Medina,D., Fassler,R., Thiery,J.P., and Glukhova,M.A. (2008). Beta1 integrin deletion from the basal compartment of the mammary epithelium affects stem cells, *Nat. Cell Biol.* 10,6.,(716-722),

Taddei,I., Faraldo,M.M., Teuliere,J., Deugnier,M.A., Thiery,J.P., and Glukhova,M.A. (2003). Integrins in mammary gland development and differentiation of mammary epithelium, *J. Mammary. Gland. Biol. Neoplasia.* 8,4.,(383-394),

Trumpp,A., Essers,M., and Wilson,A. (2010). Awakening dormant haematopoietic stem cells, *Nat. Rev. Immunol.* 10,3.,(201-209),

Tysnes,B.B. and Bjerkvig,R. (2007). Cancer initiation and progression: involvement of stem cells and the microenvironment, *Biochim. Biophys. Acta* 1775,2.,(283-297),

Vazin,T. and Schaffer,D.V. (2010). Engineering strategies to emulate the stem cell niche, *Trends Biotechnol.* 28,3.,(117-124),

Verstappen,J., Katsaros,C., Torensma,R., and Von den Hoff,J.W. (2009). A functional model for adult stem cells in epithelial tissues, *Wound. Repair Regen.* 17,3.,(296-305),

Wang,J.C. and Dick,J.E. (2005). Cancer stem cells: lessons from leukemia, *Trends Cell Biol.* 15,9.,(494-501),

Wertheim,J.A., Forsythe,K., Druker,B.J., Hammer,D., Boettiger,D., and Pear,W.S. (2002). BCR-ABL-induced adhesion defects are tyrosine kinase-independent, *Blood.* 99,11.,(4122-4130),

White,D.E., Rayment,J.H., and Muller,W.J. (2006). Addressing the role of cell adhesion in tumor cell dormancy, *Cell Cycle* 5,16.,(1756-1759),

Wilson,A., Murphy,M.J., Oskarsson,T., Kaloulis,K., Bettess,M.D., Oser,G.M., Pasche,A.C., Knabenhans,C., Macdonald,H.R., and Trumpp,A. (2004). c-Myc controls the balance between hematopoietic stem cell self-renewal and differentiation, *Genes Dev.* 18,22.,(2747-2763),

Xu,R., Boudreau,A., and Bissell,M.J. (2009). Tissue architecture and function: dynamic reciprocity via extra- and intra-cellular matrices, *Cancer Metastasis Rev.* 28,1-2.,(167-176),

Yang,L., Jackson,E., Woerner,B.M., Perry,A., Piwnica-Worms,D., and Rubin,J.B. (2007). Blocking CXCR4-mediated cyclic AMP suppression inhibits brain tumor growth in vivo, *Cancer Res.* 67,2.,(651-658),

Yang,X.F. (2007). Immunology of stem cells and cancer stem cells, *Cell Mol. Immunol.* 4,3.,(161-171),

Yin,G., Chen,R., Alvero,A.B., Fu,H.H., Holmberg,J., Glackin,C., Rutherford,T., and Mor,G. (2010). TWISTing stemness, inflammation and proliferation of epithelial ovarian cancer cells through MIR199A2/214, *Oncogene* 29,24.,(3545-3553),

Yoganathan,N., Yee,A., Zhang,Z., Leung,D., Yan,J., Fazli,L., Kojic,D.L., Costello,P.C., Jabali,M., Dedhar,S., and Sanghera,J. (2002). Integrin-linked kinase, a promising cancer therapeutic target: biochemical and biological properties, *Pharmacol. Ther.* 93,2-3.,(233-242),

Yoshida,Y., Takahashi,K., Okita,K., Ichisaka,T., and Yamanaka,S. (2009). Hypoxia enhances the generation of induced pluripotent stem cells, *Cell Stem Cell* 5,3.,(237-241),

Zhang,J., Niu,C., Ye,L., Huang,H., He,X., Tong,W.G., Ross,J., Haug,J., Johnson,T., Feng,J.Q., Harris,S., Wiedemann,L.M., Mishina,Y., and Li,L. (2003). Identification of the haematopoietic stem cell niche and control of the niche size, *Nature* 425,6960.,(836-841).

12

Cancer Stem Cells Promote Tumor Neovascularization

Yi-fang Ping, Xiao-hong Yao, Shi-cang Yu,
Ji Ming Wang and Xiu-wu Bian
The Third Military Medical University
China

1. Introduction

Tumor growth and metastasis depend on neovascularisation, which has been recently believed promoted by cancer stem cells (CSCs), a special subpopulation of tumor cells. The cancer stem cell theory can be traced back to the first mention by Furth and Kahn in 1937, when their results revealed a single leukaemic cell capable of transmitting the systemic disease in mice [1]. However, it was not until the 1990s that CSCs were identified and well-characterized in acute myeloid leukaemia (AML). Among cancer cells isolated from AML patients, only a small fraction of them exhibiting the hematopoietic stem cell surface phenotype, i.e. $CD34^+$ and $CD38^-$, were capable of initiating leukaemia in mice similar to that of the original patient. These cells were then known as SCID leukemia-initiating cells with potentials to self-renew, proliferate and differentiate in vivo [2, 3]. Since then, CSCs from various types of cancer such as breast cancer and malignant glioma have been well characterized, and then the existence of CSCs in solid tumors has been gradually accepted [4-10]. The studies promote a common recognition of the accurate definition for CSCs reached by an American Association for Cancer Research (AACR) workshop in 2006, that CSCs are a small subset within a cancer that constitute a reservoir of self-sustaining cells with the exclusive abilities to self-renew and to cause the heterogeneous lineages of cancer cells that comprise the tumor [11].

Investigation on CSCs provides a new insight into our understanding for tumorigenesis, recurrence and metastasis of cancer as well as development of new strategies for cancer treatment. Due to up-regulation of drug resistance and anti-apoptotic genes as well as greater DNA-repair responses, CSCs are more resistant to chemo- and/or radiotherapies than differentiated cancer cells [12-17]. Recent studies suggest that CSCs existing in the tumor are highly invasive, indicating their crucial role in invasion and metastasis of cancer [18]. Therefore, eradication of CSCs is of great importance in preventing cancer recurrence and metastasis.

The increasing awareness of neovascularization holding a master switch of tumor development and progression indicates that vascularization plays a crucial role in the stage of tumor progression [19]. It is generally thought that vascularization is initiated by microenvironmental changes such as hypoxia followed by tumor outgrowing its blood supply limitation. This process is further promoted by angiogenic factors derived from tumor cells and infiltrating inflammatory/immune cells into tumor tissues [20-22]. Tumor vasculatures are mainly developed through angiogenesis by sprouting from pre-existing vessels and vasculogenesis via recruitment of endothelial progenitor cells (EPCs) [23, 24]. Both of the processes are initiated and promoted by angiogenic factors [20, 22, 25] such as vascular endothelial growth factor (VEGF) and basic fibroblast growth factor (bFGF) produced by cancer cells and stromal cells [22, 26, 27]. Interestingly, cancer cells exhibit heterogeneity in their production of angiogenic factors.

CSCs have been more recently identified as initiating cells of tumor neovascularization [28-33], but many doubts still challenge CSC theory. In this review, we provide the evidence for the role of CSCs in tumor vascularization and discuss the potential therapeutic significance based on the interaction between CSCs and their vascular niches.

2. CSCs produce angiogenic factors

CSCs play a predominant role in tumor angiogenesis through producing high levels of pro-angiogenic factors. Evidence from our laboratory and others has indicated that CSCs produce preferentially higher levels of angiogenic factors, for instance, VEGF and interleukin 8 (IL-8). Ponti et al identified a subpopulation of sphere-forming cells with CSC properties, named MCF-S, from an established breast carcinoma cell line MCF-7 [28]. It was found that MCF-S cells expressed higher levels of VEGF mRNA compared with MCF-7. Meanwhile, higher amounts of VEGF protein were measured in the MCF-S culture medium, indicating CSCs might possess stronger pro-angiogenic capability than differentiated tumor cells. Bao et al found that hypoxia could induce glioma stem cells to produce higher levels of angiogenic factor VEGF [29]. CSC-enriched neurospheres derived from the GL261 murine glioma cell line and rat glioma cell line C6 express more VEGF compared with adherent, CSC-low cultures [30, 31]. Compared with adherent C6 cells, sphere-forming C6 cells induced higher levels of proliferation and tubulogenesis of endothelial cells in vitro. Accordingly, xenografts derived from sphere-forming C6 cells exhibited increased microvessel density and blood perfusion and induced increased mobilization and tumor recruitment of bone marrow-derived endothelial progenitor cells (EPCs). When VEGF was blocked, all aspects of angiogenesis observed in sphere-forming C6 cells and xenografts, including microvessel density, perfusion, EPC mobilization/recruitment, and stimulation of endothelial cell activity, were reduced to levels comparable with those observed in either adherent C6 cells or their implanted tumors [31]. Furthermore, CSC-enriched CD133+ fraction derived from the U87 human glioblastoma cell line and primary human gliomas also had a significantly stronger capacity of promoting angiogenesis than the CSC-depleted CD133- fraction. Accordingly, CD133+ glioma cells generated highly vascularized tumors when implanted in mice, whereas the matched CD133 populations were rarely tumorigenic and gave rise to poorly vascularized tumors. The proangiogenic capacity of CD133+ fraction was attributable to VEGF activity [29, 32]. The evidence of in vivo pro-angiogenic effects of CSCs was further proved by Oka and the colleagues [33]. Transfecting glioma stem cells with a retrovirus vector expressing VEGF promoted vascular formation and tumor-associated hemorrhage. The blood vessels adjacent to and within the tumors derived from VEGF-expressing glioma stem cells exhibited much higher density and more complexity of neovascularization. The newly formed vessels had functional walls and lumens when they were stained with anti-CD31 antibody and PAS histochemistry demonstrated central lumens and new basement membrane. Taken together, VEGF appears to be an important mediator for CSC contribution to tumor neovascularization.

Chemokines and their receptors are believed to be involved in CSCs-mediated production of angiogenic factors. For instance, CXCR4, a chemokine receptor that plays an important role in tumor angiogenesis, was preferentially expressed in glioma stem cells [16, 34-36]. Meanwhile, stromal derived factor-1 (SDF-1) or CXCL12, the sole ligand for CXCR4, can be detected in glioma stem cell culture medium, indicating that CXCR4 expressed by glioma stem cells can be activated in an autocrine manner. Using a rat aortic ring assay, Salmaggi and the colleagues found glioma stem cells induced apparently longer and thinner neo-vessels compared with control group. They further documented high expression of CXCR4 and release of CXCL12 by glioma stem cells might be the underlying mechanism [34]. In our recent studies, we also found that CD133+ glioma stem cells had significantly higher CXCR4 mRNA and protein expression levels, as well as higher chemotactic response to its ligand CXCL12 as compared to CD133 negative cells [37]. In addition to chemokine receptor CXCR4, formylpeptide receptor (FPR), a classic chemoattractant receptor, was also found to induce VEGF production by glioma stem cells [32]. This G-protein coupled receptor mediates neutrophils to participate in inflammation, and we previously found its promotion of tumor growth and invasion through its activation by binding its stimulator from necrotic tumor cells. We recently reported this receptor expressed on glioma stem cells was functional and its activation promotes stem cells production of angiogenic factors such as VEGF and IL-8/CXCL8, resulting in initiation of angiogenesis. When transplanting human CSCs into nude mice, the CSCs produced in situ angiogenic factors and generated a higher density of microvessels to promote tumor growth. These results strongly suggest that chemoattractants and their receptors, at least in part, are among the major signals to promote CSC-mediated tumor angiogenesis by stimulating VEGF production.

Although a greater contribution of CSCs to tumor angiogenesis than their differentiated counterparts within a tumor has been supported by many studies, contradictory phenomenons have also been observed. Salmaggi et al found non-sphere-forming cells from GBM could induce more vessels than glioma stem cells using the aortic ring assay. They observed that the pro-angiogenic capacity varied among different passages of glioma stem cells. Pro-angiogenic ability of glioma stem cells increased after serial passages in culture concomitant with elevated VEGF and CXCL12 production [34]. Consequently, VEGF mRNA was increased in the secondary tumor spheres acquired from primary tumorospheres of xenografts [34]. Recently, Sakariassen et al observed angiogenesis-dependent and angiogenesis-independent patterns in glioma stem cell-derived xenografts [38]. Great differences were seen in gene expression profiles and signaling pathways between the glioma stem cells with two different tumor generation patterns. These results indicate that CSCs are actually heterogeneous in their contribution to neovascularization. Further studies are still needed to elucidate the exact subclones preferentially contributing to tumor angiogenesis for more effective targeting to angiogenesis-initiating stem cells.

3. CSCs transdifferentiate into endothelial cells

Endothelial cells (ECs) not only interact with cancer cells through aberrant growth factors, but also share genetic abnormality with cancer cells, which might suggest a link in their common origin [39-41]. Streubel et al investigated 27 cases of lymphoma and found 15% to 85% of the microvascular ECs harbored the same lymphoma-specific genetic aberrations. In vitro assays also showed that the ECs isolated from primary human lymphoma presented the lymphoma-specific genetic aberrations [39]. In multiple myeloma patients with the 13q14 deletion, a significant proportion of circulating ECs carried the same chromosome aberration as the neoplastic plasma cells, and presented the same immunoglobulin gene rearrangement as multiple myeloma plasma cells. In addition, most circulating ECs presented EPC features as they expressed CD133, a marker gradually lost during endothelial differentiation and absent on mature ECs [40]. Renal tumor-derived ECs but not normal ECs expressed paired-box 2 (Pax2) proteins and mRNA, which were restricted to the developing kidney in the embryo [41]. These results suggest that cancer cells and ECs might derive from common multipotent progenitor cells, or possibly CSCs.

More evidence supports that CSCs might generate or transdifferentiate into ECs for neovascularization. Pezzolo et al investigated the origin of the microvascular ECs in MYCN-amplified nephroblastoma and found that 20%-78% of the ECs identified by CD105 expression exhibited amplification of the oncogene MYCN, the tumor marker of this tumor at stage 3 and 4. This finding strongly implicates the possible cancer cell origin of ECs in MYCN amplification nephroblastoma. Furthermore, microvessels formed by the ECs were functional because they contained erythrocytes and were covered with a layer of pericytes. They further studied a cell line HTLA-230 from human stage 4 nephroblastoma with MYCN amplification and injected the cells into immunodeficient mice to investigate the origin of ECs in the xenografts. It was found that the xenografts contained approximately 80% of human ECs and 20% murine ECs, suggesting the nephroblastoma cells directly transdifferentiating to tumor ECs [42, 43].

More direct evidence of the potential transdifferentiation of CSCs to ECs has been reported in recent years. In a study with the injecting fluorescence-labeled human cutaneous metastatic melanoma cells into the ischemic hind limbs of nude mice, it was found that after five days, the vessels consisted of human melanoma-derived cells adjacent to and overlapping with mouse ECs in a linear arrangement were formed and provided blood for the ischemic limbs [44]. A CD133+ cell population, which is negative for the endothelial marker CD34, but positive for the renal embryonic marker Pax-2, derived from human renal carcinomas was also able to differentiate into ECs. When injected subcutaneously in SCID mice, they formed functional vessels which integrated with the mouse vasculature. Among the tumor vasculature, vessels of human origin accounted for 85% and were mainly located within the tumors [45]. Kusumbe et al isolated a non-tumorigenic CD133+ population in ovarian cancer and termed them as endothelial stem cells (EnSCs) based on their capacity of differentiating into ECs. A unique feature of these EnSCs is the continual expression of the surface molecule CD44 at all the steps of the hierarchy [46]. In the two reports, the authors did not detect the cellular karyotypes, thus we cannot know whether these cells are normal or abnormal in their phenotype. However, the expression of Pax-2 or CD44 suggested that they are not hematopoietic cells or endothelial cells. As they were isolated from tumors, it can be hypothesized that this CD133+ population might be a committed lineage that derived from CSCs and could differentiate into ECs but not tumor cells. This was confirmed by Shen and his colleagues who found precancerous stem cells (pCSCs), representing the early stage of developing CSCs, can not only initiate tumors but also generate most of the tumor vasculature [47, 48]. More recently, Bussolati and the colleagues isolated and cloned a population of breast CSCs, which were able to differentiate into the endothelial lineage acquiring endothelial markers and the ability to organize in Matrigel into capillary-like structures when cultured in the presence of VEGF. The capacity of in vivo endothelial differentiation was proven by vessels of human origin in the transplanted tumors, formed by these cells [49]. Evidence from the studies of CSCs in human renal carcinomas and ovarian cancers also confirmed the capacity of CSCs to transdifferentiate into endothelial cells. CD105+ tumor-initiating cells isolated from human renal carcinomas acquired an endothelial phenotype when cultured in endothelial differentiating medium containing VEGF and generated ECs of human origin in the central of SCID xenografts [50]. Ovarian cancer cells with stem-like properties can also transdifferentiate into ECs both in intro and in vivo. Interestingly, this transdifferentiating process was shown to be VEGF-independent, but IKKβ-dependent [51], suggesting either VEGF-dependent or VEGF-independent mechanisms are involved in the trans-endothelial differentiation of CSCs.

4. CSCs contribute to vasculogenic mimicry

It is a widely-accepted paradigm that tumor vasculature is mostly composed of non-malignant endothelial cells originating from pre-existing blood vessels sprouting into tumor mass and recruitment of circulating endothelial progenitor cells (EPCs) mediated by angiogenic growth factors produced by host or tumor cells [52]. However, classical patterns of angiogenesis and vasculogenesis have been challenged by clinical investigation of tumor tissues because tumor vasculature can also be formed by vasculogenic mimicry (VM) [53].
VM is a structure through which tumor tissues nourish themselves, mimicking the pattern of embryonic vascular network. Tumor cells with high degree of differentiation plasticity may contribute to the de novo formation of tumor cell-lined blood channels [54]. These extracellular matrix-rich vasculogenic tumor cell networks were shown to conduct fluid. An interesting observation was that VM was most frequently observed in the boundary regions between the tumor and surrounding normal tissues [55]. Thus, VM may also play a role in tumor invasion by supplying immediate nutrition. Furthermore, angiogenesis inhibitors abrogate new vessels formed by human vascular endothelial cells in vitro, while under the same conditions did not affect tumor cell tuber network formation, and even induced the formation of VM as an escape route by tumor tissue for progressive growth [56]. Therefore, VM might represent an important survival mechanism contributing to the failure of current antiangiogenic therapy aimed to fully deprive tumors of blood supply [57]. Despite its clinical importance, the cellular and molecular events underlying the formation of VM are not well understood. Recent discovery of cancer stem cells (CSCs), with the capability of self-renewal and multi-potency of differentiation, has stimulated great interest in re-defining tumor initiation and progression [58]. However, whether CSC theory can be applied to the formation of tumor cell-associated vasculogenesis, especially in respect to VM, remains unclear. Based on the present findings that most vessels in tumor may be originated from tumor cell themselves through the process of vasculogenesis [59], as well as that CSCs were able to serve as precursors of tumor stromal components such as tumor vasculogenic stem/progenitor cells (TVPCs) regulated by signals from microenvironment/niche surrounding these cells [60], it is plausible that CSC compartment of a tumor may be involved in VM formation, by differentiating/transdifferentiating into endothelial-like cells. Such a potential function of CSCs might represent one of the

mechanisms by which CSCs initiate neoplastic formation and promote tumor progression [61]. In this review, we will focus on the possible role of CSCs in VM formation and how the niche surrounding CSCs may affect VM formation.

4.1 Current understanding of tumor VM

In 1999, Maniotis et al. first described VM in aggressive melanoma with tumor cells expressing endothelial phenotype pasted on the surface of the basement membrane in tubular structure [62]. VM in the tumor mass is connected with host vessels for blood supply. Periodic acid-Schiff (PAS) staining is commonly utilized to identify VM. PAS-positive channels were lined externally by tumor cells, lacking an inner lining of endothelial cells [63]. Although the functionality and contribution of VM channels to circulation were criticized initially, Frenkel et al. [64] demonstrated that blood circulated in VM tube with laser scanning confocal angiography in a patient with a choroidal melanoma. Therefore, VM is a new pattern that provides tumor mass with nutrition independent of conventional angiogenesis and vasculogenesis. Zhang et al. [65] proposed three-stage blood supply patterns in tumor including VM, mosaic vessels (MV) and endothelium-dependent vessels, in which all three patterns provide blood supply. The model proposes that VM is the dominant blood supply pattern in the early stage characterized by rapid tumor growth. Consequently, to maintain expansion of tumor mass, endothelial cells differentiate and proliferate, and the mosaic vessels appeared as a transitional pattern. Endothelium-dependent vessels then replace VM and mosaic vessels to become a major pattern of blood supply in the late stage of tumor growth. Thus, VM may be the main source of blood supply at the early stage of rapid tumor growth, when endothelium-dependent vessels, which require the sprouting and recruitment of endothelial cells, are insufficient to sustain aggressive tumor growth. Based on PAS staining, VM are divided into seven categories: straight channels, parallel straight pattern, parallel straight pattern with cross link, arcs (not closed), arcs with branching, closed loops, and networks [66].

VM has been detected in melanoma, breast carcinoma, prostate carcinoma, ovarian carcinoma, astrocytoma, and Ewing sarcoma, etc.[67-70]. Microarray analysis indicates that VM-positive tumor cells of aggressive melanoma expresses elevated levels of genes associated with undifferentiated embryonic-like phenotype [54]. Intra-peritoneally implantation of human ovarian cancer cell line SKOV3ip showed that the cells, expressing CD31 and Factor VIII of vascular epithelial markers, had plasticity to engage in VM formation in vivo [71]. These findings suggest that the plasticity of cancer cells enable them to mimic the activities of endothelial cells and participate in the process of VM formation. Recent findings of "plastic" endothelial-like phenotype of tumor cells provide additional evidence for the role of tumor cells in VM formation.

There are striking parallels between tumor cells and stem cells: tumors and normal tissue are comprised of phenotypically heterogeneous cell populations, and many characteristics of stem cells, for example, stem cell plasticity, which is also pertinent to tumor growth [72]. Cellular plasticity in stem cells may facilitate the formation of primary vascular network during embryonic development. Mesodermal progenitor cells differentiate in situ into endothelial cells that are organized into a primitive network to supply nutrition for the developing early embryo [73]. The subsequent remodeling of vascular network into more complex vasculature appears through the process of angiogenesis. These processes are similar to the formation of tumor vasculature and the plasticity of tumor cells may be important for the formation of VM.

4.2 Differentiation plasticity of CSCs and VM formation

CSCs are functionally defined by their capacity to regenerate tumors in xenograft mouse models [74, 75]. Similar to normal stem cells, CSCs can reproduce the heterogeneous phenotype of the parental cancer from which they are derived in transplantation, reflecting the multipotent differentiation capacity of CSCs. Plasticity defines the capacity of stem cells to differentiate or transdifferentiate into many cell types [76]. During development, multilineage differentiation plasticity is one of the characteristics of embryonic stem cells (ESC) [77]. CSCs are characterized by their stem/progenitor properties: self-renewal and the capability of differentiation into heterogeneous tumor cell populations [11]. Therefore, the differentiation plasticity of normal stem cells is also a similar property of CSCs. Bian et al. proposed a concept of CSC plasticity (CSCP) in which CSCs possess inducible and reversible properties in self-renewal, multipotent differentiation and invasion. For CSCs, differentiation plasticity refers to the ability of tumor cells to give rise to phenotypically diverse populations including non-tumorigenic cancer cells and stromal cells. In fact, aggressive melanoma cells forming VM appear to express genes relevant to multiple cellular phenotypes and stem cells including epithelial, endothelial, muscle, neuronal, and other cell types. The multipotent, plastic, and embryonic-like phenotype of these melanoma cells has also been considered as a defined property of putative malignant melanoma stem cells (MMSCs) [78]. Therefore, melanoma stem cells possess the differentiation plasticity (transdifferentiation) and this property may play a critical role in VM. Recently, a transdifferentiative capability has been demonstrated for bone marrow macrophages, which form VM in multiple myeloma. Thus, at least in melanoma, VM channel was believed to be due to the transdifferentiation of MMSC subset inside the aggressive tumor. In a study of breast cancer, CSCs in endothelial differentiating medium were capable of differentiating into endothelial cells, which formed both vessels and tumor [79]. It is conceivable that CSCs/tumor initiating stem cells of solid tumor have the competence of differentiation plasticity, which further supports the hypothesis that CSCs/tumor initiating stem cells possess the properties of normal stem cells important for tumor growth and vascularization. Evidence for direct involvement of tumor cells in VM was also obtained in human neuroblastoma (NB) [59]. Microvessels formed by MYCN-amplified NB tumor cells displayed an open lumen and consistently contained RBCs, indicating that these vessels were functional. Moreover, these tumor cell-derived vascular endothelial-like cells were different from normal endothelial cells in phenotype and function [59]. Although the study only tested MYNC-amplified tumor cells, it is possible that formation of tumor-derived endothelial cells is a characteristic feature of a subset of cells in neuroblastoma. In addition to neuroblastoma, tumor-associated endothelial microvessels are also found in human B-cell lymphomas and multiple myeloma [80]. It is also hypothesized that precancerous stem cells (pCSCs) representing the early stage of developing CSCs may serve as tumor vasculogenic progenitor cells (TVPCs) capable of differentiating into tumor vasculogenic endothelial cells [60]. Based on observations in animal models as well as human tumor xenografts, a model for pCSC or CSC participation in tumor vasculature formation was proposed, in which firstly, CSCs and their progenies aggregate to form a mass in tumorigenic microenvironment; secondly, with the extension of aggregates, a CSC subset with properties of tumor vasculogenic endothelial cells differentiate/transdifferentiate and line up to form branching lumens and tubes, resembling vascular network; and finally, the tubes extend and elongate, and the vasculature merges with host vessels from sprouting of pre-existing blood vessels and recruitment of circulating endothelial progenitor cells surrounding tumor mass. This model emphasizes the intrinsic property of CSCs in tumor vasculogenesis, and explains why most anti-angiogenic clinical trials fail to completely eradicate tumor, because the drugs tested may be effective on normal endothelial cells but not endothelial-like cells derived from CSCs [81]. Our recent studies also observed that glioma stem cells (GSCs), isolated from primary glioma sample [82] and a human glioblastoma cell line U87 [83], are capable of multipotent differentiation. In stem cell medium, such GSCs form spheroids, and in differentiation conditions they form tumor masses that contain fissure and branching lumen as revealed by electron microscope. These novel findings support the premise that VM positive tumor cells possess a multipotent phenotype and such cells with embryonic stem cell-like properties should be considered as antiangiogenic therapeutics.

4.3 Microenvironmental niche as a regulator of VM formation

The vasculogenesis and/or angiogenesis, which are necessary for tumor development and progression, involve the interaction of tumor and other cell types in the microenvironment or niche [84]. A pertinent role of the microenvironment in VM formation has been demonstrated in melanoma [85]. Collagen matrices preconditioned by aggressive melanoma cells capable of forming VM primed the lesser aggressive melanoma cells, which are initially unable to form VM, to express vasculogenic genes and to form VM in vitro. These observations illustrate the remarkable influence of microenvironment on the phenotype of tumor cells and provide a new perspective for the formation of VM, in which factors secreted by tumor cells or other niche components play a critical role in cancer cell plasticity, including dedifferentiation and transdifferentiation. In addition, the microenvironmental niche has been demonstrated to support normal stem cells in early co-culture and transplantation studies [86]. One of the mechanisms by which microenvironmental niche determines normal stem cell fate is the control of symmetric (producing two identical daughter cells) versus asymmetric (producing one identical and one differentiated cell) division [87]. Cancer stem cells, like normal stem cells, also depend on interaction with physiologically differentiated cell types or on non-tumorigenic cancer cell populations in the same tumor microenvironment to sustain their features and destiny [88]. Tumor environment creates a niche favoring the survival, proliferation, and differentiation of CSCs. CSCs utilize a specialized microenvironment/niche termed tumor stroma, consisted of a combination of different cell lineages, i.e. epithelial, vascular, fat, glial, fibroblast, and immune cells along with extracellular matrix, enzymes, and other secreted molecules produced by these cells [89]. It has been demonstrated that endothelial cells surrounding CSCs appear to directly generate specific microvasculature niche and/or secrete factors that promote the formation and/or maintenance of brain CSCs [90]. Critical signaling molecules, such as bone morphogenic proteins (BMPs) derived from the niche that govern embryonic vascular development, have been linked to melanoma cell-driven vasculogenesis, i.e. VM [94]. In human glioblastomas, BMP4-BMPR1a signaling pathway regulates the differentiation and proliferation of CSC population [92, 93]. Based on these findings, it is plausible that the niche surrounding CSCs controls the differentiation plasticity of CSCs, which is responsible for tumor vasculogenesis including VM formation.

In addition to being conditioned by niche components, CSCs may also reciprocally influence the niche through secretion of autocrine and/or paracrine factors or through direct cell-cell contact to benefit the maintenance of their stemness including self-renewal, multipotent differentiation, and tumor-initiation. We and others have suggested that CSCs from U87 cell line and primary human brain tumors secrete higher levels of endothelial growth factor (VEGF) than their non-tumorigenic counterpart cells that promoted the formation of tumor blood vessels [94, 29]. In breast cancer model, VEGF induces CSCs to express endothelial markers in vitro and incorporate in tumor vasculature in vivo [79]. Accumulating evidence shows in addition to vascular endothelial (VE)-cadherin, laminin 5γ2 chain, and VEGF receptor (R)-2, angiogenic factors, including VEGF, angiogenin-1, and ephrinA1, also play a critical role in the formation of VM by tumor cells [95]. In healthy individuals, stimulation by VEGF, cells of the monocyte lineage (another mesodermal-derived cell) display an endothelial phenotype and form a functional capillary-like mesh permeable by blood cells, recapitulating embryonic vasculogenesis. VEGF also stimulated macrophages of a patient with active multiple myeloma to undergo phenotypic and functional adaptation, expressing markers of endothelial cells, i.e. VE-cadherin, VEGFR-2, and FVIII-RA, retained their own CD14 and CD68 markers, and these cells can form vessel-like structures on the Matrigel surface. Therefore, VEGF can induce macrophages to transdiferentiate into endothelial-like cells to form VM, which functionally, phenotypically and morphologically are similar to endothelial cells, yet maintain the expression of macrophage markers. Thus, VEGF in the niche, which may be derived mainly from CSCs, directly influences the phenotype of CSCs and promotes CSCs-associated VM formation.

There are three factors determining the formation of VM channel: the plasticity of VM-associated tumor cells, remodeling of extracellular matrix, and the connection of VM with host microcirculation [96]. The remodeling of extracellular matrix provides the space needed for VM and is regulated by matrix metalloproteinases (MMP) [97]. Matrix MMP-9 and MMP-2 play a critical role during the formation of VM in aggressive melanoma. Our recent study showed that the expression of MMP-9 and MMP-2 is up-regulated in glioma stem cells (GSCs) derived from U87 cell line [98]. The formation of VM also involves migration of VM-derived tumor cells. We observed that migration associated molecules, including two G-protein coupled chemoattractant receptors formylpeptide receptor (FPR) and CXC chemokine receptor-4 (CXCR4) were over-expressed in GSCs isolated from human glioblastoma and U87 cell line [84, 37]. FPR and CXCR4 expressed on GSCs, when activated by corresponding agonists, mediate directional migration, calcium mobilization, and production of VEGF by GSCs. Our recent observations further suggest that activation of CXCR4 on GSCs elicits phosphoinositide 3-kinase (PI3K) pathway which is an important regulator of VM through MMP-2 [99]. The relationship between CSCs and VM formation through stimulatory signals in the niche is important for differentiation plasticity of CSCs. Based on the existing observations, it is conceivable that CSCs take part in the VM formation through autocrine and/or paracrine manner thereby establishing a vessel niche suitable to protect and nourish CSCs. Therefore, VM-targeted therapies should be a new strategy aimed at eliminating CSCs.

4.4 VM-targeted therapeutic strategy: new perspectives

CSCs are considered as the root of tumor initiation, metastasis, and reoccurrence. If CSCs are proven to be critical for VM formation, there will be significant implications in the design of novel anti-tumor therapies. As discussed earlier, VM is the dominant blood supply pattern in the early stage of tumor formation and CSCs are capable of differentiating/transdifferentiating and lining up to form branching lumens and tubes, a process resembling the formation of VM. Traditional anti-angiogenesis drugs, such as angiostatin and endostatin, which target normal endothelial cells, have little effect on VM due to the absence of normal endothelial cells [100]. In contrast, VEGF-specific inhibitor Bevacizumab can conspicuously decrease the number of self-renewing cancer cells from orthotopic models of medulloblastoma and glioma, resulting in tumor growth arrest. Direct evidence was obtained from aggressive melanoma in that LY294002, a specific inhibitor of PI3K, inhibited the ability of undifferentiated embryonic melanoma cells to engage in VM on three-dimensional type I collagen matrices [100]. Furthermore, the unique structure of VM channels, in which tumor cell line up the inner surface, directly exposes tumor cells to blood vessel and facilitates the metastasis of tumor cells. VM frequently is seen in the regions between the tumor and surrounding normal tissues, and its appearance in tumor is associated with poor prognosis in clinical patients. Therefore, VM-targeted therapies may destroy the niche that maintains CSCs, block the metastasis passage of tumor cells, and reduce the recurrence of cancer.

5. Conclusion

Based on these findings, we conclude that CSCs might initiate and promote neovascularization at the early stage of tumor tumorigenesis and progression. There are at least three potential mechanisms involved in this process: (1) CSCs induce neovascularization through secreting VEGF, which is further induced by hypoxia or activation of chemokine receptors; (2) CSCs might participate in angiogenesis through transdifferentiating into endothelial cells and/or endothelial progenitor cells; (3) CSCs could generate cells that form vasculogenic mimicry and provide nutrition and oxygen directly to the tumor mass (Figure 1). On the contrary, the tumor vasculature nourishes CSCs and maintains their survival and characteristics of "stemness".

Cancer stem cell hypothesis requires elimination of CSCs for more effective treatment of cancer. If CSCs exclusively generate heterogeneous tumor cells, elimination of these cells will result in arrested tumor growth and eventual eradication. The fact that CSCs contribute greatly to tumor neovascularization indicates that restraint of CSCs would impair tumor vessels. On the other hand, vascular niches support self-renewal, proliferation and differentiation of CSCs, and protect CSCs from chemo- and radiotherapies [90, 101, 102], suggesting the necessity to interfere or deplete vascular niches of CSCs. Anti-angiogenic drugs indeed reduced markedly the MVD in xenografts and arrested tumor growth [103, 104]. Thus, a combination of targeting CSCs and their vascular niche will provide more effective therapy for tumor treatment. Furthermore, differentiation induction strategy targeting the poor-differentiated CSCs may also facilitate cancer treatment [105]. However, there is a long way to go for developing the methods targeting CSCs and their vascular niche to treat cancers.

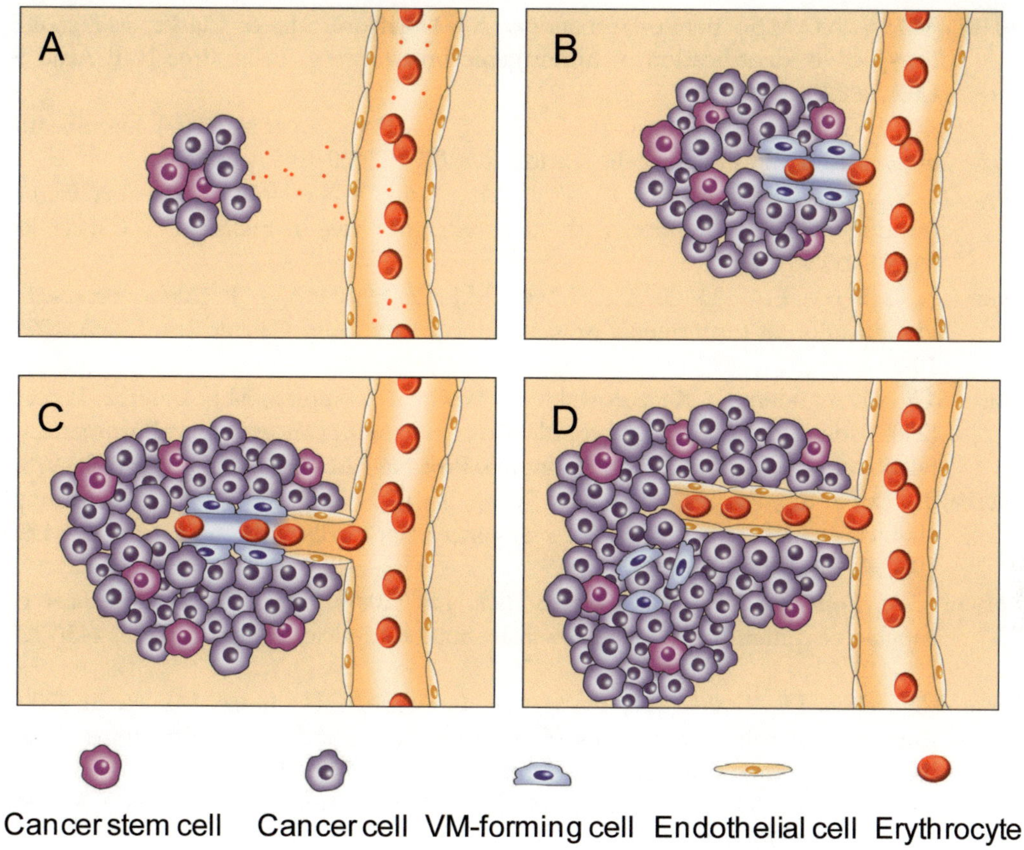

Fig. 1. Proposed mechanism of cancer stem cells (CSCs) in tumor neovascularization. CSCs self-renew and generate cancer cells (A) as well as VM-forming cells (B). The VM-forming cells can form functional lumens, incorporating with the endothelial cells either from transdifferentiation of CSCs or sprouting of endothelial cells from pre-existing vessels (known as angiogenesis), provide blood and nutrition for the tumor mass (C and D). Furthermore, proangiogenic factors produced by CSCs and cancer cells promote recruitment of circulating EPCs to the tumor tissue and integration into tumor vessels, forming new microvessels known as vasculogenesis.

6. References

Furth, J., & Kahn, M. (1937). The transmission of leukaemia of mice with a single cell. Am J Cancer, 31, 276-282.

Lapidot, T., Sirard, C., Vormoor, J., Murdoch, B., Hoang, T., Caceres-Cortes, J., et al. (1994). A cell initiating human acute myeloid leukaemia after transplantation into SCID mice. Nature, 367(6464), 645-648.

Bonnet, D., & Dick, J.E. (1997). Human acute myeloid leukaemia is organized as a hierarchy that originates from a primitive hematopoietic cell. Nat Med, 3(7), 730-737.

Al-Hajj, M., Wicha, M.S., Benito-Hernandez, A., Morrison, S.J., & Clarke, M.F. (2003). Prospective identification of tumorigenic breast cancer cells. Proc Natl Acad Sci USA, 100(7), 3983-3988.

Li, C., Heidt, D.G., Dalerba, P., Burant, C.F., Zhang, L., Adsay, V., et al. (2007). Identification of pancreatic cancer stem cells. Cancer Res, 67(3), 1030-1037.

Fang, D., Nguyen, T.K., Leishear, K., Finko, R., Kulp, A.N., Hotz, S., et al. (2005). A tumorigenic subpopulation with stem cell properties in melanomas. Cancer Res, 65(20), 9328-9337.

Collins, A.T., Berry, P.A., Hyde, C., Stower, M.J., & Maitland, N.J. (2005). Prospective identification of tumorigenic prostate cancer stem cells. Cancer Res, 65(23), 10946-10951.

Prince, M.E., Sivanandan, R., Kaczorowski, A., Wolf, G.T., Kaplan, M.J., Dalerba, P., et al. (2007). Identification of a subpopulation of cells with cancer stem cell properties in head and neck squamous cell carcinoma. Proc Natl Acad Sci USA, 104(3), 973-978.

Dalerba, P., Dylla, S.J., Park, I.K., Liu, R., Wang, X., Cho, R.W., et al. (2007). Phenotypic characterization of human colorectal cancer stem cells. Proc Natl Acad Sci USA, 104(24), 10158-10163.

O'Brien, C.A., Pollett, A., Gallinger, S., & Dick, J.E. (2007). A human colon cancer cell capable of initiating tumour growth in immunodeficient mice. Nature, 445(7123), 106-110.

Clarke, M.F., Dick, J.E., Dirks, P.B., Eaves, C.J., Jamieson, C.H., Jones, D.L., et al. (2006). Cancer stem cells-perspectives on current status and future directions: AACR workshop on cancer stem cells. Cancer Res, 66 (19), 9339-9344.

Dean, M., Fojo, T., & Bates, S. (2005). Tumour stem cells and drug resistance. Nat Rev Cancer, 5(4), 275-284.

Chalmersa, A.J. (2007). Radioresistant glioma stem cells-therapeutic obstacle or promising target? DNA Repair, 6(9), 1391-1394.

Eramo, A., Ricci-Vitiani, R., Zeuner, A., Pallini, R., Lotti, F., Sette, G., et al. (2006). Chemotherapy resistance of glioblastoma stem cells. Cell Death Differ, 13(7), 1238-1241.

Hirschmann-Jax, C., Foster, A.E., Wulf, G.G., Nuchtern, J.G., Jax, T.W., Gobel, U., et al. (2004). A distinct "side population" of cells with high drug efflux capacity in human tumor cells. Proc Natl Acad Sci USA, 101(39), 14228-14233.

Liu, G., Yuan, X., Zeng, Z., Tunici, P., Ng, H., Abdulkadir, I.R., et al. (2006). Analysis of gene expression and chemoresistance of CD133+ cancer stem cells in glioblastoma. Mole Cancer, 5, 67.

Bao, S., Wu, Q., McLendon, R.E., Hao, Y., Shi, Q., Hjelmeland, A.B., et al. (2006). Glioma stem cells promote radioresistance by preferential activation of the DNA damage response. Nature, 444(7120), 756-760.

Sheridan, C., Kishimoto, H., Fuchs, R.K., Mehrotra, S., Bhat-Nakshatri, P., Turner, CH., et al. (2006). CD44+/CD24- breast cancer cells exhibit enhanced invasive properties: an early step necessary for metastasis. Breast Cancer Res, 8(5), R59.

Narazaki, M., & Tosato G. (2006). Tumor cell populations differ in angiogenic activity: a model system for spontaneous angiogenic switch can tell us why. J Natl Cancer Inst, 98(5), 294-295.

Hanahan, D., & Folkman, J. (1996). Patterns and emerging mechanisms of the angiogenic switch during tumorigenesis. Cell, 86(3), 353-364.

Greenblatt. M., & Shubik. P. (1968). Tumor angiogenesis: transfilter diffusion studies in the hamster by the transparent chamber technique. J Natl Cancer Inst, 41(1), 111-124.

Folkman, J., & Klagsbrun. M. (1987). Angiogenic factors. Science, 235 (4787), 442-447.

Fischer, I., Gagner, J.P., Law, M., Newcomb, E.W., & Zagzag, D. (2005). Angiogenesis in gliomas: biology and molecular pathophysiology. Brain pathol, 15(4), 297-310.

Komarovaa, N.L., & Mironov, V. (2005). On the role of endothelial progenitor cells in tumor neovascularization. J Theor Biol, 235 (3), 338-349.

Bian, X.W., Chen, J.H., Jiang, X.F., Bai, J.S., Wang, Q.L., & Zhang, X. (2004). Angiogenesis as an immunopharmacologic target in inflammation and cancer. Int Immunopharmacol, 4(12), 1537-1547.

Gilad, A.A., Israely, T., Dafni, H., Meir, G., Cohen, B., & Neeman, M. (2005). Functional and molecular mapping of uncoupling between vascular permeability and loss of vascular maturation in ovarian carcinoma xenografts: the role of stroma cells in tumor angiogenesis. Int J Cancer, 117(2), 202-211.

Saarinen, N.M., Abrahamsson, A., & Dabrosin, C. (2010). Estrogen-induced angiogenic factors derived from stromal and cancer cells are differently regulated by enterolactone and genistein in human breast cancer in vivo. Int J Cancer, 127(3), 737-745

Ponti, D., Costa, A., Zaffaroni, N., Pratesi, G., Petrangolini, G., Coradini, D., et al. (2005). Isolation and in vitro propagation of tumorigenic breast cancer cells with stem/progenitor cell properties. Cancer Res, 65(13), 5506-5511.

Bao, S., Wu, Q., Sathornsumetee, S., Hao, Y., Li, Z., Hjelmeland, A.B., et al. (2006). Stem cell-like glioma cells promote tumor angiogenesis through vascular endothelial growth factor. Cancer Res, 66(16), 7843-7848.

Pellegatta, S., Poliani, P.L., Corno, D., Menghi, F., Ghielmetti, F., Suarez-Merino, B., et al. (2006). Neurospheres enriched in cancer stem-like cells are highly effective in eliciting a dendritic cell-mediated immune response against malignant gliomas. Cancer Res, 66(21), 10247-10252.

Folkins, C., Shaked, Y., Man, S., Tang, T., Lee, C.R., Zhu, Z., et al. (2009). Glioma tumor stem cell-like cells promote tumor angiogenesis and vasculogenesis via vascular endothelial growth factor and stromal-derived factor 1. Cancer Res, 69(18), 7243-7251.

Yao, X.H., Ping, Y.F., Chen, J.H., Xu, C.P., Chen, D.L., Zhang, R., et al. (2008). Glioblastoma stem cells produce vascular endothelial growth factor by activation of a G-protein coupled formlpeptide receptor FPR. J Pathol, 215(4), 369-376.

Oka, N., Soeda, A., Inagaki, A., Onodera, M., Maruyama, H., Hara, A., et al. (2007). VEGF promotes tumorigenesis and angiogenesis or human glioblastoma stem cells. Biochem Biophys Res Commun, 360(3), 553-559.

Salmaggi, A., Bolardi, A., Gelati, M., Russo, A., Calatozzolo, C., Ciusani, E., et al. (2006). Glioblastoma-derived tumorospheres identify a population of tumor stem-like cells with angiogenic potential and enhanced multidrug resistance phenotype. Glia, 54(8), 850-860.

Ehtesham, M., Mapara, K.Y., Stevenson, C.B., & Thompson, R.C. (2009). CXCR4 mediates the proliferation of glioblastoma progenitor cells. Cancer Lett, 274(2), 305-312.

Krohn, A., Song, Y.H., Muehlberg, F., Droll, L., Beckmann, C., & Alt, E. (2009).CXCR4 receptor positive spheroid forming cells are responsible for tumor invasion in vitro. Cancer Lett, 280(1), 65-71.

Ping, Y.F., Yao, X.H., Bian, X.W., Chen, J.H., Zhang, R., Yi, L., et al. (2007). Activation of CXCR4 in human glioma stem cells promotes tumor angiogenesis. Zhonghua Bing Li Xue Za Zhi. 36(3),179-183.

Sakariassen, P., Prestegarden, L., Wang, J., Skaftnesmo, K.O., Mahesparan, R., Molthoff, C., et al. (2006). Angiogenesis-independent tumor growth mediated by stem-like cancer cells. Proc Natl Acad Sci USA, 103(44), 16466-16471.

Streubel, B., Chott, A., Huber, D., Exner, M., Jager, U., Wagner, O., et al. (2004). Lymphoma-specific genetic aberrations in microvascular endothelial cells in B-cell lymphomas. N Engl J Med, 351(3), 250-259.

Rigolin, G.M., Fraulini, C., Ciccone, M., Mauro, E., Bugli, A.M., De Angeli, C., et al. (2006). Neoplastic circulating endothelial cells in multiple myeloma with 13q14 deletion. Blood, 107(6), 2531- 2535.

Fonsato, V., Buttiglieri, S., Deregibus, M.C., Puntorieri, V., Bussolati, B., & Camussi, G. (2006). Expression of Pax2 in human renal tumor-derived endothelial cells sustains apoptosis resistance and angiogenesis. Am J Pathol,168(2),706-713.

Pezzolo, A., Parodi, F., Corrias, M.V., Cinti, R., Gambini, C., & Pistoia, V. (2007).Tumor origin of endothelial cells in human neuroblastoma. J Clin Oncol, 25(4), 376-383.

Ribatti, D., Nico, B., Pezzolo, A., Vacca, A., Meazza, R., Cinti, R., et al. (2006). Angiogenesis in a human neuroblastoma xenograft model: mechanisms and inhibition by tumor-derived interferon-gamma. Br J Cancer, 94(12), 1845-1852.

Hendrix, M. J. , Seffor, R.E., Seftor, E.A., Gruman, L.M., Lee, L.M., Nickoloff, B.J., et al. (2002).Transendothelial function of human metastatic melanoma cells: role of the microenvironment in cell-fate determination. Cancer Res, 62(3), 665-668.

Bruno, S., Bussolati, B., Grange, C., Collino, F., Graziano, M.E., Ferrando, U., et al. (2006). CD133+ renal progenitor cells contribute to tumor angiogenesis. Am J Pathol, 169(6), 2223-2235.

Kusumbe, A.P., Mali, A.M., & Bapat, S.A. (2009). CD133 expressing stem cells associated with ovarian metastases establish an endothelial hierarchy and contribute to tumor vasculature. Stem cells, 27(3), 498-508.

Shen, R., Ye, Y., Chen, L., Yan, Q., Barsky, S.H., & Gao, J.X. (2008). Precancerous stem cells can serve as tumor vasculogenic progenitors. PLoS One, 3(2), e1652.

Chen, L., Shen, R., Ye, Y., Pu, X.A., Liu, X., Duan, W., et al. (2007). Precancerous stem cells have the potential for both benign and malignant differentiation. PLoS One, 2(3), e293.

Bussolati, B., Grange, C., Sapino, A., Camussi, G. (2009). Endothelial cell differentiation of human breast tumor stem/progenitor cells. J Cell Mol Med, 13(2), 309-319.

Bussolati, B., Bruno, S., Gristina, G., Ferrando, U., & Camussi, G. Identification of a tumor-initiating stem cell population in human renal carcinomas. (2008). FASEB J, 22(10), 3696-3705.

Alvero, A.B., Fu, H.H., Holmberg, J., Visintin, I., Mor, L., Marquina, C.C., et al. (2009). Stem-like ovarian cancer cells can serve as tumor vascular progenitors. Stem Cells, 27(10), 2405-2413.

Dorsam RT, Gutkind JS. G-protein-coupled receptors and cancer. Nat Rev Cancer., 2007; 7: 79-94.

Folberg R, Maniotis AJ. Vasculogenic mimicry. APMIS., 2004; 12(7-8): 508-525.

Hendrix MJ, Seftor EA, Hess AR, Seftor RE. Vasculogenic mimicry and tumour-cell plasticity: lessons from melanoma. Nat Rev Cancer,, 2003; 3:411-421.

Sun B, Zhang S, Zhao X, Zhang W, Hao X. Vasculogenic mimicry is associated with poor survival in patients with mesothelial sarcomas and alveolar rhabdomyosarcomas. Int J Oncol., 2004; 25:1609-1614.

Van Der Schaft DW, Seftor RE, Seftor EA, Hess AR, Gruman LM, Kirschmann DA, Yokoyama Y, Griffioen AW, Hendrix MJ. Effects of angiogenesis inhibitors on vascular network formation by human endothelial and melanoma cells. J Natl Cancer Inst., 2004; 96:1473–1477.

Folkman, J. Angiogenesis: an organizing principle for drug discovery? Nat Rev Drug Discov., 2007; 6(4): 273-286.

Gao JX. Cancer stem cells: the lessons from precancerous stem cells. J Cell Mol Med., 2007; 58: 267-284.

PezzoloA, Parodi F, Corrias MV, Cinti R, Gambini C, Pistoia V. Tumor origin of endothelial cells in human neuroblastoma. J Clin Oncol., 2007; 25(4): 376-383.

Shen R, Ye Y, Chen L, Yan QT, Barsky SH, Gao JX. Precancerous stem cells can serve as tumor vasculogenic progenitors. PLoS ONE, 2008; 3(2): e1652.

Bjerkvig R, Tysnes BB, Aboody KS, Najbauer J, Terzis AJA. The origin of the cancer stem cell: current controversies and new insights. Nat Rev Cancer., 2005; 5:899-904.

Maniotis AJ, Folberg R, Hess A, Seftor EA, Gardner LMG, Pe'er J, Trent JM, Meltzer PS, Hendrix MJC. Vascular channel formation by human melanoma cells in vivo and in vitro: vasculogenic mimicry. Am J Pathol., 1999; 155: 739-752.

Hendrix MJ, Seftor EA, Meltzer PS, Gardner LM, Hess AR, Kirschmann DA, Schatteman GC, Seftor RE. Expression and functional significance of VE-cadherin in aggressive human melanoma cells: role in vasculogenic mimicry. Proc Natl Acad Sci USA., 2001; 98(14): 8018-8023.

Frenkel S, Barzel I, Levy J, Lin AY, Bartsch DU, Majumdar D, Folberg R, Pe'er J. Demonstrating circulation in vasculogenic mimicry patterns of uveal melanoma by confocal indocyanine green angiography. Eye, 2008; 22(7): 948-952.

Zhang S, Guo H, Zhang D, Zhang W, Zhao X, Ren Z, Sun B. Microcirculation patterns in different stages of melanoma growth. Ocol Rep., 2006; 15(1): 15-20.

Folberg R, Hendrix MJ, Maniotis AJ. Vasculogenic mimicry and tumor angiogenesis. Am J Pathol., 2000; 156(2):361-381.

Shirakawa K, Heike Y, Watanabe I, Yanmada S, Saito K, Konishi F. Vasculogenic mimicry and pseudo-comedo formation in breast. Int J Cancer., 2002; 99(6):812-828.

Sun B, Zhang S, Zhao X, Zhang W, Hao X. Vasculogenic mimicry is associated with poor survival in patients with mesothelial sarcomas and alveolar rhabdomyosarcomas. Int J Oncol., 2004; 25(6):1609-1614.

Elzarrad K, Haroon A, Reed D, Al-Mehdi AB. Early incorporated endothelial cells as origin of metastatic tumor vasculogenesis. Clin Exp Metastasis., 2009; 26(6): 589-598.

Yue WY, Chen ZP. Does vasculogenic mimicry exist in astrocytoma? J Histochem Cytochem., 2005; 53(8):997-1002.

Su M, Feng YJ, Yao LQ, Cheng MJ, Xu CJ, Huang Y, Zhao YQ, Jiang H. Plasticity of ovarian cancer cell SKOV3ip and vasculogenic mimicry in vivo. Int J Gynecol Cancer., 2008; 18(3):476-486.

Schatton T, Frank MH. Cancer stem cells and human malignant melanoma. Pigment Cell Melanoma Res., 2008; 21(1):39-55.

Carmeliet P. Mechanisms of angiogenesis and arteriogenesis. Nat Med., 2000; 6(4): 389-395.

Galli R, Binda E, Orfanelli U, Cipelliti B, Gritti A, De Vitis S, Fiocco R, Foroni C, Dimeco F, Vescovi A. Isolation and characterization of tumorigenic, stem-like neural precursors from human glioblastoma. Cancer Res., 2004; 64(19):7011-7021.

Singh SK, Hawkins C, Clarke ID, Squire JA, Bayani J, Hide T, Henkelman RM, Cusimano MD, Dirks PB. Identification of human brain tumour initiating cells. Nature, 2004; 432(7015):396-401.

D'Amour KA, Gage FH. Genetic and functional differences between multipotent neural and pluripotent embryonic stem cells. Proc Natl Acad Sci USA., 2003; 100 (Suppl 1): 11866-11872.

Reya T, Duncan AW, Ailles L, Domen J, Scherer DC, Willert K, Hintz L, Nusse R, Weissman IL. A role for Wnt signalling in self-renewal of haematopoietic stem cells. Nature, 2003; 423(6938): 409-414.

Schatton T, Murphy GF, Frank NY, Yamaura K, Waaga-Gasser AM, Gasser M, Zhan Q, Jordan S, Duncan LM, Weishaupt C, Fuhlbrigge RC, Kupper TS, Sayegh MH, Frank MH. Identification of cells initiating human melanomas. Nature, 2008; 451:345-349.

Bussolati B, Grange C, Sapino A, Camussi G. Endothelial cell differentiation of human breast tumor stem/progenitor cells. J Cell Mol Med., 2009; 13(2):309-319.

Rigolin GM, Fraulini C, Ciccone M, Mauro E, Bugli AM, De Angeli C, Negrini M, Cuneo A, Castoldi G. Neoplastic circulating endothelial cells in multiple myeloma with 13q14 deletion. Blood, 2006; 107(6):2531-2535.

Medina MA, Munoz-Ch Puli R, Quesada AR. Challenges of antiangiogneic cancer therapy: trials and errors, and renewed hope. J Cell Mol Med., 11:378-382.

Yi L, Zhou ZH, PingYF, Chen JH, Yao XH, Feng H, Lu JY, Wang JM, Bian XW. Isolation and characterization of stem cell-like precursor cells from primary human anaplastic oligoastrocytoma. Mod Pathol., 2007; 20: 1061–1068.

Yu SC, Ping YF, Yi L, Zhou ZH, Chen JH, Yao XH, Gao L, Wang JM, Bian XW. Isolation and characterization of cancer stem cells from a human glioblastoma cell line U87. Cancer Lett., 2008; 265:124-134.

Elias AP, Dias S. Microenvironment Changes (in pH) Affect VEGF Alternative Splicing. Cancer Microenviron., 2008; 1(1):131-139.

Hendrix MJ, Seftor EA, Kirschmann DA, Quaranta V, Seftor RE. Remodeling of the microenvironment by aggressive melanoma tumor cells. Ann N Y Acad Sci., 2003; 995:151-161.

Schofield R. The relationship between the spleen colony-forming cell and the haemopoietic stem cell. Blood Cells, 1978; 4:7-25.

Morrison SJ, Kimble J. Asymmetric and symmetric stem-cell division in development and cancer. Nature, 2006; 441:1068-1074.

Scadden DT. The stem cell niche as an entity of action. Nature, 2006; 41:1075-1079.

Vermeulen L, Todaro M, de Sousa Mello F, Sprick MR, Kemper K, Perez Alea M, Richel DJ, Stassi G, Medema JP. Single-cell cloning of colon cancer stem cells reveals a multi-lineage differentiation capacity. Proc Natl Acad Sci USA., 2008; 105(36):13427-13432.

Calabrese C, Poppleton H, Kocak M, Hogg TL, Fuller C, Hamner B, Oh EY, Gaber MW, Finklestein D, Allen M, Frank A, Bayazitov IT, Zakharenko SS, Gajjar A, Davidoff A, Gilbertson RJ. A perivascular niche for brain tumor stem cells. Cancer Cell, 2007; 11(1):69-82.

Rothhammer T, Bataille F, Spruss T, Eissner G, Bosserhoff AK. Functional implication of BMP4 expression on angiogenesis in malignant melanoma. Oncogene, 2007; 26:4158–4170.

Piccirillo SG, Reynolds BA, Zanetti N, Lamorte G, Binda E, Broggi G, Brem H, Olivi A, Dimeco F, Vescovi AL. Bone morphogenetic proteins inhibit the tumorigenic potential of human brain tumour-initiating cells. Nature, 2006; 444:761-765.

Nakano I, Saigusa K, Kornblum HI. BMPing off glioma stem cells. Cancer Cell, 2008; 13(1):3-4.

Yao XH, Ping YF, Chen JH, Xu CP, Chen DL, Zhang R, Bian XW. Glioblastoma stem cells produce vascular endothelial growth factor by activation of formylpeptide receptor (FPR). J Pathol., 2008; 215(4): 369-376.

Basu GD, Liang WS, Stephan DA, Wegener LT, Conley CR, Pockaj RA, Mukherjee P. A novel role for cyclooxygenase-2 in regulating vascular channel formation by human breast cancer cells. Breast Cancer Res., 2006; 8(6): R69.

Fujimoto AOH, Mori A, Nagayama S, Yonenaga Y, Tachibana T. Tumor plasticity and extravascular circulation in ECV304 human bladder carcinoma cells. Anticancer Res., 2006; 26(1A): 59-69.

Stevens AP, Spangler B, Wallner S, Kreutz M, Dettmer K, Oefner PJ, Bosserhoff AK. Direct and tumor microenvironment mediated influences of 5'-deoxy-5'-(methylthio) adenosine on tumor progression of malignant melanoma. J Cell Biochem., 2009; 106(2):210-219.

Yu SC, Bian XW. Enrichment of cancer stem cells based on heterogeneity of invasiveness. Stem Cell Rev., 2009, 5(1): 66-71.

Hess AR, Seftor EA, Seftor RE, Hendrix MJ. Phosphoinositide 3-kinase regulates membrane Type 1-matrix metalloproteinase (MMP) and MMP-2 activity during melanoma cell vasculogenic mimicry. Cancer Res., 2003; 63(16):4757-4762.

Hillen F, Griffoen AW. Tumour vascularization: sprouting angiogenesis and beyond. Cancer Metastasis Rev., 2007; 26:489-502.

Borovski, T., Verhoeff, J.J., ten Cate, R., Cameron, K., de Vries, N.A., van Tellingen, O., et al. (2009).Tumor microvasculature supports proliferation and expansion of glioma-propagating cells. Int J Cancer, 125(5), 1222-1230.

Rak, J., Milsom, C., & Yu, J. (2008). Vascular determinants of cancer stem cell dormancy-do age and coagulation system play a role? APMIS, 116(7-8), 660-676.

Priceman, S.J., Sung, J.L., Shaposhnik, Z., Burton, J.B., Torres-Collado, A.X., Moughon, D.L., et al. (2010). Targeting distinct tumor-infiltrating myeloid cells by inhibiting CSF-1 receptor: combating tumor evasion of antiangiogenic therapy. Boold, 115(7), 1461-1471.

Koukourakis, M.I., Giatromanolaki, A., Sheldon, H., Buffa, F.M., Kouklakis, G., Ragoussis, I., et al. (2009). Phase I/II trial of bevacizumab and radiotherapy for locally advanced inoperable colorectal cancer: vasculature-independent radiosensitizing effect of bevacizumab. Clin Cancer Res, 15(22), 7069-7076.

Ito, K., Bernardi, R., Morotti, A., Matsuoka, S., Saglio, G., Ikeda, Y., et al. (2008). PML targeting eradicates quiescent leukaemia-initiating cells. Nature, 453(7198), 1072-1078.

Part 4

Signaling Pathways and Regulatory Controls

13

Potential Signaling Pathways Activated in Cancer Stem Cells in Breast Cancer

Noriko Gotoh
Division of Systems Biomedical Technology, Institute of Medical Science, University of Tokyo
Japan

1. Introduction

Accumulating evidence suggests that cancer stem cells—which make up only a small proportion of heterogeneous tumor cells—possess a greater ability to maintain tumor formation than other tumor cell types. It has been proposed that cancer stem cells have characteristics in common with normal stem cells from tumor-prone tissue. For instance, cancer stem cells can self-renew and simultaneously produce differentiated daughter cells that proliferate strongly until they reach their final differentiated state. Apparent differences also exist between cancer stem cells and normal stem cells. The latter are maintained under tight homeostatic regulation and are passively protected in the surrounding microenvironment or stem cell niche in adult tissues. However, the former may actively contribute to tumor formation. This concept was first proposed from the research of hematological malignancy, however, it is now believed that many solid tumors also have cancer stem-like cells. Although the concept of cancer stem cells greatly impacts cancer biology and evokes a reconsideration of cancer treatment, the molecular mechanisms involved in the contribution of cancer stem cells to tumorigenesis remain to be obscure. There have been many attempts to identify signaling pathways specifically activated in cancer stem cells. For example, it has been proposed that transforming growth factor (TGF)-β pathway, the epithelial-mesenchymal transition (EMT) pathway or nuclear factor-kB (NF-kB) pathway may be activated in cancer stem cells. These potential pathways may contribute to self-renewal activity of cancer stem cells or have an influence on cancer stem cell niche. In this review, I would like to summarize our present understanding about potential signaling pathways activated in cancer stem cells in solid tumors, especially focusing on breast cancer, and then describe our recent findings about potential signaling pathways in breast cancer. Finally I would like to discuss how this increasing knowledge is utilized for developing novel molecularly targeting drugs for cancer treatment.

2. Definition and characteristics of cancer stem cells

The consensus definition of a cancer stem cell is a cell within a tumor that possess the capacity to self-renew and to cause the heterogenous lineages of cancer cells that comprise the tumor. Cancer stem cells can thus only be defined experimentally by their ability to recapitulate the generation of a continuously growing tumors. The implementation of this approach explains the use of alternative terms in the literature, such as "tumor-initiating cell (TIC)" to describe putative cancer stem cells (Clarke, 2006).

Stem cells are defined by both their ability to make more stem cells, a property known as 'self-renewal", and their ability to produce cells that differentiate (Fig. 1) (Morrison and Kimble, 2006). One strategy by which stem cells can accomplish these two tasks is asymmetric cell division, whereby each stem cell divides to generate one daughter cell with a stem-cell fate and one daughter cell that differentiates. Stem cells can also use symmetric divisions to self-renew and to generate differentiate progeny. Symmetric divisions are defined as the generation of daughter cells that are destined to acquire the same fate. It is thought that stem cells use combination of both asymmetric and symmetric cell divisions to self-renew, proliferate, and differentiate. Both cancer stem cells and normal stem cells have the such similar characteristics.

Cancer stem cell shares many other properties with the normal stem cell. Normal stem cells exist properties that provide for a long lifespan such as relative quiescence, resistance to drugs and toxins through the expression of several ATP-binding cassette transporters, an active DNA-repair capacity, and a resistance to apoptosis. Many of the characteristics are shared also by cancer stem cells. Cancer stem cells have a long lifespan, and self-renewal capacity enabling them to maintain and expand the cancer cell population, although they themselves are quiescent and rarely proliferation.

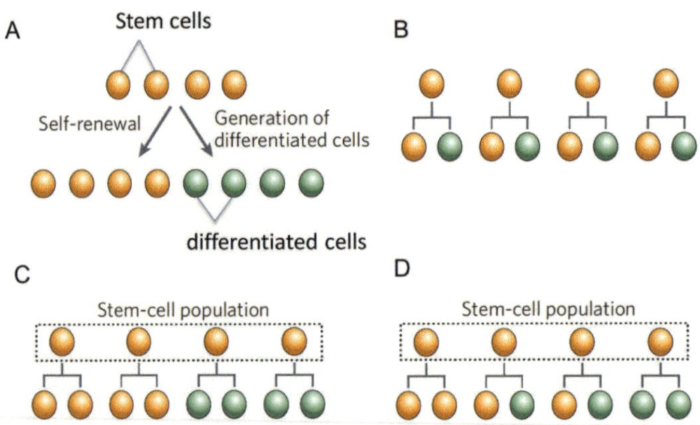

Fig. 1. Asymmetric and symmetric cell division of stem cells.
A, Stem cells self-renew and differentiate into progenitor cells.
B, Asymmetric cell division.
C, Symmetric cell division.
D, Combination of asymmetric and symmetric cell division.

An obvious question is where cancer stem cells arise; are they derived from normal stem cells or not? In hematological malignancy, it has been documented the existence of malignant stem cells in AML and CML. It has been thought that leukemic stem cells arise by mutation from normal stem cells or by mutation from progenitor cells, evoked by genomic instability in malignant cells. The mutation-prone property of malignant cells may even gives a self-renewing ability to the progenitor cells that do not have such ability originally.

Apparent differences also exist between cancer stem cells and normal stem cells. The latter are maintained under tight homeostatic regulation and are passively protected in the surrounding microenvironment or stem cell niche in adult tissues. However, the former may actively contribute to tumor formation and may use cancer stem cell niche for their own survival.

3. The impact of the cancer stem cell hypothesis on the cancer therapy

To develop more effective cancer therapies, it is critical to determine which cancer cells have the potential to contribute to tumor progression. Because it was thought that most cancer cells proliferate extensively, traditional cancer therapies aim to eliminate as many cancer cells as possible by targeting cells with increased proliferation activity. However, relapse occurs in a significant number of patients even after complete tumor resection and systemic treatment involving chemotherapy and/or radiotherapy. In these circumstances, a recently proposed hypothesis involving cancer stem cells has drawn great attention. It is hypothesized that heterogeneous tumor tissue is maintained in a hierarchical organization of rare, slowly dividing cancer stem cells; rapidly dividing progenitor cells; and differentiated tumor cells. The growth and progression of tumors are thought to be driven by such subpopulations of cancer stem cells. Therefore, it is thought that cancer stem cells are relatively resistant to conventional chemotherapy and radiotherapy and might survive after systemic treatment. These cells may remain dormant for years but eventually cause relapse. Therefore, cancer therapy should target cancer stem cells that were not targeted by conventional therapy. Although the concept of cancer stem cells greatly impacts cancer biology and evokes a reconsideration of cancer treatment, the molecular mechanisms involved in the contribution of cancer stem cells to tumorigenesis remain obscure.

Potential cancer stem cells were first identified in hematological malignancies such as leukemia. Among solid tumors, breast cancer and brain tumors were firstly shown to have cancer stem cells. Subsequently, it has been shown that many types of cancer or tumors have cancer stem cells, such as colon cancer, pancreatic cancer, prostate cancer, lung cancer and melanoma.

4. Breast cancer stem cells

The development of biomarkers to identify breast cancer stem cells as well as the validation of in vitro and mouse models has facilitated the isolation and characterization of these cells from murine and human tumors. In human breast cancers, the $CD24^{-/low}/CD44^{+}$ cell population was reported to be more highly enriched in breast cancer stem cells than was the $CD24^{high}/CD44^{+}$ cell population (Al-Hajj et al., 2003). Several groups have also identified $CD24^{-/low}/CD44^{+}$ cells as a breast cancer stem cell-enriched population in primary human breast carcinoma (Diehn et al., 2009; Shimono et al., 2009). In addition, aldehyde dehydrogenase (ALDH) expression has been used to isolate human breast cancer stem cell populations (Ginestier et al., 2007). More recently, highly pure breast cancer stem cell populations were obtained by using the lipophilic fluorescent dye PKH26, which labels relatively quiescent cells within a proliferating population (Cicalese et al., 2009). Just as primary tumors and xenografts contain cancer stem cell populations, established breast cancer cell lines may also contain cellular hierarchies driven by a population expressing cancer stem cell markers. In addition to involvement in tumor initiation, the cells also display increased metastatic potential.

5. Breast cancer cell lines as a model system of cancer stem cells

Although final proofs of cancer stem biology should be shown by experiments using tumor cells derived from human tumor tissues, it is convenient and useful if cancer cell lines are used as a model system for exploring biology. We and others found that $CD24^{-/low}/CD44^{+}$ cell populations exist in various type of breast cancer cell lines and that each cell line had various expression levels of CD24 and CD44 (Fillmore and Kuperwasser, 2008; Murohashi et al., 2010). Three cell lines, HCC1954, MCF-7 and HCC70 cells, had small population (<10 %) of the $CD24^{-/low}/CD44^{+}$ cells. This situation might be similar to the early stage breast cancer tissues in which the TIC population is assumed to be small. To determine the hierarchical organization of breast cancer cell lines, we analyzed the tumorigenic potential of the $CD24^{-/low}/CD44^{+}$ and $CD24^{+}/CD44^{+}$ cell populations of HCC1954 cell line.

The *in vivo* tumorigenicity assay is the gold standard for identifying cancer stem cells or TIC. To improve the quality of the quantitative results, we used *in vivo* bioluminescence imaging (IVIS™) to measure tumor growth (Murohashi et al. 2010). We first transduced cells with a lentiviral vector encoding luciferase or d2Venus (an improved version of yellow fluorescent protein) cDNA. We measured transduction efficiency by expression levels of d2Venus using FACS and obtained high transduction efficiency in 92.60 % for HCC1954 cells. Next, we transduced a lentiviral vector expressing luciferase into these cells. Because we used similar MOI (multiplicity of infection) levels for transduction of the lentiviral vectors expressing luciferase and d2Venus, we expected similar levels of luciferase expression in the cell line (designated HCC1954-Luc). Cells in $CD24^{-/low}/CD44^{+}$ populations were considered to be enriched for TICs and $CD24^{+}CD44^{+}$ populations were used as controls. Cells were implanted into mammary fat pads of NOD/SCID mice and tumor growth was measured by quantifying luciferase activity with the IVIS™ Imaging System (Fig. 2). Ten thousand HCC1954-Luc and MCF7-Luc cells of both populations were implanted. After 4 weeks, the analysis of luciferase activity indicated that cells in the $CD24^{-/low}/CD44^{+}$ populations of HCC1954-Luc and MCF7-Luc generated significantly larger tumors than the control populations ($p<0.05$) (Fig. 2A). Moreover, when we transplanted both populations of $1x10^2$ HCC1954-Luc, tumors were generated only by the $CD24^{-/low}/CD44^{+}$ population (n=6) (Fig. 2B).

These results indicate that $CD24^{-/low}/CD44^{+}$ populations in breast cancer cell lines have higher tumorigenicity than the control populations. It is therefore likely that $CD24^{-/low}/CD44^{+}$ cells in breast cancer cell lines may behave like TICs.

We examined the histology of tumors derived from HCC1954-Luc cells from both populations when $1x10^4$ cells of each population were implanted. The hematoxylin-eosin (HE) staining revealed that tumors derived from $CD24^{-/low}/CD44^{+}$ cells showed exclusively invasive patterns, with a variety of morphologies associated with the stromal component (Fig. 3A, B). However, tumors derived from control cells consisted of invasive and differentiated patterns, with tubular formations in association with the stromal component. The stromal component was larger in tumors derived from $CD24^{-/low}/CD44^{+}$ cells than that derived from the control cells. The fact that differentiated patterns of histology were observed only in tumors derived from the controls suggests that differentiated tumors arose from non-TICs.

Next, we assessed the cell lineage and differentiationstate of tumors derived from HCC1954-Luc cells by immunostaining for cytokeratin markers (Fig. 3C-F). The invasive lesions from $CD24^{-/low}/CD44^{+}$ cells were mostly positive for the myoepithelial marker CK-14 but were less positive for the luminal marker CK-18. On the other hand, the invasive lesions from the control cells were mostly negative for CK-14 but were positive for CK-18, suggesting that TICs contribute to the basal cell phenotype of transplanted tumors.

From these experiments, we demonstrated that cells derived from $CD24^{-/low}/CD44^{+}$ populations resulted in tumors larger than those of $CD24^{+}/CD44^{+}$ control populations. Importantly, when as few as 100 cells were implanted, only $CD24^{-/low}/CD44^{+}$ populations gave rise to tumors (Fig. 2B). This is an important criterion for TICs. Therefore,

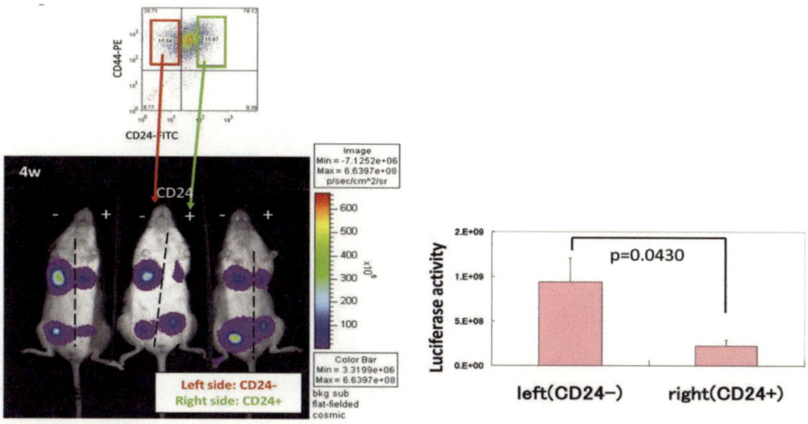

(a)

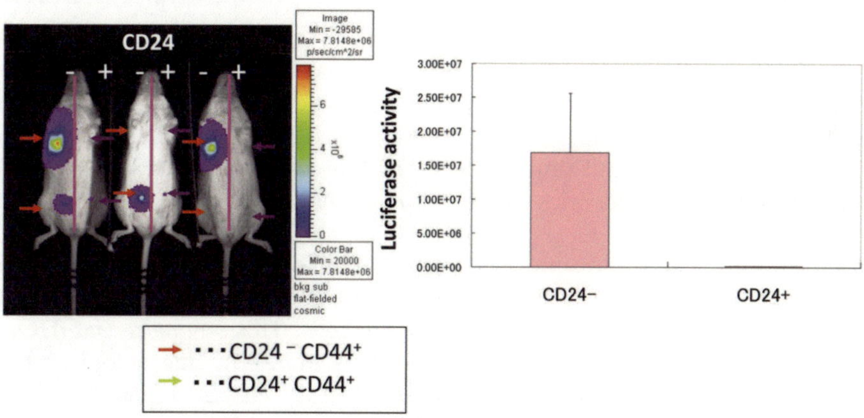

(b)

Fig. 2. Luciferase activities of $CD24^{-/low}/CD44^{+}$ cells in NOD/SCID mice.
HCC1954 cells expressing luciferase were sorted by FACS. Ten percent of the entire population, belonging to $CD24^{-/low}$ $CD44^{+}$, was selected as the TIC population ($CD24^{-}$). Ten percent of the whole population, belonging to $CD24^{+}/CD44^{+}$, was selected as the control ($CD24^{+}$). Ten thousand cells (A) or 100 cells (B) of the TIC population (left side of mice) or control population (right side of mice) cells were mixed with Matrigel and implanted in mammary fat pads of NOD/SCID mice. Luciferase activities were captured by IVIS™ after 4 weeks. Luciferase activities in implanted sites were quantified (n=6). Results are represented as the mean + SD. * $p<0.05$ (student *t*-test).

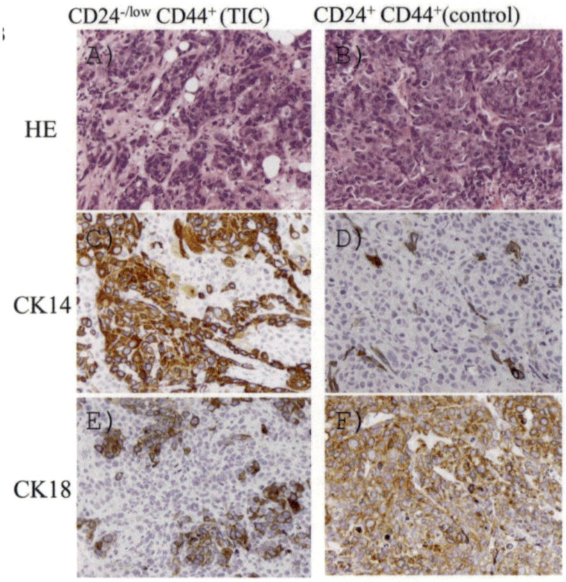

Fig. 3. Immunohistochemical analysis of tumors from HCC1954.
A, HE-stained sections of the tumors derived from $CD24^{-/low}/CD44^{+}$ cells (TICs) and $CD24^{+}/CD44^{+}$ (control) cells.
B, Immunohistochemical analysis of CK-14 expression in the TIC and control populations.
C, Immunohistochemical analysis of CK-18 expression in TIC and control cells. Brown staining represents a positive result.

$CD24^{-/low}/CD44^{+}$ populations in the cell lines may be enriched with TIC-like cells. Our results revealed heterogeneity in cell populations divided into TIC-like cells and other cells. Therefore, it is reasonable to suppose that several breast cancer cell lines are heterogeneous and that they have distinct cell populations: TIC-like cells and other cells, with both cell types preserving the characteristics of TICs and other cells in primary cancer tissues, to some extent.

We further showed that tumors derived from TIC-like cells showed a more malignant histology and contained more cells positive for CK-18, in contrast with tumors derived from control cells, which exhibited more CK-14-positive cells. This suggests that TICs may not differentiate into cells with specialized or terminal patterns in this model and raises the possibility that TICs may not need to differentiate into all cell types in tumor tissues; though, normal stem cells can generate all cell types in a specific tissue. However, we cannot exclude the possibility that this transplantation model does not recapitulate the ability of TICs to differentiate into all cell types seen in breast cancer. In order to clarify this issue, other types of *in vivo* models should be analyzed.

6. In vitro assay of breast cancer stem cells

In recent years, the in vitro mammosphere formation assay has been established as a measure for the self-renewal of breast cancer stem cells. Mammospheres are floating cell aggregations, which include cancer stem-like cells, and can be serially passaged; they are obtained by culturing breast cancer stem cells in a defined medium containing growth factors, including the epidermal growth factor (EGF) and basic fibroblast growth factor (bFGF) (Fig. 4). This medium is only a slightly modified version of the defined medium that includes the same growth factors, i.e., EGF and/or bFGF, and has been adapted for culturing neurospheres, which are aggregations of neural stem cells and their progenitors. This indicates EGF or bFGF involvement in the regulation of self-renewal of breast cancer stem cells in such in vitro culture conditions.However, little information is available regarding the regulatory mechanisms for self-renewal of breast cancer stem cells by EGF or FGF, and it is an open question whether EGF and/or FGF signaling is involved in the in vivo regulation of these cells.

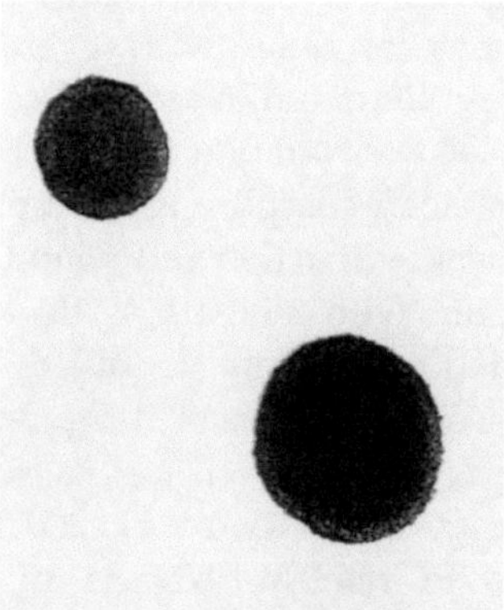

Fig. 4. Mammosphere cells derived from HCC1954 cells.

7. Inflammatory signaling pathways are potentially activated in breast cancer stem cells

Two gene expression profiling studies, comparing $CD24^{-/low}/CD44^{+}$ cell populations with other populations in primary breast cancer cells or in normal tissue presented the $CD24^{-/low}/CD44^{+}$ cell population-derived different signatures that seemed to predict poorer prognosis (Liu et al., 2007; Shipitsin et al., 2007). One study showed that TGF-β pathways appear to be activated in these cells (Shipitsin et al., 2007). It was subsequently reported that TGF-β induced the epithelial-mesenchymal transition (EMT) in mammary glands and stem-like cells in both normal mammary epithelial cells and breast cancer cells (Mani et al., 2008). Because TGF-β signaling can have positive or negative effects on tumorigenesis, additional signaling may still be needed to stimulate tumorigenesis (Massague, 2008).

The functional relationship between inflammation and cancer has been discussed since the 1860s (Coussens and Werb, 2002; Murohashi et al., 2010). Activation of several pathways involved in inflammatory responses has recently been detected in breast cancer stem cells. We and others recently discovered that NF-κB, which is one of the main regulators of the transcription of inflammatory mediators, is activated in breast cancer stem-like cells.

We used gene set enrichment analysis (GSEA) which is a recently developed analytical method of gene-expression profiling. The results are easier to interpret biologically, and the method is more accurate and robust than individual gene analysis methods, such as fold change analysis of expression levels. To identify expressed genes that were highly enriched in $CD24^{-/low}/CD44^{+}$ and control cells, we performed DNA microarray analysis using

HCC1954, MCF7, and HCC70 cell lines that have small populations of $CD24^{-}/CD44^{+}$ cells. As a control, we used $CD24^{+}/CD44^{+}$ cell populations.

We found that both TNF and IFN response gene signatures were markedly enriched in $CD24^{-/low-}/CD44^{+}$ populations (Murohashi et al.). Regarding individual genes, gene ontology (GO)-based classification revealed that genes involved in 'stemness', cell proliferation/maintenance, cell adhesion, cell motility, invasion, angiogenesis, growth factor/cytokine, immune response/suppression and metabolism were highly represented in $CD24^{-/low-}/CD44^{+}$ compared with the control cell populations. All of these genes may contribute to oncogenesis. For example, from the GSEA results, we found Notch2, a 'stemness'-related gene, LAMA3, a cell invasion- or adhesion-related gene and KLF5, EPAS1 and VEGF, angiogenesis-related genes. On the other hand, GSEA revealed that genes highly expressed in the control populations correlated with several cell-cycle-associated gene sets, which have large numbers of cell proliferation/maintenance-related genes.

One of the important effector molecules common to both TNF and INF response pathways is NF-κB. NF-κB is a transcription factor complex and is typically a heterodimer of p50, p52, p65 (RelA), RelB and c-Rel. It is usually inactive and bound to IκB, an inhibitory protein, in the cytoplasm. Upon stimulation with signals such as TNF or INF, IκB is first phosphorylated, then ubiquitinated and finally degraded. Released NF-κB translocates to the nucleus and binds to the κB sequence, where it promotes the transcription of various genes, including inflammatory cytokines. NF-κB has roles in inflammation, angiogenesis, inhibition of apoptosis, and tumorigenesis (Karin et al., 2002; Tabruyn and Griffioen, 2008).

We quantified NF-κB activities in nuclear extracts of $CD24^{-/low}/CD44^{+}$ and control populations that were sorted by FACS. We found that the activity of NF-κB was significantly higher in $CD24^{-/low}/CD44^{+}$ than in $CD24^{+}/CD44^{+}$ populations (n=4). We further examined the role of the activity of NF-κB in tumorigenesis using the mouse model. We transplanted 10^4 cells of $CD24^{-/low}/CD44^{+}$ populations into NOD/SCID mice, and treated them with DHMEQ, a specific inhibitor for NF-κB. In order to analyze the effects occurring during the course of tumorigenesis, we began inhibitor treatment two days after transplantation. We monitored tumor formation by *in vivo* imaging. We found that the luciferase activities of the tumors derived from $CD24^{-/low-}/CD44^{+}$ cell populations treated with DHMEQ were significantly decreased compared with that of untreated cell-derived tumors (Murohashi et al. 2010). These results suggest that NF-κB acts as a key effector of tumorigenesis derived from TIC-like cells.

Other reports have described that NF-κB-triggered inflammation is required for the maintenance of the epigenetic transformed phenotype and cancer stem-like cell population in the activated Src-driven breast cancer model (Iliopoulos et al., 2009). Although these observations suggest that NF-κB plays an important role in breast cancer stem cells, it is still unclear how NF-κB regulates 'stemness' of these cells. It is known that active NF-κB promotes expression of over 150 target genes. They may encode key molecules for self-renewing ability of breast cancer stem cells. Another possibility is that they encode key cytokines or chemokines, regulating the stem cell phenotype as described below.

8. Proinflammatory cytokines and chemokines and breast cancer stem cells

Several target genes of the NF-κB pathway, such as those encoding for proinflammatory cytokines and chemokines, have been identified as regulators of the breast cancer stem cell phenotype. For example, we found high interleukin-8 (IL-8) and CC chemokine ligand-5 (CCL5) expression levels in CD24$^{-/low}$/CD44^{+} breast cancer stem-like cells, and the expression of these chemokines was inhibited by treatment with an inhibitor specific for NF-κB in breast cancer stem-like cells (Murohashi et al. 2010). NF-κB activation is involved in the expression of many inflammatory cytokines/chemokines, including vascular endothelial growth factor A (VEGFA), interleukin 8 (IL8) and chemokine (C-C motif) ligand 5 (CCL5), paracrine factors associated with stroma-like activities, which are among the list of highly ranked genes. In addition, VEGFA and IL8 are important factors for angiogenesis and tumorigenesis. Among the other highly ranked genes, we also noticed Toll-like receptor 1 (TLR1), another upstream activator for NF-κB, and stromal cell-derived factor 2-like 1 (SDF2L1), which is reported to be upregulated through EMT, an important biological output of the TGF-βpathway.

Other reports showed that the IL-8 receptor CXCR1 is consistently expressed in breast cancer stem-like cell populations with high aldehyde dehydrogenase (ALDH) activity and that IL-8 increases the formation of primary and secondary mammospheres as well as that of breast cancer stem-like cell populations (Charafe-Jauffret et al., 2009). It appears that the IL-8/CXCR1 signaling pathway activates Akt and leads to nuclear translocation of β-catenin to induce complex formation with TCF for active transcription (Ginestier et al. 2010). Anther report suggests the existence of a relationship between cancer stem-like cells and interleukin-6 (IL-6) expression (Sansone et al., 2007). The results of this study suggested that IL-6 may trigger a potential autocrine/paracrine Notch-3/Jagged-1 loop to boost the self-renewal of breast cancer stem cells. Likewise, it was shown that NF-κB ensures high IL-6 levels both directly—by activation of IL-6 transcription—and indirectly—by inhibition of let-7 microRNA (Iliopoulos et al., 2009). The resulting high IL-6 levels activate NF-κB, thereby completing the positive feedback loop that maintains mammosphere formation in vitro and tumorigenesis in nude mice in the breast cancer model. These observations suggest that IL-6 is an important key molecule in breast cancer stem cell biology.

Transforming growth factor-β (TGF-β) also plays a key role in immune homeostasis (Massague, 2008). It controls the initiation and resolution of inflammatory responses through the regulation of chemotaxis and activation of peripheral leukocytes, including lymphocytes, natural killer cells, dendritic cells, macrophages, mast cells, and granulocytes.

These findings suggest that inflammatory cytokines and chemokines are critical components for the maintenance of breast cancer stem cells. However, it is still largely unknown how they maintain these cells; for example, it is equally possible that they regulate themselves in an autocrine manner or that they regulate a cancer stem cell niche in a paracrine manner.

In our findings, it is notable that genes related to stroma-like activities were highly enriched in CD24$^{-/low}$/CD44^{+} populations compared with control populations, such as inflammatory chemokines, angiogenic cytokines, SDF2L1, and TLR1. These stroma-like activities are thought to contribute to invasion, angiogenesis and immune response/suppression. Increasing evidence suggests that tumor stroma, consisting of 'cancer-associated fibroblasts' (CAF), play a major role in tumorigenesis (Kalluri and Zeisberg, 2006). CAFs secrete growth factors, cytokines, and chemokines. These, in turn, can induce inflammatory responses and angiogenesis by paracrine mechanisms. Tumor cells appear to use these activities for tumor progression. Our findings suggest that TICs behave like CAFs and contribute to tumorigenesis by producing growth factors, cytokines, and chemokines. In this sense, TICs may actively generate and maintain a microenvironment conducive to the progression of tumorigenesis, or in other words, a cancer stem cell niche (Fig. 5).

Fig. 5

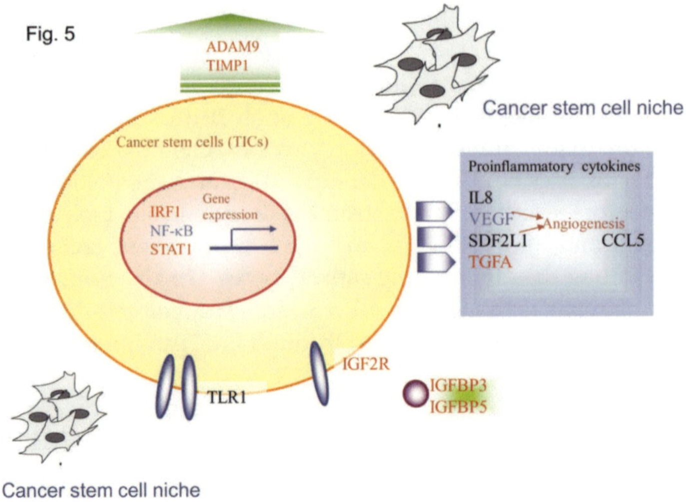

Fig. 5. Model of signaling pathways involving NF-kB in TICs.

We propose that TICs behave like CAFs, in that they actively generate and maintain the cancer stem cell niche in which NF-kB acts as a main effector that induces many secretory proteins, including cytokines and chemokines. Among GSEA-extracted genes, molecules having significantly high levels of mRNA expression or activity are shown in blue, and the others are shown in red. Molecules in black were confirmed to have significantly high levels of mRNA expression.

9. Anti-inflammatory drugs targeting cancer stem cells

Therapeutic targeting of cancer stem cells has the potential to eliminate residual disease and may become an important component of multimodality treatments. In clinical trials, it was found that several anti-inflammatory drugs reduce tumor incidence when used as prophylactics and slow down tumor progression and reduce mortality when used as therapeutics (Gupta and Dubois, 2001). These drugs include aspirin, which suppresses NF-κB transcriptional activity by preventing the binding of NF-κB to DNA(Zhang et al. 2010). Besides its well-documented preventive effects in colon cancer, several epidemiological studies have shown that aspirin reduces the incidence of breast cancer and that its use after breast cancer diagnosis is associated with a decreased risk of distant recurrence, breast cancer death, and death from any other cause (Holmes et al. 2010). Considering the recent advances in understanding inflammatory pathways in breast cancer stem cells, such findings support the possibility that the critical molecules involved in inflammatory pathways in cancer stem cells are appropriate targets for breast cancer treatment.

10. Conclusion

Our findings and others raise an intriguing possibility: TICs behave like CAFs and can actively generate and maintain the cancer stem cells and their niche, in which NF-κB acts as the main effector that can induce many secretory proteins, including cytokines and chemokines. An important avenue for future studies should be the extensive evaluation of our model, using clinical samples of breast cancer.

The discovery of the involvement of inflammatory signaling pathways in breast cancer stem cells has especially raised the possibility of developing drugs targeting molecules involved in these pathways in breast cancer stem cells. Further clarification of these mechanisms is important in order to identify critical components that could be targeted by cancer treatment. Examination of the functional roles of these molecules in normal stem cells is also important in order to avoid unnecessary side effects.

11. References

Al-Hajj, M., Wicha, M.S., Benito-Hernandez, A., Morrison, S.J., and Clarke, M.F. (2003). Prospective identification of tumorigenic breast cancer cells. Proc Natl Acad Sci U S A *100*, 3983-3988.

Charafe-Jauffret, E., Ginestier, C., Iovino, F., Wicinski, J., Cervera, N., Finetti, P., Hur, M.H., Diebel, M.E., Monville, F., Dutcher, J., *et al.* (2009). Breast cancer cell lines contain functional cancer stem cells with metastatic capacity and a distinct molecular signature. Cancer Res *69*, 1302-1313.

Cicalese, A., Bonizzi, G., Pasi, C.E., Faretta, M., Ronzoni, S., Giulini, B., Brisken, C., Minucci, S., Di Fiore, P.P., and Pelicci, P.G. (2009). The tumor suppressor p53 regulates polarity of self-renewing divisions in mammary stem cells. Cell *138*, 1083-1095.

Clarke, M.F. (2006). Cancer stem cells-AACR. Oncogene *66*, 9339.

Coussens, L.M., and Werb, Z. (2002). Inflammation and cancer. Nature *420*, 860-867.

Diehn, M., Cho, R.W., Lobo, N.A., Kalisky, T., Dorie, M.J., Kulp, A.N., Qian, D., Lam, J.S., Ailles, L.E., Wong, M., *et al.* (2009). Association of reactive oxygen species levels and radioresistance in cancer stem cells. Nature *458*, 780-783.

Fillmore, C.M., and Kuperwasser, C. (2008). Human breast cancer cell lines contain stem-like cells that self-renew, give rise to phenotypically diverse progeny and survive chemotherapy. Breast Cancer Res *10*, R25.

Ginestier, C., Hur, M.H., Charafe-Jauffret, E., Monville, F., Dutcher, J., Brown, M., Jacquemier, J., Viens, P., Kleer, C.G., Liu, S., *et al.* (2007). ALDH1 is a marker of normal and malignant human mammary stem cells and a predictor of poor clinical outcome. Cell Stem Cell *1*, 555-567.

Ginestier, C., Liu, S., Diebel, M.E., Korkaya, H., Luo, M., Brown, M., Wicinski, J., Cabaud, O., Charafe-Jauffret, E., Birnbaum, D., *et al.* (2010). CXCR1 blockade selectively targets human breast cancer stem cells in vitro and in xenografts. J Clin Invest *120*, 485-497.

Gupta, R.A., and Dubois, R.N. (2001). Colorectal cancer prevention and treatment by inhibition of cyclooxygenase-2. Nature reviews *1*, 11-21.

Holmes, M.D., Chen, W.Y., Li, L., Hertzmark, E., Spiegelman, D., and Hankinson, S.E. (2010). Aspirin intake and survival after breast cancer. J Clin Oncol *28*, 1467-1472.

Iliopoulos, D., Hirsch, H.A., and Struhl, K. (2009). An epigenetic switch involving NF-kappaB, Lin28, Let-7 MicroRNA, and IL6 links inflammation to cell transformation. Cell *139*, 693-706.

Kalluri, R., and Zeisberg, M. (2006). Fibroblasts in cancer. Nature reviews *6*, 392-401.

Karin, M., Cao, Y., Greten, F.R., and Li, Z.W. (2002). NF-kappaB in cancer: from innocent bystander to major culprit. Nature reviews *2*, 301-310.

Liu, R., Wang, X., Chen, G.Y., Dalerba, P., Gurney, A., Hoey, T., Sherlock, G., Lewicki, J., Shedden, K., and Clarke, M.F. (2007). The prognostic role of a gene signature from tumorigenic breast-cancer cells. The New England journal of medicine *356*, 217-226.

Mani, S.A., Guo, W., Liao, M.J., Eaton, E.N., Ayyanan, A., Zhou, A.Y., Brooks, M., Reinhard, F., Zhang, C.C., Shipitsin, M., *et al.* (2008). The epithelial-mesenchymal transition generates cells with properties of stem cells. Cell *133*, 704-715.

Massague, J. (2008). TGFbeta in Cancer. Cell *134*, 215-230.

Morrison, S.J., and Kimble, J. (2006). Asymmetric and symmetric stem-cell divisions in development and cancer. Nature *441*, 1068-1074.

Murohashi, M., Hinohara, K., Kuroda, M., Isagawa, T., Tsuji, S., Kobayashi, S., Umezawa, K., Tojo, A., Aburatani, H., and Gotoh, N. (2010). Gene set enrichment analysis provides insight into novel signalling pathways in breast cancer stem cells. Br J Cancer *102*, 206-212.

Sansone, P., Storci, G., Tavolari, S., Guarnieri, T., Giovannini, C., Taffurelli, M., Ceccarelli, C., Santini, D., Paterini, P., Marcu, K.B., *et al.* (2007). IL-6 triggers malignant features in mammospheres from human ductal breast carcinoma and normal mammary gland. J Clin Invest *117*, 3988-4002.

Shimono, Y., Zabala, M., Cho, R.W., Lobo, N., Dalerba, P., Qian, D., Diehn, M., Liu, H., Panula, S.P., Chiao, E., *et al.* (2009). Downregulation of miRNA-200c links breast cancer stem cells with normal stem cells. Cell *138*, 592-603.

Shipitsin, M., Campbell, L.L., Argani, P., Weremowicz, S., Bloushtain-Qimron, N., Yao, J., Nikolskaya, T., Serebryiskaya, T., Beroukhim, R., Hu, M., *et al.* (2007). Molecular definition of breast tumor heterogeneity. Cancer Cell *11*, 259-273.

Tabruyn, S.P., and Griffioen, A.W. (2008). NF-kappa B: a new player in angiostatic therapy. Angiogenesis *11*, 101-106.

Zhang, Z., Huang, L., Zhao, W., and Rigas, B. (2010). Annexin 1 induced by anti-inflammatory drugs binds to NF-kappaB and inhibits its activation: anticancer effects in vitro and in vivo. Cancer Res *70*, 2379-2388.

14

Signalling Pathways Driving Cancer Stem Cells: Hedgehog Pathway

Vanessa Medina Villaamil[1], Guadalupe Aparicio Gallego[1], Silvia Díaz Prado[1,3] and Luis Miguel Antón Aparicio[2,3]
[1]*INIBIC, A Coruña University Hospital, A Coruña*
[2]*Medical Oncology Service, A Coruña University Hospital, A Coruña*
[3]*Medicine Department, University of A Coruña, A Coruña*
Spain

1. Introduction

The hedgehog (Hh) pathway is one of the fundamental signal transduction pathways in animal development and is also involved in stem-cell maintenance and carcinogenesis. The *hedgehog* (hh) gene was first discovered in *Drosophila,* and members of the family have since been found in most metazoan. Hh proteins are composed of two domains, an amino-terminal domain HhN, which has the biological signal activity, and a carboxy-terminal autocatalytic domain HhC, which cleaves Hh into two parts in an intramolecular reaction and adds a cholesterol moiety to HhN. HhC has a sequence similarity to the self-splicing inteins, and the shared region is termed Hint. HhN is modified by cholesterol at its carboxyl terminus and by palmitate at its amino terminus in both flies and mammals. The modified HhN is released from the cell and travels through the extracellular space. On binding its receptor Patched, it relieves the inhibition that Patched exerts on Smoothened, a G-protein-coupled receptor. The resulting signalling cascade converges on the transcription factor Cubitus interruptus (Ci), or its mammalian counterparts, the Gli proteins, which activate or repress target genes. The Hh family of morphogens plays important instructional roles in the development of numerous metazoan structures (Ingham & McMahon, 2001). The Hh ligands, Sonic, Indian and Desert Hh in vertebrates and Hh in *Drosophila,* signal through binding to the membrane receptor Patched (Ptc) (Chen & Struhl, 1996), to reverse the Ptc-mediated inhibition of signalling by the trans-membrane protein Smoothened (Smo) (Alcedo et al., 1996). This allows Smo to activate the intracellular signalling components, resulting in stabilization of down-stream transcriptional activator(s) and activation of target genes (Hooper & Scott, 1989). Transcription activation is facilited through the Gli family of transcription factors in vertebrates (Ingham & McMahon, 2001). Hh signalling can initiate cellular growth, division, lineage specification, axon guidance and function as a survival factor (Cohen, 2009). Given this range of biological functions, it is not surprising that mutations in components of the Hh pathway are associated with both developmental defects and tumor progression (Cohen, 2009). Disruption of PTC, which functions as a negative regulator of the pathway, is implicated in cancer development in both inherited and sporadic cancers. Mutations in PTC and/or SMO trigger inappropriate activation of the Hh pathway, and have been identified in tumor types including basal cell carcinoma, rhabdomyosarcoma and medulloblastoma (Taipale & Beachy, 2001). Other studies also implicate activated hedgehog signalling as a mediating factor in small-cell lung cancer, pancreatic cancer and various digestive tract tumors (Kimberly et al., 2010; Brabletz et al., 2009). For the increasing types of cancer that are associated with Hh signalling, understanding signal transduction will be crucial for identifying potential drug targets and devising new therapies. The first purpose of this chapter is review the Hedgehog signalling pathway, analyze its components and describe mutations and gene overexpression that involve Hh signalling network. The last section addresses the study of Hh pathway as a pathological player in the growth of a group of human cancers.

2. Description of the signalling network

EVOLUTIONARY ORIGINS

Hh signal transduction has startling parallels with Wnt signalling, despite the different structures of the ligands and the largely distinct components that are dedicated to the separate pathways (Nusse, 2003). As both pathways are found throughout the animal kingdom, a common ancestral pathway must have been present in the earliest Metazoans. Ptc and Hh have distinct evolutionary origins. The Hh protein is comprised of a N-terminal signalling domain and a C-terminal catalytic domain. The N-terminal domain is structurally related to zinc hydrolases (Hall et al., 1995). The C-terminal catalytic domain of Hh is related to inteins, a family of self-splicing proteins (Hall et al., 1995). Hh protein probably arose when an intein was appended to the signalling domain; release of the signalling domain requires cleavage from the intein and is therefore subject to tight control. In animals, the gene for the NPC1 pump was probably duplicated and then diverged to affect the activity of a Smo ancestor. The acquisition of loops that bind Hh converted the pump into a signal-regulated pump. All of these threads woven together indicate that the Hh pathway emerged by integration of primordial pathways that are involved in protein splicing, vesicular trafficking and nuclear entry.

SIGNALLING IN VERTEBRATES

Hh signalling in vertebrates shares many features with that in *D. melanogaster* (McMahon et al., 2003), although clear distinctions have emerged. First, mammalian gene families take the place of single genes in *D. melanogaster*. There are three *hh* genes in mammals, sonic, Indian and desert hedgehog (*Shh, Ihh* and *Dhh*); two *ptc* genes (*Ptc1* and *Ptc2)*; and three *ci* homologues (*Gli1, Gli2* and *Gli3*). The three *hh* genes are expressed in different tissues and at different stages of development, and might also have different biological activities. The expression and function of *Ptc1* is similar to that of *D. melanogaster ptc* whereas *Ptc2* expression is more restricted and few phenotypes are associated with its loss (Rahnama et al., 2004). The post-translational regulation of Ci (*D. melanogaster)* and the GLI proteins is similar. Each resides in a cytoplasmic pool. In the absence of Hh, each is retained in the cytoplasm by Cos2 (KIF7 in vertebrates) and Sufu to limit transcriptional activation (Merchant et al., 2004; Rahnama et al., 2004; Paces-Fessy et al., 2004) . Ci, GLI3, and probably also GLI2, require PKA and a SCF E3 ubiquitin ligase for processing to a transcriptional repressor. However, each GLI protein also has unique roles: GLI3 functions mainly as a transcriptional repressor, GLI2 is mainly a transcriptional activator and GLI1 functions only as a transcriptional activator. The transcription of *Gli1* is induced by Hh signals, which creates a positive-regulatory loop that heightens Hh responses.

The most important differences between the *D.melanogaster* and vertebrate Hh pathways centre on Smo: its regulators and its effectors. The sequence of the cytoplasmic tail of Smo is highly divergent between vertebrates and *D. melanogaster*. The entire KIF7 protein from zebrafish has some sequence similarity to Cos2, and KIF7 can bind GLI1. Like Cos2, KIF7 is required for repression of SHH responses, although it might differ from Cos2 in the degree to which it is required for full activation of Hh responses. Another kinesin and two ciliary proteins (KIF3a and the intraflagellar transport proteins IFT88 and IFT172) also mediate Cos2-like functions in vertebrates, participating in both full repression and full activation of Hh responses (Huangfu et al., 2003). Although it is likely that some, or all, of these four proteins fulfil the biochemical role(s) of Cos2, this remains to be tested. Some vertebrate Hh pathway genes have no known orthologues in *D. melanogaster*; some have orthologues, the role of which in Hh signalling has not been explored; and some have known orthologues with other functions. Missing in metastasis (MIM), which is also known as BEG4, is an actin-binding protein that potentiates GLI dependent transcriptional activation (Callahan et al., 2004). Positive vertebrate regulators of the Hh signalling pathway that have no known orthologues in flies include megalin, which belongs to the low-density lipoprotein (LDL)-receptor-related family and binds SHH41, and iguana, a zinc-finger protein that promotes the nuclear localization of GLI1 (Wolff et al., 2004). Negative regulatory factors distinguish vertebrate Hh signalling as well: FKBP8 is a transcription factor that antagonizes SHH action in the nervous system (Bulgakov et al., 2004), whereas SIL is a cytosolic protein that seems to functions downstream of PTC (Izraeli et al., 2001). Rab23 is a regulator of vesicular trafficking and a negative regulator of the Hh response (Eggenschwiler et al., 2001). Shifted (Shf) is a secreted protein and is the *D. melanogaster* orthologue of human Wnt inhibitory factor (WIF). Shf facilitates Hh signalling by binding Hh and heparansulphate proteoglycans, whereas WIF binds WNT proteins and facilitates Wnt signalling (Glise et al., 2005). At least some of the apparent differences between phyla are the result of the functional convergence of non-homologous genes and proteins. The mammalian membrane glycoprotein Hh-interacting protein (HIP) and *D.melanogaster* Pxb have no sequence similarity, but they might fulfil the same function. Each is a transcriptional target of Hh and each participates in a negative- feedback loop that attenuates Hh responses (HIP through direct binding to SHH) (Inaki et al., 2002). The larger question of whether the core of the signal transduction apparatus works in the same manner in the two phyla remains to be elucidated.

Hh acts to regulate the three Gli proteins in different ways. Gli1 appears to act as an activator to mediate and/or amplify the Hh response and is transcriptionally induced by Hh signalling in all context studied. The situation with Gli2 and Gli3 is more complex. Hh signalling represses both the transcription of Gli3 and the proteolytic formation of Gli3 repressors. However, the function of Gli2, and probably Gli3, can be positive or negative in relation to Hh signalling in different situations (Ingham & McMahon, 2001). Therefore, Hh pathway function relies both on Gli activating function and on inhibiting Gli repressor formation (Ruiz i Altaba, 2002).

HEDGEHOG AS A CONCENTRATION-DEPENDENT SIGNAL

One of the most intriguing questions regarding Hh signaling is how Smo signalled to the HSC to regulate Ci. Although Smo shares homology with G-Protein Coupled Receptors (GPCRs), current evidence argues against the involvement of a traditional G-protein. For example, the Smo mutants SmoC and FFS, which lack the domains one would expect to

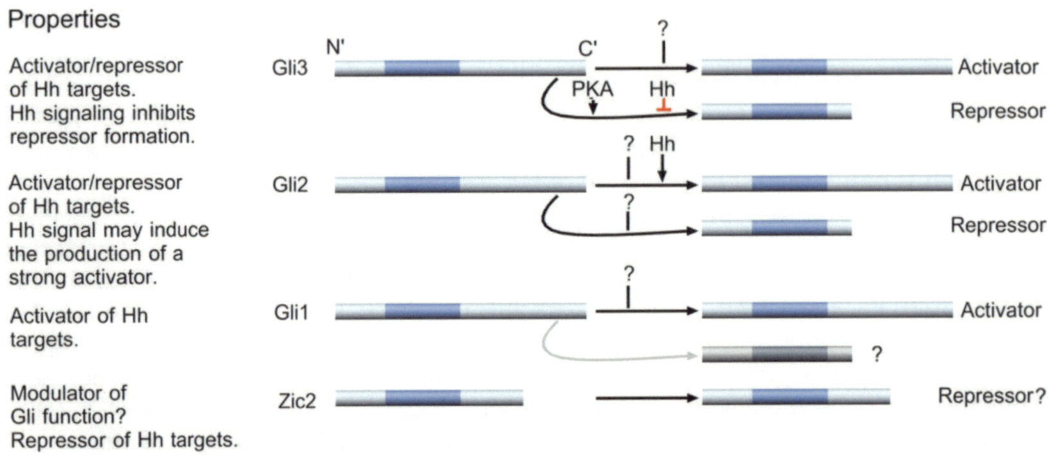

Fig. 1. Diagram schematizes the generalized regulation of the Gli proteins by proteolisis. Zic2 encodes a small protein with a GLI-type zinc-finger domain that may act as a repressor of transcription. Variations of these subjects might occur in different organs.

interact with a G-protein, are still capable of propagating Hh signalling (Hooper, 2003). Additionally, reducing the expression of all known Drosophila heterotrimeric GTP binding proteins, through use of RNA interference (RNAi), had little effect on Hh responses in cultured cells (Lum et al., 2003). This lack of compelling evidence for G-protein involvement in the Hh pathway led multiple groups to look for direct interactions between Smo and HSC components. Several recent publications, demonstrating an interaction between the carboxyl terminal tail of Smo and the cargo domain of Cos2, have begun to shed light onto the mechanistic events involved in Smo-mediated signaling to the HSC (Lum et al., 2003; Ruel et al., 2003; Jia et al., 2003; Ogden et al., 2003). In spite of there are some differences in the published studies, there seems to be a consensus on the following points: (1) Smo binds Cos2 directly; (2) the interaction is necessary for functional Hh signaling; (3) Cos2 appears to tether significant amounts of Fu to Smo, while Ci and Su(fu) binding are not as obvious. A requirement for direct Smo–Cos2 binding in signal transduction is most obvious when examining target gene expression following loss of interaction. The Smo carboxyl-terminal tail was demonstrated to contain the Cos2 interaction domain (Jia et al., 2003; Ogden et al., 2003). Over-expression of this domain appears to have a dominant negative effect, resulting in a dose dependent loss of reporter gene expression. Similarly, over-expression of Smo proteins lacking the Cos2 binding domain and/or Cos2 constructs lacking the Smo binding domain demonstrate compromised Hh responses (Lum et al., 2003; Ruel et al., 2003; Jia et al., 2003) . These results clearly demonstrate a requirement for Cos2–Smo interaction for proper Hh signal transduction. Additionally, the amount of membrane associated Hedgehog Signalling Complex (HSC) appears to decrease in response to Hh (Ruel et al., 2003). This observation is seemingly inconsistent with the model whereby the Smo/Cos2 association remains constant or even increases. To explain this apparent paradox was proposed (Ogden et al., 2004) that there may be two distinct HSCs, one involved in converting Ci into its repressor form, HSC-R, and one involved in converting Ci into its activated forms, HSC-A. In the absence of Hh, HSC-R is on and HSCA is off, while in response to maximal Hh, HSC-A is turned on and HSC-R is turned off. In between this two switch system, numerous intermediates exist.

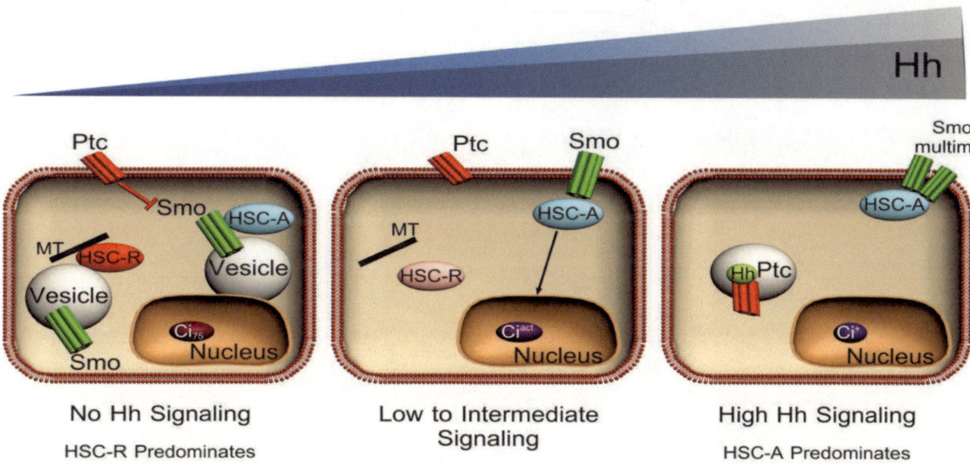

Fig. 2. Diagram shows how the Hh gradient regulates HSC activator and repressor functions. In the without Hg signalling HSC-R is producing Ci_{75} and HSC-A is inactive. In the central cell, HSC-A is producing Ci^{act}, which may be acting in presence of lower Ci_{75}. In the right cell, the greatest amount of Hh is received, HSC-A is maximally activated by Smo and HSC-R is completely silence.

It is known that graded sonic hedgehog activity patterns the ventral neural tube. Five distinct neuronal cell fates are specified in the ventral half of the neural tube in response to a gradient of SHH (Jessell, 2000). The cells of the floor plate respond to the highest concentration of SHH that is secreted by the notochord by becoming glial cells, which, in turn, begin to secrete SHH themselves. The remaining neural tube cells choose between various ventral neural fates that are specified by different thresholds of SHH signalling.

LOCALIZATION AND FUNCTION

Hh proteins are synthesized as precursor proteins (about 400-460 amino acids long) and comprise several different motifs and domains: a signal peptide for protein export, a secreted amino-terminal HhN (Hedge) domain that acts as a signalling molecule, and an autocatalytic carboxy-terminal HhC (Hog) domain that contains a Hint module. Multiple sequence alignments of the HhN and HhC domains defining the conserved residues and features have been presented in (Bürglin, 2008). HhC binds cholesterol in the sterol recognition region (SRR) (Beachy et al., 1997). The catalytic activity of the Hint module cleaves Hh into two parts and adds the cholesterol moiety to the carboxyl terminus of HhN. Figure 2 outlines the Hh signalling patway.

In the figure 2 Hh is targeted to the endoplasmic reticulum by its signal peptide, is palmitoylated at its amino terminus by Rasp/Skinny Hedgehog (Ski), and autoprocessed. Lipidated HhN (M-HhN) is released by Dispatched (Disp) and forms multimers or associates with lipoproteins (LP) in the extracellular environment (Cohen, 2003). Several molecules can interact with M-HhN and propagate or modulate its trafficking: the Dally-like protein (Dlp) that is modified by the heparan sulfate (HS) polymerases Tout-velu (Ttv), Sister of tout-velu (Sotv), and Brother of tout-velu (Botv), all members of the EXT family; the Hedgehog-interacting protein (Hip); and the Growth-arrest specific1 (Gas1) protein. Hip and Gas1 are not present in Drosophila. Megalin (Meg) is most probably involved in the

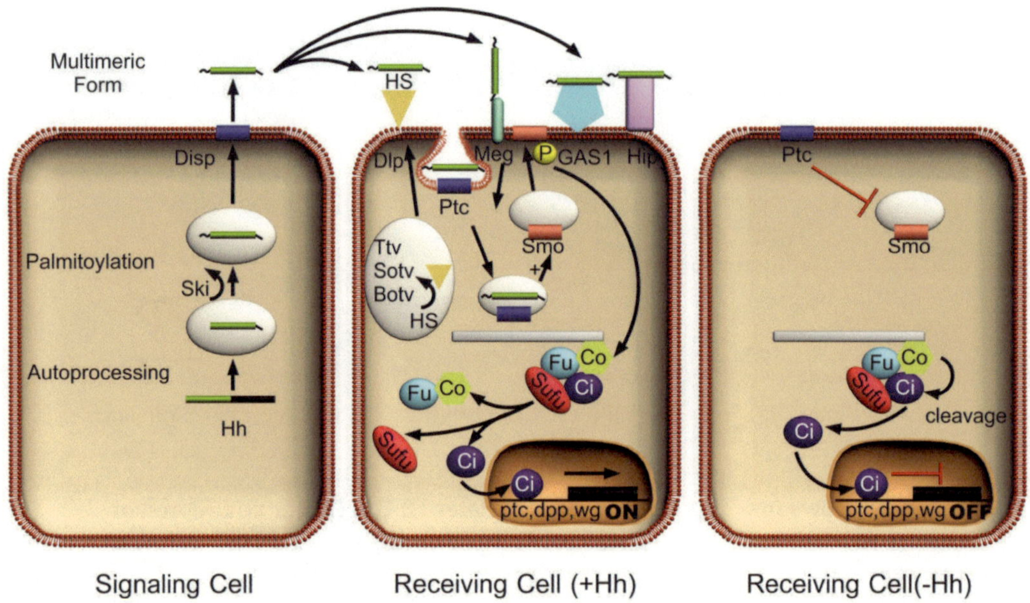

Fig. 3. A schematic Hh signalling pathway, obtained from combined Drosophila and mammalian data.

recycling of M-HhN. Ihog is thought to function as co-receptor for M-HhN. M-HhN acts as an antagonistic ligand that represses the function of the receptor Patched (Ptc), a 12-transmembrane protein related to Disp. Binding of M-HhN to Ptc results in internalization. Smoothened (Smo) is a seven-pass membrane receptor, which is the key for the transmission of the signal to the nucleus in the Hh pathway. Smo is inhibited by Ptc when not bound by M-HhN. If the inhibitory function of Ptc is released by M-HhN, Smo can translocate to the plasma membrane or - in mammals - to the primary cilium, and active Smo is phosphorylated. Ptc may secrete pro-vitamin D3 or related compounds (D3) to inhibit Smo. Conversely, oxysterols (Oxy) can indirectly activate Smo (Eaton, 2008; Rohatgi et al., 2007). The Hh pathway downstream of Smo displays some important differences between Drosophila and mammals. In Drosophila, when Smo is active, the signal passes through a complex comprising the kinesin-like molecule Costal 2 (Cos2), Fused (Fu), Suppressor of fused (Su (fu)) and Cubitus interruptus (Ci), leading to the release of Ci, which can then enter the nucleus to promote transcription. When Smo is inhibited, the Cos2/Fu/Su (fu)/Ci complex remains associated with microtubules, Ci is phosphorylated and is cleaved by Cos2. The Ci fragment now acts as a transcriptional repressor. In mammals, the targeting of Smo to primary cilia is essential for signal transduction. No obvious equivalents of Cos2 and Fu exist in mammals. Instead, Su (fu) has a more prominent role in inhibiting the pathway. Gli1, Gli2, and Gli3 are the mammalian homologs of Ci; Gli1 and Gli2 activate transcription when Smo is active, whereas Gli3 is processed and becomes a repressor when Smo is inhibited.

In animal development, the secreted M-HhN moiety functions as a morphogen. The Hh signalling pathway plays many important roles in development, including conferring segment polarity on the body segments and patterning the wing in Drosophila, and patterning the neural tube in mammals (Dessaud et al., 2008; Varjosalo & Taipale, 2008) . Hh is also required for stem-cell maintenance, and mutations in the pathway lead to cancer. Increased activity of the pathway causes basal cell carcinoma and medulloblastoma (Beachy et al., 2004; Jacob & Lum, 2007). For example, insufficient Ptc function leads to Gorlin syndrome in humans, one feature of which is an increased risk of basal cell skin cancer.

In mammals, Shh, Dhh, and Ihh have partially redundant functions. Shh is the most widely expressed of the three paralogs, and regulates development from embryo to adult. Key roles are in patterning the neural tube: Shh is first expressed in the notochord, and later in the floor plate of the neural tube, where it produces a gradient of activity in the ventral neural tube. Shh is also expressed in the zone of polarizing activity of the limb buds and is important for limb and digit formation. Other roles of Shh include inner ear, eye, taste bud, and hair follicle development. Ihh is expressed in the primitive endoderm and is required for bone growth and pancreas development. Shh and Ihh both play roles in cardiovascular development. Dhh is expressed in the gonads, and Dhh-mutant males are sterile (Bijlsma et al., 2006; Dessaud et al., 2008; Varjosalo & Taipale, 2008).

SECRETION, TRAFFICKING AND SPREADING OF HEDGEHOG

Dispatched is necessary for Hh secretion (Burke et al., 1999). Dispatched contains 12 transmembrane domains and is related to the resistance-nodulation division (RND) family of bacterial proton-driven pumps (Ma et al., 2002). Bacterial proteins of the RND family use a proton gradient to transport multiple small lipophilic molecules across the membrane bilayer. The two other metazoan members of this family include the Hh receptor Patched, and the protein encoded by the Niemann–Pick type C1 (*NPC1*) disease gene, which promotes cholesterol efflux from late endosomes. Members of the RND family: Patched, Dispatched and NPC1, contain two related copies of a signature domain with six transmembrane-spanning regions. Mutations in Dispatched which disturb conserved residues that are important for the function of bacterial transporters, also prevent Hh release (Ma et al., 2002), consistent with the hypothesis that Dispatched can transport a small molecule across the bilayer. A fragment of the signature RND domain, called a sterol-sensing domain, is also shared with other proteins that are involved in sterol metabolism. The sterol-sensing domain of HMGCoA reductase (the rate-limiting enzyme in cholesterol biosynthesis) regulates its stability in response to cholesterol. The sterol-sensing domain of SCAP [sterol-regulatory-element-binding protein (SREBP) cleavage-activating protein] responds to cholesterol levels by altering membrane trafficking and the cleavage of the membrane-associated transcription factor SREBP, which regulates the transcription of genes that are involved in sterol metabolism (Chang et al., 2006). Whether Dispatched itself responds to sterol levels is not known, and its precise function in Hh release has not yet been determined. The mechanism of Dispatched to respond to the levels of sterol and how Hh is released has not yet been determined.

Biochemical fractionation of imaginal discs from *D. melanogaster* larvae shows that, although most lipid-modified Hh will form pellets with cell membranes, Hh molecules that remain in the supernatant are almost entirely associated with lipoprotein particles (Panáková et al., 2005). It will be interesting to determine whether the cholesterol-dependent Hh multimers that are secreted by tissue-culture cells might reflect the association of Hh with serum-derived lipoproteins, or whether multimer formation is a completely distinct mechanism for Hh release. Lipoproteins comprise a phospholipid monolayer that surrounds a core of esterified cholesterol and triglyceride. Lipid modifications, such as the addition of cholesterol, palmitate and glycosyl phosphatidylinositol (GPI), that target proteins to the exoplasmic face of the plasma membrane should fit equally well into the outer phospholipid monolayer of lipoproteins. Indeed, *D. melanogaster* lipophorin particles also bind to the morphogen molecule Wingless, which is palmitoylated twice and to several GPI-linked proteins (Panáková et al., 2005; Eugster et al., 2007).

Two mechanisms are hypothesized for Hh release in wing discs: a long-range mechanism that depends on lipophorin and a shortrange mechanism that is lipophorin independent. Whether any of the mammalian Hh proteins bind to low-density lipoprotein (LDL) or high-density lipoprotein (HDL)-type particles is unknown, although this would be interesting to investigate. Cholesterol modification clearly has an important influence on Hh trafficking. The 19 kDa N-terminal Hh domain can be artificially generated in the absence of cholesterol modification by the simple expedient of stop codon insertion or C-terminal domain deletions (Porter et al., 1996). This altered protein, termed HhN, is secreted in a Dispatched-independent manner (Burke et al.,1999), does not form multimeric complexes (Gallet et al., 2006; Chen et al., 2004; Feng et al., 2004), and is distributed differently in both producing and receiving cells (Gallet et al., 2003; Callejo et al., 2006). Although HhN has been reported to spread further, it does not seem to signal as efficiently as cholesterol modified Hh (Porter et al., 1996; Gallet et al., 2006; Li et al., 2006). The anchors probably interact, either with each other (when Hh is organized as micellar multimers) or with the outer phospholipid monolayer of a lipoprotein. Interaction with heparan sulphate proteoglycans (HSPGs) provides a likely explanation for the continuing association of Hh micelles or Hh–

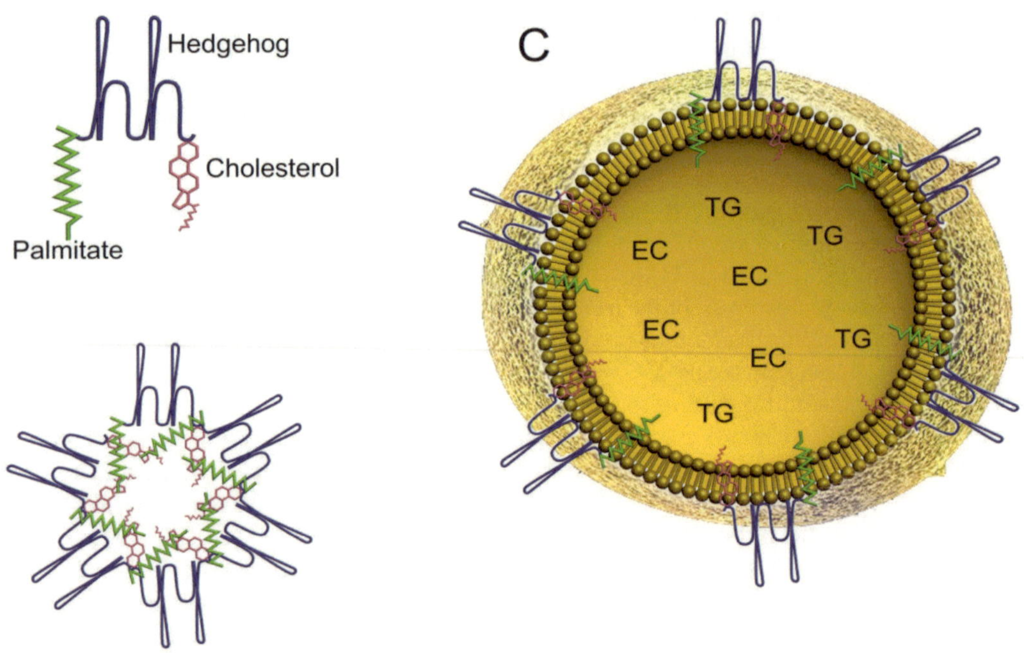

Fig. 4. Possible carriers for Hedgehog release. Hh (blue) is covalently linked to cholesterol (red) and palmitate (green). The interaction of the lipid moieties with each other promotes the formation of Hh multimers. Finally, a lipoprotein consists of an outer phospholipids monolayer (brown) that surrounds a core of sterified cholesterol (EC) and triglyceride (TG).

lipoprotein complexes with tissue. Lipid-modified Hh does not enter tissue that cannot synthesize heparan sulphate (Han et al., 2004). Recent work suggests that lipoproteins interact physically with HSPGs in *D. melanogaster* wing discs (Eugster et al., 2007). Hh that has interacted with lipoproteins through lipid anchors might therefore be restricted to tissue through these lipoprotein–heparan sulphate interactions. This would be consistent with the observation that only lipid modified Hh is dependent on HSPGs in orders to associate with tissue. Direct binding of Hh to HSPGs might also provide tissue affinity. In this case, Hh multimerization might also promote HSPG binding by increasing the local concentration of heparan sulphate-binding sites on Hh.

TRANSCRIPTIONAL REPRESSION OR ACTIVATION IN HEDGEHOG RESPONSE

Hedgehog responsive changes in gene expression are mediated by the zinc finger transcription factor Ci, which can assume repressing and activating forms. The represing form, CiR, represents an N-terminal proteolytic fragment that retains the zinc finger-mediated DNA binding specificity of Ci but lacks nuclear export signals, a cytoplasmic anchoring sequence, and a transcriptional activation domain. For some genes, such the universal Hh pathway target *ptc*, expression requires loss of CiR and the positive action of Ci. So the expression of Hh pathway targets depends on regulation of Ci processing and localization.

Formation of CiR requires phosphorylation of specific serine-threonine residues by cyclic adenosine monophosphate (cAMP) dependent protein kinase. The phosphorylated form of Ci appears to be a substrate for a proteolytic processing reaction that requires function of the proteasome and of Slimb (Slmb), an F-box-containing E3 ubiquitin ligase component. Ci phosphorylation and processing may be mediated by Cos2 scaffolding of kinases with Ci, although direct associations of these kinases with Cos2 or Ci have not yet been reported. (Lum & Beachy, 2004).

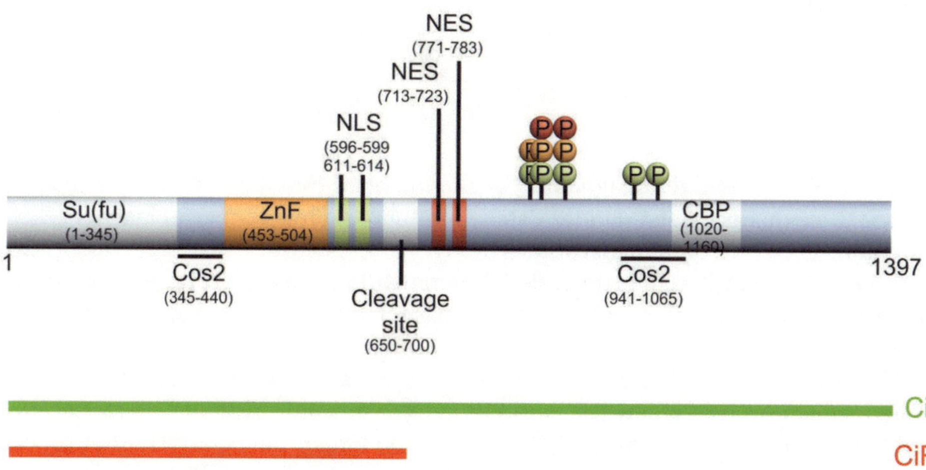

Fig. 5. Representation of Ci functional domains and motifs. They are labelled by amino acid numbers (in parenthesis). Phosphorylation sites are indicated, they are required for initiation of Ci proteolytic processing. Pathway activating functions of Ci are associated with full-length Ci (green line) whereas repressor functions are associated with the proteolytically processed form CiR (red line).

The kinase(s) that phosphorylate Fu and Cos2 remain to be identified and the significance of their phosphorylation remains to be determined. Hh also facilitates the association of a small population of Sufu molecules with the Cos2-Fu-Smo complex. A genetic analysis indicates that Fu phosphorylates Sufu, but biochemical evidence for this lacking. One possibility is that high concentrations of Hh promote Smo phosphorylation and dimerization. This activates the Fu kinase that is associated with Complex I, which then phosphorylates Sufu to release CiA. Curiously, the full spectrum oh Hh responses is seen in *D.melanogaster* in the absence of Sufu, if Cos2 regulation is normal. So there must be an alternative pathway to CiA that involves Cos2 rather than Sufu that in vertebrates remain to be determined (Lum et al., 2003; Stegman et al., 2000).

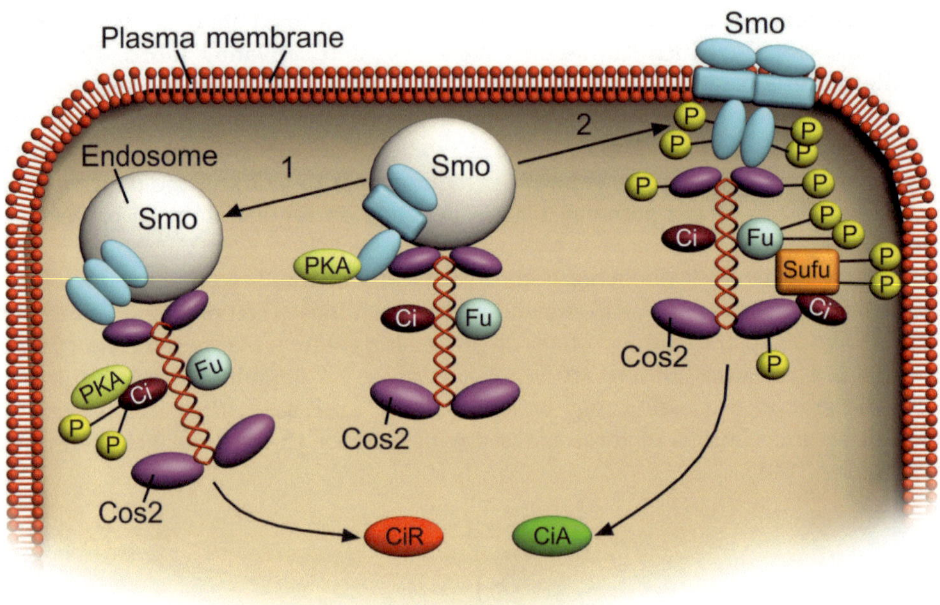

Fig. 6. Ilustration of a model for signalling by Smoothened (Smo) and Costal-2 (Cos-2). Smo can assume three distinct states. Under Patched influence, Smo adopts an inactive conformation. This form of Smo distributes between endosomes, where it can associate with Cos-2, and lysosomes, where it is degraded. The remaining Cos2 recruits protein kinase A (PKA), casein kinase I and glycogen synthase kinase-3 to Ci, which enables phosphorylation of Cubitus interruptus (Ci) and its subsequent processing to the transcriptional repressor form (CiR). When the influence of Ptc decreases, the transmembrane helices of Smo are rearranged, which exposes a new surface in its cytoplasmic tail. This surface causes PKA, CKI and GSK3 to dissociate from Cos2, so that Ci is no longer phosphorylated or processed to CiR. Smo is phosphorylated instead, and it assumes its third state. Phosphorylated Smo traffics to the surface, rather than to lysosomes for degradation. Smo concentrations rise and Smo assembles a modified signalling complex that promotes the phosphorylation of Fused (Fu) and Cos2. Phosphorylated Cos2 dissociates from membranes and recruits Fu to Sufu (Suppressor of Fused), which produces the activated form of Ci (CiA), probably through phosphorylation of Sufu phosphorylated (Ogden et al., 2004).

3. Hedgehog signalling in human disease

In addition to functioning in the embryo, Hh proteins and Hh signal-transduction components are expressed in postnatal and adult tissues, suggesting that they function in the mature organism. Defects in Hh signalling could, therefore, affect both the human embryo and the adult (Ruiz i Altaba, 2002).

THE CANCER STEM CELL THEORY

A great deal of interest has focused on mutation or aberrant regulation in stem cells as a key factor in carcinogenesis. A link between stem cells and cancer is not a new concept (Sell, 2004). Subsequently it was widely accepted that the initiation and progression of malignancy is a multi-step process, driven by numerous genetic changes that result in the transformation of normal cells into malignant cells. Environmental factors apply evolutionary pressure on the tumor, which leads to selection of clones with a greater capacity to survive, grow and metastasise. In this theory, any normal cell undergoing sufficient genetic alterations to result in its unregulated proliferation may become a tumor-initiating cell. The observed heterogeneity of many tumors is due to the development and expansion of numerous subclones. This clonal evolution theory is believed to explain the ultimate insensitivity of many tumors to chemotherapy, as clones with the ability to export the drug, or which lack key components of metabolic pathways targeted by the drug, are positively selected for their ability to evade death. The identification of stem cells in a range of tissues and organs and a greater understanding of their biology has again focused attention on the "stem cell theory of cancer" which proposes that malignancy arises from the transformation of a normal tissue stem cell. The cancer stem cell theory hypothesises that, analogous to stem cells in normal tissues, there are a small proportion of cells within tumors that have stem cell properties giving rise to progeny which may show heterogeneous patterns of differentiation and form the bulk of the tumor mass. The existence of cancer stem cells is thought to explain the failure of chemotherapy and other treatments to eradicate metastatic disease. With the continuing identification of stem-like cells within increasing numbers of malignancies, it is obviously that a new approach to treatment is required, one which directly targets the cancer stem cells in association with more traditional approaches that affect tumor bulk. These highly tumorigenic cells, also known as cancer stem cells, have the ability to self-renew and differentiate into multiple lineages. Cancer stem cells have been isolated from human tumors involving the breast, lung, colon, pancreas, prostate, skin, head/neck and brain. Experimental and clinical research indicates that cancer stem cells, as well as cells from solid tumors, are resistant to chemotherapy and radiation therapy. Therapeutic approaches are in development to block embryonic pathways that play a role in cancer stem cells, including Notch, sonic hedgehog and Wnt.

HEDGEHOG IN CANCER

Defects in Hh signalling pathway have long been known to be associated with human congenital disease with the loss of one copy of Shh resulting in holoprosencephaly (Roessler et al., 1996). More recently has been documented that aberrant Hedgehog signalling is associated with the development and progression of a wide range of human malignancies. Mutations such as Ptch1 and Smo are associated with medulloblastoma, basal cell carcinoma and rhabdomyosarcoma. Aberrant activation of Hh signalling is also suggested to play a role in other cancers that have no known mutational basis, such as glioma, breast, esophageal, gastric, pancreatic, prostate, chondrosarcoma and small-cell lung carcinoma. In these tumors the Hh pathway abnormalities are called ligand-dependent and were described first in lung (Watkins et al., 2003) and then in gastrointestinal tract and pancreatic carcinoma (Berman et al., 2003), which show no mutation in Hh pathway genes but are characterised by upregulation of the expression of Hh ligand which is also though to include autocrine and paracrine mechanism of activation. There are two proposed models to explain how Hh ligands promote tumor growth: one postulates that Hh ligands produced by cancer cells and/or their stromal environment maintain secreted stem cell renewal within the tumor (Jiang & Hui, 2008); the second proposes that Hh ligands secreted by the tumor may act on nearby stromal cells, resulting in pathway activation in the stromal microenvironment that promotes tumor growth (Yauch et al., 2008).

HEDGEHOG SIGNALLING IN CANCER STEM CELLS

Data from many human tumors including glioblastoma, breast cancer, pancreatic adenocarcinoma, multiple myeloma, and chronic myeloid leukemia (CML) have suggested that Hh signaling moderates cancer stem cells (CSC). Self-renewal of CSC is required for maintenance of the malignant clone, and reports studying mouse models of CML have provided evidence that Hh signaling regulates this property (Dierks et al., 2008; Zhao et al., 2009). Active Hh signalling pathway has also been identified in glioblastoma CSCs, and pathway inhibition with cyclopamine or siRNA directed against pathway components results in the loss of tumorigenic potential (Clement et al., 2007). In breast cancer, pathway activation in CSCs using Hh ligand and GLI1 or GLI2 expression or inhibition with cyclopamine or siRNA directed against GLI1 or GLI2 alters the expression of BMI-1 (Liu et al., 2006). In multiple myeloma, CSCs that phenotypically resemble normal memory B cells have been found to display relatively higher levels of Hh signalling than the mature plasma cells constituting the tumor bulk (Peacock et al., 2007). So, HH signalling may dictate CSC fate decisions that include self-renewal and differentiation possibly by generation of a malignant niche (LaBarge, 2010). Data from multiple myeloma demonstrate that Hh signaling can act through multiple signaling modes within the same cancer and can mediate interactions between CSCs, differentiated tumor cells and the microenvironment. Aditionally to tumor formation, CSCs have been implicated in disease progression and the development of metastasis in solid tumors (Rasheed et al., 2010), and Hh signaling may play a critical role in this process similar to the Notch and Wnt pathways in cancer. In colon carcinomas, Hh signaling has been found to be preferentially activated within CSCs as evidenced by relatively higher expression of GLI1, GLI2, PTCH1, and HIP within this cellular compartment (Varnat et al., 2009). Moreover, the relative expression of these pathway components as well as the target gene SNAIL1, which is associated with the epithelial-to mesenchymal transition (EMT) and implicated in metastasis, increases in CSCs with disease stage.

INHIBITORS OF HEDGEHOG SIGNALLING

It has been accepted that altered Hh signalling contributes to the development of up to one third of all human malignancies (Beachy et al., 2004) and so there is a great interest in therapeutic inhibition of the pathway, with a number of inhibitors in clinical trials. The first inhibitor of the Hedgehog pathway identified was cyclopamine (Cooper et al., 1998), Cyclopamine is a small molecule inhibitor of Smoothened, and a number of compounds have been identified or synthesized which have similar mechanisms of action. To inhibition of the pathway several approaches have been developed:

1. Prevention of Hh ligand binding to Ptch receptor.
2. Inhibition of Smoothened via cyclopamine and related compounds. Much of the preclinical and clinical trial work on Hh inhibitors undertaken to date focuses on inhibitors of Smo.
3. Inhibiotrs of Gli transcription.

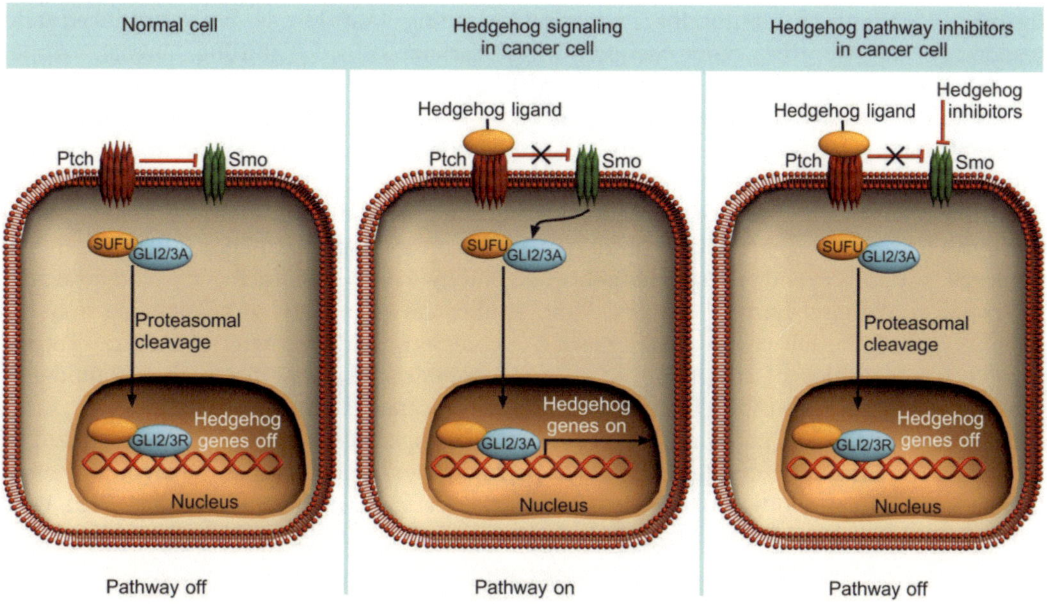

Fig. 7. Ilustration of a schematic representation of the pathway in a normal cell, a cancer cell and the action of inhibitors over the Hedgehog pathway.

DEVELOPING IMPROVED HEDGEHOG THERAPIES

In adulthood, the Hh signalling pathway is silenciated in the great majority of cells. However, there have been an increasing number of reports over the past decade documenting the implication of the Hh pathway in human diseases, such as cancer. For these reasons, Hh pathway antagonists have been sought after as potential new treatments for cancer. The theory that many tumors arise from a small number of cancer stem cells (CSCs) has recently gained strength with some landmark studies that point to the existence of a discrete population of slowly dividing tumor cells capable of self-renewal and differentiation along multiple lineages. The control of these processes in cancer stem cells is thought to be regulated by a small number of signaling pathways as Hh, Wnt, and Notch , and growing evidence suggests that some of these pathways are deregulated, allowing for their abnormal expansion and the formation of cancer.

These Hh, Wnt, and Notch pathways might be interconnected and ultimately lead to the regulation of stem-cell self-renewal via Bmi-1 transcription factor (Liu et al., 2006). These data suggest additional possible uses for inhibitors of pathway such as Hh. The outcome of Hh signaling varies according to the receiving cell type, but it can include expression of a variety of cell-specific transcription factors mediating different developmental fate response: upregulation of D-type cyclins, resulting in cell proliferation; upregulation of anti-apoptotic proteins such as Bcl-2, mediating cell survival; production of vascular endothelial growth factor (VEGF) and angiopoietins regulating angiogenesis; and transcription of SNAIL, initiating the epithelial-mesenchyme transition (EMT) in metastasis. It is, therefore, not surprising that deregulated Hh signalling can lead to a variety of cancers.

Three basic models have been proposed for Hh pathway activity in cancer (Rubin & de Sauvage, 2006). The type I cancers, which harbour pathway-activating mutations, such as basal carcinomas (BCCs), medulloblastomas, and rhabdomyosarcomas. Type II cancers, are ligand dependent and autocrine/juxtacrine, meaning that Hh is both produced and responded to by the same/neighbouring tumor cells, including breast, upper gastrointestinal tract, colorectal, prostate and lung tumors. Type III cancer, are also ligand dependent but paracrine, in that Hh produced by the tumor epithelium is received by cells in the stroma, which feed other signals back to the tumor to promote its growth or survival.

The clinical reality is that the majority of cancer patients present with locally or distant metastatic, surgically inoperable disease. Therefore, the development of more potent therapies for advanced/metastatic human cancers mandates great urgency. Multiples line of evidence support the idea that Hedgehog signalling has a role in the maintenance and progression of many human cancers. First, studies involving global sequencing analysis have identified the Hh pathway as one of the core signalling pathway of human cancers; second, the inhibition of Hh enhanced survival in genetically engineered mouse model of cancers; third, blockade of the Hh pathway eliminates cancer stem cells.

Intervention of the Hh pathway has provided a therapeutic opportunity for treatment of malignancies. Effective inhibition of the Hh pathway can be achieved at the level of ligands by using anti-Hh antibodies, or through downstream effectors molecules, such as Smo, with small-molecule antagonist (Evangelista et al., 2006).

4. References

Alcedo J.; Ayzenzon M.; Von Ohlen T. et al. (1996) The Drosophila smoothened gene encodes a seven-pass membrane protein, a putative receptor for the hedgehog signal. *Cell* 86(2):221–32

Beachy P.A.; Karhadkar S.S. & Berman D.M. (2004) Tissue repair and stem cell renewal in carcinogenesis. *Nature* 432(7015):324-331

Beachy P.A.; Cooper M.K.; Young K.E. et al. (1997) Multiple roles of cholesterol in hedgehog protein biogenesis and signaling. *Cold Spring Harb Symp Quant Biol* 62:191-204

Berman D. M.; Karhadkar S. S.; Maitra A. et al. (2003) Widespread requirement for Hedgehog ligand stimulation in growth of digestive tract tumours. *Nature* 425: 846-851

Bijlsma M.F.; Peppelenbosch M.P. & Spek C.A. (2006) Hedgehog morphogen in cardiovascular disease. *Circulation* 114:1985-1991

Bulgakov O. V.; Eggenschwiler J. T.; Hong D. H et al. (2004) FKBP8 is a negative regulator of mouse sonic hedgehog signaling in neural tissues. *Development* 131, 2149–2159

Bürglin T.R. (2008) Evolution of hedgehog and hedgehog-related genes, theirorigin from Hog proteins in ancestral eukaryotes and discovery of anovel Hint motif. *BMC Genomics* 9:127.

Burke, R. et al. *(1999)* Dispatched, a novel sterol-sensing domain protein dedicated to the release of cholesterolmodified hedgehog from signaling cells. *Cell* 99: 803–815

Callejo A.; Torroja C.; Quijada L. et al. (2006) I. Hedgehog lipid modifications are required for Hedgehog stabilization in the extracellular matrix. *Development* 133, 471–483

Chang T. Y.; Chang C. C.; Ohgami N. et al (2006) Cholesterol sensing, trafficking, and esterification. *Annu. Rev. Cell Dev. Biol.* 22, 129–157

Chen Y. & Struhl G. (1996) Dual roles for patched in sequestering and transducing Hedgehog. *Cell* 87(3):553–63

Chen M. H.; Li Y. J.; Kawakami, T. et al. (2004) Palmitoylation is required for the production of a soluble multimeric Hedgehog protein complex and long-range signaling in vertebrates. *Genes Dev.* 18, 641–659

Clement V.; Sanchez P.; de Tribolet N. et al. (2007) HEDGEHOG-GLI1 signaling regulates human glioma growth, cancer stem cell self-renewal, and tumorigenicity. *Curr Biol* 17:165–72

Cohen Jr M.M. (2003) The hedgehog signaling network. *Am J Med Genet* 123A(1):5–28.

Cooper M.K.; Porter J.A.; Young K.E. et al. (1998) Teratogen-mediated inhibition of target tissue response to Shh signalling. Science 280 (5369):1603-1607

Dessaud E.; McMahon A.P. & Briscoe J. (2008) Pattern formation in the vertebrate neural tube: a sonic hedgehog morphogen-regulated transcriptional network. *Development* 135:2489-2503

Dierks C.; Beigi R.; Guo G.R., et al. (2008) Expansion of Bcr-Abl-positive leukemic stem cells is dependent on Hedgehog pathway activation. *Cancer Cell* 14:238–49

Eaton S. (2008) Multiple roles for lipids in the Hedgehog signalling pathway. Nat Rev Mol Cell Biol. 9(6):437-45

Eggenschwiler J. T.; Espinoza E. & Anderson K. V. (2001) Rab23 is an essential negative regulator of the mouse Sonic hedgehog signalling pathway. *Nature* 412, 194–198

Eugster C.; Panakova D.; Mahmoud A. et al. (2007) Lipoprotein–heparan sulfate interactions in the Hedgehog pathway. *Dev. Cell* 13, 57–71

Evangelista M.; Tian H. & de Sauvage F.J. (2006) The hedgehog signaling pathway in cancer. *Clin Cancer Res* 12:5924

Feng J. et al. (2004) Synergistic and antagonistic roles of the Sonic hedgehog N- and C-terminal lipids. *Development* 131, 4357–4370

Gallet A.; Rodriguez R.; Ruel L. et al. (2003) Cholesterol modification of Hedgehog is required for trafficking and movement, revealing an asymmetric cellular response to Hedgehog. *Dev. Cell* 4, 191–204

Gallet A.; Ruel L.; Staccini-Lavenant L. et al. (2006) Cholesterol modification is necessary for ncontrolled planar long-range activity of Hedgehog in *Drosophila* epithelia. *Development* 133, 407–418

Glise B. et al. (2005) Shifted, the *Drosophila* ortholog of wnt inhibitory factor-1, controls the distribution and movement of hedgehog. *Dev. Cell* 8, 255–266

Hall T. M.; Porter J. A.; Beachy P. A. et al. (1995) A potential catalytic site revealed by the 1.7-Å crystal structure of the amino-terminal signalling domain of Sonic hedgehog. *Nature* 378, 212–216

Han C.; Belenkaya T. Y.; Wang B. et al. (2004) *Drosophila* glypicans control the cell-to-cell movement of Hedgehog by a dynamin-independent process. *Development* 131, 601–611

Hooper J.E. & Scott M.P. (1989) The Drosophila patched gene encodes a putative membrane protein required for segmental patterning. *Cell* 59(4): 751–65

Hooper J. E. (2003) Smoothened translates Hedgehog levels into distinct responses. *Development* 130(17):3951–63

Huangfu D. et al. (2003) Hedgehog signalling in the mouse requires intraflagellar transport proteins. *Nature* 426, 83–87

Inaki M.; Kojima T.; Ueda R. et al. (2002) Requirements of high levels of Hedgehog signaling activity for medialregion cell fate determination in *Drosophila* legs: identification of *pxb*, a putative Hedgehog signalling attenuator gene repressed along the anterior–posterior compartment boundary. *Mech. Dev.* 116, 3–18

Ingham P.W. & McMahon A.P. (2001) Hedgehog signaling in animal development: paradigms and principles. *Genes Dev* 15: 3059–87

Izraeli, S. et al. (2001) Genetic evidence that *Sil* is required for the Sonic Hedgehog response pathway. *Genesis* 31, 72–77

Jacob L. & Lum L. (2007) Deconstructing the hedgehog pathway in development and disease. Science 318:66-68

Jessell T.M. (2000) Neuronal specification in the spinal cord: inductive signals and transcriptional codes *Nature Rev. Genet.* 1:20-29

Jia J.; Tong C. & Jiang J. (2003) Smoothened transduces Hedgehog signal by physically interacting with Costal2/Fused complex through its Cterminal tail. *Genes Dev* 17(21):2709–20.

Jiang J. & Hui C.C. (2008) Hedgehog signalling in development and cancer. *Dev Cell* 15:801-812.

LaBarge M. (2010) The difficulty of targeting cancer stem cell niches. *Clin Cancer Res* 16:3121 9.

Li Y.; Zhang H.; Litingtung Y. et al. (2006) Cholesterol modification restricts the spread of Shh gradient in the limb bud. *Proc. Natl Acad. Sci. USA* 103, 6548–6553

Liu S.; Dontu G.; Mantle I.D.; et al. (2006) Hedgehog signaling and Bmi-1 regulate self-renewal of normal and malignant human mammary stem cells. *Cancer Res* 66:6063–71

Lum L.; Yao S.; Mozer B. et al. (2003) Identification of Hedgehog pathway components by RNAi in Drosophila cultured cells. *Science* 299(5615):2039–45

Lum L.; Zhang C.; Oh S. et al. (2003) Hedgehog signal transduction via Smoothened association with a cytoplasmic complex scaffolded by the atypical kinesin, Costal-2. *Mol Cell* 12(5):1261–74

Lum L. & Beachy A. (2004) The hedgehog response network: sensors, switches, and routers. *Science* 304: 1755-1759

Lum L.; Zhang C.; Oh S.; et al. (2003) Hedgehog signal transduction via Smoothened association with a cytoplasmic complex scaffolded by the atypical kinesin, Costal-2. *Mol Cell.* 12(5):1261-74.

Ma Y. et al.(2002) Hedgehog-mediated patterning of the mammalian embryo requires transporter-like function of dispatched. *Cell* 111, 63–75

McMahon A. P.; Ingham P. W. & Tabin C. J. (2003) Developmental roles and clinical significance of hedgehog signaling. *Curr. Top. Dev. Biol.* 53, 1–114

Merchant, M. et al. (2004) Suppressor of fused regulates Gli activity through a dual binding mechanism. *Mol. Cell. Biol.* 24, 8627–8641

Nusse R. (2003) Wnts and Hedgehogs: lipid-modified proteins and similarities in signaling mechanisms at the cell surface. *Development* 130, 5297–5305

Ogden S.K.; Ascano M. Jr.; Stegman M.A. et al. (2004) Regulation of Hedgehog signaling: a complex story. *Biochem Pharmacol.* 67(5):805-14

Ogden S.K.; Ascano Jr M.; Stegman M.A. et al. (2003) Identification of a functional interaction between the transmembrane protein Smoothened and the kinesin related protein Costal2. *Curr Biol* 13(22):1998–2003

Ogden S.K.; Ascano M.Jr.; Stegman M.A., et al. (2004) Regulation of Hedgehog signaling: a complex story. *Biochem Pharmacol.* 67(5):805-14

Paces-Fessy M.; Boucher D.;Petit E. et al. (2004) The negative regulator of Gli, Suppressor of fused (Sufu), interacts with SAP18, Galectin3 and other nuclear proteins. *Biochem.J.* 378: 353–362

Panáková D.; Sprong H.; Marois E. et al. (2005) Lipoprotein particles carry lipid-linked proteins and are required for long-range Hedgehog and Wingless signalling. *Nature* 435, 58–65

Peacock C.D.; Wang Q.; Gesell G.S., et al. (2007) Hedgehog signalling maintains a tumor stem cell compartment in multiple myeloma. *Proc Natl Acad Sci U S A*104:4048–53

Porter J. A. et al. (1996) Hedgehog patterning activity: role of a lipophilic modification mediated by the carboxyterminal autoprocessing domain. *Cell* 86, 21–34

Rahnama F.; Toftgard R. & Zaphiropoulos P. G. (2004) Distinct roles of PTCH2 splice variants in Hedgehog signalling. *Biochem.J.* 378, 325–334

Rasheed Z.A.; Yang J.; Wang Q., et al. (2010) Prognostic significance of tumorigenic cells with mesenchymal features in pancreatic adenocarcinoma. *J Natl Cancer Inst* 102:340–51.

Roessler E.; Belloni E.; Gaudenz K. et al. (1996) Mutations in the human Sonic Hedgehog gene cause holoprosencephaly. Nat Genet. 14:357-360

Rohatgi R.; Milenkovic L. & Scott M.P. (2007) Patched1 regulates hedgehog signalling at the primary cilium. *Science* 317:372-376

Rubin L.L. & de Sauvage F.J. (2006) Targeting the hedgehog pathway in cancer. *Nat Rev Drug Discov* 5:1026

Ruel L.; Rodriguez R.; Gallet A. et al. (2003) Stability and association of Smoothened, Costal2 and Fused with Cubitus interruptus are regulated by Hedgehog. *Nat Cell Biol* 5(10):907–13

Ruiz i Altaba A.; Sánchez P. & Dahmane N. (2002) Gli and hedgehog in cancer: tumours, embryos and stem cells. *Nat Rev Cancer.* 2(5):361-72.

Sell S. (2004). Stem cell origin of cancer and differentiation therapy. *Crit. Rev. Oncol. Hematol.* 51:1-28.

Stegman M.A.; Vallance J.E.; Elangovan G. et al. (2000) Identification of a tetrameric hedgehog signaling complex. *J Biol Chem.* 275(29):21809-12.

Taipale J. & Beachy P.A. (2001) The Hedgehog and Wnt signalling pathways in cancer. *Nature* 411 (6835):349–54.

Varjosalo M. & Taipale J. (2008) Hedgehog: functions and mechanisms. *Genes Dev* 22:2454-2472

Varnat F.; Duquet A.; Malerba M, et al. (2009) Human colon cancer epithelial cells harbour active HEDGEHOG-GLI signalling that is essential for tumour growth, recurrence, metastasis and stem cell survival and expansion. *Embo Mol Med* 1:338–51

Watkins D. N.; Berman D. M.; Burkholder S. G. et al. (2003) Hedgehog signalling within airway epithelial progenitors and in small-cell lung cancer. *Nature* 422: 313-317.

Wolff, C. et al. (2004) *iguana* encodes a novel zinc-finger protein with coiled-coil domains essential for Hedgehog signal transduction in the zebrafish embryo. *Genes Dev.* 18, 1565–1576

Yauch R.L.; Gould S.E.; Scales S.J. et al. (2008) A paracrine requeriment for hedgehog signalling in cancer. *Nature* 455: 406-410

Zhao C.; Chen A.; Jamieson C.H.; et al. (2009) Hedgehog signalling isessential for maintenance of cancer stem cells in myeloid leukaemia. *Nature* 458:776–9.

15

MicroRNAs: Small but Critical Regulators of Cancer Stem Cells

Jeffrey T. DeSano[1], Theodore S. Lawrence[1] and Liang Xu[1,2]
[1]*Department of Radiation Oncology, University of Michigan, Ann Arbor, MI*
[2]*Department of Molecular Biosciences, University of Kansas, Lawrence, KS, USA*

1. Introduction

Researchers have been attempting for decades to elucidate the molecular mechanisms at play within the cells that cause the development of cancer. There is now growing evidence that cancers may form from cancer stem cells. Somehow, a group of cells evolves that are immortal and can produce progenitor cells that can grow; however, the research community doesn't know how these cells lose control.

Recent studies have suggested the existence of a special small subpopulation of cancer cells that act as tumor-initiating cells or cancer stem cells. Cancer stem cells are implicated to maintain the self-renewal and unlimited growth capabilities of the cancer while only comprising a small fraction of the tumor. For this reason, cancer stem cells may be responsible for the tumor progression, drug/treatment resistance development, and metastasis.

Other studies have demonstrated that microRNAs (miRNAs) have a great deal to do with what genes are expressed/not expressed through their gene silencing capabilities. Interestingly, microRNAs might provide some new insight into the intricacies of cancer. These small RNA molecules could hold great potential therapeutically in the battle against cancer.

In this chapter, we discuss the functions of microRNAs and cancer stem cells and explore the link between these two topics. We also present methods to use in current and future research to study these topics and expound upon various molecular therapy options that could have implications in correcting cancer stem cell dysregulation and battling oncogenesis.

2. MicroRNAs

RNA interference is a vital system within cells that helps control which genes are active and to what extent they are activated. The two central small RNAs of RNA interference are small interfering RNA (siRNA) and microRNA (miRNA). Both are involved in gene silencing. siRNAs originate from the processing of a long, double-stranded RNAs and target mRNAs

---

Request for reprints: Liang Xu, M.D., Ph.D. Associate Professor, Department of Molecular Biosciences, University of Kansas; Departments of Urology, Radiation Oncology, University of Kansas Cancer Center, University of Kansas Medical School, Haworth Hall, Room, 4012 1200 Sunnyside Avenue, Lawrence, KS 66045-7534. e-mail: xul@ku.edu.

for degradation utilizing full complementary sequences (Zeng et al., 2003). In contrast, miRNAs are derived from the processing of short RNA hairpins and silence gene expression through mRNA degradation or translational repression of mRNAs with partially complementary target sequences (Zeng et al., 2003). However, there is a more important difference. siRNAs are often of exogenous origin, while miRNAs are endogenously encoded. Thus, miRNAs are naturally occurring in animal cells. For this reason, the use of miRNAs has interested many investigators because of their potential application to developing therapeutics to combat diseases such as cancer.

The biogenesis of miRNAs has been investigated and reviewed by many researchers and summarized in our recent review (DeSano and Xu, 2009). At the start, microRNAs are transcribed by the RNA polymerase II enzyme producing a long primary-miRNA (pri-miRNA) in the nucleus (Lee et al., 2004). Post-transcriptional modifications include a 5′ end cap structure and a 3′ end poly-adenylated tail that flank the pri-miRNAs (Cai et al., 2004). This suggests that pri-miRNAs are structurally and functionally similar to mRNAs. In addition to the 5′ cap and 3′ tail, pri-miRNAs contain specific hairpin-shaped stem-loop structures of ~70 nucleotides. These stem-loop structures are recognized and cleaved by an ~650 kDa nuclear microprocessor complex consisting of the RNase III endonuclease Drosha and the essential DiGeorge syndrome critical region gene 8 (DGCR8) binding protein, which yields a ~70 nucleotide hairpin intermediate (Qian et al., 2004). The resulting ~70 nucleotide hairpin intermediate (pre-miRNA) is transported into the cytoplasm from the nucleus by Exportin-5 and its cofactor Ran-GTP (Yi et al., 2003). While in the cytoplasm, the pre-miRNAs are further cleaved. This cleavage is carried out by a RNase III endonulease Dicer-1 and its essential transactivating response RNA binding protein (TRBP) (Haase et al., 2005). This produces a short imperfect double stranded miRNA duplex. Helicase then unwinds this imperfect miRNA duplex into a mature miRNA. Next, TRBP recruits the catalytic Argonaute 2 to the Dicer complex with the mature miRNA forming the RNA-induced silencing complex (RISC) (Chendrimada et al., 2005; Haase et al., 2005). The RISC subsequently regulates gene expression by mRNA degradation or translational repression via partially complementary sequences in the 3′-untranslated region (3′-UTR) of the targeted mRNA (Chekanova and Belostotsky, 2006; Croce and Calin, 2005; Zhang et al., 2007). In animals, microRNAs may also do this by targeting the coding regions of mRNAs (Rigoutsos, 2009). Therefore, miRNAs negatively regulate gene and protein expression via the RNA interference (RNAi) pathway.

Recently, miRNAs have been implicated to have a role in stem cell function. Stem cells are found throughout the human body and are essential to tissue development, replacement, and repair (Farnie and Clarke, 2007). This is because the level of expression of certain miRNAs is different in stem cells compared to normal tissues (Suh et al., 2004). Studies have analyzed miRNA expression profiles in undifferentiated human embryonic stem cells, partially differentiated embryoid bodies, and terminal differentiated cells. One analysis found that 104 miRNAs and 776 genes were differentially expressed among the three cells types (Ren et al., 2009). Another study found rapid regulation of certain miRNAs in response to differentiation (Stadler et al.). In addition to miRNA expression profiles, investigators have used Dicer-1 (*dcr*-1) mutants to confirm miRNAs' regulation of stem cell function. As discussed above, Dicer-1 plays an essential part in miRNA biogenesis; thus, a mutant *dcr*-1 would offer great insight into a proposed role of miRNAs in stem cells. Loss of *dcr*-1 resulted in early death in mouse models and depletion of stem cells in mouse embryos (Bernstein et al., 2003). This suggests that miRNAs do play a role in stem cell regulation because a disruption of the miRNA pathway results in a decreased stem cell population. Another study (Kanellopoulou et al., 2005) found that mutated *dcr*-1 in embryonic mouse stem cells lead to reduced miRNA expression and severe defects in stem cell differentiation *in vitro* and *in vivo*; in addition, re-expression of Dicer-1 reversed these phenotypes. These dcr-1 mutants data demonstrate that miRNAs have a fundamental role in regulating stem cell function.

MicroRNAs also can function in stem cell biology through epigenetic regulation. Epigenetic regulation, including DNA methylation and histone modification is known to play vital roles in regulating stem cell proliferation and differentiation (Szulwach et al.). A DNA methyl-CpG-binding protein (MeCP2) has been shown to epigenetically regulate specific miRNAs in adult neural stem cells (Szulwach et al.). This is a rather interesting finding because the interaction (if any) between the miRNA and epigenetic pathways is not well understood. This results demonstrates that there is specific cross talk between epigenetic regulation and the miRNA pathway (Szulwach et al.). This cross talk could be significant to modulating stem cell function and differientation. Changes in DNA methylation and histone modification also are characteristic of cancers. These epigenetic changes result in dysregulation of gene expression profiles leading to the development and progression of disease states (Sharma et al.). MicroRNAs could be affected by these epigenetic changes due to the cross talk between the two pathways. There are widespread changes in miRNA expression profiles during tumorigenesis (Sharma et al.). Therefore, microRNAs' role in stem cell regulation and cancer formation and progression are an attractive area of research.

3. Self-renewal of cancer stem cells

Stem cells are defined by their multi-lineage differentiation and their ability to undergo self-renewal (Dontu et al., 2003). This self-renewal can be either asymmetric or symmetric. Self-renewal is unique from other proliferative processes in that at least one of the progeny is identical to the initial stem cell. In all other replicative processes, the progeny of division undergo a series of differentiation events. In asymmetric stem cell self-renewal, one of the two progeny is identical to the initial stem cell, whereas the other cell is a committed progenitor cell, which undergoes cellular differentiation (Al-Hajj and Clarke, 2004). Since one stem cell is a product of asymmetrical self-renewal division, the stem cell number is maintained. However, in symmetrical self-renewal, two stem cells are produced, resulting in stem cell expansion. Both the self-renewal and differentiation of stem cells are regulated by the stem cell niche, which is the microenvironment surrounding the stem cell (Wicha, 2006).

Recently, evidence has emerged that suggests that a small subset of cancer cells in tumors have stem cell properties. The cancer stem hypothesis states that cancers are derived from a small fraction of cancer cells that constitute a reservoir of self-sustaining cells with the exclusive ability to self-renew and initiate/maintain the tumor (Papagiannakopoulos and Kosik, 2008). According to this cancer stem cell hypothesis, cancer stem cells are tumor-initiating cells that proliferate uniquely through self-renewal. Cancer stem cells are thought to only constitute a small fraction of the tumor, but may be responsible for tumor outgrowth, progression, metastasis, and treatment-resistance (Wicha, 2007). Thus, it has been hypothesized that to be maximally effective, cancer therapy should be directed against these cancer stem cells (Rich and Bao, 2007).

This self-renewal capability has also been demonstrated by examining the ability of subpopulations of tumor cells identified by cell surface markers to form tumors when transplanted into immunosuppressed NOD/SCID mice *in vivo*. This approach was first successfully used to demonstrate the existence of leukemic cancer stem cells (Bonnet and Dick, 1997). A similar approach has been utilized to identify a subpopulation of human mammary cancer cells that bear the $CD44^{+}CD24^{-}ESA^{+}$ Lineage^{-} that have the properties of breast cancer stem cells (Al-Hajj et al., 2003). After isolation from primary human breast cancer carcinomas or metastatic lesions, less than 100 of these cells are able to form tumors reproducibly, while tens of thousands of phenotypically distinct cancer cells are unable to generate tumors (Al-Hajj et al., 2003). Thus, the central feature of cancer stem cells is this relatively unlimited asymmetric self-renewal (Al-Hajj and Clarke, 2004).

In addition, an *in vitro* mammosphere assay has been developed to demonstrate that only a minority of cells in human cancers are capable of self-renewal. Using this mammosphere method, it was found that secondary mammospheres from the human breast cancer cell group bearing $Lin^{-}CD29^{H}CD24^{H}$ were larger in size and number compared with all other subpopulations of tumor cells (Zhang et al., 2008a). This suggests that these cells are tumor-initiating and undergo self-renewal. Thus, a certain subpopulation of cancer cells is able to self-renew and initiate tumor formation, supporting the term "cancer stem cells".

Self-renewal of cancer stem cells is thought to be a likely cause of the resistance seen of current cancer treatment and relapse in cancer patients. Recently, we have been provided with the first clinical evidence that implicates that a glioma stem cell/self-renewal phenotype is responsible for the treatment resistance seen in glioblastoma patients (Murat et al., 2008). Strong arguments can be made that genetic alterations cause cancer stem cell dysregulation, which results in unlimited self-renewal. It is believed that abnormal stem cell self-renewal is a likely necessity for cancer initiation, formation, and resistance to current therapies.

4. Signaling pathways of cancer stem cells

The question then becomes - How does irregular self-renewal capabilities occur in cancer stem cells? There is growing evidence that many pathways that have characteristically been connected to cancer also regulate normal stem cell development (Murat et al., 2008). This evidence suggests that these signaling pathways play a significant role in dysregulating stem cell genes in cancer stem cells leading to the formation and growth of tumors. The pathways of Bcl-2, Wnt, Hedgehog, Notch, Bmi-1, HMGA2, and CD44 have been found to be involved in the survival, self-renewal, and differentiation of cancer stem cells.

4.1 Bcl-2

Bcl-2 has been investigated rigorously because of its status as a proto-oncogene. It has been shown to be over expressed in many cancers and exhibits an anti-apoptotic effect in these cancers. Bcl-2 over-expression leads to increased number of stem cells and cancer stem cells, suggesting a role in the stem cell niche (Domen et al., 1998; Ji et al., 2009). Thus, Bcl-2 has been connected to the survival of stem cells and cancer stem cells because of its over expression in cancers.

4.2 Wnt

Wnt signaling is the next pathway. The presence of Wnt activates the Wnt receptor, causing a downstream accumulation *of β-catenin* in the cytoplasm. This accumulation of *β-catenin* is translocated to the nucleus and activates the expression of many genes associated with self-renewal. The Wnt pathway has been implicated in oncogenesis. Over-expression of *β-catenin* enlarges the pool of stem cells (Reya et al., 2003). Activation of *β-catenin* enhanced the self-renewal potential in leukemic stem cells (Jamieson et al., 2004). Therefore, Wnt signaling is involved in the self-renewal capability of cancer stem cells.

4.3 Hedgehog

The Hedgehog pathway is also important in the dysregulation of caner stem cells self-renewal potential. When Hedgehog is present, its receptor Patched is activated. This results in activation of Smoothened and later Gli transcription factors, which are translocated into the nucleus and regulates the transcription of certain genes including those that regulate self-renewal. Increased self-renewal has been shown to occur upon Hedgehog stimulation in hematopoietic stem cell populations (Bhardwaj et al., 2001). Many human cancers have activated levels of Hedgehog signal transduction (Xie et al., 1998). This suggests that dysregulation of self-renewal properties of cancer stem cells due to increased Hedgehog signaling could form cancer in humans.

4.4 Notch

The Notch pathway is significant as well. Notch is a transmembrane receptor that binds the ligand Delta. When Delta is present, an extracellular protease TACE cleaves the extracellular domain of Notch. This leads to cytoplasmic domain of Notch to be cleaved by γ-secretase. This newly liberated cytoplasmic portion of Notch is translocated into the nucleus where it binds to DNA-binding proteins of the CSL family. This activates transcription of genes utilized during development and renewal of adult tissues. Atypical Notch signaling has been demonstrated to promote self-renewal of mammary stem cells, as well as aids in the development of invasive breast cancer (Dontu et al., 2004; Farnie and Clarke, 2007). These findings suggest that Notch signaling transduction could lead to the dysregulation of self renewal in cancer stem cells.

4.5 Bmi-1

Bmi-1 signaling has been implicated in this discussion because of its effects on cancer stem cell self-renewal potential. Loss of Bmi-1 resulted in a decrease in stem cell differentiation and self-renewal (Zencak et al., 2005). Aberrant levels of Bmi-1 have also been demonstrated to generate cancers (Sparmann and van Lohuizen, 2006). Bmi-1 activation was found in $CD44^{+}CD24^{-/low}Lin^{-}$ human breast cancer stem cells (Liu et al., 2006). In addition, modulation of Bmi-1 expression alters the mammosphere-initiating cell number and size (Liu et al., 2006). This suggests a role in the dysregulation of self-renewal properties in cancer stem cells and future research is needed to gain insight into the Bmi-1 pathway.

4.6 HMGA2

HMGA2 has been associated in the self-renewal potential and survival of cancer stem cells. HMGA2 is thought to regulate gene expression by modulating macromolecule complexes that are involved in many biological processes. HMGA proteins are expressed during development; specifically, HMGA2 has been suggested to control growth, proliferation, and differentiation (Fusco and Fedele, 2007). In addition, HMGA2 has been found to be over-expressed in lung and pancreatic carcinomas and metastasis (Abe et al., 2003; Fusco and

Fedele, 2007; Meyer et al., 2007). Thus, excessive HMGA2 signaling could dysregulate cell survival and self-renewal in cancer stem cells.

4.7 CD44

CD44 is another intriguing pathway being implicated with cancer stem cells. So far, there is no specific cellular marker for CSC. We and many others have found that pancreatic cancer stem cells from cell lines or primary tumors are enriched in CD44+ population; p53 directly regulates CD44; pancreatic cancer cells lacking functional p53, especially cancer stem cells, have high *CD44*, low miR-34 and high *Bcl-2/Notch* expression. Recent studies indicate that CD44 molecules activate down-stream Nanog that in turn activate Sox2 and Rex1 (Bourguignon et al., 2008; Kasper, 2008), and these transcription factors have been implicated in stem cell maintenance. Besides being a cellular marker for CSC, CD44 has recently been functionally linked to cancer stem cell maintenance, growth and resistance (Bourguignon et al., 2008; Godar et al., 2008; Peterson et al., 2007; Pries et al., 2008). Anti-CD44 antibody treatment markedly reduced leukemic repopulation by targeting CD44+ leukemic stem cells (Jin et al., 2006). A recent study shows that CD44 downstream signaling CD44—Nanog—Sox2/Rex1 and CD44—Nanog—Stat3--MDR1/P-gp are involved in CD44+ tumor cell resistance and progression (Bourguignon et al., 2008). We have observed that anti-CD44 mAb H4C4 inhibits MiaPaCa2 tumorspheres, reduces CD44+/CD133+ CSC number and blocks tumor-initiation, accompanied by CD44 downstream signaling inhibition (Hao, et al, manuscript in preparation). Therefore, aberrant CD44 signaling could be rather important in the dysregulation seen in cancer stem cells that results in oncognesis, tumor progression, metastasis, resistance to treatments, and relapse in cancer patients.

5. Examples of MicroRNAs regulating cancer stem cells

Over the past couple of years, cancer research has focused on miRNAs and the possibilities of the cancer stem cell hypothesis. Investigators have shown that cancer stem cells have aberrant levels of specific miRNAs, which results in dysregulation of the self-renewal potential through the signaling pathways described above in these cancer stem cells. This dysregulation is a very plausible explanation to the initiation, formation, and sustainment of tumors.

MicroRNAs in cancer cells can acts as oncogenes or tumor suppressors (DeSano and Xu, 2009). Oncogenic miRNAs are often called oncomiRs. They are usually a dominant, gain-of-function mutation. As a result, they are up-regulated in cancer cells. Specific miRNAs like miR-21, miR-17-92 cluster, miR-135, and miR-294 have been shown to be oncogenic miRNAs.

5.1 miR-21

The microRNA miR-21 has been shown to be overexpressed in tumor tissues (Gao et al.). It has been shown to function as an oncogene in breast cancer through the modulation of Bcl-2 and Programmed Cell Death 4 (PDCD4) (Asangani et al., 2008; Frankel et al., 2008). It has also been shown to play a pivotal role in gastric cancer pathogenesis and progression (Zhang et al., 2008b). Thus, over-expression of miR-21 leads to dysregulation of Bcl-2 and modulation the cancer stem cell environment, which results in increased turmor growth and decreased apoptosis.

5.2 miR-17-92

The miR-17-92 cluster consists of seven miRNAs. This cluster is significantly over-expressed in lung cancers (Hayashita et al., 2005). It does act as an oncogenic miRNA. It has been shown that an introduction of miR-17-92 into hematopoietic stem cells drastically accelerates the formation of lymphoid malignancies (Hayashita et al., 2005). Interestingly, miR-17-92 is connected to the Hedgehog pathway. In engineered medulloblastomas, miR-17-92-induced tumors were found to activate the Hedgehog signaling pathway (Uziel et al., 2009). This implicates a result of increased self-renewal potential through the modulation of the Hedgehog pathway in cancer stem cells.

5.3 miR-135

The microRNA miR-135 also regulates cancer stem cells through its oncogenic properties. The miR-135a and miR-135b miRNAs were found to be greatly up-regulated in colorectal adenomas and carcinomas, functioning to down-regulate APC gene expression, which is part of the Wnt signaling pathway (Nagel et al., 2008). If APC is not expressed at the correct levels, *β-catenin* will accumulate, leading to the activation of self-renewal genes. Thus, miR-135 plays an oncogenic role in modulating Wnt signaling transduction, resulting in dysregulation of cancer stem cells.

5.4 miR-29a

Recent research has found that miR-29a plays a vital role in cancer stem cells. It has been shown that miR-29a is highly expressed in hematopoietic stem cells and acute myeloid leukemia (Han et al.). This expression of miR-29a results in the acquisition of aberrant self-renewal capacity (Han et al.). This data suggests that miR-29a initiates cancer formation through the dysregulation of self-renewing leukemia stem cells. Over-expression of these oncomiRs leads to further cancer progression and resistance to treatment.

5.5 miR-294

The microRNA miR-294 is particularly interesting because it is a representative member of the embryonic stem cells cell cycle regulating (ESCC) miRNAs. In DGCR8-/- knockouts, the introduction of miR-294 activates numerous self-renewal genes, such as *Myc*, Oct4, Sox2, Tcf3, and Nanog (Melton et al.). This data suggests that miR-294, and possibly other ESCC miRNAs, modulates the self-renewal potential through regulating many different pathways that are important in stem cells. A role in cancer stem cells needs to addressed in the future and could add some serious insight into the intricacies of cancer stem cell self-renewal and differentiation.

Nevertheless, not all miRNAs act as oncogenes. The expression of some miRNAs is decreased in cancer cells. These miRNAs are tumor suppressor miRNAs and sometimes called TSmiRs. They are usually a loss-of-function, recessive mutation. TSmiRs, when normally expressed, prevent tumor formation and development; however, in cancer, their expression is down-regulated, allowing increased disease progression.

5.6 miR-128

The first example of tumor suppressor miRNAs that play a role in cancer stem cells is miR-128. Levels of miR-128 were drastically reduced in high grade gliomas (Godlewski et al., 2008). This suggests that miR-128 is a tumor suppressor. Upon introduction of miR-128, the proliferation and growth of glioma cells were inhibited (Godlewski et al., 2008). Researchers were able to elucidate the mechanism involved. Expression of miR-128 down-regulated Bmi-1 signal transduction (Godlewski et al., 2008). Therefore, miR-128 blocked the self-renewal of glioma cancer cells via Bmi-1 modulation. This demonstrates the importance of miR-128 in regulating the self-renewal potential of cancer stem cells.

5.7 miR-199b-5p

Another intriguing miRNA is miR-199b-5p. It is a tumor suppressor miRNA. In metastatic cancer patients, its expression is lost (Garzia et al., 2009). This miR-199b-5p was discovered to down-regulate the expression of a transcription factor of the Notch signaling pathway. Upon introduction of miR-199b-5p, the Notch signaling was blocked and the subpopulation of medulloblastoma stem-cell-like cells decreased (Garzia et al., 2009). Thus, miR-199b-5p leads to a decrease of the self-renewal properties of cancer stem cells.

5.8 Let-7

Let-7 is a tumor suppressor miRNA that has garnered much interest in the cancer research community. Let-7 expression levels are reduced in various cancers relative to normal tissues (Johnson et al., 2007). Let-7 is not expressed in breast-tumor initiating cells (Yu et al., 2007). Upon expression of let-7 in breast tumor-initiating cells, it was shown that let-7 regulates the self-renewal *in vitro,* multipotent differentiation, and the ability to form tumors (Yu et al., 2007). These are the key features of cancer stem cells. It has been found to play a role in many pathways. Expression of let-7 has been shown to down-regulate HMGA2, RAS, Lin28, Sall4, and Myc (Johnson et al., 2005; Mayr et al., 2007; Melton et al.). All of these let-7 targets help regulate self-renewal. Thus, let-7 is a tumor suppressor miRNA that negatively regulates many targets in different pathways that all dysregulate the self-renewal capability of cancer stem cells.

5.9 miR-34

Another miRNA of great interest is miR-34. This TSmiR is down-regulated in various types of cancer, suggesting its tumor suppressor properties (He et al., 2007). We have researched this TSmiR rigorously. We used various assays to determine miR-34's role in cancer stem cells. In p53-deficient human gastric and pancreatic cancer cells, restoration of miR-34 inhibited cell growth and induced G1 phase block and apoptosis (Ji et al., 2008; Ji et al., 2009). This indicated that p53 function may be restored my miR-34. Restoration of miR-34 inhibited tumorsphere growth *in vitro* and tumor initiation *in vivo,* which is implicated to be correlated to the self-renewal potential of cancer stem cells (Ji et al., 2008; Ji et al., 2009). MicroR-34's mediated suppression of self-renewal seems to be through the direct modulation of its downstream targets of Bcl-2, Notch, and HMGA2 (Ji et al., 2008; Ji et al., 2009). This indicates that miR-34 is involved in the gastric and pancreatic cancer cells' self-renewal/differentiation decision making. Therefore, miR-34 is a rather significant tumor suppressor miRNA of cancer stem cells by regulating both apoptosis and self-renewal capabilities. Decreased expression of TSmiRs like these discussed above leads to cancer initiation and further tumor progression. **Figure 1** provides an overall schematic review of the stem cell miRNAs discussed concerning their interactions with stem cell signaling pathways in cancer stem cells.

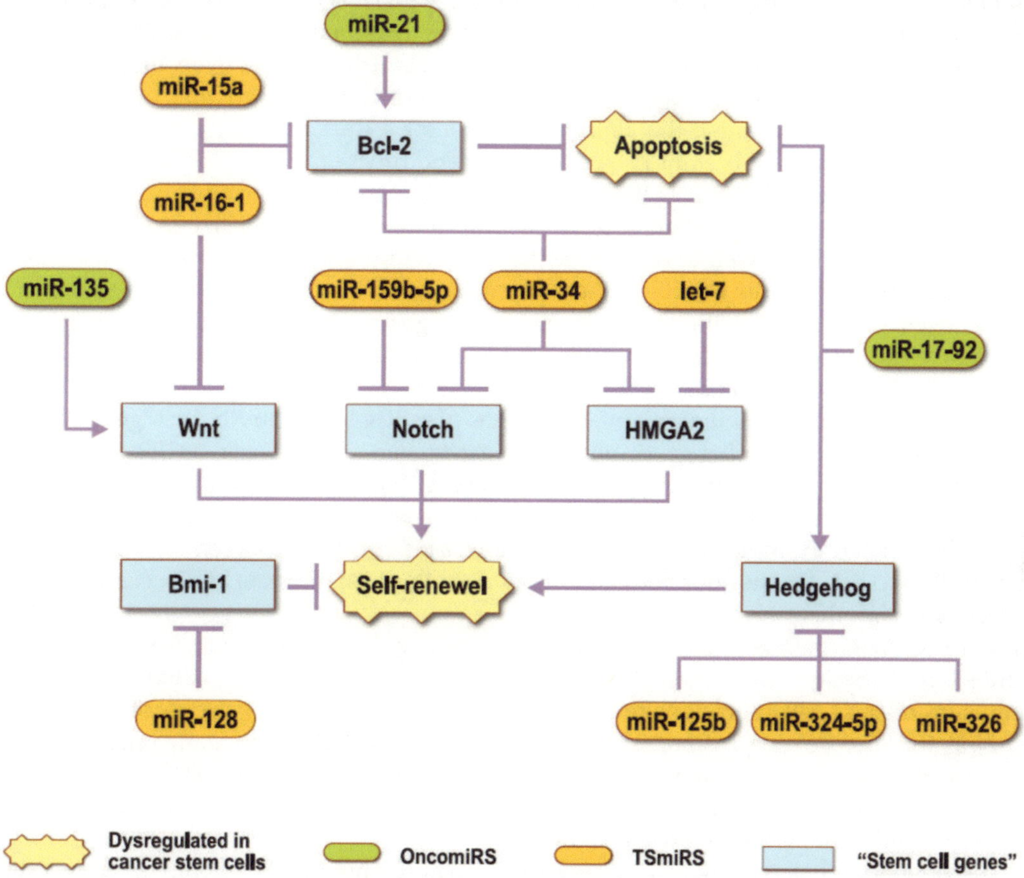

Fig. 1. **Potential "stem cell miRNAs" that modulate "stem cell genes" related to cancer stem cells.** Certain miRNAs have been shown to be aberrantly expressed in cancer. OncomiRs, which initiate cancer development, are over-expressed. TSmiRs, which prevent tumor development, are decreased. These miRNAs regulate genes that are implicated in stem cells. The aberrant expression of these potential "stem cell miRNAs" in cancer suggests that dysregulation of "stem cell genes" leads to increased levels of self-renewal and decreased levels of apoptosis within cancer stem cells. This results in further cancer progression. (Modified from DeSano and Xu, "MicroRNA regulation of cancer stem cells and therapeutic implications." AAPS J, 2009; 11(4):682-692 (DeSano and Xu, 2009). With permission.)

6. Cancer stem cells and miRNA connection in support of oncogenesis

There are aberrant expression levels of miRNAs in cancer. Tumors analyzed by miRNA profiling have been found to have significantly different miRNA profiles compared to normal cells from the same tissue (Calin et al., 2006). In addition, miRNAs have been found with rather convincing evidence to be important factors in stem cell biology. Using cDNA cloning, multiple miRNAs have been found to be uniquely expressed in human embryonic stem cells compared to their differentiated counterparts (Suh et al., 2004). Based on these findings, it is rather intriguing that undifferentiated stem cells exhibit expression profiles of miRNAs that are reminiscent of cancer cells (Papagiannakopoulos and Kosik, 2008).

Still further research has allowed us to merge this obvious parallel even further. Recent evidence shows that there is a distinct subpopulation of cancer cells acting as cancer stem cells within tumors that have the ability to self-renew - thus initiating, maintaining, and progressing the cancer. Aberrant gene expression and function are hallmark characteristics of cancer. As a result of this, it is thought that genetic alterations from acquired epigenetic abnormalities cause dysregulation of genes within cancer stem cells (Zhao et al., 2008). The cancer stem cells are allowed to escape the restrictions of the stem cell niche because of this dysregulation. This results in self-renewal potential. Microenvironmental signals or factors are believed to account for the cancer stem cells' epigenetic abnormalities, resulting in the interference or silencing of certain genes. Thus, an underlying sub-cellular process must account for the cancer stem cell dysregulation.

Knowing that cancers exhibit aberrant expressions of miRNAs and miRNAs in general work through negatively regulating gene and protein expression, miRNAs can be this sub-cellular process. It is suggested and supported by recent findings that miRNAs cause gene dysregulation in cancer stem cells that leads to oncogenesis and further disease progression. All of the miRNA examples discussed have showcased this link between cancer stem cells and miRNAs. Yet, the question remains – how does this link translate and occur within the cancer stem cells themselves?

Most researchers believed and thus previous research has focused on the conventional miRNA hypothesis – that one miRNA is up-regulated or down-regulated, leading the activation of stem cell gene signaling pathways, which results in the cancer stem cell self-renewal and disease progression. This hypothesis is supported by the many oncogenic and tumor suppressor miRNA examples outlined. It is a rather straight forward hypothesis and data has been generated that has demonstrated these effects. However, could it be this simple? Could more be going on sub-cellularly?

A new possibility has emerged from the latest research. This new possibility proposes that the dysregulation in cancer stem cells is a result of an antagonism network between different miRNAs that stabilizes the switch between self-renewal ability and differentiation (Melton et al.). These different miRNAs could have oncogenic or tumor suppressor characteristics like the conventional hypothesis states. Nevertheless, this new possibility of an antagonism network implicates that miRNAs can regulate other miRNAs, initiating downstream dysregulation of cancer stem cell self-renewal potential. Researchers have found that the let-7 and the embryonic stem cells cell cycle regulating (ESCC) miRNAs like miR-294 have opposing effects of embryonic stem cell self-renewal and proposed that these miRNAs act in self-reinforcing loops to maintain self-renewal states versus differentiated states (Melton et al.). In the self-renewing state, ESCC miRNAs indirectly increase expression of Lin28 and c-Myc, and Lin 28 functions to block the maturation of let-7 (Melton et al.). Upregulated c-Myc forms a positive feedback loop in which c-Myc, N-Myc, Oct4, Sox2, and Nanog bind and activate ESCC miRNA expression (Melton et al.). This keeps the cells in a self renewal capable state. Thus, ESCC miRNAs like miR-294 prevent co-expression of let-7 miRNAs. Oncogenic miRNAs could regulate and block co-expression of tumor suppressor miRNAs causing cancer stem cell dysregulation.

In order to differentiate, Oct4, Sox2, and Nanog expression are down-regulated, resulting in the loss of Lin28 expression (Melton et al.). Losing Lin28 expression means that let-7 expression increases. This is even enhanced by a new positive feedback loop where let-7 suppresses the expression of its own negative regulator Lin28 (Melton et al.). This causes a loss of self-renewal potential and differentiation of the stem cells. In the differentiated state, let-7's down-regulation of Myc expression prevents co-expression of the ESCC miRNAs (Melton et al.). In this instance, tumor suppressor miRNAs regulate and prevent co-expression of oncogenic miRNAs resulting in dysregulation of cancer stem cells.

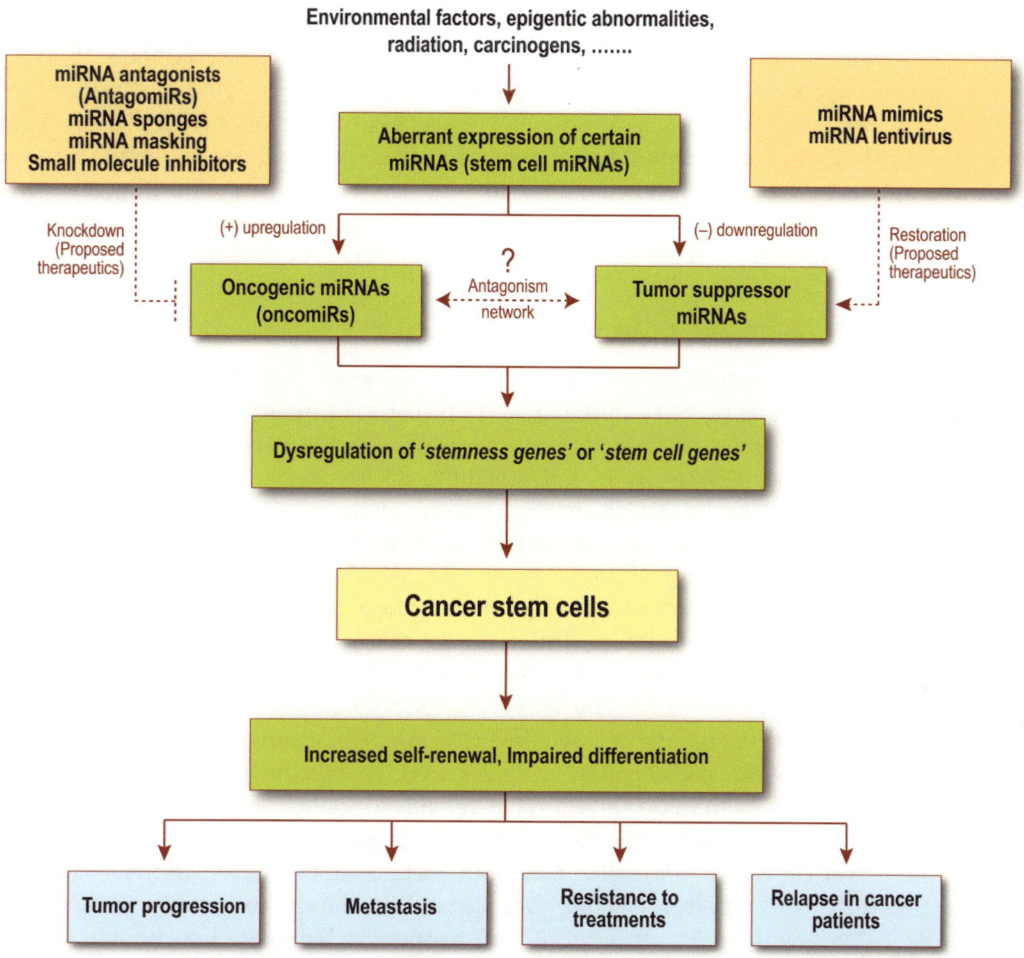

Fig. 2. **Link between miRNAs and cancer stem cells.** Aberrant expressions of miRNAs, either as oncogenic or tumor suppressor miRNAs, can lead to dysregulation of stem cell genes, causing increased self-renewal potential and impaired differentiation in cancer stem cells. This dysregulation subsequently results in carcinogenesis and oncogenesis. It is proposed that miRNA antagonists can knockdown the effects of oncogenic miRNAs, and miRNA mimics can restore the capabilities of tumor suppressor miRNAs. Therefore, miRNA could be a vital tool in addressing cancer stem cell dysregulation. MicroRNA-based molecular therapy could hold great therapeutic potential against cancer progression, resistance, and relapse. (Modified from DeSano and Xu, "MicroRNA regulation of cancer stem cells and therapeutic implications." AAPS J, 2009; 11(4):682-692 (DeSano and Xu, 2009). With permission.)

Thus, an antagonism network of miRNAs that stabilizes the switch between self-renewal and differentiation could be a possible sub-cellular mechanism that could explain the dysregulation of stem cell genes seen in cancer stem cells. This new antagonism network hypothesis is intriguing and needs to be further developed as well as the conventional miRNA hypothesis. Recent research has established and **Figure 2** outlines a rather convincing link between miRNAs and cancer stem cell dysregulation (DeSano and Xu, 2009). This dysregulation leads to increase self-renewal, resulting in tumor initiation and progression, metastasis, resistance to treatments, and relapse in cancer patients (Ji et al., 2010). Still, the underlying mechanism has evaded researchers. Studying and performing experiments that support or debunk either of these hypotheses will help the oncology community gain great insight into what is going on sub-cellularly in these terrible diseases and will allow us to attack the cancer with greater efficacy. Therefore, confronting abnormal miRNA expression levels with molecular miRNA therapy can be a promising and powerful tool to tackle oncogenesis (DeSano and Xu, 2009; Ji et al., 2009; Ji et al., 2010).

7. Potential miRNA-based molecular therapeutics

The distinct and clear connection between aberrant expression levels of certain miRNAs and dysregulation of cancer stem cells offers the scientific community an unique opportunity to fight cancer initiation and sustained development through the use of molecular miRNA therapies that target oncogenic or tumor suppressor miRNAs. In theory, molecular miRNA-based cancer therapy should eradicate the cancer stem cells' self-renewal potential, significantly reduce the cancer's resistance to current cancer treatment, and hinder relapse in sick patients.

For this reason, the development of miRNA-based molecular therapeutics has been at the forefront of oncology research recently. Still, there are many critical experimental steps that are required. The development of miRNA/RNAi-based therapeutics must include miRNA profiling of cancer compared to healthy tissue (specifically cancer stem cells compared to differentiated cells), functional analysis of dysregulated miRNAs, and *in vitro* followed by *in vivo* studies that include the use of differing RNA-based therapeutic techniques that address the aberrant miRNA expression levels (Papagiannakopoulos and Kosik, 2008). For oncogenic miRNAs, a therapeutic knockdown effect is needed because these miRNAs cause cancer when over-expressed. Potential therapies include antagomiRs, miRNA sponges, miRNA masking, and small molecule inhibitors. For tumor suppressor miRNAs, a therapeutic restoration is necessary because their expression levels are knockdown or non-existent in cancerous tissues. MicroRNA mimics or lentiviruses are possible methods that can re-establish the tumor suppressor capabilities of these miRNAs. All of these molecular therapeutic possibilities have the distinct purpose of regulating aberrant miRNA levels, which causes cancer stem cell dysregulation and disease progression. They could have a powerful impact on clinical cancer research.

For oncogenic miRNAs, an antagomiR (anti-miRNA oligonucleotide) can be used to block the effects of the oncomiR. The antagomiR uses competition to block the oncogenic interaction between the upregulated miRNA and its target mRNA, resulting in cancer suppression (Weiler et al., 2006). For example, an anti-miR-21 oligonucleotide was transfected into breast cancer MCF-7 cells and it was shown that this antagomiR suppressed cell growth in vitro and tumor growth in vivo by increasing apoptosis and decreasing cell proliferation (Si et al., 2007). Thus, antagomiRs are a promising molecular therapeutic targeting oncogenic miRNA-initiated cancer stem cell dysregulation.

Another potential therapy against oncogenic miRNAs is miRNA sponges. A miRNA sponge is a synthetic mRNA, which contains multiple binding sites for an endogenous miRNA (Li et al., 2009). The sponge, in effect, competitively "soaks" up the oncogenic miRNA. This prevents the interaction between the miRNA and its specific mRNA targets that cause cancer stem cell dysregulation through the activation of stem cell genes. A single miRNA sponge could be used to stifle an entire miRNA family because of its multiple binding sites. These miRNA sponges inhibited miRNAs as effectively as antagomiRs *in vitro* (Ebert et al., 2007). However, the efficacy of these miRNA sponges need to be evaluated *in vivo* (Li et al., 2009). Still, miRNA sponges have great potential as a molecular therapy targeted against oncogenic miRNAs.

MicroRNA masking could be used to fight cancer initiation and progression through its regulation of aberrant miRNA expression levels. Each miRNA may regulate tens if not hundreds of genes, and a single gene can be regulated by multiple miRNAs (Li et al., 2009). The potential molecular therapies discussed above are only sequence-specific, which produces many obstacles like off-target side effects and undesired toxicity that researchers must confront. MicroRNA masking is instead gene-specific. MicroRNA masking employs the strategy of designing a sequence with perfect complementarity to the binding site in the target gene for an endogenous miRNA, which can form a duplex with the target mRNA with higher affinity (Li et al., 2009; Xiao et al., 2007). This miRNA masking effectively blocks access of the miRNA to its binding site without any possible side effects because it is gene-specific instead of sequence-specific like the antagomiRs or sponges. MicroRNA masks that were complementary to cardiac pacemaker channel genes HCN2 and HCN4 significantly enhanced HCN2/HCN4 expression and function by inhibiting the suppressive actions of endogenous miR-1 and miR-133 (Xiao et al., 2007). These results demonstrate that miRNA masking can be an important molecular miRNA-interfering therapeutic strategy that is gene-specific and can be directed against aberrant oncogenic miRNA expression levels that activate self-renewal genes in cancer stem cells.

Oncogenic miRNAs can be down-regulated and even knocked out through the use of small molecule inhibitors. Since oncogenic miRNAs cause cancer stem cell dysregulation and disease progression when over-expressed, the small molecule inhibitors must block the formation or generation of these miRNAs. Thus, small molecule inhibitors that target the steps in the biogenesis of miRNAs could hold much promise. Azobenzene has been shown to be a specific and effective inhibitor of the biogenesis of miR-21 (Gumireddy et al., 2008). In an experiment that utilized miRNA array analysis, it was demonstrated that there was a rapid alteration of miRNA levels in response to the potent hydroxamic acid HDACi LAQ824 in the breast cancer cell line SKBr3 (Scott et al., 2006). In addition to blocking miRNA formation and function, small molecule inhibitors of the miRNA pathway could be promising tools used to boost patient response to existing chemo- and radiotherapies (Gumireddy et al., 2008). This can be seen in data from our lab. We have employed multiple small molecule inhibitors – Gossypol, SH-130, Celastrol, and Embelin – and demonstrated that they all can sensitize cancer cells to ionizing radiation therapy and induce apoptosis *in vitro* and *in vivo* (Dai et al., 2009; Dai et al., 2008; Lian J, 2010; Meng et al., 2008; Wu et al., 2010). Therefore, small molecule inhibitors have great potential in addressing oncogenic miRNAs that cause dysregulation of cancer stem cells. They could fight against tumor initiation and progression, metastasis, resistance to treatments, and relapse in cancer patients.

Nevertheless, not all miRNAs that cause cancer are oncogenic/up-regulated. Many tumor suppressor miRNAs are down-regulated in cancer tissues. Thus, their expression needs to be reinstated in order to fight the disease. The first way that we can therapeutically attack the down-regulated tumor suppressor miRNAs is through the introduction of miRNA mimics. MicroRNA mimics are small, chemically modified, double-stranded RNA molecules that mimic endogenous mature miRNA molecules (Li et al., 2009). These miRNA mimics are simply just re-introducing RNA molecules that can pose and fill the role of the missing endogenous miRNA molecules that were down-regulated due to mutation, etc. For example, we introduced miR-34 mimics into cancer cells by transfection. These miR-34 mimics were found to arrest the cell cycle in the G1 phase, significantly increase the activation of caspase-3 and apoptosis, and decrease the expression of its downstream targets of bcl-2, Notch, and HMGA2 (Ji et al., 2008). The use of this mimic restored miR-34 with its tumor suppressor potential and capabilities. Thus, the use of miRNA mimics as a therapy to restore the expression of tumor suppressor miRNAs could help in defeating the aberrant miRNA expression profiles that cause cancer stem cell dysregulation.

However, miRNA mimics might not be the greatest molecular therapy for tumor suppressor miRNAs because the transfection of mimics can only last a couple of days and thus, the long-term biological effects cannot be examined. Nevertheless, there are ways to overcome this obstacle. One of these ways is viral vector-based gene restoration (Li et al., 2009). Researchers have been able to engineer lentiviral vector systems. Cells can be infected with a lentivirus that expresses a certain miRNA. This infection re-establishes the tumor suppressor miRNA back into the cell, and this lentiviral vector system generates stable cells that continue to express the miRNA. These stable tumor suppressor miRNA-expressing cells can be analyzed for a long period, which solves the dilemma posed by the miRNA mimic therapy. In our lab, we infected gastric cancer cells with a lentivirus that expressed miR-34a. This produced stable cancer cells that expressed miR-34a. This lentivirus was found to inhibit cell growth and tumorsphere formation (Ji et al., 2008). These results showed the promise of the lentiviral system *in vitro* and *in vivo*. We also tested this lentiviral system in pancreatic cancer stem cells and observed the same effects (Ji et al., 2009). The lentivirus vector system was able to restore the tumor suppressor ability of miR-34. Therefore, viral vector-based miRNA restoration has potential to reinstate tumor suppressor miRNAs that have been down-regulated or knocked out, resulting in cancer stem cell dysregulation and tumor development.

8. The seemingly never solved problem – delivery, delivery, delivery

To achieve a strong therapeutic effect with any of these potential molecular therapies, we must be able to translate our research from our labs to the clinics. However, in order to be clinically ready, the miRNA-based therapeutics must be effectively, efficiently, and functionally delivered to the cancerous tumor. This has been a great challenge for researchers since the beginning of cancer therapy.

A new exciting field has emerged that has focused on nanotechnology for systemic delivery of therapeutics *in vivo*. In theory, the nanoparticle would encompass the miRNA-based therapeutic, target it to the cancerous tumor, and effectively and efficiently deliver it to the cancer cells while bypassing (and not affecting) the normal, healthy cells in the body. Nanoparticle technology could be essential to delivering a wide variety of therapies to various yet specific cells in the body. It could be a part of breakthrough treatments for many diseases that could link *in vitro* and *in vivo* studies. Researchers have tirelessly attempted to develop a nanoparticle system that would allow this to happen.

Many attempts have failed; however, some strategies have been proven to be rather successful. The human transferrin protein receptor (TFR) has been known to be up-regulated in malignant cancer cells. Using patients with metastatic melanoma, it was shown that a synthetic nanoparticle delivery system that contains a linear, cycodextrin-based polymer, a human transferrin protein (TF) targeting ligand on its exterior to engage TF receptors, a hydrophilic polymer used to promote nanoparticle stability in biological fluids, and siRNA designed to reduce the expression of RRM2, reduced RRM2 mRNA levels as well as RRM2 protein levels (Davis et al.). Tumor biopsies from melanoma patients obtained after treatment showed the presence of intracellularly localized nanoparticles in amounts that correlate with dose levels of the nanoparticles administered (Davis et al.). This is the first in-human phase I clinical trial involving the effective systemic administration of siRNA to patients with solid tumors using a targeted, nanoparticle delivery system (Davis et al.). This study demonstrates that systemic administration of siRNA to a human can produce an inhibition effect of a specific gene by an RNAi mechanism. This is rather exciting and because siRNA was successfully targeted and delievered one can infer that a systemic administration of miRNA-based therapeutics can be effectively delivered to cancer cells via nanoparticles.

We have developed a tumor-specific, ligand-targeting, self-assembled, nanoparticle-DNA lipoplex systems designed for systemic gene therapy of cancer (US Patents No. **6,749,863** and **7,479,276**) (Xu et al., 2002a; Xu et al., 2002b). These nanovector systems employ transferrin or scFv against transferrin receptors as tumor-targeting ligands (Xu et al., 2002a; Xu et al., 2002b). When using Tf as a targeting ligand, we obtained the self-assembled nanovectors at the sizes of 50-90nm, with highly compact structure and favored surface charge (Xu et al., 2002a,b). These nanovectors have novel nanostructures that resembles a virus particle with a dense core enveloped by a membrane coated with Tf molecules spiking on the surface (Xu et al., 2002a,b). This nanovector system demonstrates promising efficacy and specificity in targeted delivery of various genes and anti-sense oligonucleotides like p53 to cancer *in vivo* compared to normal tissues (Xu et al., 1997; Xu et al., 1999). This nanovector system shows promising efficiency and specificity in targeted delivery of various genes and anti-sense oligonucleotides to cancer but not normal tissues *in vivo.* In the AACR 101th Annual Meeting, Washington, DC, April 17-21, 2010, at the Late-breaking Oral Presentation session on clinical trials, Drs. Pirollo and Chang reported the success of a first-in-man, Phase I trial of this nanovector, TfRscFv-nano-p53 (SGT-53, NCT00470613, ClinicalTrials.gov). The nanovectors are well tolerated in humans and already showed early responses. The exogenous p53 expression was observed in human cancer tissues in a SGT-53 dose-dependent manner, but *not* in normal tissues. The study demonstrates that the nanovectors are safe and effective to deliver gene therapeutics to both primary tumors and metastatic lesions. These unprecedented findings in cancer gene therapy trial subjects represent a major breakthrough in the field and suggest that delivery of genes to tumors with selectivity is indeed possible (Pirollo, *et al*, LB-172, www.aacr.org). The success of these nanovectors provides a potential and rather promising tumor-targeted delivery system for novel RNAi-based therapeutics. This is a thrilling possibility because packaging miRNA-based therapeutics discussed above into nanoparticles that can be effectively and efficiently targeted and delivered to cancerous tumors could remedy aberrant miRNA expression levels that are responsible for cancer stem cell dysregulation and subsequent oncogenesis.

9. Conclusion

In this chapter, we explore the connection between microRNAs and cancer stem cells. Abnormal miRNA expression profiles of oncogenic and/or tumor suppressor miRNAs are linked to the activation of stem cell signaling pathways in cancer stem cells. This dysregulation of cancer stem cells leads to disease initiation, development, progression, metastasis, resistance to current treatments, and relapse in patients. Accordingly, the development and use molecular miRNA therapies are imperative to addressing oncogenesis. In addition and maybe more importantly, effective and efficient packaging, targeting, and delivery of these miRNA-based therapeutics needs to be addressed. Nanoparticle technology could hold the key to accomplishing this. For this reason, future research needs to be aimed at developing nanoparticle delivery systems as well as uncovering the subcellular intricacies of miRNA regulation of cancer stem cells' self-renewal potential and capabilities. Defeating cancer stem cell dysregulation through molecular miRNA therapies could aid in the fight against cancer progression, resistance, and relapse.

10. Acknowledgements

We wish to thank Mr. Steven Kronenberg for graphical support and expertise in producing the figures. This chapter was supported in part by NIH grants CA121830, CA121830S1, CA128220, CA134655 and The Fund for Cancer Research (to L. X.). J. D. is a University of Michigan Undergraduate Research Opportunity Program (UROP) student.

11. References

Abe, N., Watanabe, T., Suzuki, Y., Matsumoto, N., Masaki, T., Mori, T., Sugiyama, M., Chiappetta, G., Fusco, A., and Atomi, Y. (2003). An increased high-mobility group A2 expression level is associated with malignant phenotype in pancreatic exocrine tissue. British journal of cancer *89*, 2104-2109.

Al-Hajj, M., and Clarke, M. F. (2004). Self-renewal and solid tumor stem cells. Oncogene *23*, 7274-7282.

Al-Hajj, M., Wicha, M. S., Benito-Hernandez, A., Morrison, S. J., and Clarke, M. F. (2003). Prospective identification of tumorigenic breast cancer cells. Proceedings of the National Academy of Sciences of the United States of America *100*, 3983-3988.

Asangani, I. A., Rasheed, S. A., Nikolova, D. A., Leupold, J. H., Colburn, N. H., Post, S., and Allgayer, H. (2008). MicroRNA-21 (miR-21) post-transcriptionally downregulates tumor suppressor Pdcd4 and stimulates invasion, intravasation and metastasis in colorectal cancer. Oncogene *27*, 2128-2136.

Bernstein, E., Kim, S. Y., Carmell, M. A., Murchison, E. P., Alcorn, H., Li, M. Z., Mills, A. A., Elledge, S. J., Anderson, K. V., and Hannon, G. J. (2003). Dicer is essential for mouse development. Nat Genet *35*, 215-217.

Bhardwaj, G., Murdoch, B., Wu, D., Baker, D. P., Williams, K. P., Chadwick, K., Ling, L. E., Karanu, F. N., and Bhatia, M. (2001). Sonic hedgehog induces the proliferation of primitive human hematopoietic cells via BMP regulation. Nature immunology *2*, 172-180.

Bonnet, D., and Dick, J. E. (1997). Human acute myeloid leukemia is organized as a hierarchy that originates from a primitive hematopoietic cell. Nature medicine *3*, 730-737.

Bourguignon, L. Y., Peyrollier, K., Xia, W., and Gilad, E. (2008). Hyaluronan-CD44 interaction activates stem cell marker Nanog, Stat-3-mediated MDR1 gene expression, and ankyrin-regulated multidrug efflux in breast and ovarian tumor cells. J Biol Chem *283*, 17635-17651.

Cai, X., Hagedorn, C. H., and Cullen, B. R. (2004). Human microRNAs are processed from capped, polyadenylated transcripts that can also function as mRNAs. RNA *10*, 1957-1966.

Calin, G. A., Garzon, R., Cimmino, A., Fabbri, M., and Croce, C. M. (2006). MicroRNAs and leukemias: how strong is the connection? Leuk Res *30*, 653-655.

Chekanova, J. A., and Belostotsky, D. A. (2006). MicroRNAs and messenger RNA turnover. Methods Mol Biol *342*, 73-85.

Chendrimada, T. P., Gregory, R. I., Kumaraswamy, E., Norman, J., Cooch, N., Nishikura, K., and Shiekhattar, R. (2005). TRBP recruits the Dicer complex to Ago2 for microRNA processing and gene silencing. Nature *436*, 740-744.

Croce, C. M., and Calin, G. A. (2005). miRNAs, cancer, and stem cell division. Cell *122*, 6-7.

Dai, Y., DeSano, J. T., Meng, Y., Ji, Q., Ljungman, M., Lawrence, T. S., and Xu, L. (2009). Celastrol potentiates radiotherapy by impairment of DNA damage processing in human prostate cancer. International journal of radiation oncology, biology, physics *74*, 1217-1225.

Dai, Y., Liu, M., Tang, W., DeSano, J., Burstein, E., Davis, M., Pienta, K., Lawrence, T., and Xu, L. (2008). Molecularly targeted radiosensitization of human prostate cancer by modulating inhibitor of apoptosis. Clin Cancer Res *14*, 7701-7710.

Davis, M. E., Zuckerman, J. E., Choi, C. H., Seligson, D., Tolcher, A., Alabi, C. A., Yen, Y., Heidel, J. D., and Ribas, A. Evidence of RNAi in humans from systemically administered siRNA via targeted nanoparticles. Nature *464*, 1067-1070.

DeSano, J. T., and Xu, L. (2009). MicroRNA regulation of cancer stem cells and therapeutic implications. AAPS J *11*, 682-692.

Domen, J., Gandy, K. L., and Weissman, I. L. (1998). Systemic overexpression of BCL-2 in the hematopoietic system protects transgenic mice from the consequences of lethal irradiation. Blood *91*, 2272-2282.

Dontu, G., Al-Hajj, M., Abdallah, W. M., Clarke, M. F., and Wicha, M. S. (2003). Stem cells in normal breast development and breast cancer. Cell Prolif *36 Suppl 1*, 59-72.

Dontu, G., Jackson, K. W., McNicholas, E., Kawamura, M. J., Abdallah, W. M., and Wicha, M. S. (2004). Role of Notch signaling in cell-fate determination of human mammary stem/progenitor cells. Breast Cancer Res *6*, R605-615.

Ebert, M. S., Neilson, J. R., and Sharp, P. A. (2007). MicroRNA sponges: competitive inhibitors of small RNAs in mammalian cells. Nature methods *4*, 721-726.

Farnie, G., and Clarke, R. B. (2007). Mammary stem cells and breast cancer--role of Notch signalling. Stem cell reviews *3*, 169-175.

Frankel, L. B., Christoffersen, N. R., Jacobsen, A., Lindow, M., Krogh, A., and Lund, A. H. (2008). Programmed cell death 4 (PDCD4) is an important functional target of the microRNA miR-21 in breast cancer cells. J Biol Chem *283*, 1026-1033.

Fusco, A., and Fedele, M. (2007). Roles of HMGA proteins in cancer. Nature reviews *7*, 899-910.

Gao, W., Yu, Y., Cao, H., Shen, H., Li, X., Pan, S., and Shu, Y. Deregulated expression of miR-21, miR-143 and miR-181a in non small cell lung cancer is related to clinicopathologic characteristics or patient prognosis. Biomed Pharmacother.

Garzia, L., Andolfo, I., Cusanelli, E., Marino, N., Petrosino, G., De Martino, D., Esposito, V., Galeone, A., Navas, L., Esposito, S., *et al.* (2009). MicroRNA-199b-5p impairs cancer stem cells through negative regulation of HES1 in medulloblastoma. PLoS One *4*, e4998.

Godar, S., Ince, T. A., Bell, G. W., Feldser, D., Donaher, J. L., Bergh, J., Liu, A., Miu, K., Watnick, R. S., Reinhardt, F., *et al.* (2008). Growth-inhibitory and tumor-suppressive functions of p53 depend on its repression of CD44 expression. Cell *134*, 62-73.

Godlewski, J., Nowicki, M. O., Bronisz, A., Williams, S., Otsuki, A., Nuovo, G., Raychaudhury, A., Newton, H. B., Chiocca, E. A., and Lawler, S. (2008). Targeting of the Bmi-1 oncogene/stem cell renewal factor by microRNA-128 inhibits glioma proliferation and self-renewal. Cancer Res *68*, 9125-9130.

Gumireddy, K., Young, D. D., Xiong, X., Hogenesch, J. B., Huang, Q., and Deiters, A. (2008). Small-molecule inhibitors of microrna miR-21 function. Angewandte Chemie (International ed *47*, 7482-7484.

Haase, A. D., Jaskiewicz, L., Zhang, H., Laine, S., Sack, R., Gatignol, A., and Filipowicz, W. (2005). TRBP, a regulator of cellular PKR and HIV-1 virus expression, interacts with Dicer and functions in RNA silencing. EMBO Rep *6*, 961-967.

Han, Y. C., Park, C. Y., Bhagat, G., Zhang, J., Wang, Y., Fan, J. B., Liu, M., Zou, Y., Weissman, I. L., and Gu, H. microRNA-29a induces aberrant self-renewal capacity in hematopoietic progenitors, biased myeloid development, and acute myeloid leukemia. J Exp Med *207*, 475-489.

Hayashita, Y., Osada, H., Tatematsu, Y., Yamada, H., Yanagisawa, K., Tomida, S., Yatabe, Y., Kawahara, K., Sekido, Y., and Takahashi, T. (2005). A polycistronic microRNA cluster, miR-17-92, is overexpressed in human lung cancers and enhances cell proliferation. Cancer Res *65*, 9628-9632.

He, X., He, L., and Hannon, G. J. (2007). The guardian's little helper: microRNAs in the p53 tumor suppressor network. Cancer Res *67*, 11099-11101.

Jamieson, C. H., Ailles, L. E., Dylla, S. J., Muijtjens, M., Jones, C., Zehnder, J. L., Gotlib, J., Li, K., Manz, M. G., Keating, A., *et al.* (2004). Granulocyte-macrophage progenitors as candidate leukemic stem cells in blast-crisis CML. The New England journal of medicine *351*, 657-667.

Ji, Q., Hao, X., Meng, Y., Zhang, M., Desano, J., Fan, D., and Xu, L. (2008). Restoration of tumor suppressor miR-34 inhibits human p53-mutant gastric cancer tumorspheres. BMC Cancer *8*, 266.

Ji, Q., Hao, X., Zhang, M., Tang, W., Yang, M., Li, L., Xiang, D., Desano, J. T., Bommer, G. T., Fan, D., *et al.* (2009). MicroRNA miR-34 inhibits human pancreatic cancer tumor-initiating cells. PLoS One *4*, e6816.

Ji, Q., Karnak, D., Hao, P., Wang, R., and Xu, L. (2010). No small matter: microRNAs - key regulators of cancer stem cells. Int J Clin Exp Med *3*, 84-87.

Jin, L., Hope, K. J., Zhai, Q., Smadja-Joffe, F., and Dick, J. E. (2006). Targeting of CD44 eradicates human acute myeloid leukemic stem cells. Nat Med *12*, 1167-1174.

Johnson, C. D., Esquela-Kerscher, A., Stefani, G., Byrom, M., Kelnar, K., Ovcharenko, D., Wilson, M., Wang, X., Shelton, J., Shingara, J., *et al.* (2007). The let-7 microRNA represses cell proliferation pathways in human cells. Cancer Res *67*, 7713-7722.

Johnson, S. M., Grosshans, H., Shingara, J., Byrom, M., Jarvis, R., Cheng, A., Labourier, E., Reinert, K. L., Brown, D., and Slack, F. J. (2005). RAS is regulated by the let-7 microRNA family. Cell *120*, 635-647.

Kanellopoulou, C., Muljo, S. A., Kung, A. L., Ganesan, S., Drapkin, R., Jenuwein, T., Livingston, D. M., and Rajewsky, K. (2005). Dicer-deficient mouse embryonic stem cells are defective in differentiation and centromeric silencing. Genes Dev *19*, 489-501.

Kasper, S. (2008). Exploring the origins of the normal prostate and prostate cancer stem cell. Stem Cell Rev *4*, 193-201.

Lee, Y., Kim, M., Han, J., Yeom, K. H., Lee, S., Baek, S. H., and Kim, V. N. (2004). MicroRNA genes are transcribed by RNA polymerase II. EMBO J *23*, 4051-4060.

Li, C., Feng, Y., Coukos, G., and Zhang, L. (2009). Therapeutic microRNA strategies in human cancer. The AAPS journal *11*, 747-757.

Lian J, W. X., He F, Karnak D, Tang W, Meng Y, Xiang D, Ji M, Lawrence TS and Xu L. (2011). A natural BH3-mimetic induces autophagy in apoptosis-resistant prostate cancer via modulating Bcl-2-Beclin1 interaction at endoplasmic reticulum. *Cell Death Differ 18*, 60-71.

Liu, S., Dontu, G., Mantle, I. D., Patel, S., Ahn, N. S., Jackson, K. W., Suri, P., and Wicha, M. S. (2006). Hedgehog signaling and Bmi-1 regulate self-renewal of normal and malignant human mammary stem cells. Cancer research *66*, 6063-6071.

Mayr, C., Hemann, M. T., and Bartel, D. P. (2007). Disrupting the pairing between let-7 and Hmga2 enhances oncogenic transformation. Science *315*, 1576-1579.

Melton, C., Judson, R. L., and Blelloch, R. Opposing microRNA families regulate self-renewal in mouse embryonic stem cells. Nature *463*, 621-626.

Meng, Y., Tang, W., Dai, Y., Wu, X., Liu, M., Ji, Q., Ji, M., Pienta, K., Lawrence, T., and Xu, L. (2008). Natural BH3 mimetic (-)-gossypol chemosensitizes human prostate cancer via Bcl-xL inhibition accompanied by increase of Puma and Noxa. Molecular cancer therapeutics *7*, 2192-2202.

Meyer, B., Loeschke, S., Schultze, A., Weigel, T., Sandkamp, M., Goldmann, T., Vollmer, E., and Bullerdiek, J. (2007). HMGA2 overexpression in non-small cell lung cancer. Molecular carcinogenesis *46*, 503-511.

Murat, A., Migliavacca, E., Gorlia, T., Lambiv, W. L., Shay, T., Hamou, M. F., de Tribolet, N., Regli, L., Wick, W., Kouwenhoven, M. C., *et al.* (2008). Stem cell-related "self-renewal" signature and high epidermal growth factor receptor expression associated with resistance to concomitant chemoradiotherapy in glioblastoma. J Clin Oncol *26*, 3015-3024.

Nagel, R., le Sage, C., Diosdado, B., van der Waal, M., Oude Vrielink, J. A., Bolijn, A., Meijer, G. A., and Agami, R. (2008). Regulation of the adenomatous polyposis coli gene by the miR-135 family in colorectal cancer. Cancer Res *68*, 5795-5802.

Papagiannakopoulos, T., and Kosik, K. S. (2008). MicroRNAs: regulators of oncogenesis and stemness. BMC Med *6*, 15.

Peterson, L. F., Wang, Y., Lo, M. C., Yan, M., Kanbe, E., and Zhang, D. E. (2007). The multi-functional cellular adhesion molecule CD44 is regulated by the 8;21 chromosomal translocation. Leukemia *21*, 2010-2019.

Pries, R., Witrkopf, N., Trenkle, T., Nitsch, S. M., and Wollenberg, B. (2008). Potential stem cell marker CD44 is constitutively expressed in permanent cell lines of head and neck cancer. In Vivo *22*, 89-92.

Qian, J., Voorbach, M. J., Huth, J. R., Coen, M. L., Zhang, H., Ng, S.-C., Comess, K. M., Petros, A. M., Rosenberg, S. H., Warrior, U., and Burns, D. J. (2004). Discovery of novel inhibitors of Bcl-xL using multiple high-throughput screening platforms. Analytical Biochemistry *328*, 131-138.

Ren, J., Jin, P., Wang, E., Marincola, F. M., and Stroncek, D. F. (2009). MicroRNA and gene expression patterns in the differentiation of human embryonic stem cells. J Transl Med *7*, 20.

Reya, T., Duncan, A. W., Ailles, L., Domen, J., Scherer, D. C., Willert, K., Hintz, L., Nusse, R., and Weissman, I. L. (2003). A role for Wnt signalling in self-renewal of haematopoietic stem cells. Nature *423*, 409-414.

Rich, J. N., and Bao, S. (2007). Chemotherapy and cancer stem cells. Cell stem cell *1*, 353-355.

Rigoutsos, I. (2009). New tricks for animal microRNAS: targeting of amino acid coding regions at conserved and nonconserved sites. Cancer Res *69*, 3245-3248.

Scott, G. K., Mattie, M. D., Berger, C. E., Benz, S. C., and Benz, C. C. (2006). Rapid alteration of microRNA levels by histone deacetylase inhibition. Cancer research *66*, 1277-1281.

Sharma, S., Kelly, T. K., and Jones, P. A. Epigenetics in cancer. Carcinogenesis *31*, 27-36.

Si, M. L., Zhu, S., Wu, H., Lu, Z., Wu, F., and Mo, Y. Y. (2007). miR-21-mediated tumor growth. Oncogene *26*, 2799-2803.

Sparmann, A., and van Lohuizen, M. (2006). Polycomb silencers control cell fate, development and cancer. Nature reviews *6*, 846-856.

Stadler, B. M., Ivanovska, I., Mehta, K., Song, S., Nelson, A., Tan, Y., Mathieu, J., Darby, G. C., Blau, C. A., Ware, C., *et al.* Characterization of microRNAs Involved in Embryonic Stem Cell States. Stem Cells Dev.

Suh, M. R., Lee, Y., Kim, J. Y., Kim, S. K., Moon, S. H., Lee, J. Y., Cha, K. Y., Chung, H. M., Yoon, H. S., Moon, S. Y., *et al.* (2004). Human embryonic stem cells express a unique set of microRNAs. Dev Biol *270*, 488-498.

Szulwach, K. E., Li, X., Smrt, R. D., Li, Y., Luo, Y., Lin, L., Santistevan, N. J., Li, W., Zhao, X., and Jin, P. Cross talk between microRNA and epigenetic regulation in adult neurogenesis. J Cell Biol *189*, 127-141.

Uziel, T., Karginov, F. V., Xie, S., Parker, J. S., Wang, Y. D., Gajjar, A., He, L., Ellison, D., Gilbertson, R. J., Hannon, G., and Roussel, M. F. (2009). The miR-17~92 cluster collaborates with the Sonic Hedgehog pathway in medulloblastoma. Proc Natl Acad Sci U S A *106*, 2812-2817.

Weiler, J., Hunziker, J., and Hall, J. (2006). Anti-miRNA oligonucleotides (AMOs): ammunition to target miRNAs implicated in human disease? Gene therapy *13*, 496-502.

Wicha, M. S. (2006). Cancer stem cells and metastasis: lethal seeds. Clin Cancer Res *12*, 5606-5607.

Wicha, M. S. (2007). Breast cancer stem cells: the other side of the story. Stem Cell Rev *3*, 110-112; discussion 113.

Wu, X., Li, M., Qu, Y., Tang, W., Zheng, Y., Lian, J., Ji, M., and Xu, L. (2010). Design and synthesis of novel Gefitinib analogues with improved anti-tumor activity. Bioorg Med Chem *18*, 3812-3822.

Xiao, J., Yang, B., Lin, H., Lu, Y., Luo, X., and Wang, Z. (2007). Novel approaches for gene-specific interference via manipulating actions of microRNAs: examination on the pacemaker channel genes HCN2 and HCN4. Journal of cellular physiology *212*, 285-292.

Xie, J., Murone, M., Luoh, S. M., Ryan, A., Gu, Q., Zhang, C., Bonifas, J. M., Lam, C. W., Hynes, M., Goddard, A., *et al.* (1998). Activating Smoothened mutations in sporadic basal-cell carcinoma. Nature *391*, 90-92.

Xu, L., Frederik, P., Pirollo, K. F., Tang, W. H., Rait, A., Xiang, L. M., Huang, W., Cruz, I., Yin, Y., and Chang, E. H. (2002a). Self-assembly of a virus-mimicking nanostructure system for efficient tumor-targeted gene delivery. Human Gene Therapy *13*, 469-481.

Xu, L., Huang, C. C., Huang, W., Tang, W. H., Rait, A., Yin, Y. Z., Cruz, I., Xiang, L. M., Pirollo, K. F., and Chang, E. H. (2002b). Systemic tumor-targeted gene delivery by anti-transferrin receptor scFv-immunoliposomes. Molecular cancer therapeutics *1*, 337-346.

Xu, L., Pirollo, K. F., and Chang, E. H. (1997). Transferrin-liposome-mediated p53 sensitization of squamous cell carcinoma of the head and neck to radiation in vitro. Human gene therapy *8*, 467-475.

Xu, L., Pirollo, K. F., Tang, W. H., Rait, A., and Chang, E. H. (1999). Transferrin-liposome-mediated systemic p53 gene therapy in combination with radiation results in regression of human head and neck cancer xenografts. Human gene therapy *10*, 2941-2952.

Yi, R., Qin, Y., Macara, I. G., and Cullen, B. R. (2003). Exportin-5 mediates the nuclear export of pre-microRNAs and short hairpin RNAs. Genes Dev *17*, 3011-3016.

Yu, F., Yao, H., Zhu, P., Zhang, X., Pan, Q., Gong, C., Huang, Y., Hu, X., Su, F., Lieberman, J., and Song, E. (2007). let-7 regulates self renewal and tumorigenicity of breast cancer cells. Cell *131*, 1109-1123.

Zencak, D., Lingbeek, M., Kostic, C., Tekaya, M., Tanger, E., Hornfeld, D., Jaquet, M., Munier, F. L., Schorderet, D. F., van Lohuizen, M., and Arsenijevic, Y. (2005). Bmi1 loss produces an increase in astroglial cells and a decrease in neural stem cell population and proliferation. J Neurosci *25*, 5774-5783.

Zeng, Y., Yi, R., and Cullen, B. R. (2003). MicroRNAs and small interfering RNAs can inhibit mRNA expression by similar mechanisms. Proc Natl Acad Sci U S A *100*, 9779-9784.

Zhang, B., Pan, X., Cobb, G. P., and Anderson, T. A. (2007). microRNAs as oncogenes and tumor suppressors. Dev Biol *302*, 1-12.

Zhang, M., Behbod, F., Atkinson, R. L., Landis, M. D., Kittrell, F., Edwards, D., Medina, D., Tsimelzon, A., Hilsenbeck, S., Green, J. E., *et al.* (2008a). Identification of tumor-initiating cells in a p53-null mouse model of breast cancer. Cancer research *68*, 4674-4682.

Zhang, Z., Li, Z., Gao, C., Chen, P., Chen, J., Liu, W., Xiao, S., and Lu, H. (2008b). miR-21 plays a pivotal role in gastric cancer pathogenesis and progression. Lab Invest *88*, 1358-1366.

Zhao, R. C., Zhu, Y. S., and Shi, Y. (2008). New hope for cancer treatment: exploring the distinction between normal adult stem cells and cancer stem cells. Pharmacology & therapeutics *119*, 74-82.

16

MicroRNAs and Cancer Stem Cells in Medulloblastoma

Massimo Zollo[1,2], Immacolata Andolfo[1,2] and Pasqualino De Antonellis[2]
[1]*Dipartimento di Biochimica e Biotecnologie Mediche, Università degli Studi di Napoli "Federico II", Naples,*
[2]*CEINGE, Centro di Ingegneria Genetica e Biotecnologie Avanzate, Via Gaetano Salvatore, già Via Comunale Margherita, 482, 80131 Naples,*
Italy

1. Introduction

In this chapter, we are describing the biology of medulloblastoma influenced by several genes/pathways which concur to its pathogenesis. Of note, several levels of regulation are mediated by miRNAs functions, which we dissect their "state of art" to underline their crucial roles on controlling cancer development.
In brain tumours, literatures data, are supporting the values of Cancer Stem Cells (tumor propagating cells) and their functions for tumour recurrence for future therapeutic treatments. Thus, we link the potential use of miRNAs as "shuttle" to impair Cancer Stem Cells in medulloblastoma.

1.1 Medulloblastoma pathology and implication in medicine.

Medulloblastoma (MB) is an highly invasive embryonal tumor of the cerebellum, the most common malignant brain tumor in children and accounts for more than 25% of childhood cancer-related deaths (Wang et al., 2008). MB occurs bimodally, with peaks of incidences between 3 and 4 years and 8 and 9 years of age, even if can also arise in adults, showing the highest incidence at 20-34 years of age (Crawford et al., 2007). Patients with MB generally show symptoms of obstruction of cerebrospinal fluid flow and cerebellar disfunction including macrocephaly, vomiting and ataxia (Crawford et al., 2007). It is currently classified in several variants: classic, desmoplastic, anaplastic, large-cell and with extensive nodularity (Gilbertson and Ellison, 2008). The classic medulloblastoma is composed of small round or ellipsoid cells with a high nuclear to cytoplasmic ratio and round to oval or triangular hyperchromatic nuclei. The desmoplastic medulloblastoma is defined as having a biphasic architecture that consists of regions with dense intercellular reticulin and nodular reticulin-free zones, in which tumor cells show a neurocytic phenotype (McManamy et al., 2007). The Desmoplastic variant represents 50% of adult cases of MB and 15% of children related cancer. The original description of the large-cell medulloblastoma drew attention to the presence of large round cells with a prominent single nucleolus (Giangaspero et al., 1999). These cells occupy one end of the range of medulloblastoma cell size and have an area 2–3 times greater than the mean nuclear area of small round cells in classic tumors

(McManamy et al., 2003). The anaplastic medulloblastoma phenotype is applied to tumors dominated by combination of marked nuclear pleomorphism and high cell turnover, this phenotype is also present in a proportion of non–large-cell medulloblastomas, and accounting for almost 10%-22% of all MB tumors (McManamy et al., 2003, Brown et al., 2000, Eberhart et al., 2002). Because large-cell and anaplastic medulloblastomas share morphophenotypes and an aggressive biological behavior, are often grouped as large-cell/anaplastic (LCA) medulloblatomas, and represents the most malignant variant (Gilbertson and Ellison, 2008). Most medulloblastomas are confined to the posterior fossa, however all of the variants can metastasize and 11-43% of patients show disseminated disease either along the craniospinal axis, or, more rarely, to extraneural sites (Crawford et al., 2007). Disease dissemination rate, patient age and post-operative residual mass represent the most important prognostic markers for MB tumors. MB patients are indeed divided into risk-stratification groups with patients older than 3 years and gross or near-total surgical tumor resection assigned to the average-risk category, which accounts for 60%-70% of all MB patients; and patients with disseminated disease at presentation or greater than 1.5 cm^2 of residual tumor mass identified as high-risk category. A third stratification scheme is used for patients younger than 3 years old, who generally have worse outcomes mostly due to the increased risk of metastatic disease at presentation, increased rate of subtotal resection, and not receiving craniospinal radiation therapy (Crawford et al., 2007). Risk-adapted treatments are currently adopted in the management of the MB, including surgical tumor resection, radiotherapy and chemotherapy. Surgery represents the first approach and a fundamental part of MB treatment. It's aimed to the maximal tumor resection and has shown clear effects of survival improvement, particularly in patients with localized disease (Rutkowski et al., 2005). Addition of radiation therapy to the surgery, has allowed an overall improvement of MB patients survival. However, craniospinal axis irradiation often results in severe deleterious effects, particularly in infants, thus it is delayed or not given to children younger than 3 years (Gilbertson and Ellison, 2008). MB patients belonging to all risk-groups are also commonly treated with chemotherapeutic drugs, including vincristine, cyclophosphamide, etoposide and methotrexate. For younger patients, chemotherapy is widely used as the initial treatment, aimed to delay or avoid radiation therapy. Indeed, intensive postoperative chemotherapy alone showed promising results for treatment of young children without initial metastases (Rutkowski et al., 2005). Other therapeutic approaches include the use of myeloablative doses of chemotherapy followed by autologous stem cell rescue. Early studies have reported a survival improvement for patients with high-risk medulloblastoma; however, 15% of patients died of treatment-related toxicity (Perez-Martinez et al., 2005). Relapse of MB generally manifest within 2 years from the initial therapy in infant, and upon 5 years in adults. The management of patients with relapsing disease varies and depends on a range of factors including the age of the patient and the dissemination rate of the disease. However, surgery and possible combined use of chemotherapy and radiotherapy represent the leading therapeutic approach (Crawford et al, 2007). The employment of multimodality treatment regimens has significantly improved survival rates for MB. However, although patients belonging to the average-risk category show an overall survival rate approaching 70% to 80%, the high-risk patients are generally associated to a very poor prognosis, and MB results still incurable for more than one third of patients. Moreover, survivors commonly suffer of severe long-term side effects due to the aggressive treatments (Crawford et al., 2007, Gilbertson and Ellison, 2008).

The tumor's cell origin and the cellular pathways active in MB tumorigenesis are believed to play a crucial role in the prognosis and possibly response to therapy of MB (De Bont et al., 2008). Therefore, a better understanding of the pathology and molecular biology of medulloblastoma tumorigenesis is necessary, to identify more efficient therapeutic approaches, thereby improving survival and quality of life of MB patients.

1.2 Cancer stem cells in medulloblastoma

Once upon a time, cancer was viewed as a homogeneous mass of rapidly proliferating cells, and therapeutics were designed to eliminate highly proliferative cells. Recent studies have suggested that tumor cells are heterogeneous respect to proliferation and differentiation, and that a cell's proliferative rate may be a poor indicator of its tumorigenic potential. In several malignancies, the capacity to initiate and maintain tumor growth has been found to reside in a small population of cells called cancer stem cells (CSCs) (Al-Hajj et al.,2004, Reya et al., 2001, Wicha et al.,2006). Like normal stem cells, CSCs have the ability to self-renew and to give rise to the variety of proliferating and differentiated cells that make up the bulk of a tumor. Importantly, CSCs are often relatively quiescent and therefore may not be affected by therapies targeting rapidly dividing cells. Elevated expression of transporters that pump out chemotherapeutic agents (Donnenberg and Donnenberg, 2005) and an increased capacity to repair DNA damage (Bao et al., 2006a) may also contribute to CSCs' ability to survive conventional modes of therapy. The resistance of CSCs to conventional therapies may help explain why such therapies often fail: although they may destroy the bulk of a tumor, they cannot prevent the surviving CSCs from kicking into action and regenerating it again (Al-Hajj et al., 2004; Reya et al., 2001; Wicha et al., 2006). Moreover, the properties of CSCs appear to be influenced by both the specific genetic aberrancies in a given tumor as well as the stage of disease progression and the types of drugs used to challenge tumor growth. In some cases the number of Cancer Stem Cell able to generate a tumorigenic cascade are relatively rare, whereas in others CSCs can constitute a substantial proportion of the tumor mass. Moreover the cancer cells within a single tumor exist naturally in multiple states of differentiation that show distinct tumor-seeding properties. As suggested by Kelly, et al., 2007 and Quintana et al., 2008, CSCs representation may be a function of the cell type of origin, stromal microenvironment, accumulated somatic mutations and stage of malignant progression reached by a tumor, indeed selective pressures associated with neoplastic progression may lead to a higher frequency and to an higher variable properties of functionally defined CSCs in secondary or metastatic stages, as well inter-patient and intra-patient heterogeneity of CSCs (Kelly, et al., 2007, Quintana et al., 2008). The study of CSCs biology is predicated on the ability to accurately assess CSCs representation within cancer cell populations. However, measurements of CSCs representation are complicated by the quality of the host tissue in which tumor-initiating ability is assessed. Thus, animal hosts that offer a hospitable environment to engrafted tumor cells will yield measures of CSCs far higher than hosts that fail to do so. Indeed the use of immune-compromised mice make inaccurate the estimation of CSCs number do not taking into account that the immune system plays a pivotal role in a number of solid tumors (Bonertz et al., 2009). Another aspects of host biology that can affect cancer cell engraftment rate include vascularisation at the site of implantation, extracellular matrix constitution, growth factor availability. In light of these complexities, CSCs numbers cannot presently be stated in absolute terms, but only relative to the animal model used to measure CSC representation. (Piyush et al., 2009) In this view, the CSCs could be viewed as a parody, an abnormal deviant of tumorigenic cell influenced by environment stimuli.

In the 2004, Singh and colleagues were the first to identify prospectively isolated population of CSCs in medulloblastoma. These cells were isolated by their ability of expressing the 120-kDa 5-transmembrane cell surface protein Prominin (CD133), which marks normal human neural stem cells. Between 1% and 21% of cells in freshly resected medulloblastomas express CD133, but only few as 1000 to 5000 of these CD133+ cells are capable of forming tumors. In their experiments Singh and colleagues after cells dissociation, using magnetic bead cell sorting, separeted the CD133 positive brain tumour cells from their CD133 negative counterparts. Only prominin positive cells when were transplanted into the brains of nonobese diabetic/severe combined immunodeficient (NOD/SCID) of six-week-old mice, are able to generate a newly tumor. Moreover from analysis of mouse brains following CD133+ cells engraftment revealed that as few as 100 CD133+ cells were sufficient for the formation of human brain tumours in NOD-SCID mice that were analysed at 12–24 weeks post-injection. In the same experiment they also showed that tumor formed resembles the original patient tumour, in fact when injected cells derived from classic medulloblastomas showed small round blue cell morphology characteristic histologic structures (Homer–Wright rosettes), while CD133+ cells derived from a different MB variant, desmoplastic medulloblastoma, recapitulated the cytoarchitecture associated with this subtype.

The xenograft and the original tumour both expressed the cytoplasmic primitive intermediate filaments, neural precursor cell marker, Nestin, Vimentin, the neuronal marker βIII-tubulin (TUJI), and show a high proliferative index (MIB-1), which is further increased in the xenograft. The astrocyte cell marker GFAP appared to be also expressed in a small number of cells in the patient tumour and xenograf.

Recently Read and colleagues and Ward and colleagues have identified a rare, phenotypically primitive, multipotent, and tumorigenic population of Ptc $^{+/-}$ cells that can be propagated by espressing the neural progenitor marker Math1 and Carbohydrate antigen (Stage Specific Embrionic Antigen 1, SSEA1) CD15. They have shown that into tumors from Ptc $^{+/-}$/ P53 $^{-/-}$, an acclaimed genetic MB mouse model, CD15 positive cells are able to recapitulate the heterogeneity within the original tumor and in particular are also able to generate both CD15 positive as well as CD15 negative cells, during proliferation, suggesting that these cells may sit at the top of a hierarchy of differentiation within the tumor. Those cells retain activated Hh and Notch signaling and do not necessarily display Ptc1 loss of heterozygosity (LOH) or loss of wild-type (WT) Ptc1 gene expression. Moreover their analysis revealed that CD15 cells have a distinct gene expression profile characterized by increased expression of genes associated with proliferation and self-renewal and decreased expression of genes involved in apoptosis and differentiation. Consistent with this expression profile, they also observed that CD15+ cells are more proliferative than CD15- cells which are thought to be genetically similar to human nodular/desmoplastic medulloblastomas (Read et al., 2009, Ward et al., 2009).

1.3 Pathways involved in MB cancer stem cells maintenance

The origins of MB are intrinsically linked to the cerebellum development and MB tumor initiating cells can originate from progenitor cells and neuronal stem cells of the cerebellum (Yang et al., 2008). Pathways, such as Shh, Wnt, Notch and AKT/PI3K, regulating the normal cerebellum development, play a crucial role in the MB tumorigenesis (Marino et al.,

2005). These pathways are considered to be the master regulators of cerebellum development, and several genes belonging to these pathways are frequently mutated or deregulated in human MBs.

The hedgehog signaling (Shh) pathway is pivotal to the development of most vertebrate organs and tissues, and has been implicated in birth defects and a multitude of tumour types (McMahon et al., 2003, Riobo and Manning, 2007, Wang et al., 2007). Genomic alterations in components of the Shh signalling pathway, specifically inactivating mutations of PTCH1 and SUFU and/or activating mutations of SMO, have been found in ~15% of sporadic medulloblastomas (Pietsch et al., 1997, Raffel et al., 1997, Reifenberger et al., 1998, Taylor et al., 2002). Additionally, germline mutations in PTCH1 cause Gorlin's syndrome, a rare congenital condition that is characterized by an increased incidence of several tumour types, including medulloblastoma (Hahn et al., 1996). Shh signalling is known to drive proliferation in the granule neuron precursors of the cerebellum, and pathway dysregulation resulting from genomic alterations of its components presumably drives medulloblastoma formation through analogous downstream effects (Pomeroy et al., 2003).

Cell signaling cascades activated by Wnt proteins (the Wnt signaling pathways) have been well conserved throughout evolution. In addition to regulating cellular processes including proliferation, differentiation, motility, and survival and/or apoptosis, the Wnt signaling pathways play key roles in embryonic development and maintenance of homeostasis in mature tissues. Dysregulation of the Wnt pathway has also been linked to the development of medulloblastoma. Wnt ligand binds to its receptor frizzled (FZD) leading to the release of its downstream effector β-catenin from an inhibitory complex that includes the tumour suppressor adenomatous polyposis coli (APC) and the axin proteins. Subsequent nuclear accumulation of β-catenin is thought to mediate its tumorigenic functions, presumably through the activation of target genes such as MYC, cyclin D1 (CCND1) and Re1-silencing transcription factor (REST), which have established roles in cellular proliferation, differentiation and inhibition of apoptosis (Eberhart et al., 2000, Rossi et al., 2008). Approximately 20% of sporadic medulloblastomas harbour mutations in ApC, AXIN1, AXIN2 or CTNNB1 (which encodes β-catenin) (Baeza et al., 2003, Huang et al., 2000, Koch et al., 2007, Koch et al., 2001, Zurawe et al., 2008), and a similarly sized fraction (18%) has separately been shown to exhibit nuclear β-catenin immunostaining (Eberhart et al., 2000). Furthermore, Turcot's syndrome, which is caused by mutations in APC, is characterized by an increased incidence of medulloblastoma and other neuroepithelial tumours. Finally, medulloblastomas that are driven by increased Wnt signalling, as shown by nuclear β-catenin staining, may follow a relatively favourable clinical course (Ellison et al., 2005).

The Notch pathway is a short-range communication system in which contact between a cell expressing a membrane associated ligand and a cell expressing a transmembrane receptor sends the receptor-expressing cell (and possibly both cells) a cell fate regulatory signal. The Notch pathway has repeatedly been linked to the biology of normal neural stem cells (Wang, et al., 2009). Ligand binding to the Notch receptor results in its cleavage and the release of the Notch intracellular domain (NICD), the subsequent nuclear translocation of which activates various target genes. The Notch pathway is activated in MB (Shih et al., 2006). Furthermore, increased Notch signalling enhances the efflux of cytotoxic drugs through ABC transporters such as ABCG2, a recognized property of stem-like tumour cells that contributes to their resistance to conventional therapies (Bhattacharya et al., 2007, Fan et al., 2006). Using fluorescent Hoechst dye, which is also an ABCG2 substrate, stem cells can be effectively sorted by fluorescence-activated cell sorting (FACS) from brain tumours as a 'side population' (SP) that exhibits a lower level of fluorescence than their non-stem cell-like counterparts in the 'main population' (MP) (Fan et al., 2006,Bleau et al., 2009). NICD overexpression increases SP cell number, with Notch pathway inhibition having the opposite effect (Fan et al., 2006). Notch signaling also has been linked to MB progression by promoting a stem-like state (Jason et al., 20010, Eberhart et al., 2007). Several lines of evidence have linked Notch signaling to MB engraftment and progression. Notch pathways are upregulated in MB and increased expression of HES1, a target of both the canonical notch pathway and the non-canonical shh pathway, is associated with poor prognosis in MB patients (Fan et al., 2004, Hallahan et al., 2004, Ingram et al., 2008). Notch2 and Hes5 are overexpressed in the shh-activated SmoA1 mouse, suggesting that activation of the shh pathway is sufficient to induce notch pathway genes (Hallahan et al., 2004). Previous studies using human medulloblastoma cell lines have suggested that Notch signaling is required for maintaining subpopulations of progenitor-like cells potentially capable of re-populating tumors after initial therapy (Fan et al., 2006), and that notch pathway inhibition can limit tumor cell growth (Hallahan et al., 2004, Fan et al., 2006). Recent findings indicats that the Notch pathway is not essential for shh-driven medulloblastoma genesis or maintenance Notch signaling is not essential for the initiation, engraftment, or maintenance of sonic hedgehog pathway driven MB (Hatton et al., 2010). This interpretation is supported by the accompanying article that evaluates MB formation in the absence of RBP-J, which is a convergence point of all notch pathways (Julian et al., 20010).

The AKT/PI3K pathway has also been identified as a major effector of stem-like behaviour in malignant brain tumours. Increasing AKT signalling through PTEN loss increases SP cell number in mouse glioblastomas, at least partially through the direct activation of ABCG2 (Bleau et al., 2009). Furthermore, in mouse medulloblastoma models, activation of the PI3K–AKT–mTOR pathway seems to contribute to the relative resistance of perivascular CSCs to therapeutic irradiation (Hambardzumyan et al., 2008). Combining small molecule AKT pathway inhibitors with radiotherapy significantly decreases the survival of this resistant stem cell-like pool, indicating a promising avenue for future treatment strategies. Supporting these findings, another group has recently reported that PTEN loss and Tp53 deletion are crucial for the maintenance of self-renewal in neural stem cells and seem to mediate these effects at least in part through the induction of MYC (Zheng et al., 2008).

The cross talk among these pathways provides an interpretation for the synergy in the regulation of MB progression and in CSCs maintenance. Thus the low penetrance in medulloblastoma tumor formation in transgenic mice with single pathway deregulation would be explained by the need to target multiple pathways to achieve a high frequency of tumor formation. Shh signaling synergizes with both Notch and Wnt signaling in medulloblastoma development by controlling Notch and Wnt pathway ligand, receptor and/or target gene expression. Notch2 and the Notch target gene, HES5, were found significantly elevated in Smo-induced medulloblastoma in transgenic mice, showing that Shh pathway activation is sufficient to induce Notch pathway signaling (Hallahan et al., 2004). Expression of several components of the Notch and Wnt signaling pathways, and activation of Notch signaling were observed in medulloblastoma from Ptch mice that have elevated Shh signaling. Marked downregulation in the expression of Notch2, Jagged1, Hes1, in cerebella of developing mice with reduced Shh signaling was also observed, suggesting that Shh signaling regulates the expression of these genes (Dakubo et al., 2006). Indeed *neuronal* precursor cells in the developing cerebellum require activity of the sonic hedgehog (Shh) and phosphoinositide-3-kinase (PI3K) pathways for growth and survival. Synergy between these signaling pathways are implicated in the neuronal precursor cell cycle progression in MB. Recent studies, also show that molecular cross-talk between the beta-catenin and phosphatidylinositol 3-kinase (PI3K)/Akt signaling pathways is crucial to sustain medulloblastoma pathophysiology, in fact, constitutive activation of phosphoinositide-dependent protein kinase 1 (PDK1), Akt, and phosphorylation of GSK-3beta was detected by immunohistochemistry in all primary medulloblastomas examined. Small-molecule inhibitors targeting the PI3K/Akt signaling pathway induced beta-catenin signaling by activation of GSK-3beta, resulting in cytoplasmic retention of beta-catenin and reduced expression of its target genes cyclin D1 and c-Myc (Baryawno et al., 2009).

2. MiRNAs functions in cancer

In addition to protein-encoding genes, a second class of genes producing small noncoding RNAs (i.e. microRNAs) has been discovered over the last few years. These short RNAs (18- to 24-nucleotides) bind to cis-regulatory elements mainly present in the 3' UTR of mRNAs, resulting in translational inhibition or mRNA degradation (Bartel 2004; Hammond 2006). In mammals, miRNAs are predicted to control the activity of ~50% of all protein-coding genes. Functional studies indicate that miRNAs participate in the regulation of almost every cellular process investigated so far and that changes in their expression are associated with many human pathologies (Krol J., et al., 2010; Jeffrey T. DeSano and Liang Xu, 2009). Furthermore, microRNAs have been recently shown to be useful tools to silence cancers, they might be able to fill this gap through their control of multiple target genes. MicroRNAs have been linked to the initiation, progression, and metastasis of human malignancies, with some species displaying oncogenic and others tumor suppressive potential (Calin, Croce 2006; Chen 2005). They are often expressed aberrantly in tumors as compared to normal tissues and are likely to contribute to tumorigenesis by dysregulating critical target genes (Esquela-Kerscher and Slack 2006; Kent and Mendell 2006; Croce 2009). The case for miRNAs as tumor suppressors and oncogenes reflects their loss or gain, respectively, as a function of neoplastic transformation, their dysregulation in different tumors, the relevance of their mRNA targets to mechanisms underlying tumorigenesis and their ability to alter tumorigenesis directly in model cells and organisms (Esquela-Kerscher and Slack 2006; Kent and Mendell 2006; Croce 2009; Garzon 2009). Typically, miRNAs that serve as oncogenes are present at high levels, which inhibit the transcription of genes encoding tumor suppressors. Conversely, tumorsuppressor miRNAs are present at low levels, resulting in the overexpression of transcripts encoded by oncogenes (Esquela-Kerscher and Slack 2006).

The best characterized tumor-suppressor miRNAs are miR-15a and miR-16-1 B-cell chronic lymphocytic leukemia (CLL) (Calin, 2002). Tumor suppression by miR-15a and miR-16-1, in part, reflects inhibition of the expression of the anti-apoptotic oncogenic protein Bcl-2, which is characteristically overexpressed in CLL, promoting the survival of leukemia cells. Expression of these miRNAs inhibits cell proliferation, promotes apoptosis of cancer cells, and suppresses tumorigenicity both in vitro and in vivo. miR-15a and miR-16-1 function by targeting multiple oncogenes, including BCL2, MCL1, CCND1, and WNT3A. Down-regulation of these miRNAs has been also reported in pituitary adenomas, and prostate carcinoma (Aqeilan 2009).

Another important microRNA is the Let-7 that act as tumor suppressor gene targeting the human Ras family of proteins, oncogenes that are commonly mutated in many human tumors. Indeed, K-Ras and N-Ras expression in human cells is regulated by let-7 family members. Moreover, loss of let-7 expression in human tumors correlates with the overexpression of Ras proteins (Johnson 2005). MIR Let-7 its family members are highly conserved across species in sequence and function, and misregulation of let-7 leads to a less differentiated cellular state and the development (Roush and Slack, 2008).
The best characterized microRNA that acts as oncogenes is the cluster of miR 17 comprises a group of six miRNAs (miR-17-5p, miR-18a, miR-19a, miR-20a, miR-19b-1 and miR-92) that are overexpressed in many types of tumors, including lymphoma, colon, lung, breast, pancreas and prostate (O'Donnell et al., 2005; Mendell 2008). Expression of these miRNAs promotes cell proliferation, suppresses apoptosis of cancer cells, and induces tumor angiogenesis. New work reveals essential functions for these miRNAs not only in tumor formation but also during normal development of the heart, lungs, and immune system. The human genomic locus encoding these miRNAs, 13q31.3, undergoes amplification in several types of lymphoma and solid tumors. The best-characterized target of the miR-17 cluster is the E2F1 transcription factor and furthermore, the transcription of the miR-17-92 cluster is directly transactivated by c-Myc (O'Donnell et al., 2005; Mendell 2008).
Moreover, also miRNA-21, plays a crucial role in cancer, in fact it is overexpressed in many solid tumors, including breast, colon, lung, prostate and stomach, and in endocrine pancreas tumors, glioblastomas and uterine leiomyomas (Si et al., 2007). This miRNA is encoded at chromosome 17q23.2, a genetic locus that is frequently amplified in many tumors. The tumorigenic effects of miR-21 are mediated, in part, by targeting a number of mediators in critical cell-survival pathways. Thus, in glioblastoma cells in vitro, miR-21 modulates the expression of the common tumor suppressor PTEN, a central regulator of cell growth, proliferation and survival, which is mediated by the in phosphatidylinositol 3-kinase / Akt pathway. Also, miR-21 regulates breast cancer cell growth by reciprocally regulating apoptosis and proliferation, in part reflecting regulation of the anti-apoptotic protein, Bcl-2. In vitro studies have demonstrated that miR-21 knockdown in tumor cell lines leads to increased apoptotic cell death (Seike et al., 2009). Furthermore, miR-21 depletion reduces the growth of tumor cell lines xenografts in mice (Si et al., 2007). The transcription of miR-21 primary RNA is controlled by a conserved upstream enhancer, which has been demonstrated to be regulated by gp130-activated Stat3 in myeloma cells, and by AP-1 in promyelocitic differentiation induced by TPA (Loffler et al., 2007; Fujita et al., 2008). AP-1 activity is necessary, but not sufficient, for the induction of miR-21 triggered by Ras (Talotta et al., 2009). The miR 21 is recently been studied also in thyroid and lung tumors where it is upregulated both in vitro and in vivo by oncogenic Ras. MiR-21 regulation by Ras occurs with a delayed kinetic and requires at least two Ras downstream pathways. A screen of human thyroid cancers and non-small-cell lung cancers for the expression of miR-21 reveals that it is overexpressed mainly in anaplastic thyroid carcinomas, the most aggressive form of thyroid cancer, whereas in lung its overexpression appears to be inversely correlated with tumor progression. A LNA directed against miR-21 slows down tumor growth in mice. Consistently, a search for mRNAs downregulated by miR-21 shows an enrichment for mRNAs encoding cell cycle checkpoints regulators, suggesting an important role for miR-21 in oncogenic Ras-induced cell proliferation (Frezzetti et al., Oncogene 2010, in press).

2.1 MiRNA involved in Medulloblastoma and cancer stem cells biology

In MB, up to date, few microRNAs have been studied. MiR-17/92 is best characterized, in 6% of pediatric MBs it's found a recurrent amplification of the miR-17/92 polycistron proto-oncogene (Uziel et al., 2009). Profiling the expression of 427 mature miRNAs in a series of 90 primary human MBs revealed that components of the miR-17/92 polycistron (miR-92, miR-19a, and miR-20) are the most highly up-regulated miRNAs in MB. Expression of miR-17/92 was highest in the subgroup of MBs associated with activation of the sonic hedgehog (Shh) signaling pathway compared with other subgroups of MB. MBs in which miR-17/92 was up-regulated also had elevated levels of MYC/MYCN expression. Consistent with its regulation by Shh, the Shh treatment of primary cerebellar granule neuron precursors (CGNP), proposed cells of origin for the Shh-associated MBs, resulted in increased miR-17/92 expression. In CGNPs, the Shh effector N-myc, but not Gli1, induced miR-17/92 expression. Ectopic miR-17/92 expression in CGNPs synergized with exogenous Shh to increase proliferation and also enabled them to proliferate in the absence of Shh. MiR-17/92 is a positive effector of Shh-mediated proliferation and that aberrant expression/ amplification of this miRNA confers a growth advantage to MBs (Uziel et al., 2009). Northcutt and colleagues identified a high-level, focal amplification on chromosome 13q31.3, which mapped to the same miRNA cluster. The expression of miR-17/92 was most elevated in MBs with activated hedgehog signalling and was also associated with elevated c-Myc and n-Myc. These studies suggest that aberrant expression of miRNAs encoded by the miR-17/92 enhance the growth potential of MB and that miRNA-mediated modulation of hedgehog signaling may be an important contributing factor to MB pathogenesis (Northcutt et al., 2009).

A high throughput microRNA expression profiles was performed in human primary MB specimens to investigate microRNA involvement in MB carcinogenesis. It has been identified specific microRNA expression patterns which distinguish MB differing in histotypes (anaplastic, classic and desmoplastic), in molecular features (ErbB2 or c-Myc overexpressing tumors) and in disease-risk stratification (Ferretti et al., 2008). They proposed a role for miRNAs in modulating hedgehog signaling. In details, they showed that miR-125b, miR-326, and miR-324–5p expression was decreased in MB and that the altered expression of these miRNAs led to tumor cell proliferation through a hedgehog-dependent mechanism. Furthermore, they used high-throughput screening to examine miRNA expression profiles in 34 patients with MB. They identified 78 miRNAs with altered expression in MB, compared with normal adult and fetal cerebellar cells. Several of the identified miRNAs have been implicated in other cancer types including glioblastoma (Ciafrè et al., 2005). The majority of these miRNAs were downregulated in MB, supporting a role for miRNAs as tumor suppressors. Additionally, they found increased expression of miR-9 and miR-125a and that increased expression of these miRNAs was capable of decreasing proliferation, augmenting apoptosis, and ultimately promoting arrest of tumor growth. The proapoptotic effect was mediated by miR-9 and miR- 125a targeting of the t-TrkC receptor, which was found in this study to be upregulated in MB cells. The authors also found that miR-let7g, miR-19a, miR-106b, and miR-191 were significantly upregulated in anaplastic compared with desmoplastic MBs; miR-let7g and miR-106b were differentially expressed in desmoplastic compared with classic MBs. Changes in expression of Her2 (ErbB2) and c-Myc have been demonstrated to impact biological activity and clinical features of MB. (Gilbertson et al., 1997; Grotzer et al., 2001; Herms et al., 2000). Ferretti et al. examined miRNA expression from MBs overexpressing either Her2 or c-Myc and identified an miRNA signature in each group of MBs. Expression of miR-10b, miR-135a, miR-135b, miR-125b and miR-153 was altered in Her2-overexpressing tumors, whereas c-Myc overexpressing MBs had expression changes in miR-181b, miR-128a, and miR-128b. Additionally, the amount of expression change of 2 miRNAs correlated with disease risk. Though miR-31 and miR-153 were downregulated in all MBs, the group found that the degree of change was directly proportional to disease severity (Ferretti et al., 2009). Although, these data of Ferretti et al., are of interest, miRNAs signature is sicking of validation in a large tumors cohorts analysis.

MiR-124, is another miRNA, preferentially expressed in differentiating and mature neurons and in external granule cells of cerebellum that are thought to be cells of origins of MBs (Pierson et al., 2008). MiR-124 deregulation is common in MBs, and restoration of its function inhibits cell proliferation, suggesting that it may act as a growth suppressor. Two target of miR-124 have been studied: cyclin dependent kinase 6 (CDK6) that was identified as an adverse prognostic marker in MB and SLC16A1 that may represent a novel therapeutic target for treatment of malignant MBs (Pierson J. et al., 2008). SLC16A1, solute carrier family 16, functions to efflux lactic acid during aerobic glycolysis, and its inhibition resulted in a decrease of intracellular pH to a lethal level. This study demonstrates that miR-124 deregulation is common in medulloblastomas, and restoration of its function inhibits cell proliferation, suggesting that miR-124 may act as a growth suppressor, raising the possibility that the miR-124/SLC16A1 pathway may represent a novel therapeutic target for treatment of malignant medulloblastomas (Li et al., 2009).

A recent work, demonstrated that miR-30b and miR-30d are amplified in MB and are putative oncogenic target(s) of a novel recurrent medulloblastoma amplicon at 8q24.22-q24.23 (Lu Y. et al., 2009). Furthermore, miR-128a, inhibits growth of medulloblastoma cells by targeting the Bmi-1 oncogene. This miRNA alters the intracellular redox state of the tumor cells and promotes cellular senescence. MiR-128a has growth suppressive activity in medulloblastoma and this activity is partially mediated by targeting Bmi-1. This data has implications for the modulation of redox states in cancer stem cells, which are thought to be resistant to therapy due to their low ROS states (Venkataraman S, et al., 2010). A complete list of miRNAs implicated in MB biology with their function is showed in table 1.

Our research represents the first work that discovers a microRNA that regulate the Notch pathway and depletes the tumor stem cells compartment by using an in vivo therapeutic approach using an adenovirus type 5 as carrier, indicating the possibility for the targeting of these cells in brain tumors (Garzia et al., 2009). We identified miR199b-5p as targeting HES1, the principal Notch effector. We started our study by an in-silico analysis of the mirBase targets database (Griffiths-Jones, 2004) towards identification of miRNAs potentially targeting HES1. To determine whether HES1 is a target of miR-199b-5p, the HES1 3′ untraslated region (UTR) was cloned downstream of a luciferase reporter gene vector; pre-miR-199b-5p was also cloned in a mammalian expression vector. HEK-293 cells were then transfected with the relative luciferase activity showing that miR-199b-5p co-transfection decreased reporter gene activity, thus indicating binding with the 3′UTR and destabilisation of productive translation of luciferase mRNA. To determine the role of miR-199b-5p in MB cell biology, the miR-199b-5p expression construct was transfected into Daoy cells, and several stable clones over-expressing miR-199b-5p were selected. These effects of miR-199b-5p on HES1 protein expression were not restricted to the stable clones or Daoy cells, as D283MED cells transiently transfected with the expression construct for miR-199b-5p also showed reduced HES1 levels. Furthermore, we silenced the expression of the miRNA 199b-5p by 2-ossy-methyl antisense ribonucleotide in daoy cell line overexpressing the miRNA 199b-5p and we demonstrated that HES1 levels were restored, suggesting 2-OM block of HES1 repression by miR-199b-5p, providing further confirmation that miR-199b-5p targets HES1 directly. The clones overexpressing the miRNA 199b-5p had reduced proliferation rates under standard culture conditions, when compared to the control clone. The clones also showed a decreased in S-phase fractions, and an increase in cells in G0-G1 as compared to the empty vector clone suggesting that exit from the cell cycle has a role in the reduced proliferation of miRNA 199b-5p stable clones.

We then evaluated the effects of the induction of miR-199b-5p on molecular markers of proliferation and differentiation by a real time approach. MAP2, which is mostly expressed in mature neurons, was up-regulated in the miR 199b-5p stable clones. Similarly, GFAP levels were increased. Among the other genes, GABRA6, a marker of cerebellar granule cell differentiation, was also significantly over-expressed in the stable clones. A fine-tuned cascade of positive and negative bHLH transcription factors is central to neurogenesis, with genes such as MASH1, MATH3 and NGN2 inducing neurogenesis. Both miR-199b-5p stable clones showed increases in expression of pro-neural bHLH. In agreement with their reduction in proliferation rate, the proliferation markers c-Myc and cyclin D1 were decreased demonstrating that these stable clones had an impairment in proliferation rate and on the other hand they acquired markers of cerebellar differentiation. We next examined in a standard clonogenic assay, if the anchorage independent growth was affected by miR-199b-5p. There was a significatively reduction in colony formation potential in miR 199b-5p stable clones, compared to the empty-vector clone.

The Notch pathway has been linked to the fraction of MB tumor cells that harbour precursor stem-cell markers (Fan et al., 2006), and HES1 has a role in self-renewing of multipotent progenitor cells (Nakamura et al., 2000). This side population (SP) of tumor cells has a role in the engrafting of a tumor in animal models (Kondo et al., 2004). We thus examined the influence of miR-199b-5p on the population of tumor cells that exclude the Hoechst 33342 dye, a strategy to identify these SP cells. This was determined by flow cytometry in the Daoy cell line, the SP was decreased in miR 199b-5p overexpressing clones, as compared with the empty vector clones. It is also known that central nervous system tumor stem cells express the CD133 antigen, and that these cells are uniquely capable of tumor formation in NOD-SCID mice (Singh et al., 2004; Singh et al., 2004). Additionally, the Notch pathway has a central role in the self renewing process, with its inhibition leading to depletion of CD133-positive (CD133+) Daoy cells via induction of apoptosis of progenitor-like cells (Fan et al., 2006). Recently it was shown that CD133+ Daoy cells promote tumor growth in the flank of nude mice, while CD133 - cells do not (Eberhart 2007). For these reasons, we evaluated the CD133 positivity of Daoy cells as compared to the miR 199b-5p stable clones showing the significatively reduction of the CD133+ cells. This thus demonstrated a role for miR-199b-5p in negative regulation of this fraction of tumor-initiating cells. We demonstrate that the miR 199b-5p depletes the side population compartment in the Daoy cell line and negatively regulates MB tumor stem-cell populations positive to CD133 antigen, that are the uniquely capable of tumor formation in NOD-SCID mice.

We further study the role of miRNA 199b-5p in an in vivo tumor model stabilizing the previous clones overexpressing miR 199b-5p and control clone with an expression vector carrying luciferase cDNA. These stable obtained, were then injected into the left and right flanks, respectively, of five athymic nude/nude mice. Tumor growth was evaluated by weekly in-vivo bioluminescence imaging (BLI) of injected mice. Overall, after 8 weeks a significant difference in tumor volumes between control flanks and miR-199b-5p flanks was seen and also the bioluminescence measurements showed significant reductions in emission for the miR-199b-5p sides during tumor growth, as compared with the control sides. MiR-199b-5p thus can impair tumor formation in vivo in athymic nude mice. To further investigate the ability of miR-199b-5p to regulate MB growth, we injected the stable clones orthotopically into the fourth ventricle of nude mice of 5 weeks of age. After four weeks of in vivo non-invasive monitoring tumor growth by BLI, in mice injected with the clone overexpressing the miR 199b-5p, the tumor growth was considerably lower than that observed in the control cells injected side. As further confirmation of these effects, we also injected the daoy cells infected with an adenovirus coding for miR-199b-5p: in agreement with the previous findings, these mice also showed reduced BLI after 4 weeks. Hematoxylin-eosine staining of frozen tissues showed tumor mass in the cerebellum of the injected animals. Serial parallel frozen histological sections were examined by fluorescence microscopy for endogenous green fluorescence protein (GFP) expressed by adenovirus-infected cells. Then, we evaluated HES1 protein expression by immunohistochemistry staining of other paraffin-embedded tissues, using an anti-HES1 antibody. Overall, we assessed the levels of persistence of adenovirus expression in infected cells, as the down-regulation of HES1 expression due to miR199b-5p carrying the adenovirus expression, thus following tumor growth over time by BLI. Then, two additional nude mice underwent PET-CT studies at 12 weeks post-injection, to assess tumor proliferative activity. The BLI data were showed also by 3D reconstruction of the orthotopic engraftment. These analyses showed significant reduction of tumor mass in the animal injected with the cells infected with an adenovirus carrying the miR 199b-5p, as compared to the control mice, with PET-CT analyses also providing tumor volumes (0.024 cm3 versus 0.044 cm3, respectively). Overall, these data indicate a beneficial effect of over-expression of miR199b-5p, as a negative regulator of tumor growth of MB cells in this orthotopic xenograft nude-mouse model.

We focus our attention on the expression of the miRNA 199b-5p in human cerebella tissues and human MB tissues. We used 13 control samples obtained from the NICHD Brain and Tissue Bank for Developmental Disorders, at the University of Maryland, USA. We measured miR-199b-5p expression, comparing five cerebellum samples obtained from 0–1-year-old children with six from 13–16- year-old children by miRNAs PCR real time TaqMan assay. MiR-199b-5p showed greater expression in the explants from the younger healthy controls. To determine whether miR-199b-5p expression has a role in human MB, samples from a cohort of 61 MB patients were analysed. Indeed, it has already been shown that HES1 protein levels correlate with negative outcome in MB patients (Fan et al., 2004). The whole patient population (n= 61) was then divided into two groups, as low versus high miR- 199b-5p expression, based on the overall median. The distribution of miR-199b-5p expression between non-metastatic (M0) and metastatic (M1, M2 and M3) cases showed that miR-199b-5p expression in the non-metastatic cases was significantly higher than in the metastatic cases. In the subset of patients where follow-up information was available (n= 45), the survival curve for the patients who expressed miR-199b-5p at high levels showed a positive trend, with better overall survival than the low-expressing patients. These data showing down-regulation of miR-199b-5p in metastatic MBs indicates a mechanism of silencing through epigenetic or genetic alterations. We thus tested expression of miR-199b-5p by real-time PCR TaqMan assay in a panel of MB cell lines following induction of de-methylation with 5-aza-deoxycytidine. Indeed, two cell lines (Med8a and UW228) showed significant upregulation of miR-199b-5p, thus supporting the hypothesis of epigenetic control of miR-199b-5p expression. We can conclude that the expression levels of miR-199b-5p in M0 and M+ patients, might be due to genetic and epigenetic regulation during carcinogenesis. In patients with moderate or high expression of the miRNA 199b-5p, an increase in miR-199b-5p expression represses HES1, which then leads to an increase in pro-neural bHLHs gene expression, driving the cell towards differentiation processes. In patients with moderate or low miR-199b-5p expression the genetic or epigenetic control mechanisms, silenced the miRNA 199b-5p expression and then HES1 is over-expressed, leading to cell proliferation and induction of the SP and hence an increase in CD133+ cancer stem cells. As for many other transcription factors, HES1 is a point of integration between and among different signal transduction pathways, and its balance of expression determines fundamental cell decisions, such as whether or not to start a differentiation program. With this scenario, miR-199b-5p can be seen as part of the complex Notch signal-transduction pathway, as a fine regulator of expression levels of the HES1 bHLH transcription factor. These phenomena could be considered to occur in a variety of tissues and cancers where an activated Notch pathway is involved.

The novelties of our work are the finding of a new mechanism of regulation of Notch pathway (a fundamental signal transduction in MB development) mediated by a miRNA. The miRNA 199b-5p inhibits the Hes1 expression by binding to its 3'UTR, it is known that HES1 plays a crucial role in MB biology because high levels of Hes1 protein expression correlate with negative outcome in MB patients by negatively influence on their survival rate (Fan et al., 2004). Furthermore, the other novelty is the role of the miRNA 199b-5p in the impairing of the MB cancer stem cells by decreasing both SP cells and CD133+ cells. In MB, the expression of the neural stem cell marker CD133 has been associated with both tumour initiation capacity and radioresistance, so it is of fundamental the expression of the miRNA 199b-5p in directly target of these cells.

It is well know that one miRNA can target more than hundred of target genes (Peter, 2010), this enhance the need to study the so called "off target effect" to exclude possible unwanted side effects. We used an *in vivo* xenographt model performed by Daoy cell line, we can further use another cell line of classic histotype to confirm the same data as we evaluated *in vitro* with UW228 and D283 cell lines. Moreover, the miRNA 199b-5p function can be evaluated in MB genetic mouse models as $Ptc1^{+/-}/p53^{-/-}$ through a direct injection of the adenovirus carrying the miRNA 199b-5p in the cerebellum of mouse. Moreover, the survival analysis can be extend in a larger cohort of MB patients with consistent time of follow-up data to verify the implication of this miRNA on survival rate.

2.2 Future research

We are proceeding with the study of miRNA 199b-5p role in MB, particularly we are evaluating the finely regulation mechanism of this miRNA by its target and by other genetic and epigenetic changes. Furthermore, we are studying its possible regulation of the other marker CD15 of MB Cancer Stem Cells. The multiple effects of this miRNA function can be due to the inhibition of multiple pathways involved in MB progression, for this reason, we are studying all the other possible targets.

Finally, other miRNAs involved in medulloblastoma pathogenesis and in the impairing of MB Cancer Stem Cells are under investigation. One of this, is miRNA 34a, another regulator of the Notch pathway (Li et al., 2009) by targeting several pathways/genes of potential interests for its therapeutic application.

3. Conclusion

The study of miRNAs in medulloblastoma and in the other brain tumors is still at the beginning, but there is strong evidence of miRNAs involvement in medulloblastoma tumor development and progression also by regulation of Cancer Stem Cells. We shows our hypotesis by a schematic model pictured in figure 1, in which we underline the crucial role of miRNAs that impaired the CSCs in MB. These miRNAs act by a directly hit of the CSCs that are responsible of the origin and the progression of MB (Fig.1). It is becoming clear that miRNAs are essential regulators of many of the key pathways implicated in tumor pathogenesis. While adding another layer of complexity, the discovery of the role miRNAs in brain tumors has also revealed a new category of therapeutic targets. As miRNA research continues to evolve, novel therapeutic targets for the treatment of brain tumors will continue to emerge in the near future.

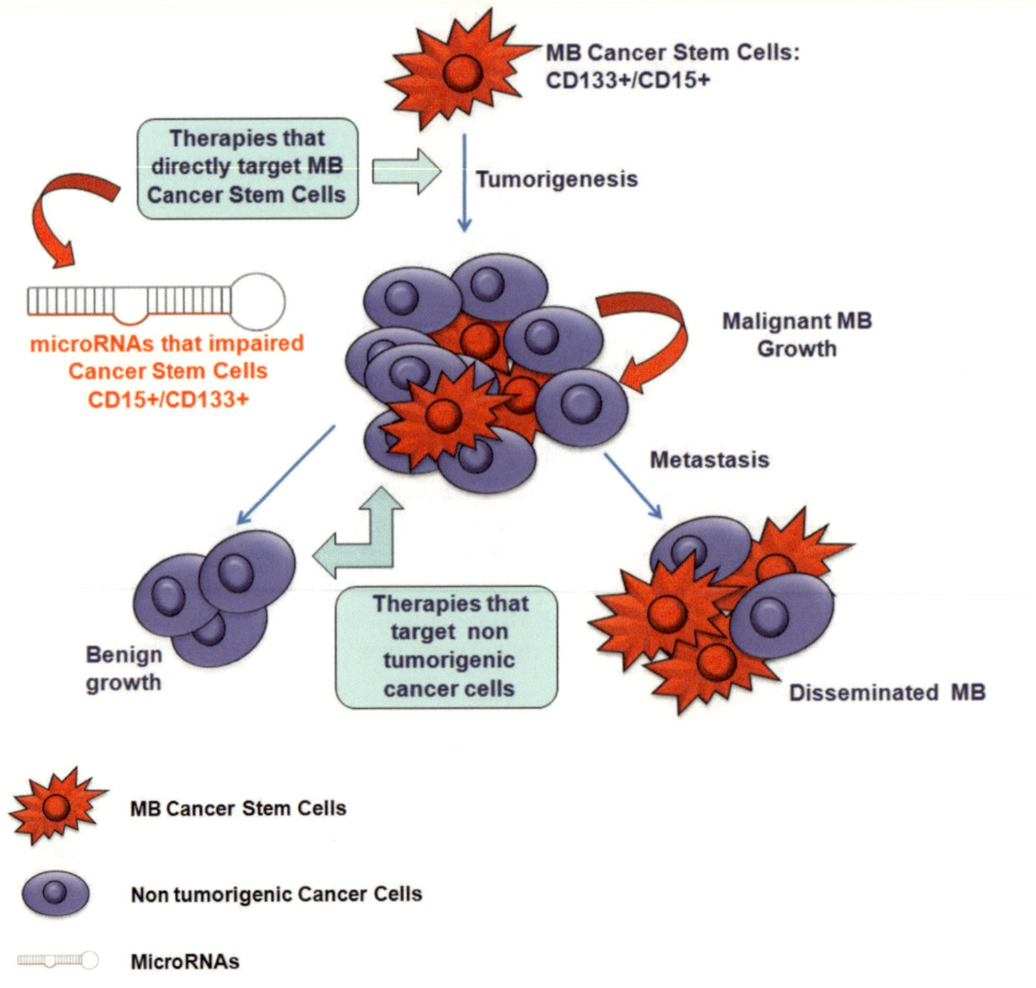

Fig. 1. Schematic model of microRNAs function in MB Cancer Stem Cells.

MiRNAs ID	MIRNAs function in MB	References
miR-124	Regulation of cell cycle by CKD6	Pierson J, et al., 2008
miR-199b-5p	Impairement of Cancer stem cells CD133+ by Notch inhibition	Garzia et al., 2009
miR-let7g, miR-9, miR-106b, miR-125a-b, miR-191	Regulation of proliferation and apoptosis of MB cells	Ferretti et al., 2009
miR-324-5p, miR-326, miR-19a, miR-20. miR-92	Hedgehog dependent proliferation	Ferretti E., et al., 2008
miR-17-92	Over-expressed in the subgroup of MBs associated with activation of the sonic hedgehog (Shh) signaling pathway and elevated levels of MYC/MYCN expression	Uziel T.et al., 2009; Northcutt PA. et al., 2009
miR128	Inhibition of medulloblastoma cells growth by targeting Bmi-1	Venkataraman S, et al., 2010
miR30b, miR30d	Target of a novel recurrent medulloblastoma amplicon at 8q24.22-q24.23	Lu Y. et al., 2009

Table 1. MiRNAs involved in MB biology

4. References

Al-Hajj M, Becker MW, Wicha M, Weissman I, Clarke MF. Therapeutic implications of cancer stem cells. Curr Opin Genet Dev. 2004 Feb;14(1):43-7.

Aqeilan RI, Calin GA, Croce CM. miR-15a and miR-16-1 in cancer: discovery, function and future perspectives. Cell Death Differ. 2010 Feb;17(2):215-20. Epub 2009 Jun 5.

BA Hatton, EH Villavicencio, J Pritchard, M LeBlanc, S Hansen. Notch signaling is not essential in sonic hedgehog-activated medulloblastoma. Oncogene. 2010 Jul 1;29(26):3865-72. Epub 2010 May 3.

Baeza, N., Masuoka, J., Kleihues, P. & Ohgaki, H. AXIN1 mutations but not deletions in cerebellar medulloblastomas. Oncogene 22, 632–636 (2003).

Bao S, Wu Q, McLendon RE, Hao Y, Shi Q, Hjelmeland AB, et al. Glioma stem cells promote radioresistance by preferential activation of the DNA damage response. Nature. 2006 Dec 7;444(7120):756-60.

Bartel DP (2004) MicroRNAs: genomics, biogenesis, mechanism, and function. Cell 116: 281–297.

Bhattacharya, S., Das, A., Mallya, K. & Ahmad, I. Maintenance of retinal stem cells by Abcg2 is regulated by notch signaling. J. Cell Sci. 120, 2652–2662 (2007).

Bleau, A. M. et al. PTEN/PI3K/Akt pathway regulates the side population phenotype and ABCG2 activity in glioma tumor stem-like cells. Cell Stem Cell 4, 226–235 (2009).

Bonertz A, Weitz J, Pietsch DH, et al. Antigen-specific Tregs control T cell responses against a limited repertoire of tumor antigens in patients with colorectal carcinoma. J Clin Invest 2009;119.:3311–21.

Boon K, Eberhart CG, Riggins GJ. Genomic amplification of orthodenticle homologue 2 in medulloblastomas, Cancer Res. 65 (2005), pp. 703–707.

Brown HG, Kepner JL, Perlman EJ, Friedman HS, Strother DR, et al. 2000. "Large cell/anaplastic" medulloblastomas: a Pediatric Oncology Group Study. J. Neuropathol. Exp. Neurol. 59:857–65.

Calin GA, Croce CM (2006) MicroRNA signatures in human cancers. Nat Rev Cancer 6: 857–866

Calin GA, Dumitru CD, Shimizu M, Bichi R, Zupo S, et al. (2002) Frequent deletions and down-regulation of micro- RNA genes miR15 and miR16 at 13q14 in chronic lymphocytic leukemia. Proc Natl Acad Sci U S A 99: 15524–15529.

Chen CZ (2005) MicroRNAs as oncogenes and tumor suppressors. N Engl J Med 353, 1768–1771.

Ciafrè SA, Galardi S, Mangiola A, Ferracin M, Liu CG, et al: Extensive modulation of a set of microRNAs in primary glioblastoma. Biochem Biophys Res Commun 334:1351–1358, 2005

Crawford JR, MacDonald TJ, Packer RJ (2007) Medulloblastoma in childhood: new biological advances. Lancet Neurol 6: 1073-1085

Croce CM. Causes and consequences of microRNA dysregulation in cancer. Nat Rev Genet. 2009 Oct;10(10):704-14.

Dakubo GD, Mazerolle CJ, Wallace VA. 2006. Expression of Notch and Wnt pathway components and activation of Notch signaling in medulloblastomas from heterozygous patched mice. J Neurooncol 79:221–227.

de Bont, J. M. Packer, R. J. Michiels, E. M. den Boer, M. L. Pieters, R. 2008 Biological background of pediatric medulloblastoma and ependymoma: a review from a translational research perspective Neuro Oncol

Di C, Liao S, Adamson DC, Parrett TJ, Broderick DK, et al., Identification of OTX2 as a medulloblastoma oncogene whose product can be targeted by all-trans retinoic acid, Cancer Res. 65 (2005), pp. 919–924.

Diehn Maximilian, Robert W. Cho, and Michael F. Clarke. Therapeutic Implications of the Cancer Stem Cell Hypothesis. Semin Radiat Oncol. 2009 April ; 19(2): 78–86. doi:10.1016/j.semradonc.2008.11.002.

Donnenberg VS, Donnenberg AD. Multiple drug resistance in cancer revisited: the cancer stem cell hypothesis. J Clin Pharmacol. 2005 Aug;45(8):872-7.

Eberhart CG (2007) In search of the medulloblast: neural stem cells and embryonal brain tumors. Neurosurg Clin N Am 18: 59–69, viii–ix.

Eberhart CG, Kepner JL, Goldthwaite PT, Kun LE, Duffner PK, et al. 2002. Histopathologic grading of medulloblastomas: a Pediatric Oncology Group study. Cancer 94:552–60

Eberhart, C. G., Tihan, T. & Burger, P. C. Nuclear localization and mutation of beta-catenin in medulloblastomas. J. Neuropathol. Exp. Neurol. 59, 333–337 (2000).

Ellison D. Classifying the medulloblastoma: insights from morphology and molecular genetics, Neuropathol. Appl. Neurobiol. 28 (2002), pp. 257–282.

Ellison, D. W. et al. β-catenin status predicts a favorable outcome in childhood medulloblastoma: the United Kingdom Children's Cancer Study Group Brain Tumour Committee. J. Clin. Oncol. 23, 7951–7957 (2005)

Esquela-Kerscher A & Slack FJ (2006) Oncomirs - microRNAs with a role in cancer. Nat Rev Cancer 6, 259–269.

Fan X, Matsui W, Khaki L, Stearns D, Chun J, et al. (2006) Notch pathway inhibition depletes stem-like cells and blocks engraftment in embryonal brain tumors. Cancer Res 66: 7445–7452.

Fan X, Mikolaenko I, Elhassan I, Ni X, Wang Y, et al. (2004). Notch1 and notch2 have opposite effects on embryonal brain tumor growth. Cancer Res 64: 7787–7793.

Fan, X. et al. Notch pathway inhibition depletes stemlike cells and blocks engraftment in embryonal brain tumors. Cancer Res. 66, 7445–7452 (2006).

Ferretti E, De Smaele E, Miele E, Laneve P, Po A, et al. Concerted microRNA control of Hedgehog signalling in cerebellar neuronal progenitor and tumour cells. EMBO J. 2008 Oct 8;27(19):2616-27.

Ferretti E, De Smaele E, Po A, Di Marcotullio L, Tosi E, et al. MicroRNA profiling in human medulloblastoma. Int J Cancer. 2009 Feb 1;124(3):568-77.

Frezzetti D, MD Menna, P Zoppoli C Guerra, A Ferraro et al.. Upregulation of miR-21 by Ras in vivo and its role in tumor growth. Oncogene (2010), 1-11.

Fujita S, Ito T, Mizutani T, Minoguchi S, Yamamichi N, et al. (2008). MiR-21 Gene expression triggered by AP-1 is sustained through a double-negative feedback mechanism. J Mol Biol 378: 492–504.

Garzia L, Andolfo I, Cusanelli E, Marino N, Petrosino G, et al. (2009) MicroRNA-199b-5p Impairs Cancer Stem Cells through Negative Regulation of HES1 in Medulloblastoma. PLoS ONE 4(3): e4998. doi:10.1371/journal.pone.0004998

Garzon R, Calin GA, Croce CM. MicroRNAs in Cancer. Annu Rev Med. 2009;60:167-79.

Giangaspero F, Rigobello L, Badiali M, Loda M, Andreini L, et al. 1992. Large-cell medulloblastomas. A distinct variant with highly aggressive behavior. Am. J. Surg. Pathol. 16:687–93

Gilbertson RJ, Ellison DW (2008) The origins of medulloblastoma subtypes. Annu Rev Pathol 3: 341-365.

Gilbertson RJ, Perry RH, Kelly PJ, Pearson AD, Lunec J. Prognostic significance of HER2 and HER4 coexpression in childhood medulloblastoma. Cancer Res 57:3272–3280, 1997.

Griffiths-Jones S (2004) The microRNA Registry. Nucleic Acids Res 32: D109–111.

Grotzer MA, Hogarty MD, Janss AJ, Liu X, Zhao H, et al: MYC messenger RNA expression predicts serviva outcome in childhood primitive neuroectodermal tumor/medulloblastoma. Clin Cancer Res 7:2425–2433, 2001

Hahn H, Wicking C, Zaphiropoulous PG, Gailani MR, Shanley S et al. Mutations of the human homolog of Drosophila patched in the nevoid basal cell carcinoma syndrome. Cell 85, 841–851 (1996).

Hallahan AR, Pritchard JI, Hansen S, Benson M, Stoeck J, et al. 2004. The SmoA1 mouse model reveals that notch signaling is critical for the growth and survival of sonic hedgehog-induced medulloblastomas. Cancer Res 64:7794–7800.

Hambardzumyan, D. et al. PI3K pathway regulates survival of cancer stem cells residing in the perivascular niche following radiation in medulloblastoma in vivo. Genes Dev. 22, 436–448 (2008).

Hammond SM (2006) MicroRNAs as oncogenes. Curr Opin Genet Dev 16: 4–9.

Herms J, Neidt I, Lüscher B, Sommer A, Schürmann P, et al: C-MYC expression in medulloblastoma and its prognostic value. Int J Cancer 89:395–402, 2000

Huang, H. et al. APC mutations in sporadic medulloblastomas. Am. J. Pathol. 156, 433–437 (2000).

Huse Jason T. and Eric C. Holland. Targeting brain cancer: advances in the molecular pathology of malignant glioma and medulloblastoma. Nature reviews cancer. Volume 10, May 2010.

Ingram WJ, McCue KI, Tran TH, Hallahan AR, Wainwright BJ. (2008). Sonic Hedgehog regulates Hes1 through a novel mechanism that is independent of canonical Notch pathway signalling. Oncogene 27: 1489–1500.

Jason T. Huse and Eric C. Holla. Targeting brain cancer: advances in the molecular pathology of malignant glioma and medulloblastoma. Nature Reviews, volume 10, may 2010

Jeffrey T. DeSano and Liang Xu. MicroRNA Regulation of Cancer Stem Cells and Therapeutic Implications. The AAPS Journal, Vol. 11, No. 4, December 2009.

Johnson SM, Grosshans H, Shingara J, Byrom M, Jarvis R, et al. (2005) RAS is regulated by the let-7 microRNA family. Cell 120, 635–647.

Julian E, Dave R, Robson J, Hallahan AR, Wainwright BJ. (2010). Canonical notch signaling is not required for the growth of hedgehog pathway induced medulloblastoma. Oncogene. 26 April 2010; doi:10.1038/onc.2010.101.

Kelly PN, Dakic A, Adams JM, Nutt SL, Strasser A. Tumor growth need not be driven by rare cancer stem cells. Science. 2007 Jul 20;317(5836):337.

Kenney AM, Cole MD, Rowitch DH. Nmyc upregulation by sonic Hedgehog signaling promotes proliferation in developing cerebellar granule neuron precursors, Development 130 (2003), pp. 15–28.

Kent OA & Mendell JT (2006) A small piece in the cancer puzzle: microRNAs as tumor suppressors and oncogenes. Oncogene 25, 6188–6196.

Koch, A. et al. Mutations of the Wnt antagonist AXIN2 (Conductin) result in TCF-dependent transcription in medulloblastomas. Int. J. Cancer 121, 284–291 (2007).

Koch, A. et al. Somatic mutations of WNT/wingless signaling pathway components in primitive neuroectodermal tumors. Int. J. Cancer 93, 445–449 (2001).

Kondo T, Setoguchi T, Taga T (2004) Persistence of a small subpopulation of cancer stem-like cells in the C6 glioma cell line. Proc Natl Acad Sci U S A 101: 781–786.

Krol J, Loedige I, Filipowicz W. The widespread regulation of microRNA biogenesis, function and decay. Nat Rev Genet. 2010 Sep;11(9):597-610. Epub 2010 Jul 27. Review.

Leung C, Lingbeek M, Shakhova O, Liu J, Tanger E et al., Bmi1 is essential for cerebellar development and is overexpressed in human medulloblastomas, Nature 428 (2004), pp. 337–341.

Li KK, Pang JC, Ching AK, Wong CK, Kong X, et al. miR-124 is frequently down-regulated in medulloblastoma and is a negative regulator of SLC16A1.. Hum Pathol. 2009 May 6.

Loffler D, Brocke-Heidrich K, Pfeifer G, Stocsits C, Hackermu¨ ller J, et al. (2007). Interleukin-6 dependent survival of multiple myeloma cells involves the Stat3-mediated induction of microRNA-21 through a highly conserved enhancer. Blood 110: 1330–1333.

Lu Y, Ryan SL, Elliott DJ, Bignell GR, Futreal PA, et al. Amplification and overexpression of Hsa-miR-30b, Hsa-miR-30d and KHDRBS3 at 8q24.22-q24.23 in medulloblastoma.. PLoS One. 2009 Jul 7;4(7):e6159

McManamy CS, Lamont JM, Taylor RE, Cole M, Pearson AD, et al. 2003. Morphophenotypic variation predicts clinical behavior in childhood nondesmoplastic medulloblastomas. J. Neuropathol. Exp. Neurol. 62:627–32

McManamy CS, Pears J, Weston CL, Hanzely Z, Ironside JW, et al. 2007. Nodule formation and desmoplasia in medulloblastomas: defining the nodular/desmoplastic variant and its biological behaviour. Brain Pathol. 17:151–64

ME Peter. Targeting of mRNAs by multiple miRNAs: the next step.. Oncogene (2010) 29, 2161–2164.

Mendell Joshua T.. miRiad roles for the miR-17-92 cluster in development and disease Cell. 2008 April 18; 133(2): 217–222.

Nakamura Y, Sakakibara S, Miyata T, Ogawa M, Shimazaki T, et al. (2000) The bHLH gene hes1 as a repressor of the neuronal commitment of CNS stem cells. J Neurosci 20: 283–293.

Northcott PA, Fernandez-L A, Hagan JP, Ellison DW, Grajkowska W, et al. The miR-17/92 polycistron is up-regulated in sonic hedgehog-driven medulloblastomas and induced by N-myc in sonic hedgehog-treated cerebellar neural precursors. Cancer Res. 2009 Apr 15;69(8):3249-55. Epub 2009 Apr 7.

O'Donnell KA, Wentzel EA, Zeller KI, Dang CV, Mendell JT (2005) c-Myc regulated microRNAs modulate E2F1 expression. Nature 435: 839–843.

Perez-Martinez, A. Lassaletta, A. Gonzalez-Vicent, M. Sevilla, J. Diaz, M. A. Madero, L. 2005. High-dose chemotherapy with autologous stem cell rescue for children with high risk and recurrent medulloblastoma and supratentorial primitive neuroectodermal tumors. J Neurooncol.

Pierson J, Hostager B, Fan R, Vibhakar. Regulation of cyclin dependent kinase 6 by microRNA 124 in medulloblastoma. R. J Neurooncol. 2008 Oct;90(1):1-7.

Pietsch T, Waha A, Koch A, Kraus J, Albrecht S. et al. Medulloblastomas of the desmoplastic variant carry mutations of the human homologue of Drosophila patched. Cancer Res. 57, 2085–2088 (1997).

Piyush B Gupta. Cancer Stem Cell: mirage or relity. nature medicine 2009

Pomeroy, S. L. & Sturla, L. M. Molecular biology of medulloblastoma therapy. Pediatr. Neurosurg. 39, 299–304 (2003).

Quintana E, Shackleton M, Sabel MS, Fullen DR, Johnson TM, Morrison SJ. Efficient tumour formation by single human melanoma cells. Nature. 2008 Dec 4;456(7222):593-8.

Raffel C, Jenkins RB, Frederick L, Hebrink D, Alderete B, et al. Sporadic medulloblastomas contain PTCH mutations. Cancer Res. 57, 842–845 (1997).

Rao G, Pedone CA, Coffin CM, Holland EC, Fults DW. et al., c-Myc enhances sonic hedgehog-induced medulloblastoma formation from nestin-expressing neural progenitors in mice, Neoplasia 5 (2003), pp. 198–204.

Read TA, Fogarty MP, Markant SL, McLendon RE, Wei Z, Ellison DW, Febbo PG, Wechsler-Reya RJ. Cancer Res. 2009 Jun 1;69(11):4682-90. Identification of CD15 as a marker for tumor-propagating cells in a mouse model of medulloblastoma. Cancer Cell. 2009 Feb 3;15(2):135-47.

Reifenberger J, Wolter M, Weber RG, Megahed M, Ruzicka T et al. Missense mutations in SMOH in sporadic basal cell carcinomas of the skin and primitive neuroectodermal tumors of the central nervous system. Cancer Res. 58, 1798–1803 (1998).

Reya T, Morrison SJ, Clarke MF, Weissman IL. Stem cells, cancer, and cancer stem cells. Nature. 2001 Nov 1;414(6859):105-11. Review

Rossi, A., Caracciolo, V., Russo, G., Reiss, K. & Giordano, A. Medulloblastoma: from molecular pathology to therapy. Clin. Cancer Res. 14, 971–976 (2008).

Roush S, Slack FJ. Trends Cell Biol. 2008 Oct;18(10):505-16. Epub 2008 Sep 4. The let-7 family of microRNAs.

Rutkowski, S. Bode, U. Deinlein, F. Ottensmeier, H. Warmuth-Metz, et al. 2005. Treatment of early childhood medulloblastoma by postoperative chemotherapy alone N Engl J Med

Seike M, Goto A, Okano T, Bowman ED, Schetter AJ, et al. (2009). MiR-21 is an EGFR-regulated anti-apoptotic factor in lung cancer in never-smokers. Proc Natl Acad Sci USA 106: 12085–12090.

Shih, A. H. & Holland, E. C. Notch signaling enhances nestin expression in gliomas. Neoplasia 8, 1072–1082 (2006).

Si ML, Zhu S, Wu H, Lu Z, Wu F & Mo YY (2007) miR-21-mediated tumor growth. Oncogene 26, 2799– 2803.

Singh SK, Clarke ID, Hide T, Dirks PB (2004) Cancer stem cells in nervous system tumors. Oncogene 23: 7267–7273.

Singh SK, Hawkins C, Clarke ID, Squire JA, Bayani J, et al. (2004) Identification of human brain tumour initiating cells. Nature 432: 396–401.

Talotta F, Cimmino A, Matarazzo MR, Casalino L, De Vita G, et al. (2009). An autoregulatory loop mediated by miR-21 and PDCD4 controls the AP-1 activity in RAS transformation. Oncogene 28: 73–84.

Taylor MD, Liu L, Raffel C, Hui CC, Mainprize TG et al. Mutations in SUFU predispose to medulloblastoma. Nature Genet. 31, 306–310 (2002).

Uziel T, Karginov FV, Xie S, Parker JS, Wang YD, et al. The miR-17~92 cluster collaborates with the Sonic Hedgehog pathway in medulloblastoma.. Proc Natl Acad Sci U S A. 2009 Feb 24;106(8):2812-7.

Venkataraman S, Alimova I, Fan R, Harris P, Foreman N, Vibhakar R. MicroRNA 128a increases intracellular ROS level by targeting Bmi-1 and inhibits medulloblastoma cancer cell growth by promoting senescence. PLoS One. 2010 Jun 21;5(6):e10748

Wang Q, Li H, Liu N, Chen XY, Wu ML, et al. (2008) Correlative analyses of notch signaling with resveratrol-induced differentiation and apoptosis of human medulloblastoma cells. Neurosci Lett 438: 168-173.

Wang, Z., Li, Y., Banerjee, S. & Sarkar, F. H. Emerging role of Notch in stem cells and cancer. Cancer Lett. 279, 8–12 (2009).

Ward RJ, Lee L, Graham K, Satkunendran T, Yoshikawa K, Ling E, Harper L, Austin R, Nieuwenhuis E, Clarke ID, Hui CC, Dirks PB. Multipotent CD15+ cancer stem cells in patched-1-deficient mouse medulloblastoma. Cancer Res. 2009 Jun 1;69(11):4682-90.

Wicha MS, Liu S, Dontu G. Cancer stem cells: an old idea--a paradigm shift. Cancer Res. 2006 Feb 15;66(4):1883-90; discussion 1895-6.

Yang ZJ, Ellis T, Markant SL, Read TA, Kessler JD, Bourboulas M, et al. Medulloblastoma can be initiated by deletion of Patched in lineage-restricted progenitors or stem cells. Cancer Cell. 2008 Aug 12;14(2):135-45

Yunqing Li, Fadila Guessous,Ying Zhang, Charles DiPierro, Benjamin Kefas,et al. MicroRNA-34a Inhibits Glioblastoma Growth by Targeting Multiple Oncogenes. Cancer Res 2009; 69: (19). October 1, 2009

Zheng, H. et al. p53 and Pten control neural and glioma stem/progenitor cell renewal and differentiation. Nature 455, 1129–1133 (2008).

Zurawel, R. H., Chiappa, S. A., Allen, C. & Raffel, C. Sporadic medulloblastomas contain oncogenic β-catenin mutations. Cancer Res. 58, 896–899 (1998).

Part 5

Diagnosis, Targeted Therapeutics, and Prognosis

17

The Rocky Road from Cancer Stem Cell Discovery to Diagnostic Applicability

Paola Marcato and Patrick W. K. Lee
Dalhousie University
Canada

1. Introduction

Since the discovery of the discretely isolatable highly tumorigenic tumor population with self renewal and differentiation properties (i.e. cancer stem cells, CSCs), it has been theorized that their quantification in tumor tissues would have significant prognostic value. Based on their increased tumorigenicity and stem cell like qualities, it is postulated that patients with elevated levels of CSCs would more likely suffer from an aggressive form of disease that is comparatively resistant to currently employed therapeutics. The results of the studies evaluating the prognostic value of CSC markers have been mixed, and cancer and marker dependant. Herein we review the currently known CSC markers for the more common cancers and their respective prognostic potential. In conclusion we will discuss what this data potentially reveals about the role of CSCs in tumor progression.

2. Leukemia

2.a Identified leukemia stem cell markers

Acute myeloid leukemia (AML) is the result of malignant transformation of hematopoietic progenitor cells. These altered cells proliferate and lead to the accumulation of AML blasts. Only a minority population of all AML cells are capable of proliferating *in vitro* and *in vivo*. This suggests that AML cells are potentially organized in a hierarchy, with only the most primitive of these cells capable of maintaining the leukemic clone. This hypothesis was the basis for identifying the AML initiating cell and the CSC theory that arose from the subsequent studies. As such, CSCs were first identified in AML in 1990's by John Dick's group in Toronto, Canada (Bonnet and Dick, 1997; Lapidot et al., 1994). AML cells that were CD34+CD38- possessed stem cell like characteristics and *de novo* leukemia repopulating properties in immunocompromised mice (Bonnet and Dick, 1997). While leukemia initiating cells (LSCs) are in the range of 0.00002 to 0.02% of all unsorted mononuclear blood cells, LSCs were in the range of 0.02 to 2% in the CD34+CD38- sorted cells of tested patient samples (sorting resulting in approximate 100-1000 fold enrichment of the CSC population). In further similarity to normal stem cells, CD34+CD38- expression is also a unique identifier for hematopoietic stem cells (HSCs). Since then, other leukemic stem cell (LSC) markers have been identified.

In 1997 and 1998, Blair et al. explored the use of other known HSC markers for the isolation of AML initiating cells and found that AML cells that are $CD34^{+}$/$HLA\text{-}DR^{-}$/$CD71^{-}$ and $Thy1^{-}$

(CD90) had the CSC phenotype (Blair et al., 1997; Blair et al., 1998). Later that same group added lack of expression of c-kit (CD117) to the list of potential AML CSC markers, as AML cells from patients that were $CD34^{+}c\text{-}kit^{-}$ were enriched for the CSC population (Blair and Sutherland, 2000). In 2000, Jordan et al., identified a cell surface molecule, interleukin-3 receptor alpha chain (CD123) as being uniquely expressed on AML CSCs, but not HSCs (Jordan et al., 2000), allowing for a potential method of distinction between LSCs and HSCs.

Other than the above described cell surface markers used for the isolation of CSCs, "functional markers" have been explored more recently. The functional marker strategy is based on stem cell characteristics, but does not rely on cell surface adhesion molecules for the viable isolation of a specific cell-subset. For example, Stemcell Technologies developed the aldefluor assay for the isolation of live hematopoietic stem cells based on increased expression of a cytoplasmic enzyme, aldehyde dehydrogenase (ALDH) isoform 1A1. ALDH1A1 is one of 19 ALDH isoforms expressed in humans, and it is a critical detoxifying enzyme responsible for oxidizing aldehydes to carboxylic acids (Marchitti et al., 2008). While, predominantly expressed in the epithelium of testis, brain, eye, liver, and kidney, ALDH1A1, is also found in high levels in hematopoietic and neural stem cells (Armstrong et al., 2004; Chute et al., 2006; Marchitti et al., 2008). ALDH1A1 is proposed to play a role in the differentiation of hematopoietic and neural stem cells via the oxidation of retinal to retinoic acid (Collins, 2008). Retinoic acid activates nuclear retinoic acid receptors (RARs) and RARs subsequently regulate the transcription of genes with RAREs (retinoic acid response elements). Furthermore, ALDH1A1 is known to metabolize and detoxify chemotherapeutics like cyclophosphamide (Magni et al., 1996), and is therefore thought to contribute to the innate chemotherapeutic resistance properties of hematopoietic stem cells. Using the aldefluor assay, Cheung et al., were the first to show that it was possible to isolate the LSCs based on the increased ALDH activity (Cheung et al., 2007). The researchers detected a population of $ALDH^{+}$ AML cells in 14 of 43 patient samples. In the remaining 29 samples an ALDH+ population was rare or unidentifiable. The $ALDH^{+}$ AML cells in most cases co-expressed $CD34^{+}$ (the previously identified marker) and engrafted significantly better than the $ALDH^{-}$ AML cells in immunocompromised mice. As discussed later, ALDH activity would become one of the few markers discovered that has applicability across a wide range of cancers. It can be said that ALDH activity is a universal CSC marker.

2.b LSC markers as prognostic indicators

Since the identification of a LSC population using cell surface markers it has been postulated that these markers could be used for diagnostic purposes, where patients with comparatively increased CSC numbers would theoretically suffer poorer outcomes. The results of the studies for leukemia are summarized in Table 1. Many of the cell surface markers had been evaluated separately for prognostic value prior to their discovery as potential CSC markers. For example as early as 1989, studies were being completed evaluating the prognostic value CD34 in AML (Borowitz et al., 1989; Campos et al., 1989). By 2000, a study by Kanda et al., summarized the results from the then 22 completed independent studies on the prognostic relevance of CD34 for AML (Kanda et al., 2000). The authors' review of the literature revealed a wide heterogeneity of results, with 12 studies concluding that increased CD34+ was associated with worse outcome, while the other 10 studies failed to show the relevance of CD34 expression in predicting patient outcome (summarized in Table 1) (Kanda et al., 2000). Kanda et al., concluded that given the wide variability of conclusions from the reports, CD34 expression could not be employed reliably as a prognostic marker (Kanda et al., 2000).

Similar disparity was seen for CD38 prognostic studies. For example, in 1993, Koehler et al. reported that CD38 expression failed to significantly correlate with the outcomes of 325 patients of childhood acute lymphoblastic leukemia (ALL) (Koehler et al., 1993). In 2000, Keyhani et al. evaluated the levels of CD38 expression in the blasts of 304 AML and 138 ALL patients (Keyhani et al., 2000). Patients with the higher percentages of $CD38^+$ cancer cells had the best outcomes, experiencing both longer times between remission and relapse and improved overall survival. Their results infer that patients with increased $CD38^-$ (LSC marker) cancer cells experienced the worse outcomes. However, lack of CD38 expression was only a significant independent risk factor for the AML patients, not ALL patients. In 2003, Repp et al. assessed the prognostic value of a panel of 33 different CD molecules for AML (Repp et al., 2003). Among the panel, expression of CD38 and CD34 was quantified singly in 783 patient samples. As the CSC theory would predict, patients with increased CD34 expression or decreased CD38 expression had poorer overall outcomes.

Other LSC markers have also been tested for their prognostic value individually. In a 1994 immunophenotyping AML prognostic study (Bradstock et al., 1994), LSC proposed markers CD34, c-kit (CD117) and HLA-DR (Blair et al., 1998; Blair and Sutherland, 2000) were among the panel of CD antigens tested. CD34, c-kit and HLA-DR expression failed to correlate with patient outcome (Bradstock et al., 1994). A more recent study concluded that increased c-kit (CD117) expression correlated with worse outcomes for AML patients (Advani et al., 2008). This result was in direct disagreement with the CSC theory since it is the lack of c-kit expression in combination with CD34 expression that was used to identify LSCs (Blair and Sutherland, 2000).

The above described studies suggest that the prognostic potential of LSC markers is not promising and clinically irrelevant. However, as discussed below, employed in combination, the prognostic potential of LSC markers becomes more apparent and the results therefore lend support to the CSC theory. In 2005, van Rhenen et al., quantified the frequency of $CD34^+CD38^-$ cancer cells in 92 AML patients at time of diagnosis and reported worse outcomes for patients with increased $CD34^+CD38^-$ cancer cells (van Rhenen A. et al., 2005). Patients with increased $CD34^+CD38^-$ cancer cell frequency (>3.5%) relapsed on average 5.6 months post remission, while patients with lower $CD34^+CD38^-$ cancer frequency relapsed on average 16 months post remission. The prognostic value of $CD34^+CD38^-$ has also been observed in other leukemias. Recently, Ebinger et al. quantified the frequency of $CD34^+CD38^-$ leukemia blasts in 42 childhood ALL cases (Ebinger et al., 2010). The researchers found that increased $CD34^+CD38^-$ cancer cells was associated with increased minimal residual disease and thus poorer prognosis for this leukemia sub-type as well. Although future studies will be required for confirmation, it appears that using the CSC markers in combination is more relevant as a prognostic tool than their application as singly applied markers.

Finally, with the more recent discovery that ALDH activity can be used as marker to isolate LSC (Cheung et al., 2007), ALDH activity is also being tested for prognostic value. Cheung et al. reported that increased ALDH activity in AML patient samples correlated significantly with the cytogenetic changes previously associated with unfavourable prognosis (Cheung et al., 2007). In 2009, Ran et al. compared the outcomes of 40 AML patients with higher percentages of ALDH+ cancer cells (>0.36%) to 28 patients with lower frequencies of ALDH+ cells ($\leq$0.36%) (Ran et al., 2009). Increased frequency of $ALDH^+$ cells correlated significantly with decreased survival probability. We await the results of future studies that will test the prognostic potential of ALDH activity combined with the LSC cell surface markers.

LSC marker	Patient sample size	Prognostic correlation: worse outcome	no correlation	improved outcome	Publication
$CD34^+$	145	X			(Campos et al., 1989)
$CD34^+$	75	X			(Borowitz et al., 1989)
$CD34^+$	96	X			(Geller et al., 1990)
$CD34^+$	27	X			(Guinot et al., 1991)
$CD34^+$	154	X			(Solary et al., 1992)
$CD34^+$	126	X			(Lee et al., 1992)
$CD34^+$	38	X			(Myint and Lucie, 1992)
$CD34^+$	150	X			(Campos et al., 1992)
$CD34^+$	70		X		(Selleri et al., 1992)
$CD34^+$	80		X		(Ciolli et al., 1993)
$CD34^+$	60	X			(Fagioli et al., 1993)
$CD34^+$	52	X			(te Boekhorst et al., 1993)
$CD34^+$	62		X		(Lamy et al., 1994)
$CD34^+$	168		X		(Bradstock et al., 1994)
$CD34^+$	481		X		(Sperling et al., 1995)
$CD34^+$	99		X		(Fruchart et al., 1996)
$CD34^+$	42		X		(Arslan et al., 1996)
$CD34^+$	517		X		(Porwit-MacDonald et al., 1996)
$CD34^+$	62	X			(Dalal et al., 1997)
$CD34^+$	141	X			(Raspadori et al., 1997)
$CD34^+$	37	X			(Kyoda et al., 1998)
$CD34^+$	783	X			(Repp et al., 2003)
$CD38^-$	325		X		(Koehler et al., 1993)
$CD38^-$	442	X			(Keyhani et al., 2000)
$CD38^-$	783	X			(Repp et al., 2003)
c-kit$^-$	168		X		(Bradstock et al., 1994)
c-kit$^-$	152			X	(Advani et al., 2008)
HLA-DR$^-$	96			X	(Geller et al., 1990)
HLA-DR$^-$	154			X	(Solary et al., 1992)
HLA-DR$^-$	168		X		(Bradstock et al., 1994)
$CD34^+CD38^-$	92	X			(van Rhenen A. et al., 2005)
$CD34^+CD38^-$	42	X			(Ebinger et al., 2010)
$ALDH^+$	65	X			(Ran et al., 2009)

Table 1. Summary of results from immunohistological prognostic studies of LSC markers

3. Breast cancer

3.a Identified breast CSC markers

Breast cancer was the first solid tumor identified to have a population of tumor cells with an inherent highly tumorigenic quality. These cells were termed tumor propagating cells at the time, and are now more commonly known as breast CSCs. In 2003, Al-Hajj et al. performed experiments akin to the leukemia studies discussed above (Bonnet and Dick, 1997; Lapidot et al., 1994), and isolated sub-tumor cell populations based on cell surface marker expression (Al-Hajj et al., 2003). The group showed that as few as 10^2 $CD24^{-/low}CD44^{+}$ breast tumor cells could re-capitulate the tumor with much of its original heterogeneity (Al-Hajj et al., 2003). The authors proposed that not all $CD24^{-/low}CD44^{+}$ cells were CSCs but that the breast $CD24^{-/low}CD44^{+}$ population was enriched for CSCs. It was hypothesized that if additional breast CSC markers were identified it may be possible to isolate and even more highly tumorigenic cells and initiate a tumor in xenograft from only one cell. This led to the pursuit of the identification of additional markers, both cell surface and functional.

Using the same functional marker approach previously employed for leukemia (Cheung et al., 2007), Ginestier *et al.* were the first to isolate CSCs from a solid tumor based on increased ALDH activity (Ginestier et al., 2007). The researchers showed that as few as 10^2 ALDH+ breast cancer cell isolated from patients could induce tumors in immunocompromised mice. Further, in a proof of principle experiment, the researchers isolated $CD24^{-/low}CD44^{+}ALDH^{+}$ breast cancer cells and were able to induce tumors in immunocompromised mice with as few as 20 injected cells. This experiment combining mulitple markers for the isolation of highly tumorigenic cells provided supportive evidence to the proposed hypothesis that identifying additional markers would lead to further enrichment of the CSC population.

In another more recent approach using a functional markers to identify novel breast CSCs, Pece et al. isolated the human normal mammary stem cells (hNMSCs) from mammary reduction surgeries by retention of a lipophillic fluorescent dye, PKH26 (Pece et al., 2010). PKH26 stains quiescent cells, allowing for the isolation of relatively non-dividing cells from a mixed population of proliferating cells (Lanzkron et al., 1999). From these isolated putative stem cells, Pece et al. identified a unique gene expression signature, the hNMSC signature, and applied it to published breast cancer gene expression data sets (Pece et al., 2010). This analysis revealed that many of the genes upregulated in normal mammary stem cells were also upregulated in higher grade, aggressive breast cancers. When the authors picked a few of these upregulated genes (i.e.CD49+, $DLL1^{high}$, $DNER^{high}$) and used them as cell surface markers, they were able to identify and isolate a sub-population of highly tumorigenic cancer initiating cells from breast tumors. As such, PKH26 stain retention and $CD49+DLL1^{high}DNER^{high}$ are the most recent breast CSC markers identified. Interestingly, CD49 is a previously known normal mammary stem cell marker, and DLL1 and DNER have been connected to normal stem cell function.

3.b Breast CSC markers as prognostic indicators

CSC quantification is a proposed prognostic indicator for breast cancer. Translating this to clinical application requires immunohistological methods for identification of CSCs in fixed tumor tissue and in this respect, the data is less convincing and is summarized in Table 2. First, for $CD24^{-/low}CD44^{+}$ the published studies have been mixed. In 2005, Abraham et al. were the first to publish a study on the prognostic applicability of the then newly identified breast CSC markers (Abraham et al., 2005). The authors double stained an archived panel of 122 fixed breast cancer patient tumor samples for the prevalence of $CD24^{-/low}CD44^{+}$. They failed to find a correlation between increased abundance of these cells and tumor progression or worse outcome, but they did note a tendency towards the development of distant metastases (Abraham et al., 2005). Subsequently, in 2008, Honeth et al. stained a panel of 240 breast cancer patient samples for $CD24^{-/low}CD44^{+}$ cells and found an association between basal-like and BRCA1 hereditary breast cancer and the presence of $CD24^{-/low}CD44^{+}$ cells (Honeth et al., 2008). Also in 2008, Mylona et al. stained a panel of 155 fixed patient tumor samples and reported that the prevalence of $CD24^{-/low}CD44^{+}$ cells did not significantly correlate with worse prognosis. In fact, in disagreement with the CSC theory they found the opposite. Surprisingly, patient tumors with increased $CD24^{-/low}CD44^{+}$ cells tended to manifest increased disease-free survival (Mylona et al., 2008).

Cultured cell experiments indicate that $CD24^{-/low}CD44^{+}$ breast cancer cells are relatively more resistant to currently used therapeutics (Phillips et al., 2006). This suggests that prevalence of $CD24^{-/low}CD44^{+}$ cells in patient tumors is a potential measure of the susceptibility of breast cancer to certain therapeutics. If this hypothesis is true, then one would predict that post treatment, the percentage of these cells would increase as the overall bulk of the tumor is decreased. In a recent neoadjuvant immunohistological study of an archived panel of patient tumor samples before and after treatment, Aulmann et al. failed to show an increase in the frequency of $CD24^{-/low}CD44^{+}$ cells post treatment (Aulmann et al., 2010). In contrast, in a challenge to the theory CSC of the therapeutic resistance of these cells, the authors found that post treatment, the percentage of $CD24^{-/low}CD44^{+}$ tumor cells decreased relative to pretreatment (Aulmann et al., 2010). Further, the prevalence of these cells in a tumor did not correlate with the patient's response to treatment or eventual outcome (Aulmann et al., 2010). However, in agreement with results by Abraham et al. who noted that patient tumors with higher percentages of $CD24^{-/low}CD44^{+}$ tumor cells tended to develop distant metastases (Abraham et al., 2005), Aulmann et al. reported that patient tumors with higher percentages of $CD24^{-/low}CD44^{+}$ cells tended to develop bone metastases with greater frequency (Aulmann et al., 2010).

The results from the above described immunohistological studies evaluating the prevalence of $CD24^{-/low}CD44^{+}$ cells in breast tumors as a readout for predicting the relative aggressiveness of a breast cancer do not support their use as prognostic indicators. This is surprising considering that the prevalence of $CD44^{+}$ cells alone in fixed breast tumor cells was discovered to be predictive of more aggressive disease long before CD44 was identified as CSC marker (Al-Hajj et al., 2003). CD44 is a recognized predictor of breast cancer tumor grade (a histoclinical assessment of tumor cells and accepted clinical prognostic indicator (Dalton et al., 2000)), where patients with tumor cells expressing higher levels of CD44 membrane proteins have worse outcomes (Joensuu et al., 1993; Looi et al., 2006; McSherry et al., 2007). In light of the undisputed correlation between $CD44^{+}$ tumors and worse outcome for breast cancer patients, it seems that at least employing $CD44^{+}$ as a CSC marker agrees with the proposed role of CSC in mediating cancer progression. Where the hypothesis fails is in the inclusion of CD24 as a CSC marker. Perhaps the inclusion of $CD24^{-/low}$ as a criterion is not necessary and may be detrimental, at least from a diagnostic perspective. In fact, even prior to its use as a selection criterion for breast CSC isolation, increased (not decreased!) CD24 expression had been correlated with worse outcome for breast cancer patients (Athanassiadou et al., 2009; Kristiansen et al., 2003).

With the revelation that breast CSCs could also be identified by increased ALDH activity, expression of ALDH1A1 prevalence in breast cancer tumors was assessed for prognostic applicability (Ginestier et al., 2007). In this first analysis, ALDH1A1 expression was detected in only 30% of fixed breast cancer tumor samples (Ginestier et al., 2007). Immunohistological staining of 577 fixed tumor specimens revealed a significant correlation between ALDH1A1 expression and higher tumor grade. While these patients also had worse outcome overall, ALDH1A1 positivity failed to correlate with cancer stage and metastasis at the time of diagnosis (Ginestier et al., 2007). Later, in contrast, for a rare highly aggressive form of breast cancer, inflammatory breast cancer (one to five percent of all breast cancers), Charafe-Jauffret et al. found a significant correlation between ALDH1A1 expression and development of metastasis and worse outcome (Charafe-Jauffret et al., 2010). However, despite this positive correlation with a rare breast cancer, others have failed to show a significant correlation with ALDH1A1 prevalence and higher tumor grade, metastasis, therapeutic resistance or outcome with breast cancer in general (Morimoto et al., 2009; Neumeister et al., 2010; Neumeister and Rimm, 2009; Resetkova et al., 2009). In 2009, Morimoto et al. double immunohistochemical stained a panel of 203 fixed breast cancer tumor sample for the prevalence of ALDH1A1 along with estrogen receptor (ER), Ki67 and HER2 receptor status (Morimoto et al., 2009). The authors failed to find a correlation between ALDH1A1 prevalence and metastasis, but did note a non-significant trend with higher grade tumors. As well, ALDH1A1^{+} tumors were more likely to be ER^{-}, Ki67^{-}, and HER2^{+} (Morimoto et al., 2009). Also in 2009, Resetkova et al. immunostained four panels of fixed breast cancer patient panels, an adjuvantly treated series of 245 samples, a neoadjuvantly treated series of 34 samples and two series of 58 and 44 ER-PR-HER2-carcinoma samples. ALDH1A1 expression correlated significantly with basal-like HER2^{+} cancers, but not with other important indicators like metastasis. Interestingly, this result for ALDH1A1 was similar to the study on CD24$^{-/low}$CD44^{+} prevalence published by Honeth et al. who described a similar correlation between basal like breast cancers and CD24$^{-/low}$CD44^{+} abundance. This would suggest that there is an overlap between ALDH1A1^{+} and CD24$^{-/low}$CD44^{+} cells and supports the notion that both markers identify at least some of the same cell population (i.e. CSCs). The neoadjuvantly stained data set failed to show an enrichment of ALDH1A1^{+} cells post treatment, therefore not supporting the hypothesis that CSC population is resistant to currently employed therapeutics (Resetkova et al., 2009). Interestingly, however, the authors noted an increased expression of ALDH1A1^{+} in the stromal tissue post treatment, but overall higher expression in the stroma was associated with better outcomes. Most recently, Neumeister et al stained a panel of 639 breast cancer for ALDH1A1, CD44 and cytokeratin (Neumeister et al., 2010). While the prevalence of all three markers together was associated with worse outcome, staining the cohort of samples for ALDH1A1 alone failed to correlate with any of the prognostic indicators (e.g. tumor grade, lymph node metastasis), nor patient outcome (Neumeister et al., 2010). Overall, the published data does not lend strong support toward the prognostic potential of ALDH1A1 or CD24$^{-/low}$CD44^{+}. This has led to the suggestion that other breast CSC marker need to be identified, and has resulted in some scepticism as to the validity of the existing identified markers (Neumeister and Rimm, 2009). However, it is noted that when employed in combination, CD44 and ALDH1A1 prevalence did predict outcome for breast cancer patients (Neumeister et al., 2010), suggesting that the key may be using the CSC markers in combination.

Breast CSC marker	Patient sample size	Prognostic correlation: worse outcome	no correlation	improved outcome	Publication
$CD24^{-/low}$	201			X	(Kristiansen et al., 2003)
$CD24^{-/low}$	70			X	(Athanassiadou et al., 2009)
$CD44^{+}$	198	X			(Joensuu et al., 1993)
$CD44^{+}$	70	X			(Ozer et al., 1997)
$CD44^{+}$	152	X			(Bankfalvi et al., 1998)
$CD44^{+}$	135	X			(Schneider et al., 1999)
$CD44^{+}$	60	X			(Looi et al., 2006)
$CD24^{-/low}CD44^{+}$	122		X		(Abraham et al., 2005)
$CD24^{-/low}CD44^{+}$	240		X		(Honeth et al., 2008)
$CD24^{-/low}CD44^{+}$	155			X	(Mylona et al., 2008)
$CD24^{-/low}CD44^{+}$	50		X		(Aulmann et al., 2010)
$ALDH1A1^{+}$	577	X			(Ginestier et al., 2007)
$ALDH1A1^{+}$	203		X		(Morimoto et al., 2009)
$ALDH1A1^{+}$	381		X		(Resetkova et al., 2009)
$ALDH1A1^{+}$	109	X			(Charafe-Jauffret et al., 2010)
$ALDH1A1^{+}$	639		X		(Neumeister et al., 2010)
$ALDH1A1^{+}CD44^{+}cytokeratin^{+}$	639	X			(Neumeister et al., 2010)

Table 2. Summary of results from immunohistological prognostic studies of breast CSC markers

4. Brain cancer

4.a Identified brain CSC markers

Soon after breast CSCs were identified based on CD24$^{-/low}$CD44^{+} expression, similar studies conducted by Sing et al. identified a sub-tumor population of glioblastoma (most common brain cancer) cancer cells that were highly tumorigenic. As few as 10^2 glioblastoma cancer cells expressiong neural stem cell marker CD133^{+} (prominin 1) (Uchida et al., 2000) induced tumors in immunocompromised mice (Singh et al., 2003; Singh et al., 2004). In contrast to the CD133^{+} brain tumor cells, the CD133^{-} cells did not induce tumors, even when 10^5 cells were injected in the mice (Singh et al., 2004). As well, CD133^{+} cells exhibited the self-renewal differentiation properties characteristic of CSCs (Singh et al., 2004). Interestingly, as discussed later, CD133 would become a prominent CSC marker used for the isolation of highly tumorigenic cells in a number of cancers. However, like in other cancers, additional markers have been explored for brain cancer as well.

Again taking cues from discoveries made from normal neural stem cell research, Ogdent et al. and Tchoghandjian et al. found that glioblastoma CSCs could be identified by increased expression A2B5 (Ogden et al., 2008; Tchoghandjian et al., 2010). A2B5 is a ganglioside expressed specifically on the cell surface of neural progenitor cells (Nunes et al., 2003). Unexpectedly, CD133^{+} and A2B5^{+} potentially identify separate populations of brain tumor cells that do not necessarily overlap, in a patient dependant manner. This finding challenges the CSC theory, which predicts the existence of a cancer initiating tumor cell population that is identifiable based on a universally expressed combination of markers.

In 2007, Barraud et al. found that stage-specific embryonic antigen 4 (SSEA4), a known cell surface pluripotent human embryonic stem cell marker could also be used to enrich for the neural stem cells (Barraud et al., 2007). Subsequently, Son et al. found that the same marker could be used to isolate brain tumor cells with the CSC phenotype (increased tumorigenicity, self-renewal/differentiation properties) (Son et al., 2009). Almost all patient samples tested contained a SSEA4^{+} population, in agreement with the CSC theory (Son et al., 2009).

As of yet ALDH activity has not been explored as a marker for the isolation of brain CSCs. Given its applicability in a number of cancers (as discussed above and below), it would be surprising to find that it is not a relevant brain CSC marker.

4b. Brain CSC markers as prognostic indicators

There have been a number of studies addressing prognostic applicability of the first brain/glioblastoma CSC marker identified, CD133^{+} (summarized in Table 3). First, in 2008, Zeppernick et al. performed immunohistochemical analysis on 95 patient glioma samples of varied tumor grade and histology (Zeppernick et al., 2008). The authors report that CD133^{+} prevalence and clustering was associated significantly with worse outcome and survival. Further, CD133^{+} was a risk factor for tumor regrowth and metastasis, independent of tumor grade. Later that year, Beier et al., quantified a set of 36 high grade oligodendroglial tumors (less than 10% of all neural cancers) for their CD133 positivity (Beier et al., 2008). The authors reported that CD133 prevalence was a more accurate predictor of worse outcome for the patients than histological grading. In another 2008 study, Pallini et al. analysed a cohort of 44 glioblastoma patient tumor samples for prevalence of CD133^{+} and Ki67^{+} cells (Pallini et al., 2008). While CD133+ expression alone failed to predict patient oucome, coexpression of CD133/Ki67 was a highly significant independent prognostic risk factor with prevalence of $CD133^{+}Ki67^{+}$ tumor cells being correlative with quickened disease progression and poor clinical outcome. In 2008, Zhang et al. stained a panel of 125 low and high grade glioblastoma patient tumor samples for coexpression of CD133 and nestin (Zhang et al., 2008). The authors reported that $CD133^{+}nestin^{+}$ was associated with worse outcome and survival, and could potentially be used as independent prognostic indicators. Finally, in 2010, Sato et al. assessed if $CD133^{+}$ prevalence was associated with spread of the cancer in glioblastoma (Sato et al., 2010). The authors assessed 26 patient samples (16 cases of which the disease had disseminated) and reported that CD133 expression was significantly higher in disseminated disease cases. In summary, these studies agree that initial CD133 expression, especially when assessed in combination with an additional marker, is associated with more aggressive brain cancer and worse outcome. Therefore, the studies provide supportive evidence for the CSC theory postulation that CSCs are the initiators and mediators of cancers. We now await the results of studies evaluating the prognostic potential of the more recently discovered brain CSC markers (i.e. A2B5 and SSEA4) alone and in combination with CD133.

Most recently, the effect of therapy on the CSC population has been evaluated. In 2010, Pallini et al. quantified the frequency of CD133 pre and post radiochemotherapy on 37 paired glioblastoma patient samples (Pallini et al., 2010). In support of the CSC theory that proposes CSCs are resistant to currently employed therapeutics, the researchers noted a significant increase (average 4.6 fold) in $CD133^{+}$ cells post treatment. However, their analysis further revealed that the increased $CD133^{+}$ frequency post treatment was surprisingly associated with improved survival, not worse. The authors' following experiments revealed that not all $CD133^{+}$ cells quantified in the tumors were in actuality tumor cells. The non-tumor cell $CD133^{+}$ population might potentially have confounded their assessment of CSC frequency pre and post treatment and the effect on patient survival (Pallini et al., 2010). Furthermore, this revelation that not all $CD133^{+}$ cells are tumor cells may explain their earlier results where $CD133^{+}$ alone did not predict patient outcome, but $CD133^{+}Ki67^{+}$ did (Pallini et al., 2008). These results highlight the importance of employing multiple markers in the accurate identification of a CSC population in illustrating its potential prognostic applicability.

Brain CSC marker	Patient sample size	Prognostic correlation			Publication
		worse outcome	no correlation	improved outcome	
$CD133^{+}$	95	X			(Zeppernick et al., 2008)
$CD133^{+}$	36	X			(Beier et al., 2008)
$CD133^{+}$	44		X		(Pallini et al., 2008)
$CD133^{+}$	26	X			(Sato et al., 2010)
$CD133^{+}$	37			X	(Pallini et al., 2010)
$CD133^{+}Ki67^{+}$	44	X			(Pallini et al., 2008)
$CD133^{+}nestin^{+}$	125	X			(Zhang et al., 2008)

Table 3. Summary of results from immunohistological prognostic studies of brain CSC markers

5. Colon cancer

5.a Identified colon CSC markers

In early 2007, two groups identified a small percentage of highly tumorigenic $CD133^+$ colon cancer (colorectal carcinoma) with the renewal/differentiation properties of CSCs (O'Brien et al., 2007; Ricci-Vitiani et al., 2007). Ricci-Vitiani et al. estimated that CD133+ tumor cells made up 2.5% of total colon tumor cells, and O'Brien further calculated that only 1 in approximately 57,000 colon cancer cells was a CSC, but 1 in 262 CD133+ colon cancer cells was a CSC. Therefore while CD133 was one potential colon CSC marker, there remained others to be identified for the further enrichment of the CSC population. The following year, Shmelkov et al., reported that colon cancer initiating cells (CSCs) were found in both $CD133^+$ and $CD133^-$ tumor cell populations, high-lighting the importance of identifying additional markers (Shmelkov et al., 2008).

Dalerba et al., successfully identified and isolated colon CSCs based on expression of cell surface molecules other than CD133 (Dalerba et al., 2007). The researchers showed that $EpCAM^+CD44^+$ colon cancer cells ranged from 0.03% to 38% (mean = 5.4%) of total colon cancer cells and were highly tumorigenic in immunocompromised mice. In addition, the authors identified another cell surface adhesion molecule, CD166, which could be used for the isolation of colon CSCs. CD166 could be used independently of EpCAM/CD44 or synergistically with these other two markers to further enrich for the CSC population. In 2008, Haraguchi et al. reported that $CD133^+$ colon cancer varied in frequency from 0.3 – 82.5% (mean 35.5%) and that the cancer initiating cell could be further enriched for by isolating cells that were positive for both CD133 and CD44 (Haraguchi et al., 2008). $CD133^+CD44^+$ colon cells were more tumorigenic than $CD133^+$ or $CD44^+$ isolated colon cancer cells. Interestingly, in 2009 another group showed that $CD44^+$ isolated colon cells were highly tumorigenic, but failed to show similar tumorigenicity results when CD133 was used as the selection criterion (Chu et al., 2009).

Spheroid cultured colon CSCs were analysed for their celluar antigen expression profile and were found to be positive for CD133, CD166, CD44, CD29, CD24, Lgr5 and nuclear β-catenin (Vermeulen et al., 2008). All of these were previously known as normal colon stem cell markers, and some had been previously identified as colon CSC markers. The authors further showed that cells identified as $CD133^+CD24^+$ were further enriched for CSCs, but that co-expression of the other identified cell surface markers (CD44, CD166, or CD29) with CD133 failed to further enrich for the CSC population.

With the identification that ALDH activity could be used to isolate breast CSCs (Ginestier et al., 2007), ALDH activity was also assessed as a CSC marker for other solid tumors, including colon cancer. Colon cancer cells isolated based on increased ALDH activity by the aldefluor assay were shown to be more tumorigenic by a number of groups (Carpentino et al., 2009; Chu et al., 2009; Huang et al., 2009). Huang et al. first showed that as few as 25 $ALDH^+$ colon cancer cells could induce tumors in immunocompromised mice, and suggested that ALDH activity may be a more stringent selection marker than CD133 or CD44 for the selection of a colon CSC population (Huang et al., 2009). Undoubtedly, future studies will reveal if $ALDH^+$ combined with expression of these cell surface molecules will lead to further enrichment of the colon CSC population.

5.b Colon CSC markers as prognostic indicators

The data evaluating the use of currently known colon CSC markers as prognostic indicators is mixed and summarized in Table 4. For example, CD133 expression analyses are plentiful and do not reflect the molecule's prognostic value. We will first review the positive studies. In 2008, Horst et al. performed an immunohistological study of 77 fixed patient tumor samples and found that increased CD133 expression was indicative of worse outcome for patients (Horst et al., 2008). Later in 2009, the same group assessed if expression of CD133 combined with β-catenin had significant prognostic value in a panel of 162 patient samples (Horst et al., 2009a). CD133 and b-catenin stained distinct, partially overlapping cell populations and increased percentages of $CD133^{+}b\text{-catenin}^{+}$ was a stronger predictor of poor outcome than either marker alone (Horst et al., 2009a). The same group also compared the prognostic value of colon CSC markers CD133, CD44 and CD166 together and alone in a panel of 110 colorectal adenocarcinomas (Horst et al., 2009b). CD133 had the best prognostic potential of the three markers and correlated significantly with worse outcome (Horst et al., 2009b). However, patients with increased $CD133^{+}CD44^{+}CD166^{+}$ tumor cells fared the worse, illustrating again the value of using the markers in combination. In a study by another group, CD133 expression was quantified in 189 colorectal carcinomas and was predictive of worse outcome when specified to patients with well- and moderately-differentiated adenocarcinomas (Kojima et al., 2008). In a final example, increased CD133 expression in a panel of 104 stage IIIB colon carcinoma patient samples correlated with worse prognosis (Li et al., 2009).

In contrast to above described positive results, Choi et al. performed immunohistological assessments on 523 patient samples, that represented the complete range of histoclinical diagnoses, to determine the prognostic value of colon CSC markers CD133, CD44 and CD24 (Choi et al., 2009). Interestingly while expression of CD adhesion molecules correlated with some of the histoclinical prognostic indicators, none were significant prognostic predictors of survival (Choi et al., 2009), disagreeing with the findings of Horst et al. (Horst et al., 2008; Horst et al., 2009a; Horst et al., 2009b). Specifically, the authors determined that CD133 expression correlated with stage, CD24 with degree of differentiation and CD44 with tumor size (Choi et al., 2009). In 2010, Lugli et al., failed to correlate increased CD133 expression with tumor progression or survival time of patients when they probed a large panel of 1420 colorectal cancers by tissue microarray (Lugli et al., 2010). The cohort of samples was also probed for other implicated colon CSC markers; CD166, CD44 and EpCAM, and in contradiction of the CSC theory, their loss of expression, not gain, was associated with increased tumor progression and survival time. This trend was even more evident when the markers were combined (e.g. $CD166^{-}CD44^{-}$).

Independent of the discoveries implicating CD44, CD166, and CD24 as potential colon CSC markers (Dalerba et al., 2007; Vermeulen et al., 2008), the expression of the CD molecules has been previously assessed for predicting the outcome for colorectal cancer patients. For example, expression of certain splice variants of CD44 has been associated with worse outcome for colorectal cancer patients as early as the 1990s. In 1994, Mulder et al., stained 64 patient panel samples and for CD44v6 reported that increased expression of the CD variant was associated with increased tumor-related death (Mulder et al., 1994). However, another study by Weg-Remers et al., failed to detect a correlation between expression of CD44, standard or variants, and patient outcome or tumor progression (Weg-Remers et al., 1998). CD166 expression had been associated with reduced survival, despite not being correlative with tumor grade, stage or nodal involvement (Weichert et al., 2004). The same group later stained a cohort of 147 colon cancer patient samples for CD24 expression and made the distinction between membrane and cytoplasmic CD24 (Weichert et al., 2005). Interestingly, patients with high levels of cyoplasmic CD24 fared significantly worse, being more likely to have higher grade tumors, and develop metastases.

Colon CSC marker	Patient sample size	Prognostic correlation worse outcome	no correlation	improved outcome	Publication
CD133+	77	X			(Horst et al., 2008)
CD133+	189	X			(Kojima et al., 2008)
CD133+	110	X			(Horst et al., 2009b)
CD133+	523		X		(Choi et al., 2009)
CD133+	104	X			(Li et al., 2010a)
CD133+	1420		X		(Lugli et al., 2010)
CD24+	147	X			(Weichert et al., 2005)
CD24+	523		X		(Choi et al., 2009)
CD44+	83		X		(Weg-Remers et al., 1998)
CD44+	110		X		(Horst et al., 2009b)
CD44+	523		X		(Choi et al., 2009)
CD44+	1420			X	(Lugli et al., 2010)
CD166+	111	X			(Weichert et al., 2004)
CD166+	110		X		(Horst et al., 2009b)
CD166+	1420			X	(Lugli et al., 2010)
EpCam+	1420			X	(Lugli et al., 2010)
CD166+CD44+	1420			X	(Lugli et al., 2010)
CD133+b-catenin+	162	X			(Horst et al., 2009a)
CD133+CD44+CD166+	110	X			(Horst et al., 2009b)
ALDH1A1+	1420		X		Lugli, 2010 442 /id}

Table 4. Summary of results from immunohistological prognostic studies of colon CSC markers

Our analysis of the literature reveals a large disparity in the prognostic potential of the identified cell surface colon CSC markers. Potentially, differences in the results between groups could be explained by the varied methods and cut-offs used in tissue staining and scoring (Zlobec et al., 2007). For example Choi et al. scored the stained tissue samples as either positive or negative for expression of the CD molecules, whereas in the studies by Horst et al., the degree of staining was graded as none, low or high (Choi et al., 2009; Horst et al., 2008; Horst et al., 2009a; Horst et al., 2009b). Undoubtedly however, this can only be part of the explanation and it is more likely that the disagreement between groups is potentially an indication of the overall insignificant or poor prognostic value of these CSC markers for colon cancer when employed alone.
With the 2009 discovery that ALDH activity is also specific to colon CSCs (Carpentino et al., 2009; Chu et al., 2009; Huang et al., 2009), the potential of ALDH1A1 as a prognostic indicator is also being evaluated. In the recent study by Lugli et al., described above, who probed a panel of 1420 colorectal carcinomas for currently known cell surface colon CSC markers, the authors also assessed if ALDH1A1 expression had prognostic value (Lugli et al., 2010). The researchers detected ALDH1A1 in less than 25% of samples and failed to correlate patient outcome or disease progression with expression of the protein. Increased ALDH1A1 expression did however correlate with tumor grade (Lugli et al., 2010). In the coming years, the results of more immunohistological studies will clarify the potential prognostic power of ALDH1A1 for colorectal cancer.

6. Prostate cancer

6.a Identified prostate CSC markers

The currently known prostate CSC markers are based on the unique cell surface molecules and functional characteristics of normal prostate stem cells. Combining previously identified prostate stem cell markers $CD44^+$, $\alpha 2\beta 1^{high}$, $CD133^+$, Collins et al. isolated prostate cancer cells from patient tumor samples that had the *in vitro* self-renewal and differentiation properties of CSCs (Collins et al., 2005). Later in 2006, Patrawala isolated $CD44^+$ prostate cancer cells from cultures and tumors and showed that these cells possessed increased tumorigenicity *in vivo* and had stem cell like qualities (Patrawala et al., 2006). In 2005, using a murine prostate cancer model, Xin et al. showed that prostate cancer cells expressing stem cell antigen-1 (sca-1) were comparatively highly tumorigenic and possessed stem cell like characteristic (Xin et al., 2005). More recently, ALDH activity was also explored as a CSC marker for prostate cancer (Li et al., 2010b; van den Hoogen et al., 2010). Prostate cancer cells with increased ALDH activity were highly tumorigenic and possessed stem cell like characteristics (Li et al., 2010b; van den Hoogen et al., 2010). Interestingly, $ALDH^+$ cancer cells were also positive for CD44 and $\alpha 2\beta 1$ integrin, but not CD133 (van den Hoogen et al., 2010).

6.b Prostate CSC markers as prognostic indicators

The prognostic potential of currently known prostate CSC markers is ambiguous at best at this time (summarized in Table 5). CD44 has been assessed as a prognostic marker for prostate cancer since the 1990's, long before it was identified as a prostate CSC marker (Patrawala et al., 2006). In 1996, Nagabhushan et al. quantified the prevalence of CD44 in 74 fixed prostate cancer patient samples and noted that CD44 expression correlated inversely with tumor grade (Nagabhushan et al., 1996). A similar inverse relationship was detected in a subsequent study (Noordzij et al., 1997). Then again, 1999 and 2000, the same group published that CD44 expression decreased in patients with metastatic disease (Noordzij et al., 1999) and the loss of CD44 expression was an independent prognostic predictor of clinical reoccurrence (Vis et al., 2000). In 2001, Aaltomaa et al. analysed 209 prostate cancer samples and found that decreased CD44 expression correlated with metastasis and worse outcome (Aaltomaa et al., 2001). The results of these studies are in clear agreement with the prognostic potential of CD44 for prostate cancer. Unfortunately, from a CSC point of view, they are opposite to the predictions of the CSC theory, whereby an increase in CD44 would be expected to be associated with worse, not better outcomes.

The recent discoveries that ALDH activity could be employed to isolate prostate CSCs were also accompanied by prognostic data. van den Hoogen et al., failed to detect ALDH1A1 in 30 tissue microarray samples and 10 fixed primary tumor samples (van den Hoogen et al., 2010). The authors then decided to evaluate if expression of some of the other ALDH isoforms correlated significantly with clinical pathological determinants. While expression of isoform ALDH7a1 was detected in the majority patient samples, its expression failed to correlate significantly with Gleason score or tumor grade. These findings are in contrast to results published by Li et al. who report that increased ALDH1A1 expression correlated significantly with Gleason score, disease stage, and worse survival (Li et al., 2010b). Future immunohistological studies should resolve the discrepancy between the two groups with regards to the prognostic importance of ALDH1A1.

The greater prognostic potential of employing the CSC markers in combination remains to be shown for prostate cancer. Collins et al. who first discovered that the approximate 0.1%of $CD44^+\alpha2\beta1^{high}CD133^+$ of all prostate tumor cells had stem cell like characteristics, also reported that prevalence of these potential CSCs did not correlate with tumor grade (Collins et al., 2005). Perhaps future studies combining cell surface and functional markers (e.g. ALDH activity) may reveal a potential prognostic role for prostate CSC markers.

Prostate CSC marker	Patient sample size	Prognostic correlation: worse outcome	no correlation	improved outcome	Publication
$CD44^+$	74			X	(Nagabhushan et al., 1996)
$CD44^+$	97			X	(Noordzij et al., 1997)
$CD44^+$	46			X	(Noordzij et al., 1999)
$CD44^+$	209			X	(Aaltomaa et al., 2001)
$CD44^+\alpha2\beta1^{high}CD133^+$	40		X		(Collins et al., 2005)
$ALDH1A1^+$	40		X		(van den Hoogen et al., 2010)
$ALDH1A1^+$	163	X			(Li et al., 2010b)

Table 5. Summary of results from immunohistological prognostic studies of prostate CSC markers

7. Lung cancer

7.a Identified lung CSC markers

Initially, a side population (SP) of lung cancer cells identified by exclusion of Hoechst 33342 stain were shown to have stem cell like characteristics and overexpression of ABC transporters like ABCG2 was thought to mediate the innate chemo-resistance of stem cells (Hirschmann-Jax et al., 2004). The findings suggested the potential presence of a CSC population in lung cancer. Later, In 2008, Chen et al. isolated CD133$^+$ and $^-$ cancer cell populations from lung cancer cell lines and non-small cell lung cancer patients and reported that CD133$^+$ lung cancer cells had *in vitro* CSC and stem cell like qualities (Chen et al., 2008). This work provided the first indication that CD133 could potentially be used as a lung CSC marker. Later in 2009, Bertolini et al. proved that CD133 was a lung CSC marker (Bertolini et al., 2009). The researchers showed that patient isolated CD133$^+$ (and stained with epithelial-specific antigen to eliminate contaminating cells) lung cancer cells were highly tumorigenic compared to CD133$^-$ cancer cells and had stem cell characteristics (Bertolini et al., 2009). Similar results using CD133 as a lung CSC marker were published by another group later that year, solidifying CD133's recognition as an important lung CSC marker (Tirino et al., 2009).

ALDH activity has also been tested for the isolation of lung CSCs (Jiang et al., 2009; Ucar et al., 2009). Jiang et al. showed it was possible to isolate ALDH$^+$ lung cancer cells from cultured cell lines that were more tumorigenic in immunocompromised mice and displayed stem cell like qualities (i.e. self renewal/differentiation and resistance to chemotherapeutics). As of yet ALDH activity and CD133 have not been employed in combination to potentially isolate a further CSC-encriched population of cells.

7.b Lung CSC markers as prognostic indicators

The data evaluating the use of currently known lung CSC markers as prognostic indicators is mixed and summarized in Table 6. In addition to illustrating the increased tumorigenicity of CD133$^+$ lung cancer cells, Bertolini et al., assessed if CD133 had prognostic value for lung cancer patients (Bertolini et al., 2009). The researchers stained a panel of 42 fixed tumor samples for CD133 expression and showed that patients with CD133$^+$ tumors tended to have a shorter progression-free survival. However, the outcome difference between CD133$^+$ and CD133$^-$ tumors was not statistically significant. Tirino et al. also evaluated the prognostic potential of CD133 for lung cancer (Tirino et al., 2009). Their study of 89 patient samples failed to find a correlation between CD133 expression and the clinical pathological assessments of disease aggressiveness (e.g. tumor size, stage). However they noted a non-significant trend toward shorter disease progression times in the CD133$^+$ patient samples. In a another study of 88 patient samples conducted by Salnikov et al., CD133$^+$ prevalence failed to significantly correlate with tumor size, cancer stage, local metastasis or overall survival (Salnikov et al., 2010). Potentially if a larger sample size was employed in the studies statistical significance may have been reached for some parameters.

The above studies suggest that presence of CD133 alone does not appear to be a strong predictor of disease progression and outcome for lung cancer. However, recent studies employing CD133 in combination with other markers appear more promising. In 2010, Li et al. showed that combination of CD133 with the ABC transporter, ABCG2, was a much more powerful prognostic tool than either marker alone (Li et al., 2010a). The researchers stained a panel of 145 lung cancer patient samples, and when used alone neither marker correlated significantly with clinical pathological assessment of disease or disease progression. However, when the prevalence of CD133+ABCG2+ was quantified, increased frequency of CD133+ABCG2+ cancer cells correlated significantly with shorter times to reoccurrence, illustrating the prognostic power of combining CSC markers.

Finally with their recent discovery that ALDH activity could be employed to isolate lung CSCs, Jiang et al. also determined if ALDH1A1 positivity in lung cancer patient samples was a potential prognostic indicator (Jiang et al., 2009). ALDH1A1 expression correlated significantly with higher tumor grade, disease stage and poor clinical outcome (Jiang et al., 2009). Interestingly, in these immunohistochemical analyses ALDH1A1 positive samples were also CD133+ (60% of patient samples). In contrast, patient samples that were negative for ALDH1A1 expression also lacked CD133 expression. This suggests that potentially CD133+ and ALDH+ can be combined to isolate a more tumorigenic population of lung cancer cells. Future studies will reveal if CD133 combined with ALDH1A1 is a superior and potentially powerful prognostic tool for lung cancer.

Lung CSC marker	Patient sample size	Prognostic correlation: worse outcome	Prognostic correlation: no correlation	Prognostic correlation: improved outcome	Publication
CD133+	42		X		(Bertolini et al., 2009)
CD133+	89		X		(Tirino et al., 2009)
CD133+	88		X		(Salnikov et al., 2010)
CD133+	145		X		(Li et al., 2010a)
ABCG2+	145		X		(Li et al., 2010a)
CD133+ABCG2+	145	X			(Li et al., 2010a)
ALDH1A1+	60	X			(Jiang et al., 2009)

Table 6. Summary of results from immunohistological prognostic studies of lung CSC markers

8. Conclusions

CSCs have become a universal cancer concept. Using *in vitro* and *in vivo* experimental models, this sub-population of highly tumorigenic tumor cells has been shown to exist in most cancers and is resistant to chemo- and radiation therapy. As such, CSCs are believed to be the initiators of cancer, propagators of metastasis and mediators of therapeutic resistance. What is needed is conclusive proof of the importance of CSCs from clinical patient data. As reviewed here, there already exists much clinical data that support or refute the CSC theory from a cancer progression and reoccurrence point of view. Based on publised data thus far, it appears that using a combination of CSC markers, and eliminating the least relevant proposed CSC markers, is the most logical approach not only for accurate identification of CSCs but also for revelation of their important roles in cancer development. With the inevitable future discovery of new CSC markers and their combined use with valid ones previously discovered, the empirical proof that CSCs are the key to both the cause and cure of cancer may be a foregone conclusion.

9. References

Aaltomaa,S., Lipponen,P., la-Opas,M., and Kosma,V.M. (2001). Expression and prognostic value of CD44 standard and variant v3 and v6 isoforms in prostate cancer. Eur. Urol. *39*, 138-144.

Abraham,B.K., Fritz,P., McClellan,M., Hauptvogel,P., Athelogou,M., and Brauch,H. (2005). Prevalence of CD44+/CD24-/low cells in breast cancer may not be associated with clinical outcome but may favor distant metastasis. Clin. Cancer Res *11*, 1154-1159.

Advani,A.S., Rodriguez,C., Jin,T., Jawde,R.A., Saber,W., Baz,R., Kalaycio,M., Sobecks,R., Sekeres,M., Tripp,B., and Hsi,E. (2008). Increased C-kit intensity is a poor prognostic factor for progression-free and overall survival in patients with newly diagnosed AML. Leuk. Res. *32*, 913-918.

Al-Hajj,M., Wicha,M.S., ito-Hernandez,A., Morrison,S.J., and Clarke,M.F. (2003). Prospective identification of tumorigenic breast cancer cells. Proc. Natl. Acad. Sci. U. S. A *100*, 3983-3988.

Armstrong,L., Stojkovic,M., Dimmick,I., Ahmad,S., Stojkovic,P., Hole,N., and Lako,M. (2004). Phenotypic characterization of murine primitive hematopoietic progenitor cells isolated on basis of aldehyde dehydrogenase activity. Stem Cells *22*, 1142-1151.

Arslan,O., Akan,H., Beksac,M., Ozcan,M., Koc,H., Ilhan,O., Konuk,N., and Uysal,A. (1996). Lack of prognostic value of CD34 in adult AML. Leuk. Lymphoma *23*, 185-186.

Athanassiadou,P., Grapsa,D., Gonidi,M., Athanassiadou,A.M., Tsipis,A., and Patsouris,E. (2009). CD24 expression has a prognostic impact in breast carcinoma. Pathol. Res. Pract. *205*, 524-533.

Aulmann,S., Waldburger,N., Penzel,R., Andrulis,M., Schirmacher,P., and Sinn,H.P. (2010). Reduction of CD44(+)/CD24(-) breast cancer cells by conventional cytotoxic chemotherapy. Hum. Pathol. *41*, 574-581.

Bankfalvi,A., Terpe,H.J., Breukelmann,D., Bier,B., Rempe,D., Pschadka,G., Krech,R., and Bocker,W. (1998). Gains and losses of CD44 expression during breast carcinogenesis and tumour progression. Histopathology *33*, 107-116.

Barraud,P., Stott,S., Mollgard,K., Parmar,M., and Bjorklund,A. (2007). In vitro characterization of a human neural progenitor cell coexpressing SSEA4 and CD133. J. Neurosci. Res. *85*, 250-259.

Beier,D., Wischhusen,J., Dietmaier,W., Hau,P., Proescholdt,M., Brawanski,A., Bogdahn,U., and Beier,C.P. (2008). CD133 expression and cancer stem cells predict prognosis in high-grade oligodendroglial tumors. Brain Pathol. *18*, 370-377.

Bertolini,G., Roz,L., Perego,P., Tortoreto,M., Fontanella,E., Gatti,L., Pratesi,G., Fabbri,A., Andriani,F., Tinelli,S., Roz,E., Caserini,R., Lo,V.S., Camerini,T., Mariani,L., Delia,D., Calabro,E., Pastorino,U., and Sozzi,G. (2009). Highly tumorigenic lung cancer CD133+ cells display stem-like features and are spared by cisplatin treatment. Proc. Natl. Acad. Sci. U. S. A *106*, 16281-16286.

Blair,A., Hogge,D.E., Ailles,L.E., Lansdorp,P.M., and Sutherland,H.J. (1997). Lack of expression of Thy-1 (CD90) on acute myeloid leukemia cells with long-term proliferative ability in vitro and in vivo. Blood *89*, 3104-3112.

Blair,A., Hogge,D.E., and Sutherland,H.J. (1998). Most acute myeloid leukemia progenitor cells with long-term proliferative ability in vitro and in vivo have the phenotype CD34(+)/CD71(-)/HLA-DR-. Blood *92*, 4325-4335.

Blair,A. and Sutherland,H.J. (2000). Primitive acute myeloid leukemia cells with long-term proliferative ability in vitro and in vivo lack surface expression of c-kit (CD117). Exp. Hematol. *28*, 660-671.

Bonnet,D. and Dick,J.E. (1997). Human acute myeloid leukemia is organized as a hierarchy that originates from a primitive hematopoietic cell. Nat. Med. *3*, 730-737.

Borowitz,M.J., Gockerman,J.P., Moore,J.O., Civin,C.I., Page,S.O., Robertson,J., and Bigner,S.H. (1989). Clinicopathologic and cytogenic features of CD34 (My 10)-positive acute nonlymphocytic leukemia. Am. J. Clin. Pathol. *91*, 265-270.

Bradstock,K., Matthews,J., Benson,E., Page,F., and Bishop,J. (1994). Prognostic value of immunophenotyping in acute myeloid leukemia. Australian Leukaemia Study Group. Blood *84*, 1220-1225.

Campos,L., Guyotat,D., Archimbaud,E., Calmard-Oriol,P., Tsuruo,T., Troncy,J., Treille,D., and Fiere,D. (1992). Clinical significance of multidrug resistance P-glycoprotein expression on acute nonlymphoblastic leukemia cells at diagnosis. Blood *79*, 473-476.

Campos,L., Guyotat,D., Archimbaud,E., Devaux,Y., Treille,D., Larese,A., Maupas,J., Gentilhomme,O., Ehrsam,A., and Fiere,D. (1989). Surface marker expression in adult acute myeloid leukaemia: correlations with initial characteristics, morphology and response to therapy. Br. J. Haematol. *72*, 161-166.

Carpentino,J.E., Hynes,M.J., Appelman,H.D., Zheng,T., Steindler,D.A., Scott,E.W., and Huang,E.H. (2009). Aldehyde dehydrogenase-expressing colon stem cells contribute to tumorigenesis in the transition from colitis to cancer. Cancer Res. *69*, 8208-8215.

Charafe-Jauffret,E., Ginestier,C., Iovino,F., Tarpin,C., Diebel,M., Esterni,B., Houvenaeghel,G., Extra,J.M., Bertucci,F., Jacquemier,J., Xerri,L., Dontu,G., Stassi,G., Xiao,Y., Barsky,S.H., Birnbaum,D., Viens,P., and Wicha,M.S. (2010). Aldehyde dehydrogenase 1-positive cancer stem cells mediate metastasis and poor clinical outcome in inflammatory breast cancer. Clin. Cancer Res. *16*, 45-55.

Chen,Y.C., Hsu,H.S., Chen,Y.W., Tsai,T.H., How,C.K., Wang,C.Y., Hung,S.C., Chang,Y.L., Tsai,M.L., Lee,Y.Y., Ku,H.H., and Chiou,S.H. (2008). Oct-4 expression maintained cancer stem-like properties in lung cancer-derived CD133-positive cells. PLoS. ONE. *3*, e2637.

Cheung,A.M., Wan,T.S., Leung,J.C., Chan,L.Y., Huang,H., Kwong,Y.L., Liang,R., and Leung,A.Y. (2007). Aldehyde dehydrogenase activity in leukemic blasts defines a subgroup of acute myeloid leukemia with adverse prognosis and superior NOD/SCID engrafting potential. Leukemia *21*, 1423-1430.

Choi,D., Lee,H.W., Hur,K.Y., Kim,J.J., Park,G.S., Jang,S.H., Song,Y.S., Jang,K.S., and Paik,S.S. (2009). Cancer stem cell markers CD133 and CD24 correlate with invasiveness and differentiation in colorectal adenocarcinoma. World J. Gastroenterol. *15*, 2258-2264.

Chu,P., Clanton,D.J., Snipas,T.S., Lee,J., Mitchell,E., Nguyen,M.L., Hare,E., and Peach,R.J. (2009). Characterization of a subpopulation of colon cancer cells with stem cell-like properties. Int. J. Cancer *124*, 1312-1321.

Chute,J.P., Muramoto,G.G., Whitesides,J., Colvin,M., Safi,R., Chao,N.J., and McDonnell,D.P. (2006). Inhibition of aldehyde dehydrogenase and retinoid signaling induces the expansion of human hematopoietic stem cells. Proc. Natl. Acad. Sci. U. S. A *103*, 11707-11712.

Ciolli,S., Leoni,F., Caporale,R., Pascarella,A., Salti,F., and Rossi-Ferrini,P. (1993). CD34 expression fails to predict the outcome in adult acute myeloid leukemia. Haematologica *78*, 151-155.

Collins,A.T., Berry,P.A., Hyde,C., Stower,M.J., and Maitland,N.J. (2005). Prospective identification of tumorigenic prostate cancer stem cells. Cancer Res *65*, 10946-10951.

Collins,S.J. (2008). Retinoic acid receptors, hematopoiesis and leukemogenesis. Curr. Opin. Hematol. *15*, 346-351.

Dalal,B.I., Wu,V., Barnett,M.J., Horsman,D.E., Spinelli,J.J., Naiman,S.C., Shepherd,J.D., Nantel,S.H., Reece,D.E., Sutherland,H.J., Klingemann,H.G., and Phillips,G.L. (1997). Induction failure in de novo acute myelogenous leukemia is associated with expression of high levels of CD34 antigen by the leukemic blasts. Leuk. Lymphoma *26*, 299-306.

Dalerba,P., Dylla,S.J., Park,I.K., Liu,R., Wang,X., Cho,R.W., Hoey,T., Gurney,A., Huang,E.H., Simeone,D.M., Shelton,A.A., Parmiani,G., Castelli,C., and Clarke,M.F. (2007). Phenotypic characterization of human colorectal cancer stem cells. Proc. Natl. Acad. Sci. U. S. A *104*, 10158-10163.

Dalton,L.W., Pinder,S.E., Elston,C.E., Ellis,I.O., Page,D.L., Dupont,W.D., and Blamey,R.W. (2000). Histologic grading of breast cancer: linkage of patient outcome with level of pathologist agreement. Mod. Pathol. *13*, 730-735.

Ebinger,M., Witte,K.E., Ahlers,J., Schafer,I., Andre,M., Kerst,G., Scheel-Walter,H.G., Lang,P., and Handgretinger,R. (2010). High frequency of immature cells at diagnosis predicts high minimal residual disease level in childhood acute lymphoblastic leukemia. Leuk. Res. *34*, 1139-1142.

Fagioli,F., Cuneo,A., Carli,M.G., Bardi,A., Piva,N., Previati,R., Rigolin,G.M., Ferrari,L., Spanedda,R., and Castoldi,G. (1993). Chromosome aberrations in CD34-positive acute myeloid leukemia. Correlation with clinicopathologic features. Cancer Genet. Cytogenet. *71*, 119-124.

Fruchart,C., Lenormand,B., Bastard,C., Boulet,D., Lesesve,J.F., Callat,M.P., Stamatoullas,A., Monconduit,M., and Tilly,H. (1996). Correlation between CD34 expression and chromosomal abnormalities but not clinical outcome in acute myeloid leukemia. Am. J. Hematol. *53*, 175-180.

Geller,R.B., Zahurak,M., Hurwitz,C.A., Burke,P.J., Karp,J.E., Piantadosi,S., and Civin,C.I. (1990). Prognostic importance of immunophenotyping in adults with acute myelocytic leukaemia: the significance of the stem-cell glycoprotein CD34 (My10). Br. J. Haematol. *76*, 340-347.

Ginestier,C., Hur,M.H., Charafe-Jauffret,E., Monville,F., Dutcher,J., Brown,M., Jacquemier,J., Viens,P., Kleer,C.G., Liu,S., Schott,A., Hayes,D., Birnbaum,D., Wicha,M.S., and Dontu,G. (2007). ALDH1 Is a Marker of Normal and Malignant Human Mammary Stem Cells and a Predictor of Poor Clinical Outcome. Cell Stem Cell *1*, 555-567.

Guinot,M., Sanz,G.F., Sempere,A., Arilla,M.J., Jarque,I., Gomis,F., and Sanz,M.A. (1991). Prognostic value of CD34 expression in de novo acute myeloblastic leukaemia. Br. J. Haematol. *79*, 533-534.

Haraguchi,N., Ohkuma,M., Sakashita,H., Matsuzaki,S., Tanaka,F., Mimori,K., Kamohara,Y., Inoue,H., and Mori,M. (2008). CD133+CD44+ population efficiently enriches colon cancer initiating cells. Ann. Surg. Oncol. *15*, 2927-2933.

Hirschmann-Jax,C., Foster,A.E., Wulf,G.G., Nuchtern,J.G., Jax,T.W., Gobel,U., Goodell,M.A., and Brenner,M.K. (2004). A distinct "side population" of cells with high drug efflux capacity in human tumor cells. Proc. Natl. Acad. Sci. U. S. A *101*, 14228-14233.

Honeth,G., Bendahl,P.O., Ringner,M., Saal,L.H., Gruvberger-Saal,S.K., Lovgren,K., Grabau,D., Ferno,M., Borg,A., and Hegardt,C. (2008). The CD44+/CD24- phenotype is enriched in basal-like breast tumors. Breast Cancer Res. *10*, R53.

Horst,D., Kriegl,L., Engel,J., Jung,A., and Kirchner,T. (2009a). CD133 and nuclear beta-catenin: the marker combination to detect high risk cases of low stage colorectal cancer. Eur. J. Cancer *45*, 2034-2040.

Horst,D., Kriegl,L., Engel,J., Kirchner,T., and Jung,A. (2008). CD133 expression is an independent prognostic marker for low survival in colorectal cancer. Br. J. Cancer *99*, 1285-1289.

Horst,D., Kriegl,L., Engel,J., Kirchner,T., and Jung,A. (2009b). Prognostic significance of the cancer stem cell markers CD133, CD44, and CD166 in colorectal cancer. Cancer Invest *27*, 844-850.

Huang,E.H., Hynes,M.J., Zhang,T., Ginestier,C., Dontu,G., Appelman,H., Fields,J.Z., Wicha,M.S., and Boman,B.M. (2009). Aldehyde dehydrogenase 1 is a marker for normal and malignant human colonic stem cells (SC) and tracks SC overpopulation during colon tumorigenesis. Cancer Res. *69*, 3382-3389.

Jiang,F., Qiu,Q., Khanna,A., Todd,N.W., Deepak,J., Xing,L., Wang,H., Liu,Z., Su,Y., Stass,S.A., and Katz,R.L. (2009). Aldehyde dehydrogenase 1 is a tumor stem cell-associated marker in lung cancer. Mol. Cancer Res. *7*, 330-338.

Joensuu,H., Klemi,P.J., Toikkanen,S., and Jalkanen,S. (1993). Glycoprotein CD44 expression and its association with survival in breast cancer. Am. J. Pathol. *143*, 867-874.

Jordan,C.T., Upchurch,D., Szilvassy,S.J., Guzman,M.L., Howard,D.S., Pettigrew,A.L., Meyerrose,T., Rossi,R., Grimes,B., Rizzieri,D.A., Luger,S.M., and Phillips,G.L. (2000). The interleukin-3 receptor alpha chain is a unique marker for human acute myelogenous leukemia stem cells. Leukemia *14*, 1777-1784.

Kanda,Y., Hamaki,T., Yamamoto,R., Chizuka,A., Suguro,M., Matsuyama,T., Takezako,N., Miwa,A., Kami,M., Hirai,H., and Togawa,A. (2000). The clinical significance of CD34 expression in response to therapy of patients with acute myeloid leukemia: an overview of 2483 patients from 22 studies. Cancer *88*, 2529-2533.

Keyhani,A., Huh,Y.O., Jendiroba,D., Pagliaro,L., Cortez,J., Pierce,S., Pearlman,M., Estey,E., Kantarjian,H., and Freireich,E.J. (2000). Increased CD38 expression is associated with favorable prognosis in adult acute leukemia. Leuk. Res. *24*, 153-159.

Koehler,M., Behm,F., Hancock,M., and Pui,C.H. (1993). Expression of activation antigens CD38 and CD71 is not clinically important in childhood acute lymphoblastic leukemia. Leukemia *7*, 41-45.

Kojima,M., Ishii,G., Atsumi,N., Fujii,S., Saito,N., and Ochiai,A. (2008). Immunohistochemical detection of CD133 expression in colorectal cancer: a clinicopathological study. Cancer Sci. *99*, 1578-1583.

Kristiansen,G., Winzer,K.J., Mayordomo,E., Bellach,J., Schluns,K., Denkert,C., Dahl,E., Pilarsky,C., Altevogt,P., Guski,H., and Dietel,M. (2003). CD24 expression is a new prognostic marker in breast cancer. Clin. Cancer Res. *9*, 4906-4913.

Kyoda,K., Nakamura,S., Hattori,N., Takeshima,M., Nakamura,K., Kaya,H., Matano,S., Okumura,H., Kanno,M., Ohtake,S., and Matsuda,T. (1998). Lack of prognostic significance of CD34 expression in adult AML when FAB M0 and M3 are excluded. Am. J. Hematol. *57*, 265-266.

Lamy,T., Goasguen,J.E., Mordelet,E., Grulois,I., Dauriac,C., Drenou,B., Chaperon,J., Fauchet,R., and le Prise,P.Y. (1994). P-glycoprotein (P-170) and CD34 expression in adult acute myeloid leukemia (AML). Leukemia *8*, 1879-1883.

Lanzkron,S.M., Collector,M.I., and Sharkis,S.J. (1999). Hematopoietic stem cell tracking in vivo: a comparison of short-term and long-term repopulating cells. Blood *93*, 1916-1921.

Lapidot,T., Sirard,C., Vormoor,J., Murdoch,B., Hoang,T., Caceres-Cortes,J., Minden,M., Paterson,B., Caligiuri,M.A., and Dick,J.E. (1994). A cell initiating human acute myeloid leukaemia after transplantation into SCID mice. Nature *367*, 645-648.

Lee,E.J., Yang,J., Leavitt,R.D., Testa,J.R., Civin,C.I., Forrest,A., and Schiffer,C.A. (1992). The significance of CD34 and TdT determinations in patients with untreated de novo acute myeloid leukemia. Leukemia *6*, 1203-1209.

Li,C.Y., Li,B.X., Liang,Y., Peng,R.Q., Ding,Y., Xu,D.Z., Zhang,X., Pan,Z.Z., Wan,D.S., Zeng,Y.X., Zhu,X.F., and Zhang,X.S. (2009). Higher percentage of CD133+ cells is associated with poor prognosis in colon carcinoma patients with stage IIIB. J. Transl. Med. *7*, 56.

Li,F., Zeng,H., and Ying,K. (2010a). The combination of stem cell markers CD133 and ABCG2 predicts relapse in stage I non-small cell lung carcinomas. Med. Oncol.

Li,T., Su,Y., Mei,Y., Leng,Q., Leng,B., Liu,Z., Stass,S.A., and Jiang,F. (2010b). ALDH1A1 is a marker for malignant prostate stem cells and predictor of prostate cancer patients' outcome. Lab Invest *90*, 234-244.

Looi,L.M., Cheah,P.L., Zhao,W., Ng,M.H., and Yip,C.H. (2006). CD44 expression and axillary lymph node metastasis in infiltrating ductal carcinoma of the breast. Malays. J. Pathol. *28*, 83-86.

Lugli,A., Iezzi,G., Hostettler,I., Muraro,M.G., Mele,V., Tornillo,L., Carafa,V., Spagnoli,G., Terracciano,L., and Zlobec,I. (2010). Prognostic impact of the expression of putative cancer stem cell markers CD133, CD166, CD44s, EpCAM, and ALDH1 in colorectal cancer. Br. J. Cancer *103*, 382-390.

Magni,M., Shammah,S., Schiro,R., Mellado,W., la-Favera,R., and Gianni,A.M. (1996). Induction of cyclophosphamide-resistance by aldehyde-dehydrogenase gene transfer. Blood *87*, 1097-1103.

Marchitti,S.A., Brocker,C., Stagos,D., and Vasiliou,V. (2008). Non-P450 aldehyde oxidizing enzymes: the aldehyde dehydrogenase superfamily. Expert. Opin. Drug Metab Toxicol. *4*, 697-720.

McSherry,E.A., Donatello,S., Hopkins,A.M., and McDonnell,S. (2007). Molecular basis of invasion in breast cancer. Cell Mol. Life Sci. 64, 3201-18.

Morimoto,K., Kim,S.J., Tanei,T., Shimazu,K., Tanji,Y., Taguchi,T., Tamaki,Y., Terada,N., and Noguchi,S. (2009). Stem cell marker aldehyde dehydrogenase 1-positive breast cancers are characterized by negative estrogen receptor, positive human epidermal growth factor receptor type 2, and high Ki67 expression. Cancer Sci. *100*, 1062-1068.

Mulder,J.W., Kruyt,P.M., Sewnath,M., Oosting,J., Seldenrijk,C.A., Weidema,W.F., Offerhaus,G.J., and Pals,S.T. (1994). Colorectal cancer prognosis and expression of exon-v6-containing CD44 proteins. Lancet *344*, 1470-1472.

Myint,H. and Lucie,N.P. (1992). The prognostic significance of the CD34 antigen in acute myeloid leukaemia. Leuk. Lymphoma *7*, 425-429.

Mylona,E., Giannopoulou,I., Fasomytakis,E., Nomikos,A., Magkou,C., Bakarakos,P., and Nakopoulou,L. (2008). The clinicopathologic and prognostic significance of CD44+/CD24(-/low) and CD44-/CD24+ tumor cells in invasive breast carcinomas. Hum. Pathol. *39*, 1096-1102.

Nagabhushan,M., Pretlow,T.G., Guo,Y.J., Amini,S.B., Pretlow,T.P., and Sy,M.S. (1996). Altered expression of CD44 in human prostate cancer during progression. Am. J. Clin. Pathol. *106*, 647-651.

Neumeister,V., Agarwal,S., Bordeaux,J., Camp,R.L., and Rimm,D.L. (2010). In situ identification of putative cancer stem cells by multiplexing ALDH1, CD44, and cytokeratin identifies breast cancer patients with poor prognosis. Am. J. Pathol. *176*, 2131-2138.

Neumeister,V. and Rimm,D. (2010). Is ALDH1 a good method for definition of breast cancer stem cells? Breast Cancer Res. Treat. 123, 109-11.

Noordzij,M.A., van Steenbrugge,G.J., Schroder,F.H., and van der Kwast,T.H. (1999). Decreased expression of CD44 in metastatic prostate cancer. Int. J. Cancer *84*, 478-483.

Noordzij,M.A., van Steenbrugge,G.J., Verkaik,N.S., Schroder,F.H., and van der Kwast,T.H. (1997). The prognostic value of CD44 isoforms in prostate cancer patients treated by radical prostatectomy. Clin. Cancer Res. *3*, 805-815.

Nunes,M.C., Roy,N.S., Keyoung,H.M., Goodman,R.R., McKhann,G., Jiang,L., Kang,J., Nedergaard,M., and Goldman,S.A. (2003). Identification and isolation of multipotential neural progenitor cells from the subcortical white matter of the adult human brain. Nat. Med. *9*, 439-447.

O'Brien,C.A., Pollett,A., Gallinger,S., and Dick,J.E. (2007). A human colon cancer cell capable of initiating tumour growth in immunodeficient mice. Nature *445*, 106-110.

Ogden,A.T., Waziri,A.E., Lochhead,R.A., Fusco,D., Lopez,K., Ellis,J.A., Kang,J., Assanah,M., McKhann,G.M., Sisti,M.B., McCormick,P.C., Canoll,P., and Bruce,J.N. (2008). Identification of A2B5+CD133- tumor-initiating cells in adult human gliomas. Neurosurgery *62*, 505-514.

Ozer,E., Canda,T., and Kurtodlu,B. (1997). The role of angiogenesis, laminin and CD44 expression in metastatic behavior of early-stage low-grade invasive breast carcinomas. Cancer Lett. *121*, 119-123.

Pallini,R., Ricci-Vitiani,L., Banna,G.L., Signore,M., Lombardi,D., Todaro,M., Stassi,G., Martini,M., Maira,G., Larocca,L.M., and De,M.R. (2008). Cancer stem cell analysis and clinical outcome in patients with glioblastoma multiforme. Clin. Cancer Res. *14*, 8205-8212.

Pallini,R., Ricci-Vitiani,L., Montano,N., Mollinari,C., Biffoni,M., Cenci,T., Pierconti,F., Martini,M., De,M.R., and Larocca,L.M. (2010). Expression of the stem cell marker CD133 in recurrent glioblastoma and its value for prognosis. Cancer.

Patrawala,L., Calhoun,T., Schneider-Broussard,R., Li,H., Bhatia,B., Tang,S., Reilly,J.G., Chandra,D., Zhou,J., Claypool,K., Coghlan,L., and Tang,D.G. (2006). Highly purified CD44+ prostate cancer cells from xenograft human tumors are enriched in tumorigenic and metastatic progenitor cells. Oncogene *25*, 1696-1708.

Pece,S., Tosoni,D., Confalonieri,S., Mazzarol,G., Vecchi,M., Ronzoni,S., Bernard,L., Viale,G., Pelicci,P.G., and Di Fiore,P.P. (2010). Biological and molecular heterogeneity of breast cancers correlates with their cancer stem cell content. Cell *140*, 62-73.

Phillips,T.M., McBride,W.H., and Pajonk,F. (2006). The response of CD24(-/low)/CD44+ breast cancer-initiating cells to radiation. J. Natl. Cancer Inst. *98*, 1777-1785.

Porwit-MacDonald,A., Janossy,G., Ivory,K., Swirsky,D., Peters,R., Wheatley,K., Walker,H., Turker,A., Goldstone,A.H., and Burnett,A. (1996). Leukemia-associated changes identified by quantitative flow cytometry. IV. CD34 overexpression in acute myelogenous leukemia M2 with t(8;21). Blood *87*, 1162-1169.

Ran,D., Schubert,M., Pietsch,L., Taubert,I., Wuchter,P., Eckstein,V., Bruckner,T., Zoeller,M., and Ho,A.D. (2009). Aldehyde dehydrogenase activity among primary leukemia cells is associated with stem cell features and correlates with adverse clinical outcomes. Exp. Hematol. *37*, 1423-1434.

Raspadori,D., Lauria,F., Ventura,M.A., Rondelli,D., Visani,G., de,V.A., and Tura,S. (1997). Incidence and prognostic relevance of CD34 expression in acute myeloblastic leukemia: analysis of 141 cases. Leuk. Res. *21*, 603-607.

Repp,R., Schaekel,U., Helm,G., Thiede,C., Soucek,S., Pascheberg,U., Wandt,H., Aulitzky,W., Bodenstein,H., Sonnen,R., Link,H., Ehninger,G., and Gramatzki,M. (2003). Immunophenotyping is an independent factor for risk stratification in AML. Cytometry B Clin. Cytom. *53*, 11-19.

Resetkova,E., Reis-Filho,J.S., Jain,R.K., Mehta,R., Thorat,M.A., Nakshatri,H., and Badve,S. (2010). Prognostic impact of ALDH1 in breast cancer: a story of stem cells and tumor microenvironment. Breast Cancer Res. Treat. 123, 97-108.

Ricci-Vitiani,L., Lombardi,D.G., Pilozzi,E., Biffoni,M., Todaro,M., Peschle,C., and De,M.R. (2007). Identification and expansion of human colon-cancer-initiating cells. Nature *445*, 111-115.

Salnikov,A.V., Gladkich,J., Moldenhauer,G., Volm,M., Mattern,J., and Herr,I. (2010). CD133 is indicative for a resistance phenotype but does not represent a prognostic marker for survival of non-small cell lung cancer patients. Int. J. Cancer *126*, 950-958.

Sato,A., Sakurada,K., Kumabe,T., Sasajima,T., Beppu,T., Asano,K., Ohkuma,H., Ogawa,A., Mizoi,K., Tominaga,T., Kitanaka,C., and Kayama,T. (2010). Association of stem cell marker CD133 expression with dissemination of glioblastomas. Neurosurg. Rev. *33*, 175-183.

Schneider,J., Pollan,M., Ruibal,A., Jimenez,E., Lucas,A.R., Nunez,M.I., Sanchez,J., and Tejerina,A. (1999). Histologic grade and CD44 are independent predictors of axillary lymph node invasion in early (T1) breast cancer. Tumour. Biol. *20*, 319-330.

Selleri,C., Notaro,R., Catalano,L., Fontana,R., Del,V.L., and Rotoli,B. (1992). Prognostic irrelevance of CD34 in acute myeloid leukaemia. Br. J. Haematol. *82*, 479-481.

Shmelkov,S.V., Butler,J.M., Hooper,A.T., Hormigo,A., Kushner,J., Milde,T., St,C.R., Baljevic,M., White,I., Jin,D.K., Chadburn,A., Murphy,A.J., Valenzuela,D.M., Gale,N.W., Thurston,G., Yancopoulos,G.D., D'Angelica,M., Kemeny,N., Lyden,D., and Rafii,S. (2008). CD133 expression is not restricted to stem cells, and both CD133+ and C. J. Clin. Invest *118*, 2111-2120.

Singh,S.K., Clarke,I.D., Terasaki,M., Bonn,V.E., Hawkins,C., Squire,J., and Dirks,P.B. (2003). Identification of a cancer stem cell in human brain tumors. Cancer Res. *63*, 5821-5828.

Singh,S.K., Hawkins,C., Clarke,I.D., Squire,J.A., Bayani,J., Hide,T., Henkelman,R.M., Cusimano,M.D., and Dirks,P.B. (2004). Identification of human brain tumour initiating cells. Nature *432*, 396-401.

Solary,E., Casasnovas,R.O., Campos,L., Bene,M.C., Faure,G., Maingon,P., Falkenrodt,A., Lenormand,B., and Genetet,N. (1992). Surface markers in adult acute myeloblastic leukemia: correlation of CD19+, CD34+ and CD14+/DR--phenotypes with shorter survival. Groupe d'Etude Immunologique des Leucemies (GEIL). Leukemia *6*, 393-399.

Son,M.J., Woolard,K., Nam,D.H., Lee,J., and Fine,H.A. (2009). SSEA-1 is an enrichment marker for tumor-initiating cells in human glioblastoma. Cell Stem Cell *4*, 440-452.

Sperling,C., Buchner,T., Creutzig,U., Ritter,J., Harbott,J., Fonatsch,C., Sauerland,C., Mielcarek,M., Maschmeyer,G., Loffler,H., and . (1995). Clinical, morphologic, cytogenetic and prognostic implications of CD34 expression in childhood and adult de novo AML. Leuk. Lymphoma *17*, 417-426.

Tchoghandjian,A., Baeza,N., Colin,C., Cayre,M., Metellus,P., Beclin,C., Ouafik,L., and Figarella-Branger,D. (2010). A2B5 cells from human glioblastoma have cancer stem cell properties. Brain Pathol. *20*, 211-221.

te Boekhorst,P.A., de,L.K., Schoester,M., Wittebol,S., Nooter,K., Hagemeijer,A., Lowenberg,B., and Sonneveld,P. (1993). Predominance of functional multidrug resistance (MDR-1) phenotype in CD34+ acute myeloid leukemia cells. Blood *82*, 3157-3162.

Tirino,V., Camerlingo,R., Franco,R., Malanga,D., La,R.A., Viglietto,G., Rocco,G., and Pirozzi,G. (2009). The role of CD133 in the identification and characterisation of tumour-initiating cells in non-small-cell lung cancer. Eur. J. Cardiothorac. Surg. *36*, 446-453.

Ucar,D., Cogle,C.R., Zucali,J.R., Ostmark,B., Scott,E.W., Zori,R., Gray,B.A., and Moreb,J.S. (2009). Aldehyde dehydrogenase activity as a functional marker for lung cancer. Chem. Biol. Interact. *178*, 48-55.

Uchida,N., Buck,D.W., He,D., Reitsma,M.J., Masek,M., Phan,T.V., Tsukamoto,A.S., Gage,F.H., and Weissman,I.L. (2000). Direct isolation of human central nervous system stem cells. Proc. Natl. Acad. Sci. U. S. A *97*, 14720-14725.

van den Hoogen,C., van der,H.G., Cheung,H., Buijs,J.T., Lippitt,J.M., Guzman-Ramirez,N., Hamdy,F.C., Eaton,C.L., Thalmann,G.N., Cecchini,M.G., Pelger,R.C., and van der,P.G. (2010). High aldehyde dehydrogenase activity identifies tumor-initiating and metastasis-initiating cells in human prostate cancer. Cancer Res. *70*, 5163-5173.

van Rhenen A., Feller,N., Kelder,A., Westra,A.H., Rombouts,E., Zweegman,S., van der Pol,M.A., Waisfisz,Q., Ossenkoppele,G.J., and Schuurhuis,G.J. (2005). High stem cell frequency in acute myeloid leukemia at diagnosis predicts high minimal residual disease and poor survival. Clin. Cancer Res. *11*, 6520-6527.

Vermeulen,L., Todaro,M., de Sousa,M.F., Sprick,M.R., Kemper,K., Perez,A.M., Richel,D.J., Stassi,G., and Medema,J.P. (2008). Single-cell cloning of colon cancer stem cells reveals a multi-lineage differentiation capacity. Proc. Natl. Acad. Sci. U. S. A *105*, 13427-13432.

Vis,A.N., Noordzij,M.A., Fitoz,K., Wildhagen,M.F., Schroder,F.H., and van der Kwast,T.H. (2000). Prognostic value of cell cycle proteins p27(kip1) and MIB-1, and the cell adhesion protein CD44s in surgically treated patients with prostate cancer. J. Urol. *164*, 2156-2161.

Weg-Remers,S., Anders,M., von,L.B., Riecken,E.O., Schuder,G., Feifel,G., Zeitz,M., and Stallmach,A. (1998). Decreased expression of CD44 splicing variants in advanced colorectal carcinomas. Eur. J. Cancer *34*, 1607-1611.

Weichert,W., Denkert,C., Burkhardt,M., Gansukh,T., Bellach,J., Altevogt,P., Dietel,M., and Kristiansen,G. (2005). Cytoplasmic CD24 expression in colorectal cancer independently correlates with shortened patient survival. Clin. Cancer Res. *11*, 6574-6581.

Weichert,W., Knosel,T., Bellach,J., Dietel,M., and Kristiansen,G. (2004). ALCAM/CD166 is overexpressed in colorectal carcinoma and correlates with shortened patient survival. J. Clin. Pathol. *57*, 1160-1164.

Xin,L., Lawson,D.A., and Witte,O.N. (2005). The Sca-1 cell surface marker enriches for a prostate-regenerating cell subpopulation that can initiate prostate tumorigenesis. Proc. Natl. Acad. Sci. U. S. A *102*, 6942-6947.

Zeppernick,F., Ahmadi,R., Campos,B., Dictus,C., Helmke,B.M., Becker,N., Lichter,P., Unterberg,A., Radlwimmer,B., and Herold-Mende,C.C. (2008). Stem cell marker CD133 affects clinical outcome in glioma patients. Clin. Cancer Res. *14*, 123-129.

Zhang,M., Song,T., Yang,L., Chen,R., Wu,L., Yang,Z., and Fang,J. (2008). Nestin and CD133: valuable stem cell-specific markers for determining clinical outcome of glioma patients. J. Exp. Clin. Cancer Res. *27*, 85.

Zlobec,I., Terracciano,L., Jass,J.R., and Lugli,A. (2007). Value of staining intensity in the interpretation of immunohistochemistry for tumor markers in colorectal cancer. Virchows Arch. *451*, 763-769

18

Drugs that Kill Cancer Stem-like Cells

Renata Zobalova,[1,2] Marina Stantic,[1] Michael Stapelberg,[1]
Katerina Prokopova,[2] Lanfeng Dong,[1] Jaroslav Truksa[2] and Jiri Neuzil[1,2]
[1]*Apoptosis Research Group. School of Medical Science and Griffith Health Institute, Griffith University, Southport, Qld,*
[2]*Molecular Therapy Group, Institute of Biotechnology, Academy of Sciences of the Czech Republic, Prague,*
[1]*Australia,*
[2]*Czech Republic*

1. Introduction

The hallmarks of cancer include processes like self-sufficiency for growth signals, insensitivity to growth-inhibitory (anti-growth) signals, evasion of programmed cell death (apoptosis), unlimited replicative potential, sustained angiogenesis, and tissue invasion and metastasis (Hanahan & Weinberg, 2000). Recent research dictates that these definitions, while valid, ought to be enriched. That is, we should also consider tumours as a heterogeneous 'collection of cancer cells' with a hierarchy. This 'hierarchical hypothesis' tells us that tumours contain a minute (sometimes very small) sub-set of cells with distinct properties from the bulk of the tumour mass (D'Amour & Gage, 2002; Visvader & Lindeman, 2008; Visvader, 2009). These cells feature certain characteristics inherent to stem cells, including the capacity of self-renewal, asymmetric division and differentiation. They have also a very high propensity to form tumours. Therefore these cells are referred to as cancer stem cells (CSC) or cancer stem-like cells or, better, tumour-initiating cells (TICs). The terminology, while not too important, may be misleading though, since the term 'cancer stem cells' implies that we are dealing with true stem cells, which is not possible to reconcile with at this stage, perhaps even more so, since the origin of CSCs is not exactly known.

Recent evidence, rather circumstantial, indicates that CSCs may have developed during the stage of tumour immunoediting (Dunn *et al.*, 2002, 2004a). According to this concept, the immune system is actively involved in tumour initiation as well as progression, and this became known as the principle of 'three Es', involving the phases of 'elimination', 'equilibrium' and 'escape' (Dunn *et al.*, 2004b). The elimination phase of the process of immunoediting is responsible for the detection and elimination of cells that became malignant, usually due to the failure of their tumour suppressor mechanisms (Smyth *et al.*, 2002). The selection of such CSCs is depicted schematically in Figure 1. Here, certain cells, possibly with slightly different properties than the bulk of the cell population, survive the pressure of the immune system, while most of the cells are eliminated by the cells of the immune system such as the cytotoxic T lymphocytes (CTLs) (Schreiber *et al.*, 1983; Bancroft *et al.*, 1991; Smyth *et al.*, 2001; Takeda *et al.*, 2001; Hayakawa *et al.*, 2002). These cells then give rise to a tumour. Upon therapeutic intervention, many cells of the tumour are induced into apoptosis and die, while some survive and give rise to 'second-line' tumours with acquired resistance to the 'first-line' treatment, vastly complicating further therapy and making the prognosis very grim (Neuzil *et al.*, 2007; Visvader & Lindeman, 2008; Alison *et al.*, 2010; McDermott & Wicha, 2010).

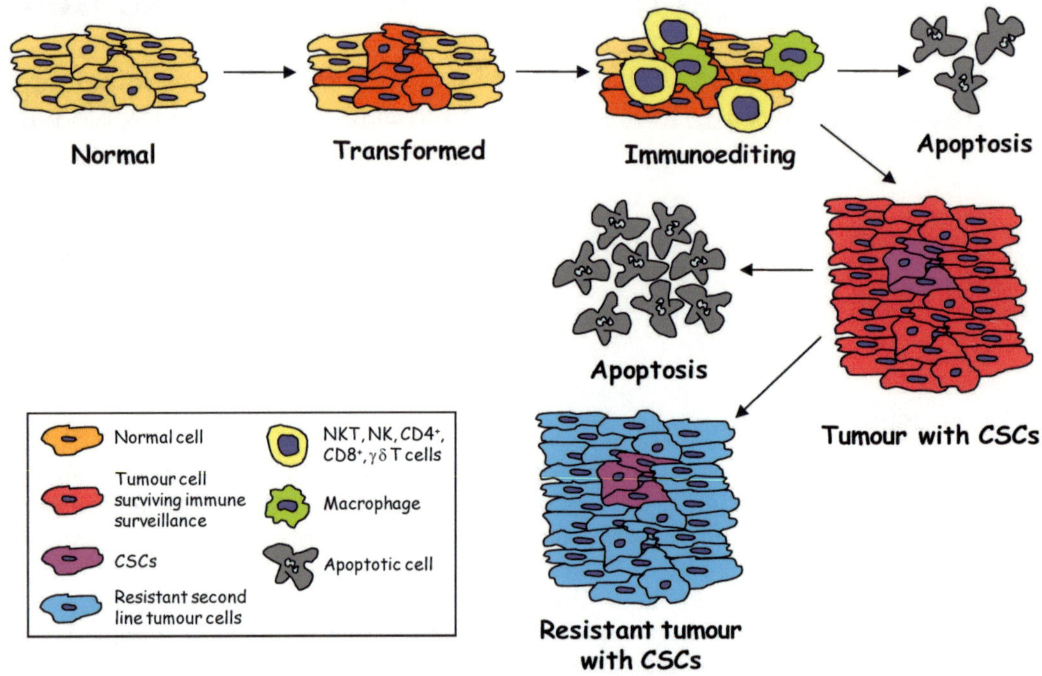

Fig. 1. Possible selection of CSCs during cancer cell immunoediting and their contribution to the resistance of tumours to therapy. During the process of malignant conversion, several cells that carry mutations escape the elimination phase of the process of immunoediting, which involves a variety of cells of the immune system, such as natural killer cells, natural killer T cells, cytotoxic T cells or macrophages. These 'selected' cells form a tumour with relatively low number of CSCs. Upon challenge of the tumour with anti-cancer drugs, majority of the cells are killed via apoptosis, while the CSCs survive. They then start differentiating and proliferating to give rise to 'second-line' tumours with higher resistance to therapy, making them very hard to eliminate. The percentage of CSCs in the 'second-line' tumours is similar to that in the primary tumour.

2. Identification of cancer stem-like cells

CSCs have been, thus far, identified in a great number of tumours. Thus, CSCs have been described in multiple myelomas (Park *et al.*, 1971) and in leukemias (Lapidot *et al.*, 1994; Bhatia *et al.*, 1998), after which they were also discovered in the neoplastic diseases of the nervous system (Singh *et al.*, 2003; Piccirillo *et al.*, 2006), colon cancer (Ricci-Vitiani *et al.*, 2007), prostate cancer (Collins *et al.*, 2005), hepatocarcinomas (Yin *et al.*, 2007), breast cancer (Al-Hajj *et al.*, 2003), melanomas (Fang *et al.*, 2005; Schatton *et al.*, 2008) and osteosarcomas (Gibbs *et al.*, 2005), and we have recently identified CSCs in the context of malignant mesotheliomas (Neuzil *et al.*, unpublished data).

One of the most vexing problems in the study of CSCs is their identification. A number of markers of CSCs or the combination thereof, varying, more-or-less, from cancer type to cancer type, have been described. Of the 'markers' used to define CSCs, many are cell surface proteins that endow the sub-set of CSCs with specific properties, and some have been involved in functional differences of CSCs when compared to the fast-proliferating, more differentiated cancer cells. However, different markers or their combinations have been proposed to characterize CSCs even within the same type of tumour. For example, breast cancer CSCs have been typified by the genotype $CD44^+/CD24^-$/ALDH (Ginestier *et al.*, 2007; Charafe-Jauffret *et al.*, 2009). We found breast cancer CSCs also upregulating CD133, while the CD24 status varies (Neuzil *et al.*, unpublished data). Similarly, ovarian carcinoma stem cells have been described as $CD44^+/CD117^+$ (Zhang *et al.*, 2008) or $CD133^+$ (Baba *et al.*, 2009).

Probably the most frequently used markers of CSCs are the surface proteins CD24, CD44, CD47, CD133, the level of expression of aldehyde dehydrogenase (ALDH), and the presence of the so-called 'side-population'. These markers have been used to characterize CSCs from a variety of tumour types, although the use of some of these markers has been challenged. This controversy has been proposed, for example, for the probably most frequently used CSC marker CD133, with Shmelkov *et al.* (2008) having reported that metastatic colon cancer cells exert comparable tumour-initiating capacity regardless of the CD133 status.

While the glycoprotein CD24 has been shown to be downregulated in CSCs of some types of breast cancer, CD44 appears to be consistently upregulated in breast cancer CSCs (Al-Hajj *et al.*, 2003; Ginestier *et al.*, 2007; Charafe-Jauffret *et al.*, 2009) as well as CSCs of prostate (Collins *et al.*, 2005), pancreatic (Patrawala *et al.*, 2006; Li *et al.*, 2007), ovarian (Zhang *et al.*, 2008; Alvero *et al.*, 2009), colorectal (Du *et al.*, 2008) and liver cancer (Yang *et al.*, 2008). CD44 has been earlier identified as a receptor for hyaluronic acid, whose engagement may result in the activation of TGFβ signalling, promoting the pro-survival, anti-apoptotic pathways (Shipitsin *et al.*, 2007).

Over the last few years, CD133 has been utilized most frequently as a marker of CSCs (Corbeil *et al.*, 2001; Miraglia *et al.*, 2007; Neuzil *et al.*, 2007; Tang *et al.*, 2007). The types of tumours that are typified by CSCs that exert high level of CD133 include such diverse neoplasias as breast cancer, colon cancer, tumours of the nervous system, etc. It is rather surprising that not too much is known about the function of the protein. CD133, also known as prominin-1, was first discovered in hematopoietic stem cells (Corbeil *et al.*, 2001; Miraglia *et al.*, 2007). It was shown that $CD133^+$ cells have the propensity to form tumours in NOD/SCID mice even when low numbers of such cells were xenografted (Ricci-Vitiani *et al.*, 2007; Yin *et al.*, 2007; O'Brian *et al.*, 2007; Wright *et al.*, 2008). Even though Shmelkov *et al.* (2008) reported that in their hands, $CD133^-$ cells are also capable of tumour initiation in immunocompromised mice, they showed that $CD133^+$ colon cancer cells exert much greater metastatic potential than their $CD133^-$ counterparts. Thus, regardless the reports doubting the usefulness of CD133 as a stem cell marker, prominin-1 can be used as a marker for the increase in the 'stemness' of the cell subpopulation, in particular in combination with other markers, such as CD44 and CD24.

A considerable problem in studying CSCs is, besides their identification, their maintenance in culture. For example, we studied $CD133^+$ Jurkat cells from 'mixed' pre-separation population of the cells following their separation by immunomagnetic sorting, and found that the $CD133^{high}$ sub-population (over 60% CD133 positivity) reverted to the 'mixed' population phenotype with some 20% CD133-positive cells within several days after placing the sorted cells to the serum-containing medium (Zobalova *et al.*, 2009). This gives only a relatively short time window for subsequent studies, and the results obtained with such cells are difficult to interpret.

Probably the best option for studying CSCs of solid tumours *in vitro* is maintaining cancer cells in spheres, growing them under conditions that prevent their adhesion. The basic feature of such conditions is the absence of serum and supplementation of the medium with growth factors, including FGF2 and EGF (Vescovi *et al.*, 2006). Keeping cells in such a medium maintains their stem-like properties for extended periods of time, and we have found that such conditions result in sphere cell phenotype for breast and prostate cancer as well as mesotheliomas (Neuzil *et al.*, unpublished data). Using microarray analysis approach, we confirmed an overall increase in the 'stemness signature' of such cultures, i.e. enrichment in markers of several types of stem cells, including the hematopoietic, embryonic and neural stem cell gene sets (Ramalho-Santos *et al.*, 2002; Ivanova *et al.*, 2002; Fortunel *et al.*, 2003). This approach also makes it possible to characterise in a global as well as more focused manner the features of CSCs, including the pathways that become activated. For example, we found that for breast and prostate cancer as well as mesothelioma spheres, the tryptophan pathway was the most activated of all pathways whose activation was common to the three types of CSCs, indicating a mechanism how such cells may survive for prolonged periods of time in the niche (Neuzil *et al.*, unpublished data). This also suggests that inhibitors of indoleamine-2,3-dioxygenase (IDO), a key enzyme in the conversion of tryptophan to N-formyl kynurenin, may be useful for promoting killing of CSCs (see below).

3. Compounds that kill cancer stem-like cells

Numerous studies have documented resistance of CSCs to established therapeutic modalities, including radiation therapy as well as chemotherapy. The reasons are multiple and include altered expression of genes that are important for initiation, progression and execution of apoptosis, activation of the survival pathways, and upregulation of trans-membrane proteins that promote survival as well as activation of the DNA repair machinery. Increased resistance has been shown for many types of CSCs, including leukemic (Essers & Trumpp, 2010), brain (Bao *et al.*, 2006; Liu *et al.*, 2006; Hambardzumyan *et al.*, 2006; Dirks 2010), pancreatic (Lonardo *et al.*, 2010), breast (McDermott & Wicha, 2010), melanoma (Frank *et al.*, 2003, 2005) as well as colon CSCs (Boman & Huang, 2008).

Liu *et al.* (2006) found that $CD133^+$ glioblastoma cells isolated from primary tumours were highly enriched in the products of genes that provide cells with survival advantage, which includes the anti-apoptotic genes Bcl-2, Bcl-x_L, four members of the IAP family (c-IAP2, XIAP, NIAP and survivin) and, most notably the protein FLIP, while the expression of the apoptosis-promoting Bax was decreased. The caspase-8 inhibitor FLIP was upregulated up to 300-fold, pointing to its importance. The pattern of genes over-expressed in the CSCs suggests that the cells are well protected from induction and execution of both the intrinsic apoptosis mechanism (Bcl-2, Bcl-x_L) as well as against the extrinsic pathway (FLIP). Moreover, the IAP family proteins inhibit the possible activation of multiple caspases. We found that $CD133^{high}$ cells, both Jurkat and MCF7, featured high level of expression of FLIP. This conferred their resistance to the immunological inducer of apoptosis TRAIL, which could be overcome by knocking down the FLIP protein using siRNA (Zobalova *et al.*, 2008). Several types of CSCs have been reported to upregulate ABC pumps that make them resistant to various chemotherapeutics. For example, ABCG5 has been shown to be upregulated in melanoma CSCs (Frank *et al.*, 2003, 2005). Cells with high level of expression of members of the ABC pumps are classified as the so-called 'side-population', and these cells have been shown to possess a high re-populating activity when injected into NOD/SCID mice (Bhatia *et al.*, 1998).

Finding efficient modalities to kill CSCs is undoubtedly of paramount importance and is a focus of intensive research. Thus far, the results are not particularly encouraging, although several potentially promising agents have been described (Table I). The first and probably best characterized is the sesquiterpene lactone parthenolide, a natural product isolated from medicinal plants including *Tanacetum parthenium* (feverfew) that has been initially found to inhibit the transcription factor NFκB (Bork *et al.*, 1997), by way of inhibiting activation of the inhibitory components of the transcription factor (Hehner *et al.*, 1998). However, it has been suggested that induction of apoptosis by parthenolide may be independent of inhibition of NFκB activation (Anderson & Bejcek, 2008). Since parthenolide proved efficient in suppressing the proliferation and inducing apoptosis of leukemia stem cells (Guzman *et al.*, 2005a,b, 2007), a number of sesquiterpene lactones have been synthesized and tested as anti-cancer drugs (Ghantous *et al.*, 2010). Parthenolide as a compound efficient in killing leukemia stem cells was confirmed using high-throughput, *in silico* screening (Hassane *et al.*, 2008). The drug is now in Phase I clinical trial for several types of leukemia (http://www.globenewswire.com/newsroom/news.html?d=158480). Recently, breast CSCs as well as prostate CSCs have been reported as targets for parthenolide (Liu *et al.*, 2008; Zhou *et al.*, 2008; Kawasaki *et al.*, 2009).

The mechanism(s) by which parthenolide kills CSCs is still obscure. Guzman *et al.* (2005b, 2007) reported that an analogue of parthenolide, dimethylamino-parthenolide, was very efficient in killing primary leukemic stem cells, which was replicated in pre-clinical models. It was found that induction of apoptosis in leukemia CSCs included generation of reactive oxygen species (ROS), inhibition of NFκB activation and activation of p53. An effect on NFκB was also proposed for inhibition of breast cancer CSCs by parthenolide as well as by other known inducers of the transcription factor, including pyrrolidinedithiocarbamate, using the mammosphere model of CSCs (Zhou *et al.*, 2008). In prostate CSCs, parthenolide has been shown to exert also other activities than inhibition of NFκB or generation of ROS, which include inhibition of a variety of non-receptor and receptor tyrosine kinases as well as a number of transcription factors, such as C/EBPα, FRA-1, HOXA-4, c-Myb, Snail, SP1, etc. (Kawasaki *et al.*, 2009). Of considerable clinical interest is combination of parthenolide with established anti-cancer agents. To this effect, Liu *et al.* (2008) reported that the combination of long-circulating (stealth) liposomes carrying parthenolide with those containing vinorelbine fully inhibited xenografts derived in immunocompromised mice from MCF7 cells. In cultured MCF7 cells sorted for the 'side-population' with high tumour-initiating potential, the combination of the two drugs exerted a very good anti-proliferative effect.

High-throughput *in silico* screening has been used recently in a search for compounds that would efficiently kill breast CSCs. This resulted in discovery of the well known agent salinomycin as an anti-CSC drug (Gupta *et al.*, 2009), with a potential clinical application (Rowan, 2009). This agent was some 100-fold more efficient in lowering the proportion of CSCs in the cancer cell population than the established anti-cancer agent paclitaxel. Analysis of breast tumour xenografts in mice treated with salinomycin reveled that the agent promoted differentiation of the tumour cells and down-regulation of the breast CSC marker

Name	Structure	Type of tumour	Mechanism of action	Reference
Parthenolide	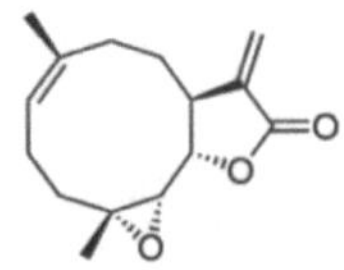	Leukemia Breast cancer Prostate cancer	Inhibition of NFκB	Guzman et al., 2005b, 2007; Hassane et al., 2008; Liu et al., 2008; Zhou et al., 2008; Kawasaki et al., 2009
Salinomycin	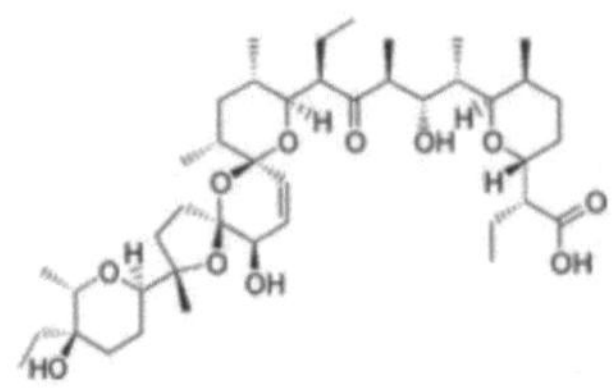	Breast cancer	Potassium ionophore	Gupta et al., 2009; Fuchs et al., 2009, 2010; Riccioni et al., 2010
Metformin	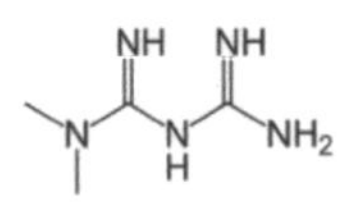	Breast cancer	Effect on energy metabolism	Hirsch et al., 2009; Vazquez-Martin et al., 2010a,b; Martin-Castillo et al., 2010
Lapatinib	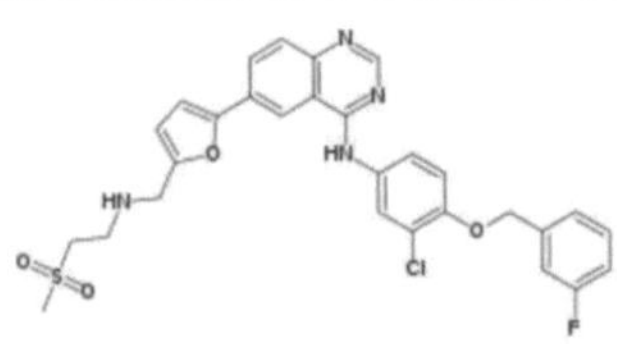	Breast cancer	Dual inhibitor of receptor tyrosine kinases	Korkaya et al., 2009; Magnifico et al., 2009; Diaz et al., 2010o
MitoVES	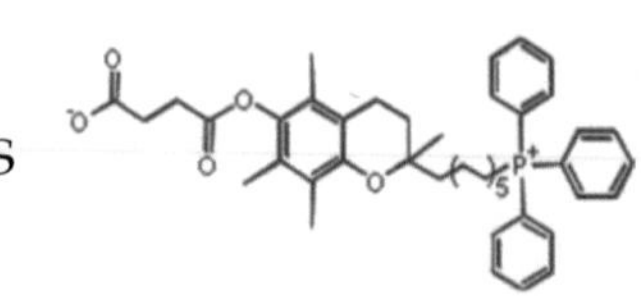	Breast cancer, mesothelioma	Generation of ROS by targeting complex II	Neuzil et al., unpublished

Table I. Small molecules killing cancer stem-like cells.

genes. A follow-up publication documented that salinomycin induces apoptosis in resistant cells, such as those expressing high levels of Bcl-2 and p-glycoprotein (Fuchs *et al.*, 2009). Similar findings were also reported by Riccioni *et al.* (2010). Multidrug resistance, mediated by the ABC transporter proteins, was overcome by salinomycin in leukemic stem-like cells, inducing the resilient cells into apoptosis (Fuchs *et al.*, 2010). Salinomycin, a potassium ionophore, is a product of the bacterium *Streptomyces albus* (Miyazaki *et al.*, 1974), and has been used for a long time in poultry industry. A potential problem with the clinical application of the agent is its relatively high toxicity (Li *et al.*, 2010) that may jeopardize its use in human medicine, quelling somewhat the enthusiasm for the future use of the agent.

Metformin is an oral anti-diabetic drug from the biguanide class, which has been used clinically as an efficient first-line agent against type 2 diabetes (Crandall *et al.*, 2008). Recently this drug was reported to target breast CSCs and, when combined with doxorubicin, prevent growth of tumours as well as their remission (Hirsch *et al.*, 2009). Another study documented that metformin could efficiently inhibit proliferation of breast CSCs refractory to the HER2-targeting agent Herceptin (trastuzumab) as well as their self renewal (Vazquez-Martin *et al.*, 2010a). Since metformin acts by interfering with the energy metabolism of cells, it may inhibit self-maintenance of mitotically competent cells acting as a caloric restriction mimetic (Martin-Castillo *et al.*, 2010; Vazquez-Martin *et al.*, 2010b; Nguyen *et al.*, 2010).

A considerable problem in cancer management is encountered in the case of HER2-high breast cancer (Slamon *et al.*, 1989). To this effect, the agent lapatinib has been applied as a drug of choice for Herceptin-resistant, metastatic breast cancer cells (Burris *et al.*, 2005). This dual receptor tyrosine kinase inhibitor (suppressing the activation of HER2/erbB2 and EGFR) has been suggested to suppress the growth of CSCs in the context of HER2-high breast and lung tumours (Magnifico *et al.*, 2009; Korkaya and Wicha, 2009; Diaz *et al.*, 2010).

Several of the above agents reported to suppress tumour growth and, in some cases, prolong the remission-free period in experimental animals, act by inducing generation of ROS. In this context, we have been studying a class of anti-cancer drugs from the group of vitamin E analogues, epitomized by the redox-silent α-tocopheryl succinate (α-TOS) (Figure 2B) (Neuzil *et al.*, 2001; Weber *et al.*, 2002). This agent acts by targeting the mitochondrial complex II (CII), whereby causing generation of high levels of ROS, which then induce apoptosis by destabilizing the mitochondrial outer membrane (Dong *et al.*, 2008, 2009), by promoting the formation of the Bak channel in mitochondria (Prochazka *et al.*, 2010; Valis *et al.*, in press). To enhance the activity of the vitamin E analogue, we modified the agent by its tagging with the positively charged triphenylphosphonium (TPP^+) group, as suggested for a variety of redox-active compounds (Smith & Murphy, 2005; Biassutto *et al.*, 2010), generating mitochondrially targeted vitamin E succinate (MitoVES) (Figure 2B). As indicated in Figure 2A, such TPP^+-modified compounds move across most biological membranes. Upon crossing the mitochondrial inner membrane (MIM) with the negative potential on the matrix face, the agent is trapped and gradually accumulates in this compartment so that its local concentration is considerably increased. In the case of MitoVES, with its target CII within the MIM, such approach can be expected to maximize its biological activity. Indeed, we found that MitoVES was 1-2 log more efficient in killing cancer cells than the untargeted counterpart (α-TOS), which was paralleled by an effect on experimental cancer, including colon cancer and HER2-high breast cancer (Dong et al., 2011). We have recently found that MitoVES is very efficient in apoptosis induction in a breast cancer CSC model represented by mammospheres, which feature cells with enhanced level of stemness and which can be characterized as $CD44^{high}/CD133^{high}/CD24^{low}/Jagged\text{-}1^{high}$ (Figure 3A,B). In fact, MitoVES was more efficient in killing the mammosphere cells than did the untargeted α-TOS and than parthenolide, probably thus far the best characterized agent toxic to CSCs (Figure 3C) (Neuzil *et al.*, unpublished data). While the mechanism is not clear at this stage and much more work needs to be done, agents like MitoVES may present a substantial promise for the development of compounds that will efficiently eradicate not only the bulk of the tumour cells but, more importantly, also the highly recalcitrant CSCs, whereby minimizing the probability of tumour remission.

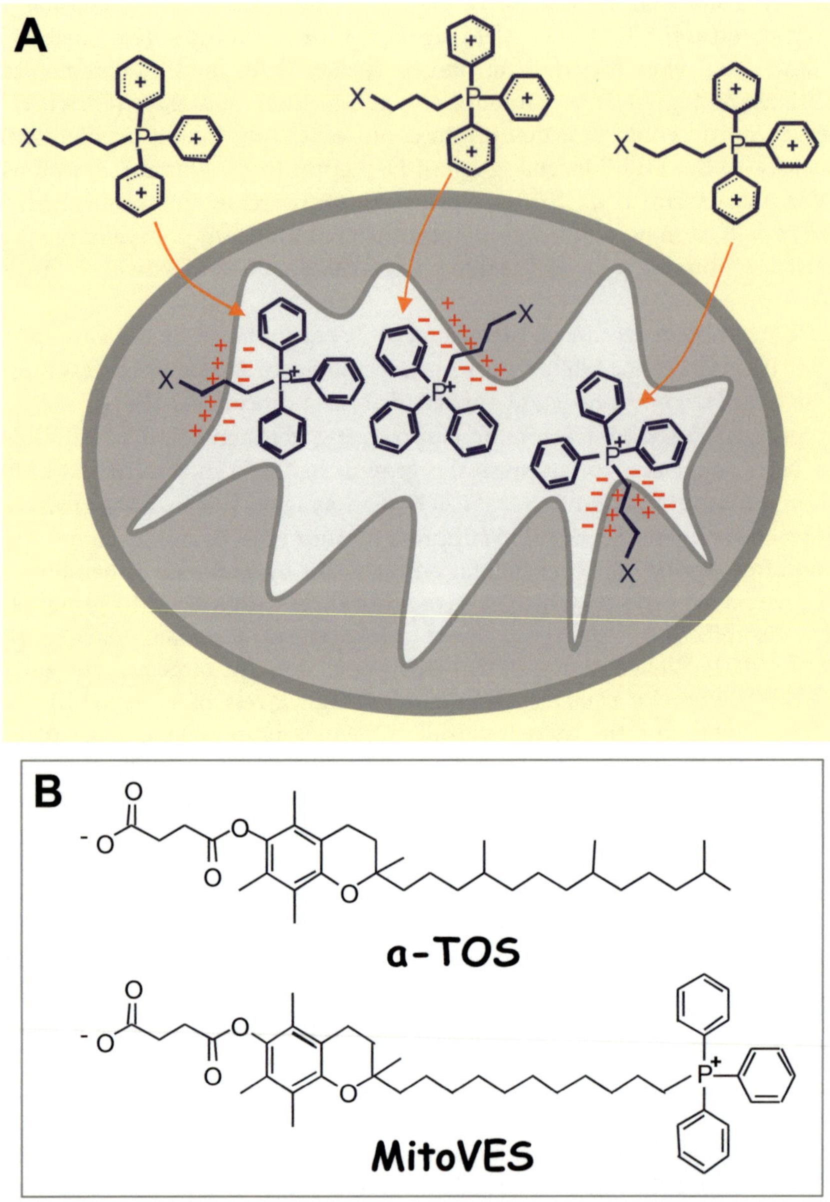

Fig. 2. **Principle of mitochondrial targeting.** A. Addition of a cationic, triphenylphosphonium (TPP^+) group to hydrophobic compounds, with the charge on the phosphorus delocalised on the flanking phenyl groups, causes their relatively free movement across biological membranes. Once in the mitochondrial matrix with the negative potential on the matrix face of the mitochondrial inner membrane (MIM), the TPP^+ group anchors the compound at the matrix-MIM interface, with increased concentration of the agent in this compartment. This is important for enhancing the bioactivity of agents, whose target is in the proximity of the interface. B. The structures are shown of the untargeted α-tocopheryl succinate (α-TOS) and the mitochondrially targeted vitamin E succinate (MitoVES).

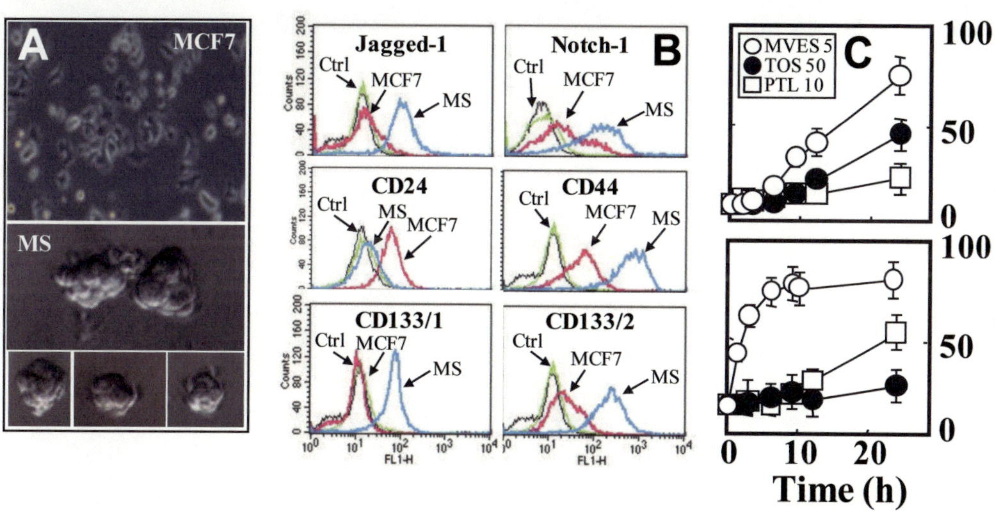

Fig. 3. **MitoVES is efficient in killing mammosphere cells.** A. The breast cancer cells (line MCF7) were cultured as adherent cells (MCF7) or as mammospheres (MS). B. Flow cytometric analysis characterized the adherent MCF7 cells as $CD24^{high}/CD44^{low}/CD133^{low}$, while the MS cells were $CD24^{low}/CD44^{high}/CD133^{high}$. We also found MCF7 cells low in expression of the stemness marker Jagged-1, which was increased in the MS cultures. Both CD133 isotypes were analysed here. C. The adherent MCF7 cells (top panel) and their mammosphere counterparts (lower panel) were exposed to 50 μM α-tocopheryl succinate (TOS), 10 μM parthenolide (PTL) or 5 μM mitochondrially targeted vitamin E succinate, MitoVES (MVES), for the time periods indicated and the cells analysed for apoptosis level.

4. Conclusions

Cancer is now number one reason for the demise of human patients, having surpassed the number of deaths linked to cardiovascular diseases (Twombly, 2005), and the trend appears rather grim (Jemal *et al.*, 2010). A factor contributing to this negative outlook is undoubtedly the hierarchical structure of tumours with a subset of cells with tumour-initiating properties. These cells share some features with stem cells, while they are tumour cells in that they are malignant. Experiments, in which CSCs were isolated from xenografts and used to give rise to a tumour in a serial manner, documented that, although more-or-less pure CSCs were used to initiate the tumour, the percentage of cells with stem-like properties were kept very similar in each subsequent experimental animal. This suggests that tumours are endowed with a level of plasticity and 'memory', which dictates that cells are always present in the tumour whose role is to make sure that the total population of cancer cells will not be eradicated. This 'memory', however, also includes additional mutations such that the 'second-line' tumours, derived from the CSCs that survived the therapeutic intervention, is resistant to the 'first-line' treatment, which considerably jeopardizes any therapeutic modalities applicable to such patients.

While every tumour has different properties, cancer cells also share many features. This may well be true also for CSCs from different types of tumours. Finding such common traits may help discover the Achilles' heel of CSCs and, subsequently, devise efficient therapeutic

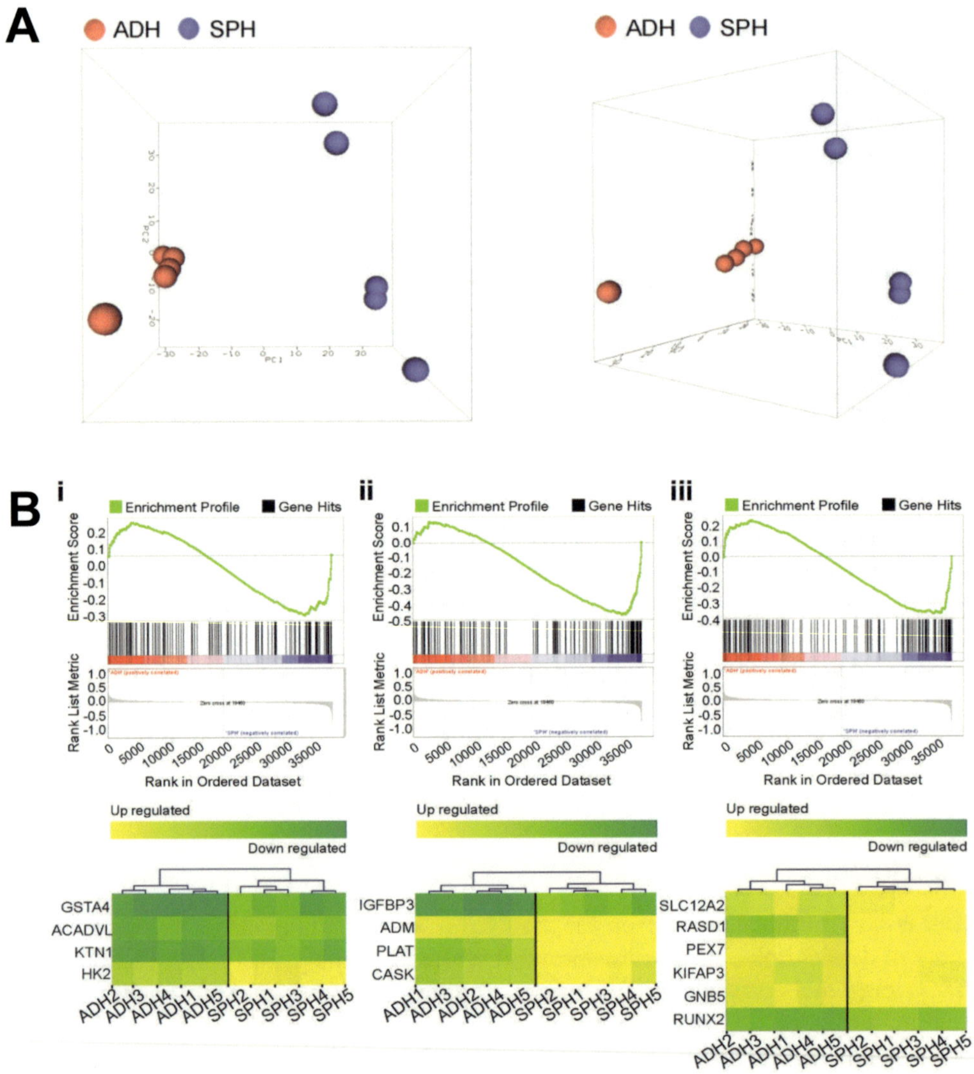

Fig. 4. **Microarray data characterise mammospheres as a phenotype with increased stemness.** A. Principle components analysis (PCA) of adherent (ADH) and mammosphere (SPH) MCF7 cell cultures shows that each phenotype clusters together. PCA projections are represented in 2D (left) and 3D (right) manner. B. Gene set enrichment analysis (GSEA) plots show enrichment of (i) embryonic stem cell (ESC) *(p = 0.044, FDR = 0.046)*, (ii) neuronal stem cell (NSC) *(p = 0.001, FDR = 0.006)* and (iii) hematopoietic stem cell (HSC) *(p = 0.075, FDR = 0.085)* gene sets in mamosphere but not adherent cultures. Each vertical line on the enrichment plot represents a probe in the corresponding gene set. The left to right position of vertical lines indicates the relative position genes from ESC, NSC and HSC gene sets within the rank-ordered list of the 37,805 probes present on the HumanHT-12 BeadChip. The first probe on the left represents the most upregulated probe in adherent samples and the last on the right represents the most upregulated probe in the sphere-forming samples. Probes in the middle are not differentially expressed.

approaches. There are studies that attempted to characterize the global difference of gene expression in fast-proliferating tumour cells and the corresponding CSCs, and such studies have been useful for confirming the stemness features of the cells (Ivanova *et al.*, 2002; Ramalho-Santoz *et al.*, 2002; Fortunel *et al.*, 2003) or to characterize specific properties of CSCs (Birnie *et al.*, 2008).

We have attempted to use microarray analysis to characterize the stemness of several types of cancer cells grown as spheres, including breast and prostate cancer as well as malignant mesotheliomas (Figure 4) (Neuzil *et al.*, unpublished data). Using this approach, we identified increased stemness in all three types of cancer. Moreover, the tools of bioinformatics allow us to search for features that are shared by the different types of model CSC cultures. We found that the three types of CSCs share certain pathways, including glycolysis and oxidative phosphorylation, which suggests that the use of agents like MitoVES (*c.f.* Figure 3) may be a way how to kill such cells. Further and probably most intriguingly, we found that of all the shared pathways that are upregulated in the three types of CSCs, tryptophan metabolism (represented by increased expression of IDO) is the most activated pathway. This is a highly interesting result, which suggests that CSCs are endowed with activity that results in lowering the level of tryptophan in their 'neighborhood'. Depletion of tryptophan (especially due to upregulation of IDO) is one way how cancer cells may protect themselves from the immune surveillance, providing the cancer cells with both passive and active defense mechanisms (Munn & Melor, 2008; Löb *et al.*, 2009), and inhibitors of IDO, such as brassinin or 1-methyl tryptophan, are being considered as anti-cancer drugs (Gaspari *et al.*, 2006; Hou *et al.*, 2007).

It is therefore very tempting to speculate that a highly efficient way to eradicate tumour cells, including the fast-proliferating ones and the resistant CSCs, may be the combination of agents like MitoVES that would kill the bulk of the tumour cells, while the IDO inhibitor would allow for the cells of the immune system to attack the remaining tumour cells, likely those with higher level of 'stemness'. Although a lot of work remains to be done, we propose that such a strategy may be potentially developed and applied in the clinic to minimize the probability of cancer relapse.

5. References

Al-Hajj, M., Wicha, M.S., Benito-Hernandez, A., Morrison, S.J. & Clarke, M.F. (2003) Prospective identification of tumourigenic breast cancer cells. *Proc Natl Acad Sci USA* 100, 3983-3988.

Alison, M.R., Islam, S. & Wright, N.A. (2010) Stem cells in cancer: instigators and propagators? *J Cell Sci* 123, 2357-2368.

Alvero, A.B., Chen, R., Fu, H.H., Montagna, M., Schwartz, P.E., Rutherford, T., Silasi, D.A., Steffensen, K.D., Waldstrom, M., Visintin, I. & Mor, G. (2009) Molecular phenotyping of human ovarian cancer stem cells unravels the mechanisms for repair and chemoresistance. *Cell Cycle* 8, 158-166.

Anderson, K.N. & Bejcek, B.E. (2008) Parthenolide induces apoptosis in glioblastomas without affecting NF-κB. *J Pharmacol Sci* 106, 318-320.

Baba, T., Convery, P.A., Matsumura, N., Whitaker, R.S., Kondoh, E., Perry, T., Huang, Z., Bentley, R.C., Mori, S., Fujii, S., Marks, J.R., Berchuck, A. & Murphy, S.K. (2009) Epigenetic regulation of CD133 and tumourigenicity of $CD133^+$ ovarian cancer cells. *Oncogene* 28, 209-218.

Bancroft, G.J., Schreiber, R.D. & Unanue, E.R. (1991) Natural immunity: A T-cell independent pathway of macrophage activation, defined in the scid mouse. *Immunol Rev* 124, 5-24.

Bao, S., Wu, Q., McLendon, R.E., Hao, Y., Shi, Q., Hjelmelad, A.B., Dewhirst, M.W., Bigner, D.D. & Rich, J.N. (2006) Glioma stem cells promote radioresistance by preferential activation of the DNA damage response. *Nature* 444, 756-760.

Bhatia, M., Bonnet, D., Murdoch, B., Gan, O.I. & Dick, J.E. (1998) A newly discovered class of human hematopoietic cells with SCID-repopulating activity. *Nat Med* 4, 1038-1045.

Biassutto, L., Dong, L.F., Zoratti, M. & Neuzil, J. (2010) Mitochondrially targeted anti-cancer drugs. *Mitochondrion* 10, 670-681.

Birnie, R., Bryce, S.D., Roome, C., Dussupt, V., Droop, A., Lang, S.H., Berry, P.A., Hyde, C.F., Lewis, J.L., Stower, M.J., Maitland, N.J. & Collins, A.T. (2008) Gene expression profiling of human prostate cancer stem cells reveals a pro-inflammatory phenotype and the importance of extracellular matrix interactions. *Genome Biol* 9, R83.

Boman, B.M. & Huang, E. (2008) Human colon cancer stem cells: a new paradigm in gastrointestinal oncology. *J Clin Oncol* 26, 2828-2838.

Bork, P.M., Schmitz, M.L., Kuhnt, M., Escher, C. & Heinrich, M. (1997) Sesquiterpene lactone containing Mexican Indian medicinal plants and pure sesquiterpene lactones as potent inhibitors of transcription factor NF-κB. *FEBS Lett* 402, 85-90.

Burris, H.A., Hurwitz, H.I., Dees, E.C., Dowlati, A., Blackwell, K.L., O'Neil, B., Marcom, P.K., Ellis, M.J., Overmoyer, B., Jones, S.F., Harris, J.L., Smith, D.A., Koch, K.M., Stead, A., Mangum, S. & Spector, N.L. (2005) Phase I safety, pharmacokinetics, and clinical activity study of lapatinib (GW572016), a reversible dual inhibitor of receptor tyrosine kinases, in heavily pretreated patients with metastatic carcinomas. *J Clin Oncol* 23, 5305-5313.

Charafe-Jauffret, E., Ginestier, C., Iovino, F., Wicinski, J., Cervera, N., Finetti, P., Hur, M.H., Diebel, M.E., Monville, F., Dutcher, J., Brown, M., Viens, P., Xerri, L., Bertucci, F., Stassi, G., Dontu, G., Birnbaum, D. & Wicha, M.S. (2009) Breast cancer cell lines contain functional cancer stem cells with metastatic capacity and a distinct molecular signature. *Cancer Res* 69, 1302-1313.

Collins, A.T., Berry, P.A., Hyde, C., Stower, M.J. & Maitland, N.J. (2005) Prospective identification of tumourigenic prostate cancer stem cells. *Cancer Res* 65, 10946-10951.

Corbeil, D., Roper, F., Fargeas, C.A., Joester, A. & Huttner, W.B. (2001) Prominin: a story of cholesterol, plasma membrane protrusions and human pathology. *Traffic* 2, 82-91.

Crandall, J.P., Knowler, W.C., Kahn, S.E., Marrero, D., Florez, J.C., Bray, G.A., Haffner, S.M., Hoskin, M. & Nathan, D.M. (2008) The prevention of type 2 diabetes. *Nat Clin Pract Endocrinol Metab* 4, 382-393.

D'Amour, K.A. & Gage, F.H. (2002) Are somatic stem cells pluripotent or lineage-restricted? *Nat Med* 8, 213-214.

Diaz, R., Nguewa, P.A., Parrondo, R., Perez-Stable, C., Manrique, I., Redrado, M., Catena, R., Collantes, M., Penuelas, I., Diaz-Gonzalea, J.A. & Calvo, A. (2010) Antitumour and antiangiogenic effect of the dual EGFR and HER-2 tyrosine kinase inhibitor lapatinib in a lung cancer model. *BMC Cancer* 10, 188.

Dirks, P.B. (2010) Brain tumour stem cells: The cancer stem cell hypothesis writ large. *Mol Oncol* 4, 420-430.

Dong, L.F., Freeman, R., Liu, J., Zobalova, R., Marin-Hernandez, A., Stantic, M., Rohlena, J., Rodriguez-Enriquez, S., Valis, K., Butcher, B., Goodwin, J., Brunk, U.T., Witting, P.K., Moreno-Sanchez, R., Scheffler, I.E., Ralph, S.J. & Neuzil, J. (2009) Suppression of tumour growth *in vivo* by the mitocan α-tocopheryl succinate requires respiratory complex II. *Clin Cancer Res* 15, 1593-1600.

Dong, L.F., Low, P., Dyason, J., Wang, X.F., Prochazka, L., Witting, P.K., Freeman, R., Swettenham, E., Valis, K., Liu, J., Zobalova, R., Turanek, J., Spitz, D.R., Domann, F.E., Scheffler, I.E., Ralph, S.J. & Neuzil, J. (2008) α-Tocopheryl succinate induces apoptosis by targeting ubiquinone-binding sites in mitochondrial respiratory complex II. *Oncogene* 27, 4324-4335.

Dong, L.F., Jameson, V.J.A., Tilly, D., Cerny, J., Mahdavian, E., Marín-Hernández, A., Hernández-Esquivel, L., Rodríguez-Enríquez, S., Witting, P.K., Stantic, B., Rohlena, J., Truksa, J., Kluckova, K., Dyason, J.C., Salvatore, B.A., Moreno-Sánchez, R., Coster, M.J., Ralph, S.J., Smith, R.A.J., & Neuzil, J. (2011) Mitochondrial targeting of vitamin E succinate enhances its pro-apoptotic and anti-cancer activity via mitochondrial complex II. *J Biol Chem* 286, 3717-3728.

Du, L., Wang, H., He, L., Zhang, J., Ni, B., Wang, X., Jin, H., Cahuzac, N., Mehrpour, M., Lu, Y. & Chen, Q. (2008) CD44 is of functional importance for colorectal cancer stem cells. *Clin Cancer Res* 14, 6751-6760.

Dunn, G.P., Bruce, A.T., Ikeda, H., Old, L.J. & Schreiber, R.D. (2002) Cancer immunoediting: From immunosurveillance to tumour escape. *Nat Immunol* 3, 991-998.

Dunn, G.P., Old, L.J. & Schreiber, R.D. (2004a) The immunobiology of cancer immunosurveillance and immunoediting. *Immunity* 21, 137-148.

Dunn, G.P., Old, L.J. & Schreiber, R.D. (2004b) The three Es of cancer immunoediting. *Annu Rev Immunol* 22, 329-360.

Essers, M.A.G. & Trumpp, A. (2010) Targeting leukemic stem cells by breaking their dormancy. *Mol Oncol* 4, 443-450.

Fang, D., Nguyen, T.K., Leishear, K., Finko, R., Kulp, A.N., Hotz, S., Van Belle, P.A., Xu, X., Elder, D.E. & Herlyn, M. (2005) A tumourigenic subpopulation with stem cell properties in melanomas. *Cancer Res* 65:9328-9337.

Fortunel, N.O., Out, H.H., Ng, H.H., Chen, J., Mu, X., Chevassut, T., Li, X., Joseph, M., Bailey, C., Hatzfeld, J.A., Hatzfeld, A., Usta, F., Vega, V.B., Long, P.M., & Libermann, T.A., & Lim, B. (2003) *Science* 302, 393.

Frank, N.Y., Pendse, S.S., Lapchak, P.H., Margaryan, A., Shlain, D., Doeing, C., Sayegh, M.H. & Frank, M.H. (2003) Regulation of progenitor cell fusion by ABCB5 P-glycoprotein, a novel human ATP-binding cassette transporter. *J Biol Chem* 278, 47156-47165.

Frank, N.Y., Margaryan, A., Huang, Y., Schatton, T., Waaga-Gasser, A.M., Gasser, M., Sayegh, M.H., Sadee, W. & Frank, M.H. (2005) ABCB5-mediated doxorubicin transport and chemoresistance in human malignant melanoma. *Cancer Res* 65, 4320-4333.

Fuchs, D., Daniel, V., Sadeghi, M., Opelz, G. & Naujokat, C. (2010) Salinomycin overcomes ABC transporter-mediated multidrug and apoptosis resistance in human leukemia stem cell-like KG-1a cells. *Biochem Biophys Res Commun* 394, 1098-1104.

Fuchs, D., Heinold, A., Opelz, G., Daniel, V. & Naujokat, C. (2009) Salinomycin induces apoptosis and overcomes apoptosis resistance in human cancer cells. *Biochem Biophys Res Commun* 390, 743-749.

Gaspari, P., Banerjee, T., Malachowski, W.P., Muller, A.J., Prendergast, G.C., DuHadaway, J., Bennett, S. & Donovan, A.M. (2006) Structure-activity study of brassinin derivatives as indoleamine 2,3-dioxygenase inhibitors. *J Med Chem* 49, 684-692.

Ghantous, A., Gali-Muhtasib, H., Vuorela, H., Saliba, N.A. & Darwiche, N. (2010) What made sesquiterpene lactones reach cancer clinical trials? *Drug Discov Today* 15, 668-678.

Gibbs, C.P., Kukekov, V.G., Reith, J.D., Tchigrinova, O., Suslov, O.N., Scott, E.W., Ghivizzani, S.C., Ignatova, T.N. & Steindler, D.A. (2005) Stem-like cells in bone sarcomas: implications for tumourigenesis. *Neoplasia* 7, 967-976.

Ginestier, C., Hur, M.H., Charafe-Jauffret, E., Monville, F., Dutcher, J., Brown, M., Jacquemier, J., Viens, P., Kleer, C.G., Liu, S., Schott, A., Hayes, D., Birnbaum, D., Wicha, M.S. & Dontu, G. (2007) ALDH1 is a marker of normal and malignant human mammary stem cells and a predictor of poor clinical outcome. *Cell Stem Cell* 1, 555-567.

Gupta, P.B., Onder, T.T., Jiang, G., Tao, K., Kuperwasser, C., Weinberg, R.A. & Lander, E.S. (2009) Identification of selective inhibitors of cancer stem cells by high-throughput screening. *Cell* 138, 645-659.

Guzman, M.L. & Jordan, C.T. (2005a) Feverfew: weeding out the root of leukaemia. *Expert Opin Biol Ther* 5, 1147-1152.

Guzman, M.L., Rossi, R.M., Karnischky, L., Li, X., Peterson, D.R., Howard, D.S. & Jordan, C.T. (2005b) The sesquiterpene lactone parthenolide induces apoptosis of human acute myelogenous leukemia stem and progenitor cells. *Blood* 105, 4163-4169.

Guzman, M.L., Rossi, R.M., Neelakantan, S., Li, X., Corbett, C.A., Hassane, D.C., Becker, M.W., Bennett, J.M., Sullivan, E., Lachowicz, J.L., Vaughan, A., Sweeney, C.J., Matthews, W., Carroll, M., Liesveld, J.L., Crooks, P.A. & Jordan, C.T. (2007) An orally bioavailable parthenolide analog selectively eradicates acute myelogenous leukemia stem and progenitor cells. *Blood* 110, 4427-4435.

Hambardzumyan, D., Squartro, M. & Holland, E.C. (2006) Radiation resistance and stem-like cells in brain tumours. *Cancer Cell* 10, 454-456.

Hanahan, D. & Weinberg, R.A. (2000) The hallmarks of cancer. *Cell* 100, 57-70.

Hassane, D.C., Guzman, M.L., Corbett, C., Li, X., Abboud, R., Young, F., Liesveld, J.L., Carroll, M. & Jordan, C.T. (2008) Discovery of agents that eradicate leukemia stem cells using an in silico screen of public gene expression data. *Blood* 111, 5654-5662.

Hayakawa, Y., Kelly, J.M., Westwood, J.A., Darcy, P.K., Diefenbach, A., Raulet, D. & Smyth, M.J. (2002) Cutting edge: Tumour rejection mediated by NKG2D receptor-ligand interaction is dependent upon perforin. *J Immunol* 169, 5377-5381.

Hehner, S.P., Heinrich, M., Bork, P.M., Vogt, M., Ratter, F., Lehmann, V., Schulze-Osthoff, K., Dröge, W. & Schmitz, M.L. (1998) Sesquiterpene lactones specifically inhibit activation of NF-κB by preventing the degradation of IκB-α and IκB-β. *J Biol Chem* 273, 1288-1297.

Hemmati, H.D., Nakano, I., Lazareff, J.A., Masterman-Smith, M., Geschwind, D.H., Bronner-Fraser, M. & Kornblum, H.I. (2003) Cancerous stem cells can arise from pediatric brain tumours. *Proc Natl Acad Sci USA* 100, 15178–15183.

Hirsch, H.A., Iliopoulos, D., Tsichlis, P.N. & Struhl, K. (2009) Metformin selectively targets cancer stem cells, and acts together with chemotherapy to block tumour growth and prolong remission. *Cancer Res* 69, 7507-7511.

Hou, D.Y., Muller, A.J., Sharma, M.D., DuHadaway, J., Banerjee, T., Johnson, M., Mellor, A.L., Prendergast, G.C. & Munn, D.H. (2007) Inhibition of indoleamine 2,3-dioxygenase in dendritic cells by stereoisomers of 1-methyl-tryptophan correlates with antitumour responses. *Cancer Res* 67, 792-801.

Ivanova, N.B., Dimos, J.T., Schaniel, C., Hackney, J.A., Moore, K.A. & Lemischka, I.R. (2002) A stem cell molecular signature. *Science* 298, 601-604.

Jemal, A., Siegel, R., Xu, J. & Ward, E. (2010) Cancer statistics, 2010. *CA Cancer J Clin* 60, 277-300.

Kawasaki, B.T., Hurt, E.M., Kalathur, M., Duhagon, M.A., Milner, J.A., Kim, Y.S &, Farrar, W.L. (2009) Effects of the sesquiterpene lactone parthenolide on prostate tumour-initiating cells: An integrated molecular profiling approach. *Prostate* 69, 827-837.

Korkaya, H. & Wicha, M.S. (2009) HER2, Notch, and breast cancer stem cells: targeting an axis of evil. *Clin Cancer Res* 15, 1845-1847.

Lapidot, T., Sirard, C., Vormoor, J., Haas, T.L., Diessenbacher, P., Sprick, M.R., Schön, M.P., Henkler, F., Gollnick, H., Walczak, H. & Leverkus, M (1994) A cell initiating human acute myeloid leukaemia after transplantation into SCID mice. *Nature* 367, 645-648.

Li, C., Heidt, D.G., Dalerba, P., Burant, C.F., Zhang, L., Adsay, V., Wicha, M., Clarke, M.F. & Simeone, D.M. (2007) Identification of pancreatic cancer stem cells. *Cancer Res* 67, 1030-1037.

Li, Y., Fang, J., Wu, S., Ma, K., Li, H., Yan, X. & Dong, F. (2010) Identification and quantification of salinomycin in intoxicated human plasma by liquid chromatography-electrospray tandem mass spectrometry. *Anal Bioanal Chem* 398, 955-961.

Liu, G., Yuan, X., Zeng, Z., Tunici, P., Ng, H., Abdulkadir, I.R., Lu, L., Irvin, D., Black, K.L. & Yu, J.S. (2006) Analysis of gene expression and chemoresistance of CD133^{+} cancer stem cells in glioblastoma. *Mol Cancer* 5, 1476-1498.

Liu, Y., Lu, W.L., Guo, J., Du, J., Li, T., Wu, J.W., Wang, G.L., Wang, J.C., Zhang, X. & Zhang, Q. (2008) A potential target associated with both cancer and cancer stem cells: a combination therapy for eradication of breast cancer using vinorelbine stealthy liposomes plus parthenolide stealthy liposomes. *J Control Release* 129, 18-25.

Löb, S., Königsrainer, A., Rammensee, H.G., Opelz, G. & Terness, P. (2009) Inhibitors of indoleamine-2,3-dioxygenase for cancer therapy: can we see the wood for the trees? *Nat Rev Cancer* 9, 445-452.

Lonardo, E., Hermann, P.C. & Heeschen, C. (2010) Pancreatic cancer stem cells – update and future perspective. *Mol Oncol* 4, 431-442.

Magnifico, A., Albano, L., Campaner, S., Delia, D., Castiglioni, F., Gasparini, P., Sozzi, G., Fontanella, E., Menard, S. & Tagliabue, E. (2009) Tumour-initiating cells of HER2-positive carcinoma cell lines express the highest oncoprotein levels and are trastuzumab-sensitive. *Clin Cancer Res* 15, 306-313.

Martin-Castillo, B., Vazquez-Martin, A., Oliveras-Ferraros, C. & Menendez, J.A. (2010) Metformin and cancer: Doses, mechanisms and the dandelion and hormetic phenomena. *Cell Cycle*, in press.

McDermott, S.P. & Wicha, M.S. (2010) Targeting breast cancer stem cells. *Mol Oncol* 4, 404-419.

Miraglia, S., Godfrey, W., Yin, A.H., Atkins, K., Warnke, R., Holden, J.T., Bray, R.A., Waller, E.K. & Buck, D.W. (2007) A novel five-transmembrane hematopoietic stem cell antigen: isolation, characterization, and molecular cloning. *Blood* 90, 5013-5021.

Miyazaki, Y., Shibuya, M., Sugawara, H., Kawaguchi, O. & Hirsoe, C. (1974) Salinomycin, a new polyether antibiotic. *J Antibiot* 27, 814-821.

Munn, D.H. & Mellor, A.L. (2007) Indoleamine 2,3-dioxygenase and tumour-induced tolerance. *J Clin Invest* 117, 1147-1154.

Murphy, M.P. & Smith, R. (2007) Targeting antioxidants to mitochondria by conjugation to lipophilic cations. *Annu Rev Pharmacol Toxicol* 47, 629-656.

Neuzil, J., Stantic, M., Zobalova, R., Chladova, M., Wang, X.F., Dong, L.F., Prochazka, L., Andera, L. & Ralph, S.J. (2007) Tumour-initiating cells *vs.* cancer 'stem' cells and CD133: What's in the name? *Biochem Biophys Res Commun* 355, 855-859.

Neuzil, J., Weber, T., Schröder, A., Lu, M., Ostermann, G., Gellert, N., Mayne, G.C., Olejnicka, B., Nègre-Salvayre, A., Sticha, M., Coffey, R.J. & Weber, C. (2001) Induction of apoptosis in cancer cells by α-tocopheryl succinate: Molecular pathways and structural requirements. *FASEB J* 15, 403-415.

Nguyen, N.P., Almeida, F.S., Chi, A., Nguyen, L.M., Cohen, D., Karlsson, U. & Vinh-Hung, V. (2010) Molecular biology of breast cancer stem cells: potential clinical applications. *Cancer Treat Rev* 36, 485-491.

O'Brien, C.A., Pollett, A., Gallinger, S. & Dick, J.E. (2007) A human colon cancer cell capable of initiating tumour growth in immunodeficient mice. *Nature* 445, 106-110.

Park, C.H., Bergsagel, D.E. & McCulloch, E.A (1971) Mouse myeloma tumour stem cells: a primary cell culture assay. *J Natl Cancer Inst* 46, 411-422.

Patrawala, L., Calhoun, T., Schneider-Broussard, R., Li, H., Bhatia, B., Tang, S., Reilly, J.G., Chandra, D., Zhou, J., Claypool, K., Coghlan, L. & Tang, D.G. (2006) Highly purified CD44+ prostate cancer cells from xenograft human tumours are enriched in tumourigenic and metastatic progenitor cell *Oncogene* 25, 1696-1708.

Piccirillo, S.G., Reynolds, B.A., Zanetti, N., Lamorte, G., Binda, E., Broggi, G., Brem, H., Olivi, A., Dimeco, F. & Vescovi, A.L (2006) Bone morphogenetic proteins inhibit the tumourigenic potential of human brain tumour-initiating cells. *Nature* 444, 761-765.

Prochazka, L., Dong, L.F., Valis, K., Freeman, R., Ralph, S.J., Turanek, J. & Neuzil, J. (2010) α-Tocopheryl succinate causes mitochondrial permeabilization by preferential formation of Bak channel. *Apoptosis* 15, 782-794.

Ramalho-Santos, M., Yoon, S., Matsuzaki, Y., Mulligan, R.C. & Melton, D.A. (2002) "Stemness": transcriptional profiling of embryonic and adult stem cells. *Science* 298, 597-600.

Ricci-Vitiani, L., Lombardi, D.G., Pilozzi, E., Ricci-Vitiani, L., Lombardi, D.G. & Pilozzi, E. (2007) Identification and expansion of human colon-cancer-initiating cells. *Nature* 445, 111-115.

Riccioni, R., Dupuis, M.L., Bernabei, M., Petrucci, E., Pasquini, L., Mariani, G., Cianfriglia, M. & Testa, U. (2010) The cancer stem cell selective inhibitor salinomycin is a p-glycoprotein inhibitor. *Blood Cells Mol Dis* 45, 86-92.

Rowan, K. (2009) High-throughput screening finds potential killer for cancer stem cells. *J Natl Cancer Inst* 101, 1438-1439.

Schatton, T., Murphy, G.F., Frank, N.Y., Yamaura, K., Waaga-Gasser, A.M., Gasser, M., Zhan, Q., Jordan, S., Duncan, L.M., Weishaupt, C., Fuhlbrigge, R.C., Kupper, T.S., Sayegh, M.H. & Frank, M.H. (2008) Identification of cells initiating human melanomas. *Nature* 451, 345-349.

Schreiber, R.D., Pace, J.L., Russell, S.W., Altman, A. & Katz, D.H. (1983) Macrophage-activating factor produced by a T cell hybridoma: Physiochemical and biosynthetic resemblance to γ-interferon. *J Immunol* 131, 826-832.

Shipitsin, M., Campbell, L.L., Argani, P., Weremowicz, S., Bloushtain-Qimron, N., Yao, J., Nikolskaya, T., Serebryiskaya, T., Beroukhim, R., Hu, M., Halushka, M.K., Sukumar, S., Parker, L.M., Anderson, K.S., Harris, L.N., Garber, J.E., Richardson, A.L., Schnitt, S.J., Nikolsky, Y., Gelman, R.S. & Polyak K: Molecular definition of breast tumour heterogeneity. *Cancer Cell* 11, 259-273.

Shmelkov, S.V., Butler, J.M., Hooper, A.T., Hormigo, A., Kushner, J., Milde, T., St Clair, R., Baljevic, M., White, I., Jin, D.K., Chadburn, A., Murphy, A.J., Valenzuela, D.M., Gale, N.W., Thurston, G., Yancopoulos, G.D., D'Angelica, M., Kemeny, N., Lyden, D. & Rafii, S. (2008) CD133 expression is not restricted to stem cells, and both CD133+ and CD133- metastatic colon cancer cells initiate tumours. *J Clin Invest* 118, 2111-2120.

Singh, S.K., Clarke, I.D., Terasaki, M., Haas, T.L., Diessenbacher, P., Sprick, M.R., Schön, M.P., Henkler, F., Gollnick, H., Walczak, H. & Leverkus, M. (2003) Identification of a cancer stem cell in human brain tumours. *Cancer Res* 63, 5821-5828.

Slamon, D.J., Godolphin, W., Jones, L.A., Holt, J.A., Wong, S.G., Keith, D.E., Levin, W.J., Stuart, S.G., Udove, J. & Ullrich, A. (1989) Studies of the HER-2/neu proto-oncogene in human breast and ovarian cancer. *Science* 244, 707–712.

Smyth, M.J., Cretney, E., Takeda, K., Wiltrout, R.H., Sedger, L.M., Kayagaki, N., Yagita, H. & Okumura, K. (2001) Tumour necrosis factor-related apoptosis-inducing ligand (TRAIL) contributes to interferon γ-dependent natural killer cell protection from tumour metastasis. *J Exp Med* 193, 661-670.

Smyth, M.J., Crowe, N.Y., Hayakawa, Y., Takeda, K., Yagita, H. & Godfrey, D.I. (2002) NKT cells-conductors of tumour immunity? *Curr Opin Immunol* 14, 165-171.

Takeda, K., Hayakawa, Y., Smyth, M.J., Kayagaki, N., Yamaguchi, N., Kakuta, S., Iwakura, Y., Yagita, H. & Okumura, K. (2001) Involvement of tumour necrosis factor-related apoptosis-inducing ligand in surveillance of tumour metastasis by liver natural killer cells. *Nat Med* 7, 94-100.

Tang, C., Ang, B.T. & Pervaiz, S. (2007) Cancer stem cell: target for anti-cancer therapy. *FASEB J* 21, 1-9.

Twombly, R. (2005) Cancer surpasses heart disease as leading cause of death of all but the very elderly. *J Natl Cancer Inst* 97, 330-331.

Valis, K., Prochazka, L., Boura, E., Chladova, M., Obsil, T., Rohlena, J., Truksa, J., Dong, L.F., Ralph, S.J. & Neuzil, J. Hippo/Mst1 stimulates transcription of *NOXA* in a FoxO1-dependent manner. *Cancer Res*, in press.

Vazquez-Martin, A., Oliveras-Ferraros, C., Barco, S.D., Martin-Castillo, B. & Menendez, J.A. (2010a) The anti-diabetic drug metformin suppresses self-renewal and proliferation of trastuzumab-resistant tumour-initiating breast cancer stem cells. *Breast Cancer Res Treat*, in press.

Vazquez-Martin, A., Oliveras-Ferraros, C., Cufí, S., Martin-Castillo, B. & Menendez, J.A. (2010b) Metformin and energy metabolism in breast cancer: From insulin physiology to tumour-initiating stem cells. *Curr Mol Med* 10, 674-691.

Vescovi, A.L., Galli, R., & Reynolds, B.A. (2006) Brain tumour stem cells. *Nat Rev Cancer* 6, 425-436.

Visvader, J.E. (2009) Keeping abreast of the mammary epithelial hierarchy and breast tumourigenesis. *Genes Dev* 23, 2563-2577.

Visvader, J.E. & Lindeman, G.J. (2008) Cancer stem cells in solid tumours: accumulating evidence and unresolved questions. *Nat Rev Cancer* 8, 755-768.

Weber, T., Lu, M., Andera, L., Lahm, H., Gellert, N., Fariss, M.W., Korinek, V., Sattler, W., Ucker, D.S., Terman, A., Schröder, A., Erl, W., Brunk, U., Coffey, R.J., Weber, C. & Neuzil, J. (2002) Vitamin E succinate is a potent novel anti-neoplastic agent with high tumour selectivity and cooperativity with tumour necrosis factor-related apoptosis-inducing ligand (TRAIL, Apo2L) in vivo. *Clin Cancer Res* 8, 863-869.

Wright, M.H., Calcagno, A.M., Salcido, C.D., Carlson, M.D., Ambudkar, S.V. & Varticovski, L. (2007) Brca1 breast tumours contain distinct $CD44^+/CD24^-$ and $CD133^+$ cells with cancer stem cell characteristics. *Breast Cancer Res* 10, R10.

Yang, Z.F., Ho, D.W., Ng, M.N., Lau, C.K., Yu, W.C., Ngai, P., Chu, P.W., Lam, C.T., Poon, R.T. & Fan, S.T. (2008) Significancer of CD90+ cancer stem cells in human liver cancer. *Cancer Cell* 13, 153-166.

Yin, S., Li, J., Hu, C., Chen, X., Yao, M., Yan, M., Jiang, G., Ge, C., Xie, H., Wan, D., Yang, S., Zheng, S. & Gu, J. (2007) CD133 positive hepatocellular carcinoma cells posses high capacity for tumourigenicity. *Int J Cancer* 120, 1436-1442.

Zhang, S., Belch, C., Chan, M.W., Lai, H.C., Matei, D., Schilder, J.M., Yan, P.S., Huang, T.H. & Nephew, K.P. (2008) Identification and characterization of ovarian cancer-initiating cells from primary human tumours. *Cancer Res* 68, 4311-4320.

Zhou, J., Zhang, H., Gu, P., Bai, J., Margolick, J.B. & Zhang, Y (2008) NF-κB pathway inhibitors preferentially inhibit breast cancer stem-like cells. *Breast Cancer Res Treat* 111, 419-427.

Zobalova, R., McDermott, L., Stantic, M., Prokopova, K., Dong, L.F. & Neuzil, J. (2008) CD133-positive cancer cells are resistant to TRAIL due to upregulation of FLIP. *Biochem Biophys Res Commun* 373, 567-571.

19

Cancer Stem Cells as a New Opportunity for Therapeutic Intervention

Victoria Bolós[1], Ángeles López[2] and Luis Anton Aparicio[3]
[1,2]*Pfizer Oncology, Madrid. Spain*
[3]*Medical Oncology Service CHU A Coruña*
Spain

1. Introduction

For several years, a new theory about the formation of tumors is gathering strength. This new theory sustains that, tumors, as most of adult tissues, contain a very small population of altered stem cells. These long lived tumor stem cell population through its capacity of cell renewal and differentiation would be the origin of the larger short lived population of malignant differentiated cells in the tumor. However, central questions are still pending to be solved such as; if tumors start with mutations in adult stem cells or if a more differentiated cell could acquire stem cell properties and develop and maintain the tumor bulk.

These tumor stem cells just like adult stem cells would also operate through specific signaling pathways, different to those in any other differentiated healthy cell of the adult or the tumor mass.

According to this theory, it is believed that relapses in patients treated with traditional therapeutic strategies like chemotherapy and even new anti-target agents are due to the fact that this type of treatment although having the capacity to destroy most of the tumor cells, would not affect the cancer stem cells. These residual tumor stem cells would therefore be the ones that in a shorter or longer time span would end up regenerating the tumor.

Thereby, new anti-target agents designed to block the signaling pathways that rule the activity of stem cells may be considered a new promising therapeutic strategy to avoid relapses to conventional treatments.

At the moment, large pharmaceutical companies are developing drugs that can block three signaling pathways considered critical for the maintenance of stem cells, the Notch pathway, the Wnt pathway and the Hedgehog pathway. These drugs have already shown promising efficacy and safety in clinical trials in different settings and tumor types. In this chapter we will review this issue with depth.

2. Stem cells and cancer stem cell theory

Stem Cells

In order to understand cancer stem cells a brief description of normal adult stem cells and the environment in which they live should be an indispensible requisite in this chapter.

Normal adult stem cells (SCs) are cells with the ability to continually repopulate the tissues that comprise the organ system in which they exist. One of their main properties is their differentiation capability which allows them to produce tissue-specific specialized daughter cells under certain conditions (Schöler, 2007). They also possess a self-renewal capability comprised by an asymmetric cell division in which one of the daughter cells is always a stem cell (self-renewal) while the other will be a transient amplifying precursor with high proliferative capacity which will undergo several symmetric divisions resulting in the generation of lineage-committed progenitors that will finally differentiate into non-cycling, terminally differentiated, mature cells (Bapat, 2007). Lastly, SCs have a high proliferative capacity even though they usually appear in a quiescent or slowly cycling state (Lobo et al. 2007).

SCs reside within a tissue microenvironment often described as *niche;* a stroma made up of differentiated cells which secrete a rich extracellular matrix and other factors essential for the tight regulation of the maintenance and renewal processes in organs or tissues (Fuchs et al. 2004). The niche microenvironment promotes adhesion and maintenance of the quiescent state of SC by inhibiting both proliferation and differentiation and, when needed, also regulates SC self-renewal, proliferation of the transit amplifying cell population and cell differentiation (Rizvi et al. 2005; Fuchs et al. 2004).

Cancer Stem Cell Theory

The idea of cancer being a pathology related with less mature cells was already introduced in 1858 by Rudolf Virchow. He laid the foundations for cell pathology suggesting that all cells arise from other cells ("*omnis cellula e cellula*"), and provided scientific basis for cancer through its microscopical and clinical observations which lead to the idea that cancer arises form an immature cell (Lobo et al. 2007).

Later on, in 1889, Sir S. Paget introduced the *soil and seed* hypothesis of metastasis suggesting that the distribution of metastases could not be due to chance alone and that only some tissues provide more optimal conditions for the growth of certain tumors (Paget, 1889). In his hypothesis, the *seed* would refer to the ostensible less mature tumor-initiating cell or stem cell from the primary tumor which would be the tumorigenic force behind tumor initiation, growth, metastasis and the cause of treatment resistance and relapse (reviewed in Pardal et al, 2003); while the *soil* would refer to the secondary site where the tumor would arise.

A variation of this idea was provided by the *homing* hypothesis which suggested that different organs could be able to attract different types of metastatic cells originated at the primary site through chemotactic mechanisms provided by signals secreted by cells at the future metastatic sites (Stetler-Stevenson 2001, Müller 2001, Strieter, 2001). In this hypothesis, the *seed* would produce cell surface receptors capable of recognizing secreted signals from the new site defined as the *soil*.

Although the mechanisms of tissue specificity of metastases still remains obscure, researchers have focused on small messenger molecules that may act as attractants and larger cell surface receptors which could guide the tumor-initiating cells or *seeds*. Müller (Müller et al, 2001) and Murphy (Murphy, 2001) focused on chemokines and their receptors as potential viable candidates for this *soil and seed* signaling. Murphy specifically proposes a "spatial and temporal code" made up of specific combinations of chemokines, chemokine receptors and adhesion molecules as being responsible for the neovascularization, metastasis, and immunosurveillance avoidance in tumors.

Cancer Stem Cells

Cancer Stem Cells (CSCs) are tumor cells different from the rest of the tumor bulk in that they can drive the growth and spread of a tumor (Lobo et al. 2007). They share their main characteristics with normal SCs and that is why they share a similar nomenclature. CSCs show self-renewal, certain potency as the can produce all the cell types that appear in a tumor through division and differentiation processes and have a high proliferative capacity although they usually appear in a quiescent state (Bhattacharyya et al. 2010; Lobo et al. 2007) which allows them to be more resistant to traditional anti-cancer drugs.

The main difference with SCs would be that the above processes in CSCs would be uncontrolled due to alterations in genes that encode for key signaling proteins or in the niche control and they therefore may give rise to aberrant tumorigenic tissues (Ishiguro et al. 2006; Weber et al. 2006; Clarke, 2005).

Disruption of the niche signal may also lead to either loss of SCs or malignant transformation of these SCs resulting in cancer (Bhattacharyya et al. 2010).

Several authors demonstrate that changes in the stability of the stroma lead to the induction of colorectal adenomas and invasive breast carcinomas amongst others (Ishiguro et al. 2006; Weber et al. 2006). Disruptive processes occurring in the niche during infection, inflammation, tissue damage, or chemical assault, could therefore be partly responsible of the changes that give rise to cancer stem cells (CSCs).

The discovery of tumor heterogeneity, where different cells within the tumor show different phenotypes gave rise to a CSC theory leaving behind the classical or stochastic model which stated that all neoplastic cells within a tumor have the same tumorigenic capacity but their ability to enter the cell cycle and find a permissive environment for growth would be a stochastic event that would occur with low probability (Dick, 2003; Lobo et al. 2007; Huntly & Gilliland,2005).

The CSC theory therefore suggests that a malignant tumor would be composed of a heterogeneous population of cells with different degrees of tumorigenic potential in which only a subset of cancer cells would be able to initiate and propagate the tumor. This theory arose from the fact that therapeutic approaches that aim the bulk of the tumor are not successful in avoiding relapses which must mean that not all cells in a tumor are the same. A subset of cells with different characteristics must achieve an extensive proliferation inducing the re-growth of the tumor (Reya et al. 2001). This phenomenon was proved by showing both in solid and hematological tumors that only a proportion of the tumor cells were clonogenic in culture and *in vivo* (Park et al. 1971; Fidler IJ et al. 1977).

The origin of these CSC is slightly controversial; its name suggests a SC origin although mutations in more differentiated progenitors could also give rise to CSCs (Figure 1).

The first hypothesis suggests that CSCs arise from stem cells with transforming mutations or epigenetic alterations that acquire a malignant phenotype. In a murine model of prostate cancer, a targeted suppression of the *PTEN* gene in luminal stem cells resulted in rapid formation of neoplasias and invasive carcinomas indicating a possible CSC origin in prostate cancers (Wang et al. 2009).

On the other hand, CSCs could be originated in a more committed cell progeny through maturation arrest of progenitor cells and the ability of these more differentiated cells to re-enter the cell cycle and undergo uncontrolled proliferation both mediated by mutational events that reactivate the self-renewal machinery (Bapat, 2007; Wang 2010).

In order to favor the appearance of CSCs several changes should occur such as: changes in the niche microenvironment, epigenetic deregulation and mutations in specific genes responsible for alterations in the cell cycle pattern, self-renewal, metabolism and differentiation processes and finally, amplification of these genetically altered populations (Bapat, 2007).

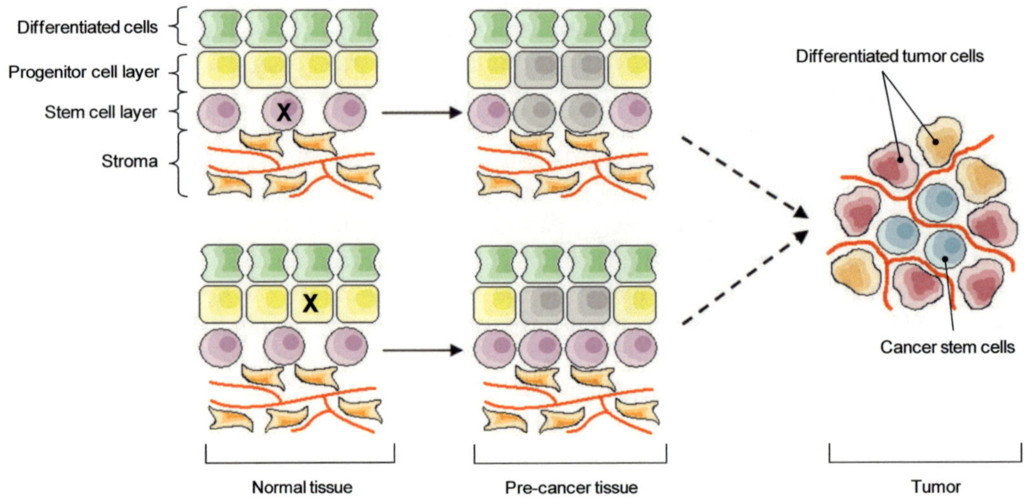

Fig. 1. Origin of CSCs.
CSCs may arise from the normal SC population due to spontaneous genetic or epigenetic changes or changes induced by disruption of the SC niche/stroma (**X**). The acquisition of malignant traits by SCs will be inherited by their progeny (grey cells). On the other hand, CSC origins could start in a more committed cell progeny through acquisition of self-renewal properties once again mediated by mutational events and giving rise to modified daughter cells (grey cells). Additional modifications of this partially modified progeny and subsequent cell divisions would then lead to the formation of CSCs and a heterogeneous tumor bulk.

3. Cancer stem cell pathways and new opportunities for therapeutic interventions

By definition, CSCs would maintain the self-renewal and differentiation capacities of SCs; thus it is likely that similarities exist in the pathways governing these processes in both normal and CSCs. Understanding the subjacent responsible molecular pathways that regulate these events in normal SCs is therefore extremely important for the design of drugs aimed to destroy CSCs and even avoid tumor relapse.

It has been suggested that specific signaling pathways such as Notch, Sonic Hedgehog (Shh) and Wingless (Wnt)-β-catenin are critical for self-renewal and differentiation in normal stem cells. In agreement with the CSC hypothesis, alterations in those genes that encode for signaling molecules belonging to these pathways have been found in human tumor samples suggesting that they are likely involved in tumor development and maintenance (Lobo et al, 2007; Sánchez-García et al. 2007). .

Hedgehog signaling pathway

The Hedgehog (Hh) signaling pathway plays a crucial role in human embryogenesis, but is largely inactive in adult tissues under normal conditions (Rubin and de Sauvage, 2006) The SHH signaling pathway is involved in the maintenance of normal adult stem cell population and expansion of progenitors (Ingham and McMahon, 2001).

The Hh gene family encodes several secreted glycoproteins such as Indian Hedgehog (IHH), Desert Hedgehog (DHH), and Sonic Hedgehog (SHH) (reviewed in Taipale & Beachy, 2001; Liu et al., 2005). The Hh pathway is unique in that the above ligands serve to relieve a series of repressive interactions between membrane receptors. In the absence of ligands, the transmembrane receptor Patched 1 (PTCH) blocks the smoothened (SMO) receptor, blocking its activity. The binding of the ligand to PTCH derepresses SMO, allowing the activation of the serine/threonine kinase Fused (Fu) which leads to the release of the transcription factor Gli from the sequestration by Suppressor of Fused (SuFu). Subsequently Gli proteins are able to translocate to the nucleus and regulate transcription of target genes involved in proliferation and differentiation such as cyclin D and c-myc (reviewed in Nybakken & Perrimon, 2002; Pasca di Magliano & Hebrok, 2003) (Figure 2).

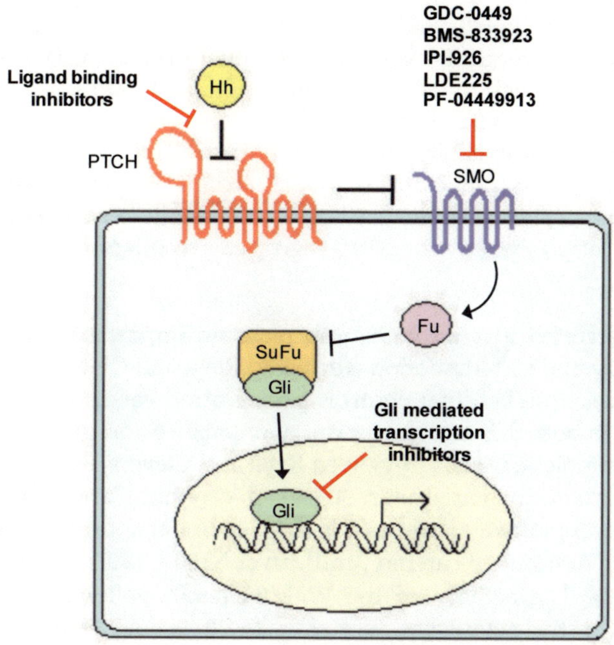

Fig. 2. Hedgehog signaling pathway.
In the absence of ligands, the receptor patched (PTCH) represses the smoothened (SMO) receptor. When the hedgehog (Hh) ligand is present, it represses PTCH which allows the serine/threonine kinase Fused (Fu) to induce the release of the transcription factor Gli from the sequestration by Suppressor of Fused (SuFu). Gli can therefore enter the nucleus and induce the transcription of target genes.
Molecules under study are being developed against the SMO receptor and against the processes of ligand binding and Gli mediated transcription.

Activation of SHH has been showed in basal cell carcinoma (BCC) of the skin (Hahn et al 1996; Bale and Yu, 2001), medulloblastome (Berman et al. 2002), pancreatic cancer (Berman et al. 2003; Kayed et al. 2004; Thayer et al. 2003), prostate cancer (Karhadkar et al. 2004; Fan et al. 2004), small cell lung cancer (Watkins et al. 2003), hepatocellular carcinoma (Sicklick et al. 2005; Patil et al. 2005) and also in hematological malignancies (Kubo et al. 2004)

Therapeutic inhibition of the Hh signaling destroys CSC, improves outcome, and even may effect a cure when is combined with gemcitabine in a direct pancreatic cancer xenograft model (Jimeno et al. 2009) suggesting the importance of combining therapeutic approaches that target CSCs with conventional drugs to improve efficacy.

Based on evidence, many inhibitors of this pathway are currently under development: (reviewed in Peukert and Miller-Moslin 2010) Although the majority of HH pathways inhibitors reported to date are SMO antagonist, drugs that block Hh ligand binding and GLI mediated transcription have been also been developed (see Figure 2, red arrows).

SMO inhibitors have already advanced to human clinical trials (reviewed in Peukert and Miller-Moslin 2010). GDC-0449 (RG3616) (Genetech) has already showed positive results in a Phase I study in patients with metastatic or locally advanced BCC (Von Hoff DD et al. 2009) that have led to an extensive clinical development as a single agent and in combination not only in BCC of the skin also in other tumor types such as colorectal, ovarian, breast, prostate, small cell lung cancer, pancreatic medulloblastoma and glioblastoma (http://www.clinicaltrials.gov/ct2/results?term=GDC-0449&pg=2).

Although less advanced in their development, other SMO inhibitors have already moved to the clinical setting: BMS-833923 (Exelixis/Bristol-Myers)
(http://www.clinicaltrials.gov/ct2/results?term=BMS-833923),
IPI-926 (infinity) (http://www.clinicaltrials.gov/ct2/results?term=IPI-926),
LDE225 (Novartis) (http://www.clinicaltrials.gov/ct2/results?term=LDE225), and
PF-04449913 (Pfizer) (http://www.clinicaltrials.gov/ct2/results?term=PF-04449913).

Wnt signaling pathway

The Wnt family of secreted glycoproteins also plays an important role in embryonic and adult stem cell biology and differentiation (reviewed Reya and Clevers, 2005). This pathway is considered as a master switch that controls proliferation versus differentiation (Van der Wetering et al. 2002) in both SCs and cancer cell maintenance and growth in intestinal, other epidermal and hematopoietic tissues (reviewed Reya and Clevers, 2005).

The Wnt pathway is subdivided into a so called canonical and a non canonical Wnt signaling. The canonical pathway (Figure 3) is the best understood and is dependent on the intracellular signaling molecule β-catenin (Cadigan & Nusse, 1997; reviewed in MacDonald, Tamai and He, 2009). The activity of the Wnt/β-catenin pathway is dependent of the amount of β-catenin in the cytoplasm. Normally the β-catenin level is kept low through continuous ubiquitin proteosome mediated degradation. In the "off state" of the pathway (absence of Wnt ligands), cells maintain low cytoplasmic and nuclear levels of β-catenin, although β-catenin is associated with the cell-cell adhesion molecule E-cadherin at the plasma membrane, an association that spares it from the degradative pathway. In the absence of Wnt ligands, cytoplasmic β-catenin is constantly degraded by the action of a destruction complex known as Axin composed by the Axin scaffolding protein, the adenomatous poliposys coli gene product (APC), casein kinase 1 (CK1) and glycogen syntase kinase 3 (GSK3). CK1 and GSK3 sequentially phosphorylate the amino terminal region of β-catenin allowing its subsequent ubiquitination and proteosomal degradation

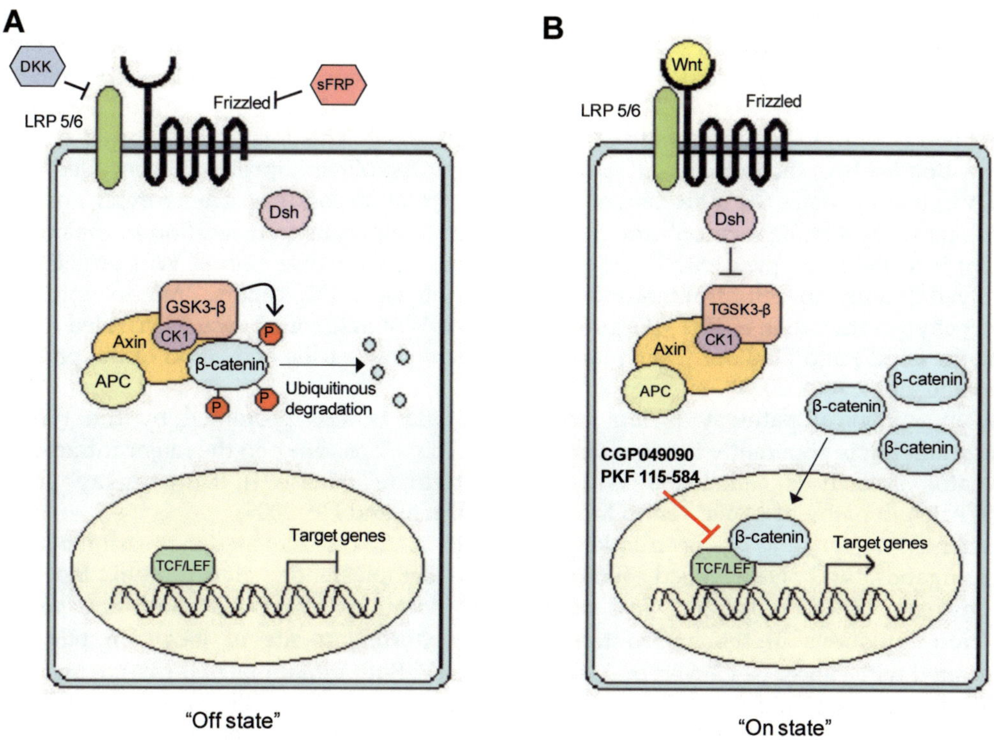

Fig. 3. Wnt canonical signaling pathway.
The "off state" of the pathway (A) takes place in absence of the Wnt ligand, The complex formed by Axin scaffolding protein, the adenomatous poliposys coli gene product (APC), casein kinase 1 (CK1) and glycogen syntase kinase 3 (GSK3) constantly induces the degradation of the molecule β-catenin due to a sequential phosphorylation that induces ubiquitination and proteosomal degradation which inhibits the translocation of β-catenin to the nucleus and transcription of target genes. In absence of β-catenin, T cell factor/ lymphoid enhancer factor (TCF/LEF) acts as a repressor of the Wnt target genes. Wnt antagonist such as Frizzled related proteins (sFRP) and Dikkopf (DKK) family members prevent the activation of the pathway.
On the "on state" of the pathway (B), Wnt binds to its receptor, Frizzled (Fz) and its co-receptor, the low density lipoprotein receptor related protein 5/6 (LRP5/6) inducing the activation of the phosphoprotein Dishevelled (DSH or DVL) and mediating the inhibition of the Axin destruction complex. The accumulation of β-catenin allows it to enter the nucleus and bind to TCF/LEF to activate transcription. Inhibitory molecules against the β-catenin/TCF interaction are currently under study.

(reviewed in MacDonald, Tamai and He, 2009). This degradation prevents the nuclear translocation of β-catenin and the subsequent expression of Wnt target genes. Thereby in absence of nuclear β-catenin, transcription factors such as DNA-bound T cell factor/ lymphoid enhancer factor (TCF/LEF) act as repressors of Wnt target genes instead of as activators (reviewed in MacDonald, Tamai and He, 2009) (Figure 3)

Activation of the pathway occurs when a Wnt ligand binds the transmembrane receptor Frizzled (Fz) and its co-receptor, the low density lipoprotein receptor related protein 5/6 (LRP5/6). In humans 19 members of the Wnt family and 10 Fz receptors have been described (reviewed in MacDonald, Tamai and He, 2009). This ligand-receptor-co-receptor interaction leads to the recruitment and activation of the phosphoprotein Dishevelled (DSH or DVL) that mediates the inhibition of the Axin destruction complex. Therefore, the on state of the pathway stabilizes cytoplasmatic β-catenin and allows its translocation to the nucleus where it forms a complex with TCF/LEF that leads to the expression of Wnt target genes involved mainly in cell proliferation (e,g c-myc, cyclcin D1, others) and in epithelial-mesenchymal transitions (EMT) (Figure 3). Secreted Wnt antagonist such as Frizzled related proteins (sFRP) and Dikkopf (DKK) family members prevent the activation of the pathway (Kawano and Kypta, 2003)

The non-canonical pathway is less understood and is also promoted by the Wnt Fz interaction but is apparently independent of β-catenin. Depending on the major intracellular mediator used it is called the Wnt/ jun N-terminal kinase (JNK) pathway or the Wnt/calcium pathway (reviewed in MacDonald, Tamai and He, 2009).

Aberrant Wnt signaling has been linked to a range of tumors. Elevated expression of some Wnt ligands and Dishevelled (DSH/DVL, a cytoplasmatic glycoprotein that acts downstream the Fz repceptor), loss of function mutations of APC or Axin and gain of function mutations in the amino terminal phosphorilation site of β-catenin has been associated with cancer (reviewed by Moon et al. 2004). Both mutations of β-catenin and APC genes are common in colorectal cancer (Kolligs et al. 1999). The APC gene is inherited or sporadic early mutated in the development of most colon tumors, which reduces the degradation of β-catenin (Van der Wetering et al. 2002). In non small cell lung cancer DSH/DVL genes are overexpressed (Uematsu et al. 2003). β-catenin accumulation has been also observed in breast cancer, melanoma, sarcoma, skin and brain tumors, and also hematological (myeloid leukemia and multiple myeloma) tumor samples (Reguart et al. 2005: Taipale & Beachy, 2001;Reya et al, 2003 ;Bastian et al, 2005; Mohinta et al, 2007; Bruxvoort et al, 2007). Furthermore, activating mutations in β-catenin have been found in endometrial (Okuda et al. 2010; Samarnthai et al. 2010), prostate (Robinson et al. 2008) and hepatocellular carcinoma (Whittaker et al. 2010) and an association of this pathway with renal cancer has been also suggested (Yamamura et al. 2010; Hirata et al. 2010)

Recently, two small molecular inhibitors, CGP049090 and PKF 115-584 (Novartis), both of them fungal derivatives, have been identified, which specifically disrupt nuclear β-catenin/TCF interaction (see Figure 3, red arrow) (Dihlmann and Von Knebel Doeberitz, 2005). These two compounds have already show anti-tumoral activity in acute myeloid leukemia cells (Minke et al. 2008), chronic lymphocytic leukemia cells (Gandhirajan et al. 2010) and in hepatocarcinoma cell lines (Wei et al. 2010) *in vivo* and *in vitro.*

Notch signaling pathway

Notch is a conserved signaling pathway that takes part in embryonic and postnatal development by regulating SC self renewal, cell fate specification and initiation of differentiation (reviewed in Bolós et al. 2007)

Four different Notch receptors (Notch 1-4) have been described in humans (Fleming, 1998). Each Notch gene encodes a single-pass transmembrane receptor that harbors an extracellular domain involved in ligand binding and a cytoplasmatic domain involved in signal transduction (Bolós et al. 2007).
There are also five Notch ligands in mammals, three Delta ligands and two Jagged ligands. These ligands are also membrane bound and they are placed in the surface of neighboring cells (Bolós et al. 2007)
Following the binding of the ligand, the receptor is activated by two consecutive proteolytic cleavages that lead to the release of its intracellular domain (NICD) (Figure 4). The first proteolytic cleavage is mediated by the metalloprotease ADAM17 (TNF-α-converting-enzyme or TACE), which cleaves Notch on the extracellular side, near the transmembrane domain. The released extracellular portion of the receptor is then transendocytosed by the cell expressing the ligand. The second cleavage occurs within the transmembrane domain and is mediated by a gamma-secretase activity whose key component is presenilin (Bolós et al. 2007). This final cleavage liberates the NICD, which subsequently translocates to the

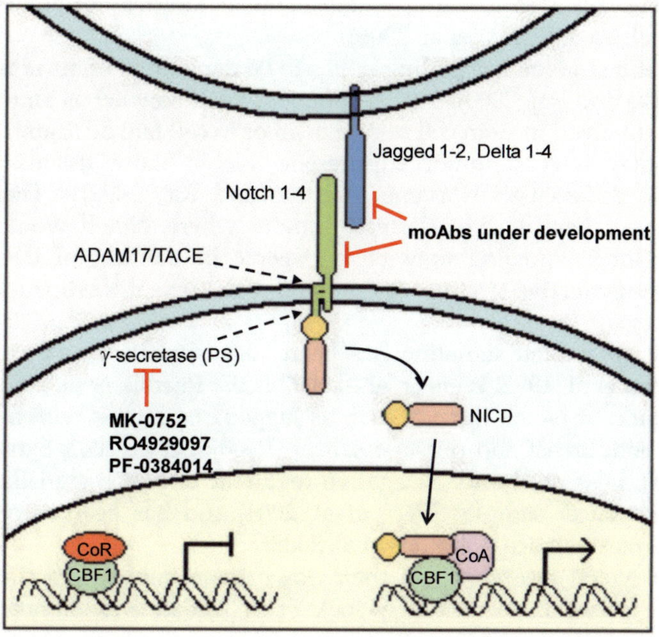

Fig. 4. Notch signaling pathway.
The binding of the Notch receptor (1-4) with its ligand Jagged (1-2) or Delta (1-4) placed in the surface of a neighbouring cell promotes the sequential cleavage of Notch by metalloprotease ADAM17 (TNF-α-converting-enzyme or TACE) and by a γ-secretase with presenilin (PS) as its key component. This cleavage liberates the NICD which translocates to the nucleus and binds to the transcription factor CBF1 displacing nuclear co-repressor proteins (CoR) and recruiting nuclear co-activator proteins (CoA) inducing the transcription of target genes.
Molecules against γ-secretase and monoclonal antibodies against Notch receptors and ligands are being developed to disrupt the Notch signaling pathway.

nucleus where it binds to the transcription factor CBF1. This interaction converts CBF1 from a transcriptional repressor into a transcriptional activator by displacing nuclear co-repressor proteins (CoR) and through the recruitment of nuclear co-activator proteins (CoA) (see Figure 4).

To date, only a few target genes have been identified; some of these genes are dependent on Notch signaling in all tissues, whereas others are tissue-specific (Bolós et al. 2007). The best-known Notch target genes are genes that encode for transcription repressors of the HES and HEY families. Genes that encode for Deltex1, the pre-T-cell receptor α and the cell cycle regulator p21 are also targets of NICD.

Deregulated expression of this pathway is observed in a growing number of hematological and solid tumors (Nickoloff et al. 2003). Aberrant Notch signaling may be necessary not only for the initiation of tumors but also for tumor maintenance (Weng et al, 2003; Roy et al,2007). Notch also has an important role in normal arteriogenesis and neo-angiogenesis, both of which are likely to be recapitulated in cancer (Rehman & Wang, 2006). In some instances, Notch signaling in endothelial cells appears to be triggered by ligands expressed on tumor cells (Zeng et al, 2005), which may contribute to the aggressive clinical behavior of those tumors expressing high levels of Notch ligands (Ridgway et al. 2006; Reedjik et a, 2005; Santagata et al, 2004; Bismar et al. 2006).

The result of alteration in Notch signaling seems to be dependent on its normal function in a given tissue (Radtke and Raj, 2003). In this context, Notch may act as an oncogene in those tissues where it is involved in stem cell self renewal or in cell fate decisions. On the contrary, Notch signaling may have a tumor suppressor role in those tissues in which Notch promotes terminal differentiation events (Radtke and Raj, 2003). Therefore, with the possible exception of keratinocyte derived tumors where Notch would have a tumor suppressor role, Notch signaling may be oncogenic in the rest of the tumors and its inhibition may be an effective strategy to combine with current therapeutic agents (Radtke and Raj, 2003).

An oncogenic role for Notch signaling has been suggested in breast and salivary gland epithelium (Jhappan et al. 1992; Weijzen et al,2002 la 38; Reedijk et al, 2005; Stylianou et al. 2006). The expression of Notch ligands such as Jagged1 correlates with a more aggressive disease course in both breast and prostate cancer (Reedjik et al, 2005; Santagata et al, 2004; Bismar et al. 2006). Loss of Numb, a negative regulator of Notch signaling, has been also observed in breast cancer samples (Pece et al. 2004) and has been associated with poor prognosis and chemoresistance (Colaluca et al. 2008)

Elevated levels of Notch receptors and their downstream targets are showed in primary human melanomas (Balint et al, 2005; Hoek et al, 2004), and enforced expression of constitutively active Notch1 promotes melanoma progression (Balint et al. 2005; Liu et al. 2006). Other neoplasias such as medulloblastoma (Marino et al. 2005; Hallahan et al. 2004), neuroblastoma (Ferrari-Toninelli et al. 2010) ovarian cancer (Park et al, 2006) and T acute cell lymphoblastic leukemia/lymphoma (T-ALL) (Weng et al. 2004; Aster, 2005) have an implication of Notch signaling in their pathogenesis.

Preclinical evidence suggest that Notch signaling may be involved in different breast cancer molecular subtypes and its inhibition may enhance the efficacy of current therapeutic agents (Rizzo et al. 2008; Osipo et al. 2008; Lee et al. 2008).A role for Notch signaling in intestinal SC biology is well established (Van Es et al. 2005; Fre et al. 2005)

Furthermore, a crosstalk between Wnt and Notch pathways has also been suggested in intestinal self-renewal and in the proliferation of adenomas and adenocarcinomas in the intestine (Van Es et al. 2005). Gamma-secretase inhibitors enhanced the action of some chemotherapeutics in colon cancer cell lines (Van Es et al. 2005).

And monoclonal antibodies that target Notch receptors have also lead to an antitumoral effect in colon cancer models (Wu et al. 2010)

Notch signaling has also played an important role in hematopoiesis (Duncan et al. 2005). In fact, one of the clearest examples of oncogenic Notch signaling is found in T-ALL (Weng et al. 2004; Aster et al. 2005 ; Van Vlierberghe et al. 2006, Chiang et al. 2006). Less than 1% of T-ALL shows a chromosome translocation that leads to the expression of a constitutively active intracellular version of Notch1 (Weng et al. 2004; Aster et al. 2005) and more than 50% of human T-ALLs, without specific chromosome translocation, also show activating mutations in *Notch-1* (Weng et al. 2004; Aster et al. 2005) Furthermore, it has been shown that Notch1 also suppresses p53 function in T-ALL cells (Beverly et al, 2005) which could promote oncogenesis through increased cell survival and genomic instability.

A tumor suppressor role for Notch has been established in Keratinocyte-derived carcinomas (Rangaranjan et al. 2001; Nicolas et al. 2003) due to its role in differentiation events in the homeostasis of the skin (Lowell et al. 2000). The tumor suppressor effect of Notch in the skin may be mediated by its action as a repressor of the Hh and Wnt pathways in this tissue, both involved in self renewal of skin stem cells (Thelu et al. 2002; Devgan et al. 2005). The tyrosine kinase receptor of the epidermal growth factor (EGFR) also acts as a main player in skin tumorigeneis. EGFR has been also showed to be a negative regulator of *Notch1* transcription in keratinocytes (Kolev et al. 2008), also supporting a tumour suppressor role for Notch1 in the skin.

The molecular mechanisms by which aberrant Notch signaling causes cancer are not fully understood. Experimentally, Notch1 could collaborate with c-myc (Girad et al, 1996; Palomero et al,2006; Sharma et al,2006), E2A-PBX1 (Rohn et al, 1996) and Ikaros (Beverly & Capobianco, 2003), whereas Notch3 would down-regulate tumour suppressive E2A activity (Talora et al, 2003). Notch1 may inhibit p53-mediated apoptosis by stimulating signaling through the PI3K-Akt-mTOR-eIF4E pathway (Mungamuri et al, 2006), and may antagonize the growth suppressive effects of the transforming growth factor beta (TGF-β) signaling pathways (Sun et al, 2005). Other researches suggest the existence of an intimate and functionally important interaction between Notch and hypoxia-inducible factor (HIF)-1α, a transcription factor that regulates many genes involved in the response to hypoxia, including factors that promote angiogenesis (Gordan & Simon, 2007). Other data suggest that HIF-1α binds and stabilizes activated Notch1, leading to enhanced Notch signaling (Gustafsson et al, 2005). Expression of HIF-1α and Notch1 are correlated in breast cancer, in which Notch1 appears to up-regulate HIF-1α expression (Soares et al, 2004). It is also possible that Notch ligands on tumor cells impact the host immune response through effects on B and T cells (Dallman et al, 2005)

Based on the role of Notch signaling in the homeostasis of adult tissues and its implication in cancer, gamma secretase inhibitors (GSIs) and monoclonal antibodies against Notch receptors and ligands are under development (see Figure 4, red arrows) by large pharmaceutical companies as a new therapeutic tools (Reviewed by Miele et al. 2006).

MK-0752 (Merck) is a GSI under clinical development in early stage and advanced breast cancer, stage IV pancreatic cancer, recurrent or refractory CNS cancer and T-ALL (http://www.clinicaltrials.gov/ct2/results?term=MK-0752). RO4929097 (La Roche) is another potent GSI (Luistro et al. 2009). Numerous Clinical trials with RO4929097 are underway in brain and CNS tumors; breast; colorectal; kidney; lung; melanoma; ovarian and pancreatic (http://www.clinicaltrials.gov/ct2/results?term=RO4929097). PF-0384014 (Pfizer) is also a GSI that have already shown antitumor and antiangiogenic effects in preclinical breast cancer models (Zhang C et al AACR 2010). A clinical trial in advancer solid tumors and in leukemia patients is underway with this drug (http://www.clinicaltrials.gov/ct2/show/NCT00878189?term=notch&rank=17).

4. Conclusions

Conventional chemotherapy and even new anti-target agents for the treatment of cancer patients in advanced stages have only yielded limited benefit in overall survival.

If a small but long lived population of tumor cells, CSCs, is involved in resistance and relapse to current anti-cancer therapies it seems of paramount importance to understand the molecular events governing these CSC in order to develop therapies specifically aimed at them.

At the moment, drugs that can block pathways considered critical for the maintenance of stem cells are under clinical development. The future will tell us if thanks to these new drugs there will be a turning point in the treatment of cancer.

5. Abbreviations

SC - stem cell
CSC - cancer stem cell
Shh - Sonic Hedgehog
Wnt - Wingless
Hh - Hedgehog
HIF - Hipoxia inducible factor

6. References

Aster JC. Deregulated NOTCH signaling in acute T-cell lymphoblastic leukemia/lymphoma: new insights, questions, and opportunities. Int J Hematol. 2005;82(4):295-301.

Bhattacharyya S and Khanduja KL. New hope in the horizon: cancer stem cells. Acta Biochim Biophys Sin 2010;42(4):237-242

Bale AE, Yu KP. The hedgehog pathway and basal cell carcinomas. Hum Mol Genet. 2001;10(7):757-62.

Balint K, Xiao M, Pinnix CC, Soma A, Veres I, Juhasz I, Brown EJ, Capobianco AJ, Herlyn M, Liu ZJ. Activation of Notch1 signaling is required for β-catenin-medaited human primary melanoma progression. J Clin Invest 2005;115:3166-3176

Bapat SA.. Evolution of cancer stem *cells.* Seminars in Cancer Biology 2007;17:204–213

Bastian PJ, Ellinger J, Wellmann A, Wernert N, Heukamp LC, Muller SC and von Ruwcker A. Diagnostic and information in prostate cancer with the help of a small set of hypermethylated gene loci. Clin Xcancer Res 2006;11:4097-4106

Berman DM, Karhadkar SS, Hallahan AR, Pritchard JI, Eberhart CG, Watkins DN, Chen JK, Cooper MK, Taipale J, Olson JM, Beachy PA. Medulloblastoma growth inhibition by hedgehog pathway blockade. Science 2002;297(5586):1559-61.

Berman DM, Karhadkar SS, Maitra A, Montes De Oca R, Gerstenblith MR, Briggs K, Parker AR, Shimada Y, Eshleman JR, Watkins DN, Beachy PA.Widespread requirement for Hedgehog ligand stimulation in growth of digestive tract tumours. Nature. 2003;425(6960):846-51

Beverly LJ, and Capobianco AJ. Perturbation of Ikaros isoform selection by MLV integration is a cooperative event in Notch(IC)-induced T cell leukemogenesis. Cancer Cell 2003:3:551-564

Beverly LJ, Felsher DW, Capobianco AJ. Sppression pf p53 by Notch in lymphomagenesis:implications for initiation and regrassion. Cancer Res 2005;65:7159-7168

Bismar TA, Demichelis F, Riva A, Kim R, Varambally S, He L, Kutok J, Aster JC, Tang J, Kuefer R, Hofer MD, Febbo PG, Chinnaiyan AM, Rubin MA. Defining aggressive prostate cancer using a 12-gene model. Neoplasia 2006;8(1):59-68

Bolos V, Grego-Bessa J, de la Pompa JL. Notch signaling in developent and cancer. Endocr Rev 2007;28:339-363

Bruxvoort KJ, Charbonneau HM, Giambernardi TA, Goolsby JC, Qian CN, Zylstra CR, Robinson DR, Roy-BurmanP, Shaw AK, Buckner-Berghuis BD, Singler RE, Resau JH, Sillivan R, Busjman W and Williams BO. Inactivation od Apc in the mouse prostate causes porostate carcinoma. Cancer Res 2007;67:2490-2496

Cadigan KM and Nusse R. Wnt signaling : a common theme in animal development. Genes Dev 1997;11:3286-3305

Clarke MF. A self-renewal assay for cancer stem cells. Cancer Chemother Pharmacol 2005; 56 suppl 1:64-68

Chiang MY, Xu ML, Histen G, Shestova O, Roy M, Nam Y, Blacklow SC, Sacks DB, Pear WS, aster JC. Ientification of a conserved negative regulatory sequence that influences the leukemogenic activity of NOTCH1. Mol Cell Biol 2006;26;6261-6271

Colaluca IN, Tosoni D, Nuciforo P, Senic-Matuglia F, Galimberti V, Viale G, Pece S, Di Fiore PP. NUMB controls p53 tumour suppressor activity. Nature 2008;451(7174):76-80

Dallman MJ, Smith E, Benson RA, Lamb JR. Notch: control of lymphocyte differentiation in the periphery. Curr Opin Immunol 2005;17:259-266

Devgan V, Mammucari C, Millar SE, Dotto GP. p21WAF1/Cip1 is a negative transcriptional regulator of Wnt4 expression downstream of Notch1 activation. Genes Dev 2005;19:1485-1495

Dick JE. Breast cancer stem cells revealed. PNAS 2003;100(7):3547-3549

Dihlmann S, von Knebel Doeberitz M. Wnt/beta-catenin-pathway as a moleculartarget for future anti-cancer therapeutics. Int J Cancer. 2005;113(4):515-24

Duncan AW, Rattis FM, DiMascio LN, Congdon KL, Pazianos G, Zhao C, Yoon K, Cook JM, Willert K, Gaiano N, Reya T. Integration of Notch and Wnt signaling in hematopoietic stem cell maintenance. Nat Immunol. 2005;6(3):314-22.

Fan L, Pepicelli CV, Dibble CC, Catbagan W, Zarycki JL, Laciak R, Gipp J, Shaw A, Lamm ML, Munoz A, Lipinski R, Thrasher JB, Bushman W. Hedgehog signaling promotes prostate xenograft tumor growth. Endocrinology 2004;145(8):3961-70.

Ferrari-Toninelli G, Bonini SA, Uberti D, Buizza L, Bettinsoli P, Poliani PL, Facchetti F, Memo M. Targeting Notch pathway induces growth inhibition and differentiation of neuroblastoma cells. Neuro Oncol. 2010 Aug 17. [Epub ahead of print]

Fidler IJ, & Kripke ML. Metastasis results from preexisting variant cells within a malignant tumor. Science 1977;197:893–895

Fleming RJ. Structural conservation of Notch receptors and ligands. Seminars in Cell and Developmental Biology 1998;9(6):599-607

Fre S, Huyghe M, Mourikis P, Robine S, Louvard D, Artavanis-Tsakonas S. Notch signals control the fate of immature progenitor cells in the intestine. Nature. 2005;435(7044):964-8.)

Fuchs E, Tumbar T and Guasch G. Socializing with the Neighbors: Stem Cells and Their Niche. Cell 2004;116:769–778

Gandhirajan RK, Staib PA, Minke K, Gehrke I, Plickert G, Schlösser A, Schmitt EK, Hallek M, Kreuzer KA. Small molecule inhibitors of Wnt/beta-catenin/lef-1 signaling induces apoptosis in chronic lymphocytic leukemia cells in vitro and in vivo. Neoplasia. 2010;12(4):326-35

Girad L, et al. Frequent provirus insertional mutagenesis of Notch1 in thymomas of MMTVD/myc transgenic mice suggests a collaboration of c-myc and Notch 1 for oncogenesis. Genes Dev 1996;10:1930-1996

Gordan JD, Simon MC..Hypoxia-inducible factors: central regulators of the tumor phenotype. Curr Opin Gene Dev 2007;17(1):71-7

Gustafsson MV, Zheng X, Pereira T, Gradin K, Jin S. Lundkvist J, Ruas JL, Poellinger L, Lendahl U, Bondeson M. Hypoxia requires notch signaling to maintain the undifferentiated cell state. Dev Cell 2005;9:617-628

Hahn H, Wicking C, Zaphiropoulous PG, Gailani MR, Shanley S, Chidambaram A, Vorechovsky I, Holmberg E, Unden AB, Gillies S, Negus K, Smyth I, Pressman C, Leffell DJ, Gerrard B, Goldstein AM, Dean M, Toftgard R, Chenevix-Trench G, Wainwright B, Bale AE. Mutations of the human homolog of Drosophila patched in the nevoid basal cell carcinoma syndrome. Cell 1996;85(6):841-51

Hallahan AR, Pritchard JI, Hansen S, Benson M, Stoeck J, Hatton BA, Russell TL, Ellenbogen RG, Bernstein ID, beachy PA et at. The SmoA1 mouse model reveals that Notch signaling is critical for the growth and survival of sonic hedgehog-induced medulloblastomas. Cancer Res 2004;64:7794-7800

Hirata H, Hinoda Y, Nakajima K, e, Kikuno N, Ueno K, Yamamura S, Zaman MS, Khatri G, Chen Y, Saini S, Majid S, e, e, Dahiya R. Wnt antagonist DKK1 acts as a tumor suppressor gene that induces apoptosis and inhibits proliferation in human renal cell carcinoma. Int J Cancer. 2010 Jun 14. [Epub ahead of print]

Hoek K, Rimm DL, Williams KR, Zhao H, Ariyan G, Lin A, Kluger HM, Berger AJ, Cheng E, Trombetta ES et al. Expression profiling reveals novel pathways in the transformation of melanocytes to melanoma. Cancdr Res 2004;64:5270-5282

Huntly BJ and Gilliland DG. Leukemia stem cells and the evolution of cancer-stem-cell research. Nat Rev Cancer 2005;5:311-321

Ingham PW, McMahon AP. Hedgehog signaling in animal development: paradigms and principles. Genes Dev. 2001;15:3059-3087

Ishiguro K, Yoshida T, Yagishita H, et al. Epithelial and stromal genetic instability contributes to genesis of colorectal adenomas. *Gut* 2006 55: 695-702

Jhappan C, Gallahan D, Stahle C, Chu E, Smith GH, Merlino G, Callahan R. Expression of an activated Notch-related int-3 transgene interferes with cell differentiation and induces neoplastic transformation in mammary and salivary glands. Genes Dev 1992;6(3):345-55

Jimeno A, Feldmann G, Suárez-Gauthier A, Rasheed Z, Solomon A, Zou GM, et al. A direct pancreatic cancer xenograft model as a platform for cancer stem cell therapeutic development. Mol Cancer Ther 2009;8(2)310-314

Kawano Y and Kypta R. Secreted antagonists of the Wnt signaling pathway. J Cell Sci 2003;116(Pt 13):2627-2634

Kayed H, Kleeff J, Keleg S, Guo J, Ketterer K, Berberat PO, Giese N, Esposito I, Giese T, Büchler MW, Friess H. Indian hedgehog signaling pathway: expression and regulation in pancreatic cancer. Int J Cancer. 2004 Jul 10;110(5):668-76.

Kolev V, Mandinova A, Guinea-Viniegra J, Hu B, Lefort K, Lambertini C, Neel V, Dummer R, Wagner EF, Dotto GP. EGFR signalling as a negative regulator of Notch1 gene transcription and function in proliferating keratinocytes and cancer. Nat Cell Biol 2008;10:902–911

Kolligs FT, Hu G, Dang CV, Fearon ER. Neoplastic transformation of RK3E by mutant beta-catenin requires deregulation of Tcf/Lef transcription but not activation of c-myc expression. Mol Cell Biol 1999;19(8):5696-706

Kubo M, Nakamura M, Tasaki A, Yamanaka N, Nakashima H, Nomura M, Kuroki S, Katano M. Hedgehog signaling pathway is a new therapeutic target for patients with breast cancer. Cancer Res 2004;64(17):6071-4

Lee CW, Raskett CM, Prudovsky I, Altieri DC. Molecular dependence of estrogen receptor-negative breast cancer on a notch-surviving signaling axis. Cancer Res 2008;68:5273–5281

Liu S, Dontu G and Wicha MA. Mammary stem cells, self-renewal pathways , and carcinogenesis. Breast Cancer Res 2005;7:86-95

Liu ZJ, Xiao M, Balint K, Smalley KS, Brafford P, Qiu R, Pinnix CC, Li X, Herlyn M. Notch1 signaling promotes primary melanoma progression by activating mitogen-activated protein kinase/phosphatidylibositol 3-kinase-Akt pathways and up-regulating N-cadherin expression. Cancer Res 2006;66:4182-4190

Lobo NA, Shimono Y, Qian D and Clarke MF. The biology of cancer stem cells. Annu Rev Cell Dev Biol 2007;23:675-699

Lowell S, Jones P, Le Roux I, Dunne J, Watt FM. Stimulation of human epidermal differentiation by delta-notch signalling at the boundaries of stem-cell
clusters. Curr Biol 2000;10:491–500

Luistro L, He W, Smith M, Packman K, Vilenchik M, Carvajal D, Roberts J, Cai J, Berkofsky-Fessler W, Hilton H, Linn M, Flohr A, Jakob-Røtne R, Jacobsen H, Glenn K, Heimbrook D, Boylan JF. Preclinical profile of a potent gamma-secretase inhibitor targeting notch signaling with in vivo efficacy and pharmacodynamic properties. Cancer Res. 2009;69(19):7672-80

MacDonald BT, Tamai K, He X. Wnt/beta-catenin signaling: components, mechanisms, and diseases. Dev Cell 2009;17(1):9-26

Marino S. Medulloblastoma: development mechanisms out of control. Trends Mol Med 2005;11:17-22

Miele L. Notch signaling. Clin Cancer Res 2006;12(4):1074-9

Minke KS, Staib P, Puetter A, Gehrke I, Gandhirajan RK, Schlösser A, Schmitt EK, Hallek M, Kreuzer KA. Small molecule inhibitors of WNT signaling effectively induce apoptosis in acute myeloid leukemia cells. Eur J Haematol. 2009;82(3):165-75

Mohinta S, Wu H, Chaurasia P, and Watabe K. Wnt pathway and breast cancer. Front Biosci 2007;12:4020-4033

Moon RT, KohnAD, De Ferrari GV and Kaykas A. WNT and β-catenin signalling: diseases and therapies Nature Reviews Genetics 5, 691-701 (September 2004) | doi:10.1038/nrg1427

Morrison SJ, Shah NM and anderson DJ. Regulatory mechanism in stem cell biology. Cell 1997;88:287-298

Müller A, Homey B, Soto H, et al. Involvement of chemokine receptors in breast cancer metastasis. Nature 2001;410:50-56

Mungamuri SK, Yang X, Thor AD, Somasundaram K. Survival signaling by Notch1: mammalian target of rapamycin (mTOR)-dependent inhibition of p53. Cancer Res 2006;66:4715-4724

Murphy PM. Chemokines and the molecular basis of cancer metastasis. N Engl J Med 2001;345:833-835

Nicolas M, Wolfer A, Raj K, Kummer JA, Mill P, van Noort M, Hui CC, Clevers H, Dotto GP, Radtke F. Notch1 functions as a tumor suppressor in mouse skin. Nat Genet 2003;33:416–421

Nickoloff BJ, Osborne BA, Miele L. Notch signaling as a therapeutic target in cancer: a new approach to the development of cell fate modifying agents. Oncogene 2003;22:6598-6608

Nybakken K and Perrimon N. Hedgehog signal transduction:recent findings . Curr Opin Genet Dev 2002;12:503-511

Okuda T, Sekizawa A, Purwosunu Y, Nagatsuka M, Morioka M, Hayashi M, Okai T. Genetics of endometrial cancers. Obstet Gynecol Int. 2010;2010:984013.

Osipo C, Patel P, Rizzo P, Clementz AG, Hao L, Golde TE, Miele L.ErbB-2 inhibition activates Notch-1 and sensitizes breast cancer cells to a gamma-secretase inhibitor. Oncogene 2008;27:5019–5032

Paget S. The distribution of secondary growths in cancer of the breast. Lancet 1889;133;571-573

Palomero T, Lim WK, Odom DT, Sulis ML, Real PJ, Margolin A, Barnes KC, O´Neil J, Neuberg D, Weng AP, et al. Notch1 directly regulates c-MYC and activates as feed-forward-loop transcriptional network promoting leukemic cell growth. Proc Natl Acad Sci USA 2006;103:18261-18266

Pardal R, Clarke MF and Morrison SJ. Applying the principles ofstem cell biology to cancer. Nat Rev Cancer 2003;3:895-902

Park CH, Bergsagel DE and McCulloch EA. Mouse myeloma tumor stem cells: a primary cell culture assay. J Natl Cancer Inst 1971;46:411–422

Park JY, Li M, Nakayama K, Mao TL, Davidson B, Zhang Z, Kurman RJ, Eberhart CG, Shih I, Wang TL. Notch3 gene amplification in ovarian cancer. Cancer Res 2006;66:6312-6318

Pasca di Magliano M, Hebrok M. Hedgehog signalling in cancer formation and maintenance Nature Reviews Cancer 2003;3:903-911 (December 2003)

Patil MA, Zhang J, Ho C, Cheung ST, Fan ST and Chen X. *Hedgehog signaling in human hepatocellular carcinoma. Proc Amer Assoc Cancer Res, 2005;46:* 3942

Pece S, Serresi M , Santolini E, Capra M, Hulleman E, Galimberti V, Zurrida S, Maisonneuve P, Viale G, Di Fiore PP. Loss of negative regulation by Numb over Notch is relevant to human breast carcinogenesis. J Cell Biol 2004;167(2):215-221

Peukert S, Miller-Moslin K. Small-molecule inhibitors of the hedgehog signaling pathway as cancer therapeutics. ChemMedChem 2010;5(4):500-12.

Radtke F, Raj K. The role of Notch in tumorigenesis: oncogene or tumor suppressor? Net Rev Cancer 2003;3:756-767

Rangarajan A, Talora C, Okuyama R, Nicolas M, Mammucari C, Oh H, Aster JC, Krishna S, Metzger D, Chambon P, Miele L, Aguet M, Radtke F, Dotto GP. Notch signaling is a direct determinant of keratinocyte growth arrest and entry into differentiation. EMBO J. 2001 Jul 2;20(13):3427-36.

Reedjik M, Odoric S, Chang L, Zhang H, Miller N, McCready DR, Lockwood G, Egan SE. High-level coexpression of JAG1 and NOTCH1 is observed in human breast cancer and is associated with poor overall survival. Cancer Res 2005;65:8530-8537

Reguart N, He B, Taron M, You L, Jablons DM, Rosell R. The role of Wnt signaling in cancer and stem cells. Future Oncol 2005;1(6):787-97

Rehman AO, Wang CY. Notch signaling in the regulation of tumor angiogenesis. Trends Cell Biol 2006;16:293-300

Reya T, Clevers H. Wnt signalling in stem cells and cancer. Nature 2005;434(7035):843-50

Reya T, Morrison SJ, Clarke MF, Weissman IL. Stem cells, cancer, and cancer stem cells. Nature 2001;414:105-111

Reya T, Duncan AW, Ailles L, Domen J, Scherer DC, Willert K, Hintz L, Nusse R, and Weissman IL. A role for Wnt signaling in self-renewal of hepatopoieic stem cells. Nature 2003;423:409-414

Ridgway J, Zhang G, Wu Y, Stawicki S, Liang WC, Chanthery Y, Kowalski J, Watts RJ, Callahan C, Kasman I, Singh M, Chien M, Tan C, Hongo JA, de Sauvage F, Plowman G, Yan M. Inhibition of Dll4 signalling inhibits tumour growth by deregulating angiogenesis. Nature. 2006;444(7122):1083-7

Rizvi AZ, Wong MH. Epithelial stem cells and their niche: there's no place like home. Stem Cells 2005;23:150–165

Rizzo P, Miao H, D'Souza G, Osipo C, Song LL, Yun J, Zhao H, Mascarenhas J, Wyatt D, Antico G, Hao L, Yao K, Rajan P, Hicks C, Siziopikou K, Selvaggi S, Bashir A, Bhandari D, Marchese A, Lendahl U, Qin JZ, Tonetti DA, Albain K, Nickoloff BJ, Miele L. Crosstalk between notch and the estrogen receptor in breast cancer suggests novel therapeutic approaches. Cancer Res 2008;68:5226–5235

Robinson DR, Zylstra CR, Williams BO. Wnt signaling and prostate cancer. Curr Drug Targets. 2008 Jul;9(7):571-80

Rohn JL, Lauring AS, Linenberg MI, and Overbaugh J. Transduction of Notch2 in feline leukemia virus-induced thymic lymphoma. J Virol 1996;70:8071-8880

Roy M, Pear WS, and Aster JC. The multifaceted role of Notch in cancer. Curr Opin Gene Dev 2007;17:52-59

Rubin LL, de Sauvage FJ. Targeting the Hedgehog pathway in cancer. Nat Rev Drug Discov. 2006;5:1026-1033;

Samarnthai N, Hall K, Yeh IT. Molecular profiling of endometrial malignancies. Obstet Gynecol Int. 2010;2010:162363.

Sánchez-García I, Vicente-Dueñas C, Cobaleda C. The theoretical basis of cancer-stem-cell-based therapeutics of cancer: can it be put into practice? Bioessays 2007;29(12):1269-80.

Santagata S, Demichelis F, Riva A, Varambally S, Hofer MD, Kutok JL, Kim R, Tang J, Montie JE, Chinnaiyan AM et al. JAGGED1 expression is associated with prostate cancer metastasis and recurrence. Cancer Res 2004;64:6854-6857

Schöler HR. "The Potential of Stem Cells: An Inventory". in Nikolaus Knoepffler, Dagmar Schipanski, and Stefan Lorenz Sorgner. Humanbiotechnology as Social Challenge 2007. Ashgate Publishing, Ltd. p. 28. ISBN 0754657558.

Sharma VM, Calvo JA, Drahein KM, Cunninham LA, Hermance N, Beverly L, Krishnamoorthy V, Bhasin M, Capobianco AJ, Kelliher MA. Notch1 contributes to mouse T-cell leukemia by directly inducing the expression of c-myc. Mol Cell Biol 2006;26:8022-8031

Sicklick K, Jayaraman A, Kannangai R, Torbenson MS, Choti MA, and Diehl AM. Hedgehog signaling correlates with hepatocellular carcinoma progression J Clin Oncol (Meeting Abstracts) 2005;23: 9610

Soares R, Balogh G, Guo S, gartner F, Russo J, Schmitt F. Evidence for the notch signaling pathway on the role of estrogen in angiogenesis. Mol Endocrinol 2004;18:2333-2343

Stetler-Stevenson WG, Kleiner DE Jr. Molecular biology of cancer: invasion and metastases. In: DeVita VT Jr, Hellman S, Rosenberg SA, eds. Cancer: principles and practice of oncology. 6th ed. Philadelphia: Lippincott Williams & Wilkins, 2001:123-36.

Strieter RM. Chemokines ; not just leukocyte chemoattractans in the promotion of cancer. Nat Immunol 2001;2:285-286

Stylianou S, Clarke RB, Brennan K. Aberrant activation of notch signaling in human breast cancer. Cancer Res. 2006;66(3):1517-25.

Sun Y, Lowther W, Kato K, Blanco C, Kenney N, Strizzi KL, Raafat D, Hirota M, Khan NI, Bargo S, et al. Notch4 intracellular tomain binding to Smad3 and inhibition of the TGF-β signaling. Oncogene 2005;24:5365-5374

Taipale J and Beachy PA. The Hedgehog and Wnt signaling pathways in cancer. Nature 2001;411:349-354

Talora C, et al. Pre-TCR-triggered ERK signaling-dependent downregulation of E2A activivty. EMBO Rep 2003;4:1067-1072

Thayer SP, di Magliano MP, Heiser PW, Nielsen CM, Roberts DJ, Lauwers GY, Qi YP, Gysin S, Fernández-del Castillo C, Yajnik V, Antoniu B, McMahon M, Warshaw AL, Hebrok M. Hedgehog is an early and late mediator of pancreatic cancer tumorigenesis. Nature. 2003;425(6960):851-6.

Thelu J, Rossio P, Favier B. Notch signalling is linked to epidermal cell differentiation level in basal cell carcinoma, psoriasis and wound healing. BMC Dermatol 2002;2:7

Uematsu K, He B, You L, Xu Z, McCormick F, Jablons DM. Activation of the Wnt pathway in non small cell lung cancer: evidence of dishevelled overexpression. Oncogene. 2003;22(46):7218-21

Van de Wetering M, Sancho E, Verweij C, de Lau W, Oving I, Hurlstone A, van der Horn K, Batlle E, Coudreuse D, Haramis AP, Tjon-Pon-Fong M, Moerer P, van den Born M, Soete G, Pals S, Eilers M, Medema R, Clevers H. The beta-catenin/TCF-4 complex imposes a crypt progenitor phenotype on colorectal cancer cells. Cell 2002;111(2):241-50

Van Es JH, van Gijn ME, Riccio O, van den Born M, Vooijs M, Begthel H, Cozijnsen M, Robine S, Winton DJ, Radtke F, Clevers H. Notch/gamma-secretase inhibition turns proliferative cells in intestinal crypts and adenomas into goblet cells. Nature. 2005;435(7044):959-63.

Van Vlierberghe P, Meijerink JP, Lee C, Ferrando AA, Look AT, van Wering ER, Beverloo HB, Aster JC, Pieters R. A new recurrent 9q34 duplication in pediatric T-cell acute lymphoblastic leukemia. Leukemia 2006;20:1245-1253

Von Hoff DD, LoRusso PM, Rudin CM, Reddy JC, Yauch RL, Tibes R, Weiss GJ, Borad MJ, Hann CL, Brahmer JR, Mackey HM, Lum BL, Darbonne WC, Marsters JC Jr, de Sauvage FJ, Low JA. Inhibition of the hedgehog pathway in advanced basal-cell carcinoma. N Engl J Med. 2009;361(12):1164-72

Wang JC. Good cells gone bad: the cellular origins of cancer.Trends Mol Med. 2010;16(3):145-51.

Wang X, Kruithof-de Julio M, Economides KD, Walker D, Yu H, Halili MV, Hu YP, Price SM, Abate-Shen C and Shen MM. A luminal epithelial stem cell that is a cell of origin for prostate cancer. Nature 2009;461:495-502

Watkins DN, Berman DM, Burkholder SG, Wang B, Beachy PA, Baylin SB. Hedgehog signalling within airway epithelial progenitors and in small-cell lung cancer.Nature 2003;422(6929):313-7

Weber F, Shen L, Fukino K, Patocs A, Mutter GL, Caldes T and Eng C. Total-Genome Analysis of *BRCA1/2*-Related Invasive Carcinomas of the Breast Identifies Tumor Stroma as Potential Landscaper for Neoplastic Initiation. Am. J. Hum. Genet. 2006;78:961–972

Wei W, Chua MS, Grepper S, So S. Small molecule antagonists of Tcf4/beta-catenin complex inhibit the growth of HCC cells in vitro and in vivo. Int J Cancer. 2010;126(10):2426-36

Weijzen S, Rizzo P, Braid M, Vaishnav R, Jonkheer SM, Zlobin A, Osborne BA, Gottipati S, Aster JC, Hahn WC, et al. Activation of Notch-1 signaling maintain the neoplastic phenotype in human Ras-transformed cells. Nat Med 2002;8:979-986

Weng AP, Ferrando AA, Lee W, Morris JP 4th, Silverman LB, Sanchez-Irizarry C, Blacklow SC, Look AT, Aster JC. Activating mutations of NOTCH1 in human T cell acute lymphoblastic leukemia. Science. 2004;306(5694):269-71.

Weng AP and Aster JC. Multiple niches for Notch in cancer: context is everything. Curr Opin Genet Dev 2004;14:48-54

Whittaker S, Marais R, Zhu AX. The role of signaling pathways in the development and treatment of hepatocellular carcinoma. Oncogene. 2010 Jul 19. [Epub ahead of print]

Wu Y, Cain-Hom C, Choy L, Hagenbeek TJ, de Leon GP, Chen Y, Finkle D, Venook R, Wu X, Ridgway J, Schahin-Reed D, Dow GJ, Shelton A, Stawicki S, Watts RJ, Zhang J, Choy R, Howard P, Kadyk L, Yan M, Zha J, Callahan CA, Hymowitz SG, Siebel CW. Therapeutic antibody targeting of individual Notch receptors. Nature 2010;464(7291):1052-7

Yamamura S, Kawakami K, Hirata H, Ueno K, Saini S, Majid S, Dahiya R. Oncogenic functions of secreted Frizzled-related protein 2 in human renal cancer. Mol Cancer Ther. 2010 Jun;9(6):1680-7

Zeng Q, Li S, Chepeha DB, Giordano TJ, Li J, Zhang H, Polverini PJ, Nor J, Kitajewski J, Wang CY. Crosstalk between tumor and endothelial cells promotes tumor angiogenesis by MAPK activation of Notch signaling. Cancer Cell 2005;8:13-2

Zhang C, Zhang Q, Painter C, Yan Z, Li W, Buckman D, Zheng X, Kuszpit K, Wong A, Affolter T, Lappin PB, Lee NV, Wei P, Qiu M, Randolph S, Smeal T, Christensen JG. γ-secretase inhibitor PF-03084014 impairs Notch signaling and induces antiangiogenic and antitumor effects in breast cancer models. AACR 2010. Abstract 5218.

Part 6

Targeting Resistance

20

Targeting Signal Pathways Active in Leukemic Stem Cells to Overcome Drug Resistance

Miaorong She MD, PhD[1] and Xilin Chen MD, PhD[2]
[1]*Department of Hematology, Guangdong General Hospital, Guangzhou*
[2]*Department of Hepatobiliary Surgery, the First Affiliated Hospital of Sun Yat-Sen University, Guangzhou*
China

1. Introduction

Acute myeloid leukemia (AML) is a serious and often lethal disease. Over the last several decades, although there have been advances in the treatment of AML, however, the survival of patients with AML has not changed significantly[1-3]. Most of patients will relapse within two years and ultimately died of the disease[4]. The scarce efficacy of current treatments indicates the resistance of leukemia cells to cytotoxic agents and even immunotherapy and survival from the treatment without major injure. Thus, there is a desperate need for new effective therapies for AML patients.

The hematopoietic system is thought to originate from pluripotent hematopoietic stem cells (HSC) capable of producing a hierarchy of downstream multilineage and unilineage progenitor cells that differentiate into mature cells[5]. HSCs have self-renewal and can differentiate into multiple lineages[6]. HSC self-renewal is either symmetrical, producing two daughter HSCs, or asymmetrical, producing an identical HSC and a progenitor with diminished self-renewal capacity but with the ability to enact clonal expansion[7]. It is also believed that leukemia is initiated and maintained by a rare population of leukemia cells with stem cell properties similar to those of normal HSCs known as leukemic stem cell (LSC). The concept that a rare population of the tissue stem cell maybe the cellular origin of cancer was proposed almost 150 years ago. Approximately 50 years ago the concept that only a small subpopulation of so-called LSCs may be connected to the maintenance and evolution of myeloid leukemia emerged. Conclusive evidences for the existence of LSCs come from the function assay using SCID-leukemia and NOD/SCID-leukemia xenotransplantation models in which mice were transplanted with leukemic cells from the bone marrow and peripheral blood of AML patients. These studies demonstrated that the leukemic grafts were highly representative of the original patients disease and the SCID/leukemia initiating cell presented at a frequency of 0.2-100/10^6 mononuclear cells[8]. More recently, this principle has also been extended to other tumors, such as breast, brain, prostate, pancreas, colon, lung, liver, and head and neck tumors[9-15]. Due to a high degree of phenotypic and functional similarity, it has been hypothesized that most human leukemias arise from transformation of HSCs. However, other studies have shown that transduction of the MLL-ENL or MOZ-TIF2 fusion genes into HSCs, common myeloid progenitors, and granulocyte-macrophage progenitors resulted in the identical leukemia. These results indicate that committed progenitors may acquire self-renewal capability and transform into LSCs[16,17].

LSCs have been reported to be the only tumorigenic population and play a central role in relapse because of the failure of current chemotherapy to eradicate them. The existence of LSC highlights the critical need for the new therapeutic strategies to directly target the LSC population for ultimately curing leukemia.

Basing on the solid evidences that leukemia is stem cell disease, the view of drug resistance changes. It is believed that LSCs are naturally resistant to conventional chemotherapy and serve as the main mediators of drug resistance[18-22]. Moreover, it is accepted that drug resistance is governed by the mutations that confer protection mechanism through modulation of cell survival factors. To that end, a number of signal pathways involved in LSCs viability and survival, namely the Hedgehog, Ras, FLT3, PI3K/AKT, NF-κB, mTOR are aberrantly regulated in LSCs. Because of their wide-ranging biological effects, deregulation one or more of these pathways may give rise to a failure of current chemotherapy. Others and we have long been interested in exploring the mechanisms of drug resistance of LSCs influenced by these cell survival pathways and molecular interaction networks. Thus we can determine the critical elements and the general rules driving the network to guide the use of specific inhibitors of a given pathway. This review will focus on the drug resistance of LSCs and the signal pathway and their potential cross-talk. (Figure1).

2. Leukemic stem cells and drug resistance

According to the hierarchy model, Leukemia consists of a heterogeneous population, within which only a rare population of LSCs sustains the disease. LSCs share some properties of normal stem cells, Such as self-renewal potential, proliferation and essential property of self-protection. The whole drug resistance concept has been revised incorporating the LSC paradigm. LSCs play the key role in the drug resistance of leukemia. LSCs present in the original tumour mass and survive chemotherapy, whereas the committed but variably differentiated cells are killed. Several mechanisms make LSCs more resistant to conventional chemotherapeutic agents. For example, LSCs exhibited higher expression of drug resistance proteins, such as lung resistance-related protein (LRP) and multiple resistance-associated proteins (MRP)[23]. Recent work from our group suggests that LSCs are resistance to mitoxantrone and daunorubicin via up-regulation of ABCG2 and MRP. Another group of investigators have demonstrated that LSCs isolated from human leukemia are predominantly in the G0 phase of the cell cycle that made it resistance to cell cycle specific chemotherapeutic agents such as Ara-c[24]. Furthermore, LSCs have capacity for DNA repair. As a result, at least some of LSCs can survive chemotherapy including DNA damage agents such as alkylating agents[25]. Moreover, LSCs are resistant to chemotherapy through impaired apoptosis pathway[26-28]. Our unpublished data show that LSCs up-regulated Bcl2 protein and Bcl2 siRNA enhanced the sensitivity of LSCs to mitoxantrone cytotoxicity. The properties of LSCs suggest that the current chemotherapy drugs will not be curative. Current studies focus on a number of signaling pathways that regulate chemoresistance of LSCs through survival pathway. We will outline some of these pathways and their potential in drug resistance.

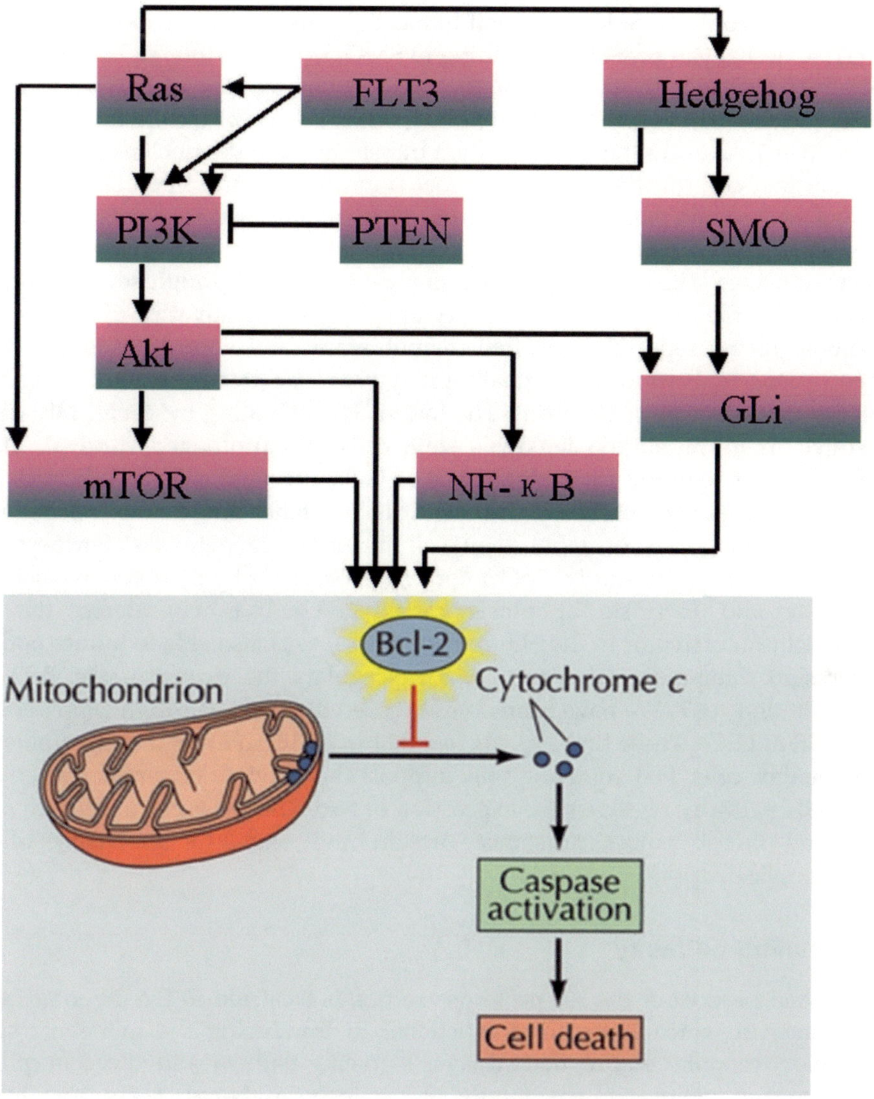

Fig. 1. Signal transduction pathways important in leukemic stem cells

3. Hedgehog pathway

'Hedgehog' (HH) molecules are secretory signaling proteins that were first discovered in Drosophila. Three HH homologs have been identified in humans including Sonic hedgehog (SHH), Indian hedgehog (IHH) and Desert hedgehog (DHH). Secreted hedgehog molecules bind to and inhibit the cell surface receptor Patched 1 protein on target cells. Smoothened is a transmembrane protein primarily located in the membrane endosomes. It is proposed that the endogenous agonist of SMO is a small intracellular molecule transported out of the cell by PTCH1, a mechanism preventing binding to SMO. Upon binding an HH ligand, PTCH1 is internalized and inactivated so that the endogenous agonist of SMO accumulates in cytoplasm and activates SMO. Activated SMO causing release of the Gli family of transcription factors (Gli-1, -2, and -3), which can then translocate into the nucleus and activate gene transcription that control the cell cycle, signal transduction, and apoptosis. HH pathway, which is one of the main pathways that control stem cell fate, self-renewal and maintenance, plays a central role in drug resistance of cancer cells[29-33].

HH pathway makes LSCs more resistance to chemotherapy through several mechanisms. First, HH controls the cell cycle fate during cell proliferation. Activation of the HH pathway may promote tumor repopulation after chemotherapy and contribute to chemotherapy resistance in cancers. Second, HH signaling may act as upstream of other signal pathway that regulate self-renewal of stem cell. The loss of HH signaling by genetically disrupting Smo resulted in the inhibition leukemic stem cells and prolonged survival. Thus, HH pathway activity is required for maintenance of leukemic stem cells and dictates LSC fate decisions[34,35]. It raises the possibility that the drug resistance and disease relapse might be avoided by targeting this essential stem cell maintenance pathway. Furthermore, HH pathway contributes to the survival of tumor progenitor cells by opposing the activation of both intrinsic and extrinsic apoptosis cascades. Gli-1 is considered the positive transcriptional transactivator in the Shh pathway. Gli-1 was also able to induce endogenous Bcl2 expression. Moreover, Hh signal also up-regulats the expression of Bcl2 through activated PI3K and AKT. We have been demonstrated that Bcl2 was high expression via up-regulation Gli in LSCs. These findings suggest that in addition to regulating proliferation of tumor progenitor cells, HH signaling may support the survival of tumor progenitor cells. Moreover, HH pathway regulates the expression of two ABC proteins, multidrug resistance protein-1 and breast cancer resistance protein and leads to the efflux of various chemotherapeutic drugs[36].

4. Ras signaling pathway

Ras, the protein product of the ras proto-oncogenes, is localized to the inner surface of the cell membrane, in which it becomes functional in tranducing the mitogenic signals of tyrosine kinase receptors that regulate diverse signaling pathways involved in cell growth, differentiation and apoptosis. The family of ras includes N-ras, K-ras, and H-ras. Ras mutations are most commonly associated with cancer including leukemia. Transplantation of highly purified hematopoietic stem cells (HSCs) and myeloid progenitors identified HSCs as the primary target for the oncogenic Kras mutation. Karyotypic analysis further indicated that secondary genetic hit(s) target lineage-specific progenitors rather than HSCs for terminal tumor transformation into leukemic stem cells. Thus, the cellular mechanism underlying oncogenic Kras-induced leukemogenesis, with HSCs as the primary target by the oncogenic Kras mutations and lineage-committed progenitors as the final target for cancer stem cell transformation[37]. Once activated, ras is able to trigger several signaling including Raf-Mek-Map kinase pathway[38], FMS-like tyrosine kinase 3 (FLT3) pathway[39], and phosphoinositide 3-kinase (PI3K)/ cytoplasmic protein kinase B (AKT) pathway. The potential relevance of the Raf-MEK-MAP kinase pathway to abnormal hematopoiesis is highlighted by the ability of a constitutively activated mutant Raf to eliminate growth factor dependence of hematopoietic cells. Ras also activates the PI3K pathway, which can result in suppression of apoptosis by directly activating AKT. The PI3K/AKT pathway is important for relaying survival signals in hematopoietic cells by Ras. Mutations of ras in LSCs result in refractory and relapse of leukemia[40].

5. FMS-like tyrosine kinase 3 signaling

The FLT3 gene, also known as fetal liver tyrosine kinase 2 (PLK2), encodes a membrane-bound receptor tyrosine kinase (RTK). FLT3 have been shown to play a role in leukemogenesis. In most examined patient cohorts, FLT3 is consistently associated with unfavorable prognosis and relapse of AML patients. In recent studies, it was also shown that FLT3 was expressed in LSCs. FLT3 activates special anti-apoptotic signal by up-regulating Bcl2 family. In additionally, FLT3 mediates drug resistance through activating PI3K/AKT survival pathway[41-43]. Interestingly, simultaneous mutations of ras and FLT3 are rare, suggesting functional overlap between the two.

6. The PI3K/AKT cell survival pathway

Oncogenic ras and FLT3 have been shown to activate PI3Ks in AML. Moreover, activating mutations of c-Kit tyrosine kinase receptor, PI3K p110β and/or δ overexpression, low levels of PP2A, autocrine/paracrine secretion of growth factors such as IGF-1 and VEGF also result in PI3K/Akt signaling up-regulation. PI3Ks are heterodimers with separate regulatory (p85) and catalytic (p110) subunits. PI3K activation may be due to the close proximity of p110 to its lipid substrates in the membrane and relief of the inhibitory effect of p85 on p110 kinase activity upon RTK-p85 interaction. Direct binding of p110 to activating ras proteins following growth factor stimulation further stimulates PI3K activity. The increasing evidences have supported that PI3K plays critical roles in the chemotherapy-resistance in LSCs. Furthermore, the downstream effector of PI3K, AKT (a subfamily of the serine/threonine protein kinases), have been associated with the cell growth and survival of cancer stem cell[44-46]. Three AKT isoforms (AKT1, AKT2, and AKT3) have been identified, all of which share an N-terminal PH domain, with central kinase domain, and a serine/threonine-rich C-terminal region. The intermediates of the PI3K/AKT survival pathway are activated in LSCs and high level of PI3K/AKT has been linked to poor prognosis and chemoresistance. Tumor suppressor gene Phosphatase and tensin homolog (PTEN) is negative regulator of AKT pathway. Mutations or losses of PTEN have been found in a large number of cancers including brain, breast, prostate and leukemia[47,48]. Loss of PTEN function results in AKT activating and cancer resistance to conventional therapy and a relapse following initial regression. Shoman etal have reported a strong correlation between down-regulation of PTEN expression and failure to respond to tamoxifen treatment in estrogen receptor-positive tumors[49]. In the hematopoietic system, recently studies show that conditional deletion of PTEN result in leukemia[47]. Thus PI3K/Akt pathway plays the critical role in the LSC resistance to a number of anti-tumor agents. PI3K/AKT pathway controls the expression of the membrane ATP binding cassette (ABC) transporter, multidrug resistance-associated protein 1 to extrude chemotherapeutic drugs. Furthermore, PI3K/AKT activating defect the apoptosis pathway of LSC to protect LSC from chemotherapy.

7. NF-κB signaling pathway

Nuclear factor of kB (NF-κB) is a family of closely related dimeric transcription factors that bind to the kB sites. NF-κB is an inducible and ubiquitously expressed transcription factor that regulates cell survival, inflammation, and differentiation. It is becoming increasingly clear that NF-κB signaling plays critical roles in cancer development and progression. Cancer cells especially poorly differentiated cancer cells show activated NF-κB in the nucleus, suggesting that activated NF-κB regulates its downstream genes to promote cancer cell growth. The exciting results have shown that NF-κB is constitutively activated in LSCs whereas it is strikingly not activated in their normal counterpart, suggesting this transcription factor is preferentially in LSCs[50]. This provides a possible that specific target the LSCs while spare the normal HSCs. More importantly, it has been well known that many chemotherapeutic agents such as neucleoside analogs and anthracyclines induce the activity of NF-κB, which causes drug resistance in cancer cells[51]. Therefore, targeting NF-κB would be promising strategy to overcome the drug resistance of LSCs.

8. Strategies to overcome drug resistance through regulating survival signal pathways of LSCs

The concept that leukemia is a stem cell disease has the potential to change the view of drug resistance. As the understanding of the signaling pathway involved in the survival and chemoresistance of LSCs, it is likely to identify new mechanism-based effective therapy directed at LSCs to cure leukemia.

9. Targeting of hedgehog pathway

As indicated above, The HH pathway is activated in LSCs and plays the central role in drug resistance. Cyclopamine is a natural steroidal alkaloid that inhibits the HH pathway by directly binding and suppressing the Smo receptor. Recent studies showed that cyclopamine inhibits various human malignancies including breast, prostate, liver, pancreas, small cell lung cancer, and glioma[52,53]. Importantly, continuous cyclopamine eliminated PC3 cancer-initiating cells. Similarly, cyclopamine treatment also counteracts the expansion of multiple myeloma (MM) stem cell and decrease the number of MM stem cell[54]. Furthermore, blocking the HH signal pathway by Gli siRNA or humanized anti-SHH antibodies has been shown to induce apoptosis in a wide variety of tumors through activation of intrinsic and extrinsic apoptosis cascades and resensitized the chemoresistant CSCs. Recently, Kobune et al showed that HH signaling is active in CD34+ leukemic cells. These CD34+ cells express the downstream effectors glioma-associated oncogene homolog Gli-1 or Gli-2, indicative of active HH signaling. Moreover, inhibition of HH signaling with the naturally derived Smoothened antagonist cyclopamine, endogenous HH inhibitor hedgehog-interacting protein or anti-hedgehog neutralizing antibody induced apoptosis of these CD34+ cells exhibited resistance to cytarabine (Ara-C). Furthermore, combination with cyclopamine significantly reduced drug resistance of CD34+ cells to Ara-C[55]. Taken together, these studies suggest that selective target HH pathway may lead to more effective cancer therapies.

10. Targeting of the ras pathway

The emerging evidences have shown that increase in ras activity may be an early step in the deveplopment of leukemia. The preclinical concept of farnesyltransferase blockade as a targeted therapy against oncogenic Ras has clearly evolved with the recognition that many proteins involved signaling pathways in tumor cells undergo farnesylation. Several farnesyltransferase inhibitors as monotherapy in cancer in vitro or in clinical trial demonstrate encouraging responses and good tolerability. BMS-214662, a cytotoxic farnesyltransferase inhibitor, previously reported to selectively kill nonproliferating subpopulation in tumor cells. Recent studies have also been shown that BMS-214662, alone or in combination with imatinib or dasatinib, effectively induced apoptosis of resistant CML stem cells and potently induced apoptosis of both proliferating and quiescent CML stem/progenitor cells with less than 1% recovery of Philadelphia-positive long-term culture-initiating cells. Normal stem/progenitor cells were relatively spared by BMS-214662[56]. Our unpublished data also showed that manumycin enhanced mitoxantrone-induced apoptosis in LSCs. These data suggest that RAS contribute to drug resistance of LSC and are potential targets for new therapeutic strategies. Farnesyltransferase inhibitor may offer potential for eradication of LSC.

11. Regulation of the PI3K/AKT pathway

The increasing evidence has shown that activated FLT3, PI3K/AKT pathway is critical for drug resistance of LSCs, therefore, downregulation of FLT3, PI3K, and AKT could sensitize LSCs to chemotherapy and overcome drug resistance. The PI3K/ AKT pathway may be inhibited with PI3K (LY294002, PX-866), PDK1 (OSU-03012, celecoxib), AKT (A-443654, perifosine, tricribine) or downstream mTOR inhibitors such as rapamycin and modified rapamycins (CCI-779 andRAD001). Inhibition of the PI3K/AKT pathway by the specific pathway inhibitors LY294002 leads to a dose-dependent decrease in survival of LSCs[57]. LY294002 also significantly reduced the survival of SP fraction within MCF7 cells and decrease cancer stem-like cells[58]. Wortmannin are able to inhibit CML and AML cell proliferation and to synergize with targeted tyrosine kinase inhibitors. Additionally, dual PI3K/PDK-1 Inhibitor BAG956 have been demonstrated effective against leukemia[59]. Recently, publication by Yilmaz and colleagues demonstrated that mammalian target of rapamycin (mTOR) inhibition with rapamycin not only depleted leukaemia-initiating cells but also restored normal HSC function[47]. In conclusion, inhibition of this pathway leads to an increase in apoptosis in LSCs, and that it potentiates the response to cytotoxic chemotherapy.

12. Targeting of NF-κB Signaling Pathway

Previous studies have demonstrated that NF-κB, a known regulator of growth and survival, is constitutively active in LSCs but not in normal hematopoietic stem cells (HSCs). These suggest that LSC-specific targeted therapy should be feasible using a variety of strategies. Guzman etal have previously shown that a combination of the proteasome inhibitor MG-132 and the anthracycline idarubicin was sufficient to preferentially ablate human LSCs in vitro while sparing normal HSCs[51]. These studies demonstrate that LSC-specific targeting can be achieved. Recently, Guzman etal also demonstrated that the single plant-derived compound parthenolide (PTL) effectively eradicates AML LSCs by inducing robust apoptosis via induce oxidative stress and inhibit NF-κB while sparing normal HSCs[60]. These properties make these compound an attractive agent for clinical evaluation. However, the poor solubility of PTL makes pharmacologic use of the compound difficult. Thus, more recently, orally bioavailable Dimethylamino- parthenolide (DMAPT) induces rapid death of primary human LSCs from both myeloid and lymphoid leukemias, and is also highly cytotoxic to bulk leukemic cell populations[61]. Servida etal also reported that PS-341 induced apoptosis in leukemia progenitor cells[62]. In an effort to expand strategies for selectively targeting LSCs, the recent study has been shown that the compound TDZD-8 (4-benzyl,2-methyl,1,2,4-thiadiazolidine, 3,5 dione), which was originally developed as a non-ATP competitive inhibitor of GSK-3β, was strongly and selectively cytotoxic to multiple types of primary leukemia cells, as well as phenotypically and functionally defined LSCs. The cytotoxicity is associated with a rapid loss of membrane integrity, induction of oxidative stress, and inhibition of several signal transduction pathways including NF-κB and FLT3[63].

13. Conclusions

Altogether, these recent investigations have revealed that leukemia originate from leukemic stem cells. The leukmic stem cells can provide critical functions in leukemic initiation and progression and recurrent disease states. LSCs are often resistant to standard chemotherapy, which make leukemia refractory and relapse. The concept of leukemia as a stem cell disease has the potential to change significantly the view of the problem of drug resistance. Research efforts to discover the specific signal pathway serving to resistance of LSCs should lead to more effective and safe leukemia therapeutic treatments for ultimately curing leukemia. Future studies will focus on the identifying and targeting of critical signal pathway to overcome the drug resistance of LSCs for improvement of the current leukemia treatments.

14. Reference

[1] Krause DS, Van Etten RA. Right on target: eradicating leukemic stem cells. Trends Mol Med. 2007;13:470-481.

[2] Kurosawa S, Yamaguchi T, Miyawaki S, et al. Prognostic factors and outcomes of adult patients with acute myeloid leukemia after first relapse. Haematologica.

[3] Kell J. Emerging treatments in acute myeloid leukaemia. Expert Opin Emerg Drugs. 2004;9:55-71.

[4] Yagi T, Morimoto A, Eguchi M, et al. Identification of a gene expression signature associated with pediatric AML prognosis. Blood. 2003;102:1849-1856.

[5] Dick JE. Stem cells: Self-renewal writ in blood. Nature. 2003;423:231-233.

[6] Reya T, Morrison SJ, Clarke MF, Weissman IL. Stem cells, cancer, and cancer stem cells. Nature. 2001;414:105-111.

[7] Bullock TE, Wen B, Marley SB, Gordon MY. Potential of CD34 in the regulation of symmetrical and asymmetrical divisions by hematopoietic progenitor cells. Stem Cells. 2007;25:844-851.

[8] Bonnet D, Dick JE. Human acute myeloid leukemia is organized as a hierarchy that originates from a primitive hematopoietic cell. Nat Med. 1997;3:730-737.

[9] Singh SK, Hawkins C, Clarke ID, et al. Identification of human brain tumour initiating cells. Nature. 2004;432:396-401.

[10] Waterworth A. Introducing the concept of breast cancer stem cells. Breast Cancer Res. 2004;6:53-54.

[11] Collins AT, Berry PA, Hyde C, Stower MJ, Maitland NJ. Prospective identification of tumorigenic prostate cancer stem cells. Cancer Res. 2005;65:10946-10951.

[12] O'Brien CA, Pollett A, Gallinger S, Dick JE. A human colon cancer cell capable of initiating tumour growth in immunodeficient mice. Nature. 2007;445:106-110.

[13] Chiba T, Kita K, Zheng YW, et al. Side population purified from hepatocellular carcinoma cells harbors cancer stem cell-like properties. Hepatology. 2006;44:240-251.

[14] Peacock CD, Watkins DN. Cancer stem cells and the ontogeny of lung cancer. J Clin Oncol. 2008;26:2883-2889.

[15] Prince ME, Ailles LE. Cancer stem cells in head and neck squamous cell cancer. J Clin Oncol. 2008;26:2871-2875.

[16] Jamieson CH, Weissman IL, Passegue E. Chronic versus acute myelogenous leukemia: a question of self-renewal. Cancer Cell. 2004;6:531-533.

[17] Huntly BJ, Shigematsu H, Deguchi K, et al. MOZ-TIF2, but not BCR-ABL, confers properties of leukemic stem cells to committed murine hematopoietic progenitors. Cancer Cell. 2004;6:587-596.

[18] Todaro M, Perez Alea M, Scopelliti A, Medema JP, Stassi G. IL-4-mediated drug resistance in colon cancer stem cells. Cell Cycle. 2008;7:309-313.

[19] Shafee N, Smith CR, Wei S, et al. Cancer stem cells contribute to cisplatin resistance in Brca1/p53-mediated mouse mammary tumors. Cancer Res. 2008;68:3243-3250.

[20] Ma S, Lee TK, Zheng BJ, Chan KW, Guan XY. CD133+ HCC cancer stem cells confer chemoresistance by preferential expression of the Akt/PKB survival pathway. Oncogene. 2008;27:1749-1758.

[21] Lu C, Shervington A. Chemoresistance in gliomas. Mol Cell Biochem. 2008;312:71-80.

[22] Eramo A, Ricci-Vitiani L, Zeuner A, et al. Chemotherapy resistance of glioblastoma stem cells. Cell Death Differ. 2006;13:1238-1241.

[23] de Figueiredo-Pontes LL, Pintao MC, Oliveira LC, et al. Determination of P-glycoprotein, MDR-related protein 1, breast cancer resistance protein, and lung-resistance protein expression in leukemic stem cells of acute myeloid leukemia. Cytometry B Clin Cytom. 2008;74:163-168.

[24] Ravandi F, Estrov Z. Eradication of leukemia stem cells as a new goal of therapy in leukemia. Clin Cancer Res. 2006;12:340-344.

[25] Bao S, Wu Q, McLendon RE, et al. Glioma stem cells promote radioresistance by preferential activation of the DNA damage response. Nature. 2006;444:756-760.

[26] Zobalova R, McDermott L, Stantic M, Prokopova K, Dong LF, Neuzil J. CD133-positive cells are resistant to TRAIL due to up-regulation of FLIP. Biochem Biophys Res Commun. 2008;373:567-571.

[27] Wei C, Guo-min W, Yu-jun L. Apoptosis resistance can be used in screening the markers of cancer stem cells. Med Hypotheses. 2006;67:1381-1383.

[28] Costello RT, Mallet F, Gaugler B, et al. Human acute myeloid leukemia CD34+/CD38- progenitor cells have decreased sensitivity to chemotherapy and Fas-induced apoptosis, reduced immunogenicity, and impaired dendritic cell transformation capacities. Cancer Res. 2000;60:4403-4411.

[29] Liu S, Dontu G, Mantle ID, et al. Hedgehog signaling and Bmi-1 regulate self-renewal of normal and malignant human mammary stem cells. Cancer Res. 2006;66:6063-6071.

[30] Clement V, Sanchez P, de Tribolet N, Radovanovic I, Ruiz i Altaba A. HEDGEHOG-GLI1 signaling regulates human glioma growth, cancer stem cell self-renewal, and tumorigenicity. Curr Biol. 2007;17:165-172.

[31] Kubo M, Kuroki S, Tanaka M. [New therapeutic target of breast cancer]. Nippon Rinsho. 2007;65 Suppl 6:142-147.

[32] Tung DC, Chao KS. Targeting hedgehog in cancer stem cells: how a paradigm shift can improve treatment response. Future Oncol. 2007;3:569-574.

[33] Vestergaard J, Lind-Thomsen A, Pedersen MW, et al. GLI1 is involved in cell cycle regulation and proliferation of NT2 embryonal carcinoma stem cells. DNA Cell Biol. 2008;27:251-256.

[34] Zhao C, Chen A, Jamieson CH, et al. Hedgehog signalling is essential for maintenance of cancer stem cells in myeloid leukaemia. Nature. 2009;458:776-779.

[35] Dierks C, Beigi R, Guo GR, et al. Expansion of Bcr-Abl-positive leukemic stem cells is dependent on Hedgehog pathway activation. Cancer Cell. 2008;14:238-249.

[36] Lou H, Dean M. Targeted therapy for cancer stem cells: the patched pathway and ABC transporters. Oncogene. 2007;26:1357-1360.

[37] Zhang J, Wang J, Liu Y, et al. Oncogenic Kras-induced leukemogeneis: hematopoietic stem cells as the initial target and lineage-specific progenitors as the potential targets for final leukemic transformation. Blood. 2009;113:1304-1314.

[38] McCubrey JA, Steelman LS, Abrams SL, et al. Targeting survival cascades induced by activation of Ras/Raf/MEK/ERK, PI3K/PTEN/Akt/mTOR and Jak/STAT pathways for effective leukemia therapy. Leukemia. 2008;22:708-722.

[39] Schessl C, Rawat VP, Cusan M, et al. The AML1-ETO fusion gene and the FLT3 length mutation collaborate in inducing acute leukemia in mice. J Clin Invest. 2005;115:2159-2168.

[40] Styczynski J, Drewa T. Leukemic stem cells: from metabolic pathways and signaling to a new concept of drug resistance targeting. Acta Biochim Pol. 2007;54:717-726.

[41] Levis M, Murphy KM, Pham R, et al. Internal tandem duplications of the FLT3 gene are present in leukemia stem cells. Blood. 2005;106:673-680.

[42] Mony U, Jawad M, Seedhouse C, Russell N, Pallis M. Resistance to FLT3 inhibition in an in vitro model of primary AML cells with a stem cell phenotype in a defined microenvironment. Leukemia. 2008;22:1395-1401.

[43] Pollard JA, Alonzo TA, Gerbing RB, et al. FLT3 internal tandem duplication in CD34+/CD33- precursors predicts poor outcome in acute myeloid leukemia. Blood. 2006;108:2764-2769.
[44] Tazzari PL, Cappellini A, Ricci F, et al. Multidrug resistance-associated protein 1 expression is under the control of the phosphoinositide 3 kinase/Akt signal transduction network in human acute myelogenous leukemia blasts. Leukemia. 2007;21:427-438.
[45] Hambardzumyan D, Becher OJ, Rosenblum MK, Pandolfi PP, Manova-Todorova K, Holland EC. PI3K pathway regulates survival of cancer stem cells residing in the perivascular niche following radiation in medulloblastoma in vivo. Genes Dev. 2008;22:436-448.
[46] Yilmaz OH, Morrison SJ. The PI-3kinase pathway in hematopoietic stem cells and leukemia-initiating cells: a mechanistic difference between normal and cancer stem cells. Blood Cells Mol Dis. 2008;41:73-76.
[47] Yilmaz OH, Valdez R, Theisen BK, et al. Pten dependence distinguishes haematopoietic stem cells from leukaemia-initiating cells. Nature. 2006;441:475-482.
[48] Yanagi S, Kishimoto H, Kawahara K, et al. Pten controls lung morphogenesis, bronchioalveolar stem cells, and onset of lung adenocarcinomas in mice. J Clin Invest. 2007;117:2929-2940.
[49] Shoman N, Klassen S, McFadden A, Bickis MG, Torlakovic E, Chibbar R. Reduced PTEN expression predicts relapse in patients with breast carcinoma treated by tamoxifen. Mod Pathol. 2005;18:250-259.
[50] Guzman ML, Neering SJ, Upchurch D, et al. Nuclear factor-kappaB is constitutively activated in primitive human acute myelogenous leukemia cells. Blood. 2001;98:2301-2307.
[51] Guzman ML, Swiderski CF, Howard DS, et al. Preferential induction of apoptosis for primary human leukemic stem cells. Proc Natl Acad Sci U S A. 2002;99:16220-16225.
[52] Kumar SK, Roy I, Anchoori RK, et al. Targeted inhibition of hedgehog signaling by cyclopamine prodrugs for advanced prostate cancer. Bioorg Med Chem. 2008;16:2764-2768.
[53] Kim Y, Yoon JW, Xiao X, Dean NM, Monia BP, Marcusson EG. Selective down-regulation of glioma-associated oncogene 2 inhibits the proliferation of hepatocellular carcinoma cells. Cancer Res. 2007;67:3583-3593.
[54] Peacock CD, Wang Q, Gesell GS, et al. Hedgehog signaling maintains a tumor stem cell compartment in multiple myeloma. Proc Natl Acad Sci U S A. 2007;104:4048-4053.
[55] Kobune M, Takimoto R, Murase K, et al. Drug resistance is dramatically restored by hedgehog inhibitors in CD34+ leukemic cells. Cancer Sci. 2009;100:948-955.
[56] Copland M, Pellicano F, Richmond L, et al. BMS-214662 potently induces apoptosis of chronic myeloid leukemia stem and progenitor cells and synergizes with tyrosine kinase inhibitors. Blood. 2008;111:2843-2853.
[57] Tabe Y, Jin L, Tsutsumi-Ishii Y, et al. Activation of integrin-linked kinase is a critical prosurvival pathway induced in leukemic cells by bone marrow-derived stromal cells. Cancer Res. 2007;67:684-694.

[58] Zhou J, Wulfkuhle J, Zhang H, et al. Activation of the PTEN/mTOR/STAT3 pathway in breast cancer stem-like cells is required for viability and maintenance. Proc Natl Acad Sci U S A. 2007;104:16158-16163.

[59] Weisberg E, Banerji L, Wright RD, et al. Potentiation of antileukemic therapies by the dual PI3K/PDK-1 inhibitor, BAG956: effects on BCR-ABL- and mutant FLT3-expressing cells. Blood. 2008;111:3723-3734.

[60] Guzman ML, Rossi RM, Karnischky L, et al. The sesquiterpene lactone parthenolide induces apoptosis of human acute myelogenous leukemia stem and progenitor cells. Blood. 2005;105:4163-4169.

[61] Guzman ML, Rossi RM, Neelakantan S, et al. An orally bioavailable parthenolide analog selectively eradicates acute myelogenous leukemia stem and progenitor cells. Blood. 2007;110:4427-4435.

[62] Servida F, Soligo D, Delia D, et al. Sensitivity of human multiple myelomas and myeloid leukemias to the proteasome inhibitor I. Leukemia. 2005;19:2324-2331.

[63] Guzman ML, Li X, Corbett CA, et al. Rapid and selective death of leukemia stem and progenitor cells induced by the compound 4-benzyl, 2-methyl, 1,2,4-thiadiazolidine, 3,5 dione (TDZD-8). Blood. 2007;110:4436-4444.

Cancer Stem Cells and Chemoresistance

Suebwong Chuthapisith MD, MSc, PhD, FRCST
Department of Surgery, Faculty of Medicine Siriraj Hospital,
Mahidol University, Bangkok
Thailand

1. Introduction

Chemoresistance is a complex mechanism, involving various biological pathways. Also, chemoresistance is a major cause of cancer treatment failure. Cancer stem cell (CSC) in solid cancer has recently identified, but its role in solid organ tumour is not clearly documented. However, research data supported that CSC may involve in carcinogenesis, invasion and metastasis, as well as resistance to various form of chemotherapy. Understanding more how CSCs involve in chemoresistance would enhance our knowledge and thus would lead us to the possibly newly developed cancer treatment.

2. Stem cells and clinical relevance to therapy

Stem cells are a small and distinct population of cells in living body. Stem cells can divide, and can produce progeny of differentiated cells with specific functions, therefore, have two major key characteristics: 1) capacity for asymmetric division or self-renewal and 2) generate a quiescent stem cell that can produce "progenitor" cells, which can differentiate into more mature and differentiated cells.

Self-renewal is a characteristic process of stem cells, thereby, ensuring that the stem cells survive a long time. All stem cells must regulate the balance between self-renewal and differentiation. The self-renewal and differentiation of stem cells is regulated by many signalling pathways, and some pathways are associated with carcinogenesis including Notch, Shh, BMI 1 and Wnt signalling pathways [Jordan, 2004]. In fact, some of these proteins (eg. Wnt) has become therapeutic target [Takahashi-Yanaga and Kahn, 2010].

In general, human stem cells can be classified broadly into embryonic, foetal and adult stem cells. Adult stem cells have limited potential for differentiation into different cell types of their tissue of origin whereas embryonic stem cells can differentiate into all cell phenotypes [Bellantuono and Keith, 2007]. Most adult tissue-specific stem cells are traditionally believed to be multipotent, but not pluripotent. However, recent data has documented that adult stem cells can show plasticity, and that the adult tissue-restricted stem cells may develop into cells resembling pluripotent stem cells [Askenasy et al., 2006;Kiger et al., 2000;Bellantuono and Keith, 2007].

Recently, stem cell research has been expanding rapidly, not only in basic scientific research but also in clinical research. Treatment of many complex diseases with stem cell is more widely used in various types of haematologic diseases, including thallasemia, aplastic anemia and other hematologic malignancies. As well, stem cell has increasing roles in the

treatment of other non-haematologic diseases including heart failure, liver dysfunctions and neurodegenerative diseases [Chang and Appasani, 2006;Dimarakis et al., 2005;Gordon et al., 2006;Burt et al., 2008].
Better understanding about stem cells has started from the studies of haematopoietic tissues. In the haematopoiectic system a wide variety of blood cells in the circulation appear to originate from the same precursors [Huntly and Gilliland, 2005]. With this observation, later identification of haematologic stem cells was achieved. The rapid further advancement in haematopoietic stem cell knowledge has later made haematopoietic stem cell transplantation become a standard treatment for various haematologic diseases, with a good and safe outcome [Ikehara, 2003]. Therefore, approval of stem cell therapy is limited primarily to haematologic diseases. Treatment of other degenerative diseases with stem cell therapy is possibly only in the research area, but with a potential expand to clinical practice in the near future. For example, recent published data has used human CD34+ adult bone marrow stem cells for the treatment of chronic liver disease and has shown an impressive outcome [Gordon et al., 2006;Levicar et al., 2008]. Haematopoietic stem cells have also being used in many clinical (Phase I) trails in the treatment of ischaemic heart disease, diabetes and other neurodegenerative diseases with an impressive preliminary outcome [Balsam and Robbins, 2005;Dimarakis et al., 2005;Levicar et al., 2007]. However, long-term outcome clinical data has still to be documented and carefully evaluated.

3. Cancer stem cells: a small population in tumours

Most cancer cells grow and divide rapidly and indefinitely, as well as stem cells. This observation has led to the possible link between cancer cell and stem cell. In fact, knowledge about cancer stem cell (CSC) become widely accepted following the work of John Dick and his colleagues in 1994 who described the presence of CSCs in haematologic malignancies [Lapidot et al., 1994]. The concepts of CSCs arose from the observations of the capacity to and comparability of self-renewal between stem cells and cancer cells. As a result, CSCs are believed to be involved in carcinogenesis, as well as in local invasion and in the metastatic process [Glinsky et al., 2005; Spillane and Henderson, 2007]. As well, there is also accumulating data supported that stem cells play an important role in chemo- and radiotherapy resistance [Dean et al., 2005].
In the seminal experiment in 1960, patients had their own tumour cells injected into their body subcutaneously. A low success rate of tumour growth occurred at the injection site (14.3%), with a large number of cancer cells (at least 1×10^6 cells) required in order to induce a tumour growth at the autotransplantation site [Southam and Brunschwig, 1960]. At that time, the explanation as to why cancer cells isolated from malignant tumours could not regenerate on reinjection was unclear. However, with the recent knowledge about CSC, an explanation for the results of the experiment may be the small percentage of CSCs in the tumour inoculations. Out of the 1×10^6 cells that implanted into his patients, less than 0.5% consisted of CSCs. This small population of stem cells was able to induce growth and form a tumour at the injection site. Thus, the reason as to why at least 1×10^6 cells were required for the implantation in order to generate a new tumour.

4. Breast cancer stem cells

The success to identify CSCs in haematologic malignancies has led to the discovery of stem cells in solid tumours, which later has enhanced our knowledge of cancer biology. Amongst the study of CSC in solid organ malignancies, breast CSC is one of the most widely investigated. In normal breast epithelium, there are two main cell types, known as luminal epithelial and myoepithelial cells. The stem cell populations reside in the luminal, but not in the myoepithelial compartment [Gudjonsson and Magnusson, 2005]. As a result of mutations in the stem/progenitor cells, normal breast stem/progenitor cells are transformed into breast CSCs/progenitor cells [Beier et al., 2007;Ricci-Vitiani et al., 2007].

Previously, identification and isolation of stem cells in solid organ tumour was not possible. Until recently, identification and isolation of CSCs from the other cell populations was succeeded due to development of newly discovered cell surface biomarkers and advancement of biomolecular technology (ie. flow cytometery). Stem cells identified from solid tumours express organ-specific cell surface markers. For example, EpCAM(high)/CD44(+)/CD166(+) is a specific marker for the human colon CSCs [Dalerba et al., 2007] and CD133 is the specific stem cell marker for human central nervous system cancers [Beier et al., 2007]. Breast CSCs were first identified by Al-Hajj *et al* (2003) who established that the CD44(+)/CD24(-) was the surface phenotypic profile of breast CSCs [Al-Hajj et al., 2003]. A small number of CD44(+)/CD24(-) cells (as few as 200 cells) were able to give rise to new tumours after injection into the mammary fat pad of NOD/SCID mice [Al-Hajj et al., 2003]. These findings have been confirmed subsequently by other research [Ponti et al., 2005].

CD44 is a 37 kDa cell adhesion molecule expressed in most cell types, including putative breast CSCs [Goodison et al., 1999]. CD24 was originally found during the early stage of B cell development and is highly expressed in neutrophils, but not in normal T cells or monocytes [Balic et al., 2006]. The gene studies of CD44+ cells, extracted from human breast tissues, have shown the expression of genes associated with self-renewal, including hedgehog signaling pathway-related genes - Gli1 and Gli2 [Shipitsin et al., 2007]. As well, the TGF-β signalling pathway, known to be important in human embryonic stem cells and promoting invasion and angiogenesis, was found to be activated in CD44(+) breast cancer cells [Shipitsin et al., 2007]. These findings have suggested that CD44 (+) expressing cells that are CD24(-) are CSCs and have supported the probable role(s) of CSCs in determination of biological aggressiveness and invasive behaviour.

In addition, recently, aldehyde dehydrogenase 1 (ALDH 1) has been used as another marker to identify breast CSCs. ALDH1 is a detoxificating enzyme responsible for the oxidation of intracellular aldehydes [Duester, 2000]. As few as 20 breast cancer cells with $CD44^{+}/CD24^{-}/ALDH^{+}$ were able to generate tumours in NOD/SCID mice [Ginestier et al., 2007].

Success in identifying and isolation of CSC in breast cancer is probably a breakthrough in cancer research and that make scientist can study further the roles of CSC in cancer biology more easily.

5. Anti-cancer chemotherapy resistance

Nowadays, treatment of cancer consists of various modalities, including surgery, radio-, chemo-therapy and others. However, in order to achieve the maximum systemic control, one of the most crucial modalities is chemotherapy. Therefore, resistance to chemotherapy is a major cause of failure in the treatment of solid organ malignancies. Mechanisms involved to resistance process are complex and not fully understood. The following mechanisms are proposed to be involved in chemotherapy resistance.

5.1 ABC transporters and multidrug resistance

Chemotherapeutic drug resistance includes the efflux/influx of drugs via the adenosine triphosphate-binding cassette (ABC) transporters. These cell membrane proteins include 3 main types - P-gp (ABCB1/multi-drug resistance (MDR) 1), MDR-associated protein (MRP1/ABCC1) and breast cancer resistance protein (BCRP/ABCG2). The ABC transporter system has been conserved across the phylogenic spectrum, from bacteria to mammals, and through evolution. The main function of ABC transporters is to excrete toxins from the liver, kidneys and gastrointestinal tract. In addition, ABC transporters act as a filter for toxins which enter certain vital structures such as the brain, placenta and testes. ABC transporters are thought to play a crucial role in chemotherapeutic agent resistance mechanisms by effluxing drugs out of tumour cells. Consequently, intracellular drug concentrations may fluctuate and be low. To date, more than 40 ABC transporter genes have been discovered and are classified into 8 subfamilies: ABCA through ABCG and ANSA (arsenite and antimonite transporter) [Mahadevan and List, 2004].

ABC transporter subfamily A (ABCA) gene consists of 13 members that have various roles in the cell membrane. ABC transporter subfamily B, also known as MDR, comprises 11 members. The best characterised is P-gp (MDR1/ABCB1), a 170 kDa glycoprotein encoded by the *MDR1* gene. The ABC transporter subfamily C is also known as MRP, with currently at least nine members (MRP1-9) having been identified and related closely to chemoresistance mechanisms [Hopper-Borge et al., 2004]. BCRP is another protein associated with chemoresistance mechanisms. It is a member of the ABC transporter subfamily G. It is named "BCRP" because it was originally isolated from the MCF-7 breast cancer cell line; it is not only found in breast cancer, but is also detected in various types of chemoresistant malignancies.

In cancer cells, over-expression of P-gp correlates with resistance to anthracyclines, vinca alkaloids, colchicines, epipodophyllotoxins and taxanes [Avendano and Menendez, 2002]. Over-expression of P-gp is associated with many chemoresistant cancers including lymphoma, acute leukaemia, breast cancer, ovarian and head and neck cancer [Sauna et al., 2001]. A study of more than 400 tumour specimens of colon, renal, adrenal, liver and pancreas, showed that patients with increased levels of MDR1 RNA tended to be more resistant to chemotherapy [Goldstein et al., 1989]. A meta-analysis review by Trock *et al* (1997) indicated that the proportion of breast tumours expressing P-gp of the various studies was 41.2%. Moreover, the same study claimed that breast cancer patients who had tumours expressing P-gp were three times more likely to be chemoresistant [Trock et al., 1997].

In the human normal cell, BCRP can be detected in the heart, ovary, kidney and foetal liver [Allikmets et al., 1998]. Cell lines selected for resistance to mitoxantrone, topotecan, doxorubicin, SN-38 (the active metabolite of irinotecan), flavopiridol and indolocarbazole topoisomerase I inhibitors, all over-expressed BCRP. However, typical substrate of P-gp such as vinca alkaloids, paclitaxel and verapamil are not transported by BCRP [Allen and Schinkel, 2002]. Expression of BCRP was seen in all tumour types, but was more common in adenocarcinomas of the GI tract, endometrium, lung, and melanoma [Diestra et al., 2002].

5.2 Detoxification enzyme involving in chemotherapy resistance

Three phases of drug detoxification are responsible for excretion of toxic substances from the cell. Phase I detoxification is usually mediated by cytochome P450 and results in eliminating OH forming free radicals. Phase II is generally involved in converting metabolites to less toxic agents. During phase II, toxic substances will conjugate with glutathione, glucuronic acid or sulphate, which will be catalyzed by glutathione S-transferase, uridine diphosphate-glucuronosyl transferase, and sulfatase. Finally, exporting the toxic drug with its metabolites out of the cells via transmembrane efflux pumps is the main activity that occurs during phase III detoxification. Therefore, impairment of detoxification process is directly linked to impairment of chemotherapeutic agent activation, thus involves to chemotherapy resistance.

5.3 Inactivation of apoptosis

The deregulation or inactivation of apoptosis in a cell is crucial to the subsequent development of cancer in that cell. This malfunction of the apoptotic process may predispose the cell to resistance to chemotherapeutic agents, as induction of apoptosis is a key element of drug-induced cancer cell death. The apoptosis is thought to be mediated by the tumour-suppressor protein p53. It prevents tumourigenesis by acting as a cellular-stress and DNA-damage sentinel. As a result of DNA damage, hypoxia or proliferating signals, p53 stabilizes causing cells to undergo cell cycle arrest (checkpoint function) temporarily or permanently, or apoptosis and death [Levine, 1997].

Most human cancers have either mutations in p53 or defects in p53 regulated pathways [Lowe et al., 1994; Vousden and Lu, 2002]. p53 null mice are very prone to developing cancers [Attardi and Donehower, 2005]. Most cancer therapies are DNA-damaging agents, thus, if the cancer cells have a disabled/deregulated apoptotic pathway (p53 mutation or over-expression of BCL-2 protein), this will prevent death of the cancer cell through drug-induced apoptosis. Therefore, there probably is a non-apoptotic dependent pathway of cell death. Clonogenic survival assays in mice have failed to reveal any differences between rates of cell death of normal and malignant cells to ionising radiation, implying that there are other pathways for cancer cell death. This suggests that those cancers carrying the Tp53 allele or over-expressing the anti-apoptotic protein BCL-2 should be more resistant to cancer drug therapy than tumour cells with intact apoptotic pathways (presence of wild type 53, low levels of BCL-2). This has not been shown to be the case for non-haematological malignancies.

In a recent review, there was no clear evidence that either the apoptotic index or levels of p53, BCL-2 or other homologous proteins are predictive of the response of solid tumours to chemotherapy or radiotherapy [Schmitt and Lowe, 1999;Brown and Wilson, 2003]. Apart from apoptosis, cells can be eliminated following DNA damage by necrosis, mitotic catastrophe (giant or multinucleated cells), autophagy (self-cell digestion) with intracellular vacuoles containing ribosomes, and premature senescence.

The precise pathway of cell death as a result of drug treatment is difficult to determine and is dependent on a range of factors, including tumour cell type and volume, drug combinations and doses used as well as activated anti-cancer host defences.

6. Role of cancer stem cells in chemoresistance

One characteristic of CSCs that differentiates them from other normal cells in the tumour is that CSCs have high levels of ABC transporter proteins. These transporter molecules are responsible for protecting cells from drug damage via the efflux pumping mechanisms. Thus, CSCs, as a result of these biological properties, are resistant to drug treatment, including chemotherapeutic drugs [Dean et al., 2005].

In clinical practice, optimal chemotherapy treatment can kill most cells within solid tumour. However, a small fraction of cells (CSCs) are drug resistant, possibly because of enrichment of ABC transporter proteins. This small fraction of CSCs remain quiescent in the G0 phase. Over a period of time and due to stimuli associated with tumour cell death, these quiescent stem cells give rise to progenitor cells and subsequently become new mature tumour cells with a chemoresistant phenotype. This is the postulated model of acquired chemoresistance in breast cancer observed in the clinic [Dean et al., 2005]. Patients at this stage will develop recurrent tumours and fail to be responsive to further chemotherapy treatment.

The high expression of ABC transporter protein in tumour stem cells results in exclusion of the fluorescent dye Hoechst 33342 and Rhodamine 123, and can be detected by flow-cytometry. The cells that are able to efflux Hoechst 33342 as detected on flow-cytometry are known as the "side population" (SP) cells. However, some drug resistant non-stem cells have these properties as well. Stem cells also have an active DNA repair capacity and a resistance to apoptosis.

In addition, as previously evidenced, CSCs are believed to have overexpression of ALDH1, a detoxification enzyme [Lugli et al., 2010;Neumeister et al., 2010]. However, ALDH1 alone is not specific marker for stem cells [Neumeister and Rimm, 2010]. For example, in a study of breast CSC, as few as 500 ALDH1 positive cells can generate a new tumour; whist as few as 20 CD44+/CD24-/lin-/ALDH1+ cells can induce a new tumour [Ginestier et al., 2007].

The linkage between CSCs and chemoresistance is an interesting and challenging area of research. The ability to identify CSCs in tumours and perhaps to kill these cells is a therapeutic strategy designed to overcome cancer chemoresistance. However, the knowledge and evidence regarding the contribution of CSCs to chemoresistance is still embryonic and requires further careful evaluation.

7. Strategies to overcome chemoresistance by targeting cancer stem cells

If the chemoresistant cells are CSCs, targeting treatment at these cells would be the way forward to overcome the chemoresistance and could improve the outcome of breast cancer treatment. The traditional approach of changing chemotherapeutic regimens, after tumours develop resistance to one chemotherapeutic regimen, may not be useful in chemoresistant breast cancers. Most current chemotherapeutic drugs are targeted on rapidly dividing cells within the tumour, but tend to spare the slowly dividing and inherently resistant CSCs and, thus, may not lead to long-term cures [Hellman et al., 2008].

CSCs may be eliminated by selectively targeted therapies against various self-renewal signalling pathways including Notch, Shh, BMI 1 and Wnt signalling pathways [Massard et al., 2006]. However, if normal stem cells and CSCs share the same pathways to maintain their self-renewal, it would be more complex to selectively target at self-renewal pathways of CSCs without any side-effects to normal stem cells. Fortunately, it appears that CSCs are more likely to be more dependent on certain putative pathways [Pardal et al., 2003].

CSCs may be protected from external toxic agents via the over-expression of ABC transporter proteins. Therefore, targeting at this protein may be an alternative strategy and, thus, a way to overcome chemoresistance. Recently, an *in vitro* study have shown the benefit of gefitinib (Iressa, AstraZeneca), a tyrosine kinase inhibitor, in reversing chemotherapy resistance in multidrug resistant breast cancer cells expressing ATP transporters [Yang et al., 2005]. Also, gefitinib has been recently reported to successfully overcome SN-38-resistance in small-cell lung cancer cells *in vitro* [Takigawa et al., 2007].

Moreover, instead of killing tumour cells with chemotherapy, biological therapy with monoclonal antibodies targeted against specific cellular surface molecules or receptors should be considered. Targeting at the apoptotic pathway could be an alternative. Cell death is generally programmed by apoptosis, including that regulated by CSCs [Baguley, 2006]. The elimination of CSCs may be feasible by increasing the ratio of pro-apoptotic to anti-apoptotic proteins and signal pathways, perhaps targeting at pro-apoptotic members of the Bcl2 family [Thompson and Thompson, 2004]. Alternatively, targeting CSCs at the niche endothelium would be a possible therapeutic strategy. CSCs niches are likely to be well endowed with a blood supply by angiogenesis [Baguley, 2006]. Therefore, blockage of action of VEGF signalling with anti-VEGF, bevacizumab (Avastin, Genetech), could be an alternative.

However, all the strategies proposed above are speculative. Published data, so far, has not yet confirmed the benefit of these approaches in chemoresistant patients where CSCs are believed to be the predominant factor. If CSCs are key molecules responsible for chemoresistance, there is an urgent need to enhance both experimental and clinical studies to support the use of these biological therapies in chemoresistant breast cancers. It is likely that additional agents, following chemotherapy, may be needed to eradicate CSCs, if a good long-term outcome is to be achieved.

8. References

Al-Hajj M, Wicha MS, Benito-hernandez A, Morrison SJ, Clarke MF (2003) Prospective identification of tumorigenic breast cancer cells. *Proc Natl Acad Sci USA* 100: 3983-3988

Allen JD, Schinkel AH (2002) Multidrug resistance and pharmacological protection mediated by the breast cancer resistance protein (BCRP/ABCG2). *Mol Cancer Ther* 1: 427-434

Allikmets R, Schriml LM, Hutchinson A, Romano-Spica V, Dean M (1998) A human placenta-specific ATP-binding cassette gene (ABCP) on chromosome 4q22 that is involved in multidrug resistance. *Cancer Res* 58: 5337-5339

Askenasy N, Yaniv I, Stein J, Sharkis SJ (2006) Our perception of developmental plasticity: esse est percipi (to be is to be perceived)? *Curr Stem Cell Res Ther* 1: 85-94

Attardi LD, Donehower LA (2005) Probing p53 biological functions through the use of genetically engineered mouse models. *Mutat Res* 576: 4-21

Avendano C, Menendez JC (2002) Inhibitors of multidrug resistance to antitumour agents (MDR). *Curr Med Chem* 9: 159-193

Baguley BC (2006) Tumor stem cell niches: a new functional framework for the action of anticancer drugs. *Recent Patents Anticancer Drug Discov* 1: 121-127

Balic M, Lin H, Young L, Hawes D, Giuliano A, McNamara G, Datar RH, Cote RJ (2006) Most early disseminated cancer cells detected in bone marrow of breast cancer patients have a putative breast cancer stem cell phenotype. *Clin Cancer Res* 12: 5615-5621

Balsam LB, Robbins RC (2005) Haematopoietic stem cells and repair of the ischaemic heart. *Clin Sci (Lond)* 109: 483-492

Beier D, Hau P, Proescholdt M, Lohmeier A, Wischhusen J, Oefner PJ, Aigner L, Brawanski A, Bogdahn U, Beier CP (2007) CD133(+) and CD133(-) glioblastoma-derived cancer stem cells show differential growth characteristics and molecular profiles. *Cancer Res* 67: 4010-4015

Bellantuono I, Keith WN (2007) Stem cell ageing: does it happen and can we intervene? *Expert Rev Mol Med* 9: 1-20

Brown JM, Wilson G (2003) Apoptosis genes and resistance to cancer therapy: what does the experimental and clinical data tell us? *Cancer Biol Ther* 2: 477-490

Burt RK, Loh Y, Pearce W, Beohar N, Barr WG, Craig R, Wen Y, Rapp JA, Kessler J (2008) Clinical applications of blood-derived and marrow-derived stem cells for nonmalignant diseases. *JAMA* 299: 925-936

Chang AI, Appasani K (2006) Stem cells & regenerative medicine: from molecular embryology to tissue engineering and therapeutics. *Regen Med* 1: 385-392

Dalerba P, Dylla SJ, Park IK, Liu R, Wang X, Cho RW, Hoey T, Gurney A, Huang EH, Simeone DM, Shelton AA, Parmiani G, Castelli C, Clarke MF (2007) Phenotypic characterization of human colorectal cancer stem cells. *Proc Natl Acad Sci U S A* 104: 10158-10163

Dean M, Fojo T, Bates S (2005) Tumour stem cells and drug resistance. *Nat Rev Cancer* 5: 275-284

Diestra JE, Scheffer GL, Catala I, Maliepaard M, Schellens JH, Scheper RJ, Germa-Lluch JR, Izquierdo MA (2002) Frequent expression of the multi-drug resistance-associated protein BCRP/MXR/ABCP/ABCG2 in human tumours detected by the BXP-21 monoclonal antibody in paraffin-embedded material. *J Pathol* 198: 213-219

Dimarakis I, Habib NA, Gordon MY (2005) Adult bone marrow-derived stem cells and the injured heart: just the beginning? *Eur J Cardiothorac Surg* 28: 665-676

Duester G (2000) Families of retinoid dehydrogenases regulating vitamin A function: production of visual pigment and retinoic acid. *Eur J Biochem* 267: 4315-4324

Ginestier C, Hur MH, Charafe-Jauffret E, Monville F, Dutcher J, Brown M, Jacquemier J, Viens P, Kleer CG, Liu S, Schott A, Hayes D, Birnbaum D, Wicha MS, Dontu G (2007) ALDH1 Is a Marker of Normal and Malignant Human Mammary Stem Cells and a Predictor of Poor Clinical Outcome. *Cell Stem Cell* 1: 555-567

Glinsky GV, Berezovska O, Glinskii AB (2005) Microarray analysis identifies a death-from-cancer signature predicting therapy failure in patients with multiple types of cancer. *J Clin Invest* 115: 1503-1521

Goldstein LJ, Galski H, Fojo A, Willingham M, Lai SL, Gazdar A, Pirker R, Green A, Crist W, Brodeur GM, . (1989) Expression of a multidrug resistance gene in human cancers. *J Natl Cancer Inst* 81: 116-124

Goodison S, Urquidi V, Tarin D (1999) CD44 cell adhesion molecules. *Mol Pathol* 52: 189-196

Gordon MY, Levicar N, Pai M, Bachellier P, Dimarakis I, Al Allaf F, M'Hamdi H, Thalji T, Welsh JP, Marley SB, Davies J, Dazzi F, Marelli-Berg F, Tait P, Playford R, Jiao L, Jensen S, Nicholls JP, Ayav A, Nohandani M, Farzaneh F, Gaken J, Dodge R, Alison M, Apperley JF, Lechler R, Habib NA (2006) Characterization and clinical application of human CD34+ stem/progenitor cell populations mobilized into the blood by granulocyte colony-stimulating factor. *Stem Cells* 24: 1822-1830

Gudjonsson T, Magnusson MK (2005) Stem cell biology and the cellular pathways of carcinogenesis. *APMIS* 113: 922-929

Hellman S, Botnick L, Mauch P (2008) Stem-cell biology and cancer therapy: the more things change. *J Clin Oncol* 26: 821-822

Hopper-Borge E, Chen Z-S, Shchaveleva I, Belinsky MG, Kruh GD (2004) Analysis of the drug resistance profile of Multidrug Resistance Protein 7 (ABCC10): Resistance to docetaxel. *Cancer Res* 64: 4927-4930

Huntly BJ, Gilliland DG (2005) Leukaemia stem cells and the evolution of cancer-stem-cell research. *Nat Rev Cancer* 5: 311-321

Ikehara S (2003) New strategies for BMT, organ transplantation, and regeneration therapy. *Hematology* 8: 77-81

Jordan CT (2004) Cancer stem cell biology: from leukemia to solid tumors. *Curr Opin Cell Biol* 16: 708-712

Kiger AA, White-Cooper H, Fuller MT (2000) Somatic support cells restrict germline stem cell self-renewal and promote differentiation. *Nature* 407: 750-754

Lapidot T, Sirard C, Vormoor J, Murdoch B, Hoang T, Caceres-Cortes J, Minden M, Paterson B, Caligiuri MA, Dick JE (1994) A cell initiating human acute myeloid leukaemia after transplantation into SCID mice. *Nature* 367: 645-648

Levicar N, Dimarakis I, Flores C, Tracey J, Gordon MY, Habib NA (2007) Stem cells as a treatment for chronic liver disease and diabetes. *Handb Exp Pharmacol* 180: 243-262

Levicar N, Pai M, Habib NA, Tait P, Jiao LR, Marley SB, Davis J, Dazzi F, Smadja C, Jensen SL, Nicholls JP, Apperley JF, Gordon MY (2008) Long-term clinical results of autologous infusion of mobilized adult bone marrow derived CD34+ cells in patients with chronic liver disease. *Cell Prolif* 41 Suppl 1: 115-125

Levine AJ (1997) p53, the cellular gatekeeper for growth and division. *Cell* 88: 323-331

Lowe SW, Bodis S, McClatchey A, Remington L, Ruley HE, Fisher DE, Housman DE, Jacks T (1994) p53 status and the efficacy of cancer therapy in vivo. *Science* 266: 807-810

Lugli A, Iezzi G, Hostettler I, Muraro MG, Mele V, Tornillo L, Carafa V, Spagnoli G, Terracciano L, Zlobec I (2010) Prognostic impact of the expression of putative cancer stem cell markers CD133, CD166, CD44s, EpCAM, and ALDH1 in colorectal cancer. *Br J Cancer* 103: 382-390

Mahadevan D, List AF (2004) Targeting the multidrug resistance-1 transporter in AML: molecular regulation and therapeutic strategies. *Blood* 104: 1940-1951

Massard C, Deutsch E, Soria JC (2006) Tumour stem cell-targeted treatment: elimination or differentiation. *Ann Oncol* 17: 1620-1624

Neumeister V, Agarwal S, Bordeaux J, Camp RL, Rimm DL (2010) In situ identification of putative cancer stem cells by multiplexing ALDH1, CD44, and cytokeratin identifies breast cancer patients with poor prognosis. *Am J Pathol* 176: 2131-2138

Neumeister V, Rimm D (2010) Is ALDH1 a good method for definition of breast cancer stem cells? *Breast Cancer Res Treat* 123: 109-111

Pardal R, Clarke MF, Morrison SJ (2003) Applying the principles of stem-cell biology to cancer. *Nat Rev Cancer* 3: 895-902

Ponti D, Costa A, Zaffaroni N, Pratesi G, Petrangolini G, Coradini D, Pilotti S, Pierotti MA, Daidone MG (2005) Isolation and in vitro propagation of tumorigenic breast cancer cells with stem/progenitor cell properties. *Cancer Res* 65: 5506-5511

Ricci-Vitiani L, Lombardi DG, Pilozzi E, Biffoni M, Todaro M, Peschle C, De Maria R (2007) Identification and expansion of human colon-cancer-initiating cells. *Nature* 445: 111-115

Sauna ZE, Smith MM, Muller M, Kerr KM, Ambudkar SV (2001) The mechanism of action of multidrug-resistance-linked P-glycoprotein. *J Bioenerg Biomembr* 33: 481-491

Schmitt CA, Lowe SW (1999) Apoptosis and therapy. *J Pathol* 187: 127-137

Shipitsin M, Campbell LL, Argani P, Weremowicz S, Bloushtain-Qimron N, Yao J, Nikolskaya T, Serebryiskaya T, Beroukhim R, Hu M, Halushka MK, Sukumar S, Parker LM, Anderson KS, Harris LN, Garber JE, Richardson AL, Schnitt SJ, Nikolsky Y, Gelman RS, Polyak K (2007) Molecular definition of breast tumor heterogeneity. *Cancer Cell* 11: 259-273

Southam CM, Brunschwig A (1960) Quantitative studies of autotransplantation of human cancer. *Cancer* 14: 971-978

Spillane JB, Henderson MA (2007) Cancer stem cells: a review. *ANZ J Surg* 77: 464-468

Takahashi-Yanaga F, Kahn M (2010) Targeting Wnt signaling: can we safely eradicate cancer stem cells? *Clin Cancer Res* 16: 3153-3162

Takigawa N, Takeyama M, Kozuki T, Shibayama T, Hisamoto A, Kiura K, Tada A, Hotta K, Umemura S, Ohashi K, Fujiwara Y, Takata S, Ichihara E, Osawa M, Tabata M, Tanimoto M, Takahashi K (2007) Combination of SN-38 with gefitinib or imatinib overcomes SN-38-resistant small-cell lung cancer cells. *Oncol Rep* 17: 983-987

Thompson JE, Thompson CB (2004) Putting the rap on Akt. *J Clin Oncol* 22: 4217-4226

Trock BJ, Leonessa F, Clarke R (1997) Multidrug resistance in breast cancer: a meta-analysis of MDR1/gp170 expression and its possible functional significance. *J Natl Cancer Inst* 89: 917-931

Vousden KH, Lu X (2002) Live or let die: the cell's response to p53. *Nat Rev Cancer* 2: 594-604

Yang CH, Huang CJ, Yang CS, Chu YC, Cheng AL, Whang-Peng J, Yang PC (2005) Gefitinib reverses chemotherapy resistance in gefitinib-insensitive multidrug resistant cancer cells expressing ATP-binding cassette family protein. *Cancer Res* 65: 6943-6949

22

Cancer Stem Cells in Drug Resistance and Drug Screening: Can We Exploit the Cancer Stem Cell Paradigm in Search for New Antitumor Agents?

Michal Sabisz and Andrzej Skladanowski
Laboratory of Molecular and Cellular Pharmacology
Gdansk University of Technology
Poland

1. Introduction

It is now evident that despite an enormous progress in our understanding of molecular mechanisms and processes which operate in tumor cells, this knowledge does not directly translate into more efficient treatment and cure of cancer patients. At the origin of the inefficiency of cancer treatment is inherent or therapy-induced resistance of tumor cells to therapeutic agents. Many different mechanisms of drug resistance have been described and characterized, including elevated expression of membrane drug transporters, changed drug activation and/or detoxification, more efficient repair of drug-induced lesions and non-functional cell death pathways. Another reason for an inefficiency of currently available cancer treatment modalities can be related to cellular heterogeneity of tumors and targeting by anticancer drugs only some tumor cells in the population, which are more sensitive to applied therapeutic agents. In this situation, anticancer treatment can lead to the selection of drug resistant tumor cells and cytostatic rather than cytotoxic effect. The origin of these more resistant cells in tumor cell population was classically perceived as a result of spontaneous or therapy-induced gene mutations, making surviving tumor cells less sensitive to anticancer agents. According to the alternative hypothesis, heterogeneity of tumor cell population, also in its response to drug treatment, can result from a clonal expansion of rare malignant stem cells which may differentiate and produce tumors.

Cancer was proposed to originate from stem cells more than 150 years ago (see Wicha et al., 2006 and references therein) and this idea re-appeared in the early sixties of the last century, first for leukemias (Bruce & van der Gaag, 1963) and later for epithelial tumors (Hamburger & Salmon, 1977). About the same time, Pierce and Wallace provided experimental evidence for the existence of cellular hierarchy in tumors, where malignant undifferentiated cells give rise to benign well-differentiated cells (Pierce & Wallace, 1971). A few years later, Potter proposed a new model of oncogenic transformation according to which tumor cells resulted from blocked differentiation of their progenitors (Potter, 1978). Collectively, a new paradigm of cancer origin was established in which malignant stem cells with de-regulated self-renewal and differentiation mechanisms are responsible for tumor initiation and growth.

Recent explosion of reports providing experimental data that confirm this hypothesis is undoubtedly associated with a growing knowledge about normal stem cells and their potential practical applications in regenerative medicine.
It is known for years that embryonic cells may spontaneously form teratocarcinomas when transplanted into mice. Secondly, when adult differentiated cells are induced by oncogenes and transcription factors to trans-differentiate into pluripotent cells (iPSCs) with stem-like features, they form tumors in experimental animal models with a relatively high frequency (for recent review see Yamanaka & Blau, 2010). Accumulating evidence show that there are remarkable similarities between the reprogramming processes and oncogenic transformation of adult somatic cells and similar factors regulate both pluripotency and tumorigenicity. For example, it was shown that cell reprogramming is regulated by p53, p16 (INK4a) and p21 (Banito et al., 2009) similarly to tumors. Both reprogramming and oncogenic transformation require specific combinations of collaborating genes, that can produce a less differentiated cell able to proliferate and self-renew indefinitely. All four factors, which were initially shown to reprogram somatic cells to iPS cells, are overexpressed in at least some types of tumor, and two of them – *c-myc* and *Klf4* – are established oncogenes. Similarly, reprogramming is less efficient in cells which are close to senescence suggesting that, similarly as in tumorigenicity, cellular senescence protects cells from induced pluripotency (Banito et al., 2009). Together, one can conclude that studies on reprogramming of adult somatic cells into iPS cells provide probably the best experimental evidence that the idea of abnormal stem cells as the origin of tumors may actually be true. It seems that today it is more and more important to delineate similarities and differences between tumor cells and iPS/stem cells as it may provide insights into cancer origin and potentially give new clues for anticancer drug screening and therapy (for recent review see Tilkorn et al., 2010).
There are many controversies related to the cancer stem cell paradigm and its importance for anticancer therapy, some of them will be presented in the following sections of this chapter. To begin with, there is a problem with terminology since the term 'cancer stem cells' (CSC), that is used quite commonly, is somewhat confusing as it relates cancer cells to true stem cells, and this is still hypothetical. Introduction of the name 'stemloids' by Blagosklonny is less ambiguous since it implies some similarity to stem cells, however, pointing to important differences (Blagosklonny, 2005). Another term that is in use, 'tumor-initiating cells', is also confusing since it suggests that these are the cells that have initiated the tumor *in vivo*. The most relevant is probably the term 'tumor-propagating cells', introduced by Kelly et al (Kelly et al., 2007) and Hong et al (Hong et al., 2008), that points to the ability of tumor cells to propagate both *in vitro* and *in vivo*. In this review, we will use the term cancer stem cells (CSCs) as it still is the most popular in the current literature.
It is still not clear as to whether the cancer stem cell paradigm can be applied to all human tumors or it is restricted to leukemias and several types of solid tumors. Moreover, cancer stem cells have been shown to be resistant to anticancer agents but molecular mechanisms, which are responsible for drug resistance phenotype of these cells, are far from being fully characterized. Finally, it is not at all clear how to include the knowledge about cancer stem cells, that we accumulated so far, into new methodologies and assays used in drug screening, both in cytotoxicity measurements *in vitro* and antitumor assays in animal models. Without these practical tools, it will be impossible to screen for new drugs and drug combinations that will allow us to eradicate CSCs and in consequence tumors.

2. Identification and quantitation of cancer stem cells in human tumors

The existence of rare stem-like cells is being experimentally confirmed in a growing number of different tumor types (for review see Reya et al., 2001; Pardal et al., 2003), including myeloid leukemia, breast carcinomas, glioblastoma, melanoma, lung and colon carcinomas (Quintana et al., 2008; Li et al., 2008; Meng et al., 2009; Yeung et al., 2010). One of the most astonishing discoveries concerning CSCs was identification of cancer cells with stem-like properties in cell populations from established tumor cell lines maintained *in vitro* (Yeung et al., 2010). This discovery has important implications as it opens a possibility to use tumor cells cultivated *in vitro* in drug screening and find new compounds which are able to kill CSCs (see section 5 of this chapter).

One of the controversial issues in the field is whether all known tumor types are heterogeneous and consist of a small fraction of CSCs that is able to produce tumors *in vivo* and differentiate to non-CSC cells. It has been shown that human colon carcinoma HCT-116 cells do not contain a hierarchy of tumor cells as concerns production of tumors in nude mice (Kai et al., 2009, Diettfeld et al., 2010). Another example is glioblastoma C6 cells where the majority of cell population formed tumors *in vivo* although these cells have only 0.4% side population (SP) cells (Zheng et al., 2007). Does it mean that in these tumor cell populations all cells have features of CSC? Is it a typical situation or rare examples between tumors of epithelial origin? Similarly, the fraction of CSCs in different human tumors is very divergent. This is at least partially related to the fact that estimations of the number of CSCs are based on several different methodologies (discussed below). Moreover, all of them assume that the CSC fraction is homogenous and can be clearly distinguished from non-CSC cells, and this has never been firmly established. In contrast, there are reasons to believe that CSC cells, with the capacity for long-term self-renewal, constitute an identifiable subpopulation of tumor cells but there is a hierarchy of stem-like cancer cells, as has been recently shown for glioblastomas (Chen et al., 2010).

The most popular strategy to identify CSCs uses specific cell surface markers, such as CD34, CD44, CD117, CD133, integrin a2b1, ESA (epithelial specific antigen) and others or their combinations. A different approach is to mark side population (SP) cells based on the exclusion of Hoechst 33342 dye, as the SP fraction is postulated to be enriched in CSCs (Hirschmann-Jax et al., 2004; Patrawala et al., 2005). However, there are reports showing that expression of membrane markers can not reliably distinguish between CSCs and non-CSCs and cells expressing specific stem cell markers can be as tumorigenic in nude mice as tumor cells which are devoid of specific stem cell markers. This has been particularly well documented for a commonly used stem cell marker CD133 in glioblastomas (Beier et al., 2007; Prestengarden et al., 2010; Chen et al., 2010) but also in colon carcinoma HCT-116 cells (Dittfeld et al., 2010).

CSCs are also frequently quantitated based on the number of cells which are tumorigenic, when transplanted into immunocompromized mice. Although most researchers of the cancer stem cell community consider the latter method as the most reliable, there are also reports suggesting that one has to be very cautious when interpreting results of these tests. It seems, for example, that one may greatly underestimate the frequency of tumorigenic cells in tumor cell population as it depends on the animal model used. Recent studies showed that the detection of tumorigenic melanoma cells injected into mice can be increased by several orders of magnitude if more highly immunocompromised NOD/SCID interleukin-2 receptor gamma chain null (Il2rg(-/-)) mice are used in the modified xenotransplanation assay and tumor cells are injected in Matrigel (Quintana et al., 2008). In these conditions, the estimated fraction of melanoma CSCs from cancer patients increased to about 25%, suggesting that these cells are much more common, at least in some human tumors. Therefore, it is possible that estimations of CSC number by tumorigenicity assay may be biased by the way this assay is performed i.e. animal model used (nude mice vs. SCID mice, or SCID mice with no residual immunity), the number of tumor cells injected into animals, etc.

Some authors postulate that human tumor cells may also differ in their ability to produce tumors in mice and this factor may also greatly influence estimations of CSCs fraction (Baker, 2008). If this is true, one may argue whether the xenotransplanation assay really detects a rare subset of cells that can propagate tumors (i.e. which are tumorigenic) or a rare subset of human tumor cells that can establish themselves in mice. It should also be noted that staining by Hoechst 33342 may be toxic for CSCs as shown for C6 glioblastoma cells and cell sorting by flow cytometry, that is based on Hoechst 33342 stainability, may considerably lower tumorigenicity and, in effect, hamper accurate estimation of CSC fractions (Shen et al., 2008).

The origin of CSCs both in *in vivo* tumor models and in tumor cell lines maintained in *in vitro* culture is another controversial issue. According to the standard CSC hypothesis, the initial CSC originates from normal stem cells or by re-programming more differentiated progenitor cells by oncogenic insults or both. Propagation of these initial CSCs is based on asymmetrical cell division and production of other CSCs and non-CSCs. However, it should be noted that other mechanisms have been proposed by which CSCs may be formed. These include epithelial to mesenchymal transition induced in non-CSC cells from mammary carcinoma that has recently been shown to be involved in CSC formation (Mani et al., 2008; Morel et al., 2008; Santisteban et al., 2009). Some other phenomena related to anticancer therapy may also be implicated in CSC formation. De-differentiation of non-CSC cells into CSCs may be favored by stress-induced factors released after drug treatment. Moreover, many anticancer drugs induce growth arrest in G2 and M phases that frequently leads to polyploidization. Drug-induced polyploidy usually leads to cells death by mitotic catastrophe (for review see Vakifahmetoglu et al., 2008) but in some situations the process of de-polyploidization may occur and result in CSC production (Erenpreisa & Craigg, 2010; Salmina et al., 2010). Polyploidy and consequently cancer stem cells may be also produced by cell-cell fusion (Rizyj et al., 2006; Dittmar et al., 2009). These effects can also explain the effect of the so-called 'oncogenic resistance', the phenomenon frequently observed in the clinical situation, where after treatment with therapeutic agents tumor cells are both more malignant and resistant to anticancer therapy, compared to untreated tumor cells. It seems that 'oncogenic resistance' can not be attributed to resistance phenotype of CSCs (discussed in Dittmar et al., 2009). One possibility is that DNA damage induced by anticancer treatment may lead to gross genomic re-arrangements (both genetic and epigenetic) that result not only in acquiring by tumor cells the stem-like phenotype but also in drug resistance. Changes in tumor cell genome may occur during de-polyploidization of polyploid cells, followed by abnormal mitotic divisions that lead to reduction of cellular DNA content. CSCs can also be generated by cell-cell fusion that is also stimulated by anticancer treatment (Dittmar et al., 2009). According to this scenario, fusion between e. g. CSC and non-CSC cells may result in tumor cells with stem properties. This approach has been used to produce pluripotent cells from adult somatic cells (discussed in Pralong et al., 2006).

3. Properties of stem cells and CSCs: similarities and differences

One of the issues concerning CSCs that needs clarification is which properties are shared between normal stem cells and cancer stem cells. This is particularly important for potential therapies directed toward CSCs that should spare normal stem cells. CSCs are defined to have three features: i) represent a minor population of a tumor (typically 0.1-2% of all cells but may be as high as 25% - see previous section); ii) have the property of self-renewal; iii) are the only cells within the tumor which are capable of immortal growth and production of the tumor *in vivo*. It follows that tumor cell population is composed of relatively rare CSCs and 'committed' or 'differentiated' non-CSC tumor cells with possibly limited life span. Important properties of normal stem cells include self-renewal, as well as pluripotency i. e. the ability of stem cells to differentiate to many functionally distinct cell types. In addition to that, stem cells are characterized by their very limited proliferation potential, as stem cells cells divide only occasionally and in response to very specific intra- and extracellular signals.

Some of these stem cell features cannot directly be applied to CSCs. Most of the available literature data show that CSCs proliferate quite rapidly, although doubling times are frequently much slower compared to the non-stem tumor population (Ropolo et al., 2009; Ishimoto et al., 2010). An extreme case can be leukemia stem cells which are commonly dormant but can be induced to proliferate by specific cytokines or anticancer agents such as arsenic oxide (Essers & Trumpp, 2010; Thomas & Cannas 2010). Secondly, one of the features of stem cells is their ability to produce more differentiated cell progeny. Accordingly, cells of many tumor types are able to differentiate reversibly or irreversibly into different cell types. For example, irreversible differentiation of myeloid leukemia HL-60 cells into monocytes or granulocytes is induced by sodium butyrate, forskolin and hexamethylene bisacetamide (Breitman et al., 1990) or re-activation of wild-type p53 (Soddu et al., 1994). Similarly, colon carcinoma HT-29 cells may be reversibly differentiated into enterocytes or mucin-producing lineages (Chakrabarty et al., 1992; Choi et al., 2000; Demers et al., 2009), and another colon carcinoma SW1222 cells differentiate into enterocytes, enteroendocrine and goblet cells (Yeung et al., 2010). Yet another classical example is breast carcinomas such as MCF-7 cells which may also be induced to differentiate by sodium butyrate and forskolin (Wasserman et al., 1987; Guilbaud et al., 1990). Conversely, nuclear transfer studies showed that the phenotype of at least some cancer cells (as shown for melanomas) can be reversed to a pluripotent state that allows apparently normal differentiation (Hochedlinger et al., 2004). Unfortunately, it is not known whether tumor cell nuclei used for nuclear transfer were from CSCs or non-CSC cells. Another example of tumor cell plasticity related to cell differentiation is the work of Kulesa et al where metastatic phenotype of melanoma cells was shown to be reversed by embryonic milieu (Kulesa et al., 2006). These data point to the important role of tumor microenvironment for the maintenance of tumor cell phenotype.

As mentioned above, there are also tumor cells e. g. HCT-116 where there is apparently no hierarchy of cells differing in tumorigenicity (Kai et al., 2009) and which have little or no capacity to differentiate, therefore, in these tumors majority (if not all) cells can be considered as CSC. This suggests the existence at least two types of tumors: these with CSC sub-population which are able to differentiate and those, which contain only cells with CSC features and no or limited differentiation capacity. An intriguing question remains whether in cells like HCT-116, differentiation of CSC cells is irreversibly blocked or it may still be activated in stress conditions imposed for example by a drug treatment. This is important given that in tumor cell populations, where no hierarchy is observed, drug response and sensitivity should be more homogenous so *in vitro* testing for cytotoxic activity gives more reliable results as for drug concentrations required to eradicate all tumor cells. In contrast, if tumors contain populations of cells, with various in their differentiation status, cytotoxic action of antitumor drugs may also be heterogeneous. In that case, drug screening with mixed tumor cell populations can provide information about overall sensitivity of tumor cells only if the cytotoxic effect is determined in such a way that distinguishes killing or not of both CSCs and more differentiated non-CSC cells.

Finally, according to a classical stem cell hypothesis differentiated non-CSC cells have a limited life span. However, very little is known about molecular mechanisms which can explain the potential limited proliferation capacity of non-stem tumor cells and the ultimate fate of non-stem tumor cells. This may be related to the fact that relatively little research activity has been devoted to non-CSC tumor cells.

It is well known that in cell culture there is always a small fraction of apoptotic cells but where the fraction of dead cells comes from, whatever low it is, is not clear. Is this slow but progressive shedding of differentiated tumor cells? It is possible that these dying 'mature' tumor cells reached the survival limit due to the number of cells divisions. Another interesting point is whether there is a 'Hayflick-like limit' for differentiated tumor cells, if it at all exists? If positive, what is the mechanism of survival limit of tumor cells if it most probably does not depend on telomere-length maintenance? Are CSCs immortal cells?

It should be remembered that molecular mechanism(s) of cell senescence-like process is still active in tumor cells as it can be induced by several different stimuli such as expression of oncogenes, stress conditions or DNA damage (Roninson, 2003). This process resembles replicative senescence but is usually not associated with telomere shortening. Surprisingly, relatively recent studies have shown that human hepatocarcinomas and immortal breast carcinoma cells both *in vitro* and in animal *in vivo* models produce spontaneously senescent progeny (Ozturk et al., 2006). It is not clear which type of cells (i.e. CSCs or non-CSCs) had limited proliferation potential and were able to undergo cellular senescence. Analysis of cell clones generated from single cells of breast carcinoma tumor cell lines *in vitro* showed that within 12 different cells lines tested there were two groups. One group (5 cell lines) produced senescent cells (positive for SA-β-Gal/negative for BrdU incorporation) with high frequency (5-40%) whereas the other group produced less that 5% of senescent cells (Mumcuoglu et al., 2010). Based on these features, the authors classified all breast cell lines studied as senescent cell progenitor (SCP) and immortal cell progenitor (ICP) cell subtypes. Interestingly, ICP cells were much more tumorigenic in immunodeficient mice compared to SCP cell lines. Even more importantly, more tumorigenic ICP cells were deficient in their ability to generate more differentiated progeny, pointing to the fundamental difference between these cell subtypes. It would be extremely interesting to find out whether these two types of cells, with different abilities to produce differentiated progeny and ability to undergo senescence-associated growth arrest, are also present in other tumor types. Equally important would be to establish whether these two types of cell clones correspond to CSC and non-CSC cells.

The presence of senescent cells in tumor cell population have been confirmed by others for prostate, head and neck squamous cell and breast carcinomas (Locke et al., 2005; Li et al., 2008). Molecular mechanism of spontaneous senescence induced in tumor cells was associated with repression of hTERT expression, that led to telomere shortening (Ozturk et al., 2006), therefore, it followed a classical replicative senescence program. These results provide an experimental evidence for the reversibility of cancer cell immortality by repression of telomerase expression. This is probably not surprising considering the fact that expression of telomerase is switched on in most tumor cells and is regulated by a number of different genes, including *SIP1*, *hSIR2*, *c-myc*, *Mad1*, *Menin*, *Rak*, and *Brit1* as well as TGF-β and SMAD pathway (Wang et al., 1998; Verschueren et al., 1999; Lin & Elledge, 2003). Therefore, the epigenetic mechanism responsible for upregulation of hTERT expression and telomerase activity in a majority of tumor cells is potentially reversible and can be turned off again.

4. Resistance of CSCs to anticancer treatment: possible molecular mechanisms

It is well established that a fraction of cells in a tumor frequently survives anticancer treatment when exposed to radiation and cytotoxic drugs. This drug resistant subpopulation of tumor cells may constitute of CSCs, and in this way, these cells may be responsible for the failure of most, if not all, anticancer therapies, as these cells are postulated to be inherently resistant to anticancer agents. Based on that, a new therapeutic strategy has been proposed in which drugs should specifically target CSCs, and this will allow us to eradicate tumors. However, finding of these CSC-specific agents is only possible if we characterize possible mechanisms responsible for resistance of CSCs to anticancer therapy (summarized in Figure 1). Another important question is whether CSCs are resistant to all therapeutic agents or there are drug-specific resistance phenotypes, associated with changes in the functioning of defined intracellular pathways in these cells. Moreover, drug resistance of CSCs may involve several mechanisms and results from changes in different intracellular pathways. It is also not clear if molecular mechanisms responsible for CSC therapeutic resistance are shared across different tumor types.

The most straightforward mechanism that can be responsible for lower activity of anticancer drugs toward CSCs is overexpression of ABC transporters. One of the methods for CSC determination is based on lower stainability of CSC-containing fraction, the so-called SP cells, to fluorescent dye Hoechst 33342 (discussed in section 2 of this chapter). Low fluorescence of SP cells after Hoechst 33342 staining is attributed to overexpression of ABC pumps by CSCs, frequently ABCG2. Since many antitumor drugs are substrates for ABC membrane transporters, this can lead to typical multidrug resistance phenotype of CSCs. It should be noted, however, that Hoechst-based assay for SP fraction may give misleading results. It has been shown that ABCC1-overexpressing cells HL-60/Adr (Marsch et al., 1986) contain more than 90% of SP cells (Patrawala et al., 2005) that is not necessarily associated with increased CSC content.

Up-regulation of ABC transporters is a typical feature of both normal stem cells and CSCs (Patrawala et al., 2005; Nakai et al., 2009; Yamamoto et al., 2009; Angelastro & Lamé, 2010; Jin et al., 2010). However, this can not be a general phenomenon as our results obtained for non-small cell lung carcinoma A549 cells showed that CSCs cells isolated after treatment with anticancer drugs (dexrazoxane, amsacrine) did not overexpress ABC transporters and had unchanged drug sensitivity (Sabisz & Skladanowski, 2009).

It is interesting that overexpression of ABC transporters in stem cells and CSCs correlates with the level of several stem cell markers such as CD133, nestin, CD117 (c-kit) (Yamamoto et al., 2009; Adhikari et al., 2010) or Notch-1 and Nanog (Patrawala et al., 2005; Bourguignon

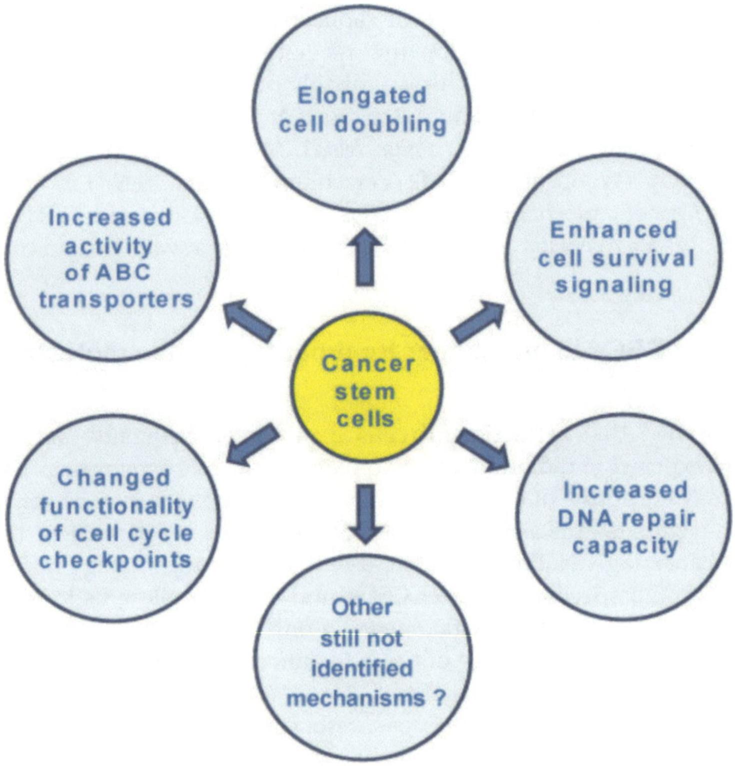

Fig. 1. The proposed mechanisms responsible for drug resistance phenotype of cancer stem cells.

et al., 2008). Inherent overexpression of ABC pumps in these cells is dependent on stem factors such as Oct4, that is present both in embryonic stem cells and CSCs (Wang et al., 2010) and may be induced by anticancer treatment (Nakai et al., 2009). Similarly, interaction between stem cell related transcription regulators STAT1/3 and Nanog leads to activation of STAT1/3 and increased expression of several genes, including ABCB1 transporter (Bourguignon et al., 2008). Given the fact that CSCs frequently overexpress ABC transporters, it is interesting to note that salinomycin, that has been shown to selectively kill mammary carcinoma CSCs (Mani et al., 2008) is the inhibitor of ABCB1 pump (Ricconi et al., 2010).

Alternative drug resistance mechanism of CSCs may be associated with lower proliferation potential of these cells compared to 'committed' non-CSC cells. In this situation, anticancer treatment that targets actively proliferating cells, such as DNA damaging agents, mitotic spindle poisons or antimetabolites, are less effective in killing CSCs than mature 'differentiated' cancer cells. Although this issue has not been systematically studied, several groups reported that CSCs isolated from gastric carcinomas and glioblastomas have either increased (Beier et al., 2008) or elongated (Ropolo M et al., 2009; Ishimoto et al., 2010; Thomas & Cannas, 2010) doubling time compared to a bulk tumor cell population or non-CSC cells. Surprisingly, changes in doubling time are not always associated with differences in the distribution between cell cycle phases (Ropolo M et al., 2009). As discussed above, in hematological malignancies, leukemia stem cells usually do not proliferate.

It is not clear whether longer doubling times are characteristic for CSCs in all types of tumors and if they result from fundamental differences in cell cycle regulation between CSCs and differentiated tumor cells. It should be noted that determination of a doubling time for CSCs and non-CSCs was performed in the artificial situation where these two cell populations grow separately, and this may influence their growth rate. The existence of a possible interaction between CSCs and non-CSC cells and other cells from tumor microenvironment can be concluded based on results obtained in colon carcinoma, glioma and leukemia models (Evers et al., 2010; Raaijmakers et al., 2010; Saito et al., 2010; Vermeulen et al., 2010). Perturbations of mechanism(s) of cross-regulation of cell growth, which potentially exist between CSCs and non-CSCs, may also influence drug sensitivity (see next paragraph).

Another mechanism that can be proposed to explain drug resistance phenotype of CSCs is related to differences between CSCs and non-CSCs in the functionality of cell cycle checkpoints and enhanced repair of drug-induced damage. However, this is controversial as there are contradictory data in the available literature concerning this issue. Defective intra-S checkpoint but intact G2 checkpoints were documented in glioblastoma CD133-positive stem-like cells isolated from patient tumor samples. These cells showed increased sensitivity to irradiation with respect to the standard glioblastoma model, established glioma cell lines (McCord et al., 2009a). Interestingly, when radiosensitivities of CD133-positive and negative cells from glioma cell lines were compared, CD133+ stem-like cells showed radioresistance (McCord et al., 2009a). Other studies have shown that glioma CSCs as well as epithelial cells with stem-like properties, preferentially activate DNA damage response and cell cycle checkpoints after treatment with ionizing irradiation both *in vivo* and *in vitro* and this can be related to their radioresistance (Bao et al., 2006; Facchino et al., 2010; Harper et al., 2010). Molecular mechanism that was responsible for lower sensitivity to irradiation of glioma CSCs involved increased activity of two intra-S and G2 checkpoint kinases, Chk1 and Chk2. Inhibition of these kinases by a selective chemical inhibitor debromohymenialdisine sensitized CSC cells to irradiation (Bao et al., 2006; Harper et al., 2010). Interestingly, increased Chk1 and Chk2 activity was also shown in untreated glioma CSCs (Ropolo et al., 2009), suggesting that enhanced basal activation of checkpoint kinases in $CD133^+$ cells may determine their cell cycle delay and contribute to their radioresistance by allowing more time for DNA repair of damages.

The role of DNA repair in radio- and chemoresistance of CSCs is less clear. In one report, no differences in DNA base excision or single-strand break repair nor in resolution of γ-H2AX nuclear foci were found in radioresistant $CD133^+$ CSCs compared with $CD133^-$ glioma cells (Ropolo et al., 2009). However, earlier study with glioma tumor cells treated with temozolomide showed increased rather than decreased sensitivity of CD133-positive CSCs (Beier et al., 2008). The drug produced essentially no cell death but a prominent growth inhibitory effect was observed specifically for glioma stem cells. In contrast, temozolomide did not inhibit the growth of progenitor and differentiated cells derived from CSC but showed a selective growth inhibitory effect toward glioma CSCs. Temozolomide is the most commonly used chemotherapeutic agent in the treatment of glioblastomas and induces DNA adducts which are repaired by the DNA repair protein O^6-methylguanine-DNA-methyltransferase (MGMT). MGMT is expressed only in a subgroup of glioblastomas since its promoter is frequently methylated in this type of tumor cells (Hegi et al., 2005). Accordingly, temozolomide concentrations required to deplete glioma CD133+ CSCs was substantially higher (about 10-fold) in tumor cells expressing MGMT. However, combination of the drug with the MGMT inhibitor 6-buthylguanine sensitized stem cell-like glioma cells with high MGMT expression to the deleterious effects of temozolomide.

Finally, radio- and chemoresistance of CSCs may be associated with the interplay between DNA damage response induced by anticancer treatment and regulated by the ATM/ATR pathway as well as survival signaling mediated by PI3K/Akt pathway (for recent review see Skladanowski et al., 2009). It was postulated that regulation of DNA damage response induced by irradiation in CSCs follows the classical ATM-dependent mechanism (Facchino et al., 2010; Golding et al., 2009). Furthermore, a specific ATM inhibitor KU-60019 reduced basal activation of Akt by downregulation of its Ser-473 phosphorylation and this led to reduced glioma cell migration and invasion (Golding et al., 2009). In this way, inhibition of DNA damage response by KU-60019 is associated with downregulation of pro-survival signaling mediated by Akt and sensitizes glioma cells to irradiation. The important role of Akt pathway in stemness and invasion but also in response to cancer treatment has been confirmed by others in gliomas (Molina et al., 2010; Wang et al., 2010), but also in lung, colon and mammary carcinomas (Sabisz & Skladanowski, 2009; Wang et al., 2010; Zhang et al., 2010). Interestingly, there may be a cross-talk between at least some stem cell markers, such as CD44, and PI3 kinase/Akt-related survival pathways, can also lead to chemotherapeutic drug resistance, as shown in breast tumor cells (Miletti-González et al., 2005). Collectively, these results raise important therapeutic implications for a concurrent combination of DNA damaging drugs and inhibitors of Akt pathway to target CSCs (Mueller et al., 2009; Sabisz & Skladanowski, 2009; Zhang et al., 2010).

5. Perspectives: can we exploit the CSC paradigm in drug screening?

There is accumulating experimental evidence that CSCs are resistant to standard anticancer therapies. This suggests that screening procedures, in which cytotoxic and antitumor effect induced by antitumor agents is evaluated, should be modified in such a way to select drugs or drug combinations which are able to target CSCs. Current *in vitro* drug screening systems, with the most widely known the NCI 60 cell line model, are based on a relatively short-term drug treatment and continuous drug exposure of tumor cells. The cytotoxic effect is evaluated using different tests which are sensitive to drug-induced changes of tumor cell number and/or viability, using typically the MTT assay (reduction of the MTT stain to formazan), chemiluminescence-based measurements of intracellular ATP content.

Several different experimental approaches were proposed for screening of CSC-specific antitumor agents (see Figure 2). In one of them the standard cytotoxicity assays are performed using CSC populations which are sorted based on the expression of membrane stem markers by e.g. flow cytometry or immunomagnetic cell sorting. The cytotoxic effect toward CSCs is then compared with that induced in non-CSCs. A simpler variant of this methodology is to sort the SP cells as a fraction of cells with high content of CSCs. This method can also be applied to evaluate antitumor effect of drugs *in vivo* using animal models.

Another way of enrichment of tumor cell populations with CSCs is the generation of cell spheres at conditions when the attachment of tumor cells to the substratum is prevented. This could be realized in several different ways, the most typical involves low attachment substrata where cell dishes are covered both by natural (e. g. agar) or synthetic polymers. In a more technically sophisticated approach, magnetic levitation is used where tumor cells are cultivated in hydrogels on magnetic iron oxide nanoparticles, with magnetic-controlled

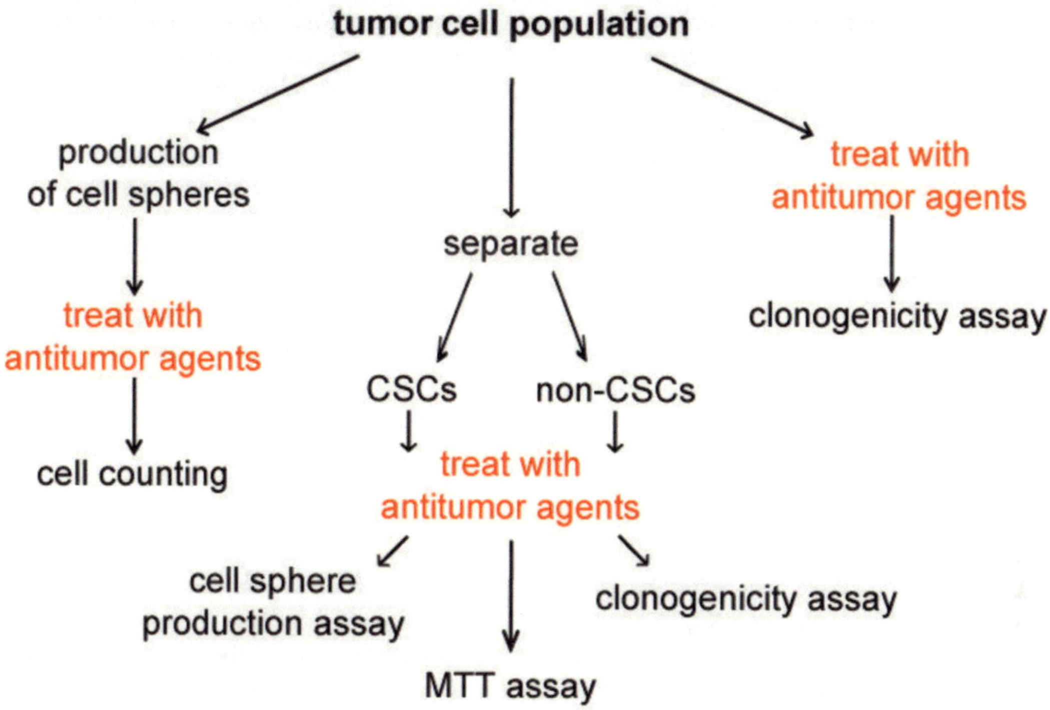

Fig. 2. Currently available strategies which can be used to screen for drugs or drug combinations with selective activity toward cancer stem cells.

levitation system (Souza et al 2010). Interestingly, magnetically levitated human glioblastoma cells showed similar protein expression profiles to those observed in human tumor xenografts (Souza et al 2010). The sphere formation models were used to determine the cytotoxic activity of antitumor drugs of different tumor types, including mammary carcinomas (mammospheres), gliomas (neurospheres) and lung carcinomas (Setoguchi et al., 2004; Patrawala et al., 2005; Levina et al., 2008; Bertolini et al., 2009). It is worth mentioning that the seminal work of Robert Kerbel and his co-workers on drug resistance of tumor cells, associated with what was at this time called the 'social effect' (Kobayashi et al 1993), can be related today to the CSC phenomenon.

Yet another possibility is to treat bulk tumor populations with different antitumor agents and the fraction of tumor cells, which are able to proliferate after drug treatment, is subsequently estimated based on the colony formation ability or production of spheres on low adherent plates by drug-treated tumor cells. The latter approach was successfully applied for lung, breast and ovarian carcinoma cells (Levina et al., 2008, Sabisz & Skladanowski, 2009). In addition, to confirm that cells surviving after drug treatment are truly CSCs, cells may be also analysed for the expression of stem markers.

The features of CSCs that were presented in this chapter suggest that there are two groups of potential problems related to the described above screening assays and possibly other screening methods aimed at the selection of anti-CSC drugs. These problems may potentially makes it very difficult to apply the CSC paradigm in search for new therapeutic strategies to kill CSCs. First group is associated with problems which we call 'technical' such as cell systems used and estimation of the cytotoxic effect of potential drugs toward CSCs.

Classical cytotoxicity assays such as MTT or ATP-based chemoluminescence tests can not be applied in sphere formation systems. In multicellular spheroids, there is a problem with the penetration of biochemical stains used in these assays and mitochondrial activity of cells present inside spheroids is greatly reduced, that underestimates the number of viable cells in spheroids. On the other hand, colony formation assays are difficult to be performed in high throughput systems where drug screening is highly automated and a very small number of cells is used. In this situation, results may be irreproducible and experimental errors may be exceedingly high. As for cell systems used to screen for anti-CSC drugs, it should be borne in mind that cell spheres are not always enriched in CSCs (Gasparini et al., 2010). In addition, there are no generally accepted stem markers of CSC that makes it very difficult to reliably separate these cells from non-CSCs very difficult (discussed in section 2 of this chapter). In addition, expression of some stem markers may be functionally inter-related and downregulation of marker 1 expression may lead to increased/decreased expression of marker 2. This kind inter-relationship in membrane marker expression has been shown in breast carcinoma cells for β1 integrin and EGFR (Wang et al 1998).

Cell growth conditions used to cultivate CSCs to be used in drug screening may also be problematic. Typical growth media containing serum may change cancer stem cell phenotype and their characteristic gene expression profile. It has been shown that maintenance of glioblastoma CSCs in media with defined growth factors such as β–FGF and EGF (stem conditions) preserve more closely stem-like phenotype of these cells but serum (differentiation conditions) induces irreversible cell differentiation (Lee et al 2006). Similarly, oxygen concentration in cell culture may be critical for the preservation of the CSC phenotype. It has been shown that the SP fraction in tumor cell population *in vivo* is increased in hypoxic regions (Das et al 2008). This effect was reproduced with the same cell system by exposure of cultured cells *in vitro* to hypoxia. The authors propose that a highly tumorigenic SP cells migrate to the area of hypoxia that may serve as a niche for the highly tumorigenic fraction of SP cells and can be induced *in vitro*. Moreover, increasing evidence suggest that hypoxia has the potential to inhibit tumor cell differentiation that leads to increased fraction of CSCs in hypoxic regions that results result in accelerated the initiation and growth of tumors (Calabrese et al 2008). An elegant study has shown that growing CD133(+) cells sorted from three GB neurosphere cultures at 7% oxygen reduced their doubling time and increased the self-renewal potential as reflected by clonogenicity (McCord et al., 2009b). Furthermore, at 7% oxygen, the cultures exhibited an enhanced capacity to differentiate along both the glial and neuronal pathways. As compared with 20%, growth at 7% oxygen resulted in an increase in the expression levels of the neural stem cell markers CD133 and nestin as well as the stem cell markers Oct4 and Sox2 (McCord et al., 2009b). Collectively, these reports point to still greatly underestimated role of hypoxia in the maintenance of the CSC properties.

Another group of problems is related to our current understanding of the CSC paradigm. It seems that the most fundamental question is whether a tumor develops from a homogenous but scarce population of CSCs, as the classical hypothesis of cancer stem cells proposes. In this case, it makes very much sense to search for the Achille's heel of such a population and use it as a drug target for selective killing of CSCs. However, an emerging picture is that CSCs do not constitute a homogenous population of cells, with defined molecular markers and cell features, as it is still widely believed. There is also accumulating evidence that the phenotype of CSCs is not stable and, at least in some situations, is reversible. In addition, differences between CSCs and 'mature' tumor non-CSC cells are frequently only quantitative not qualitative, and result from stochastic rather than deterministic processes. Drug selectivity can be a difficult problem to resolve in anti-CSCs therapies. All the already characterized drug resistance mechanisms, which are active in CSCs and responsible for their drug resistance phenotype, operate in tumor cells in general, others are characteristic for normal stem cells. For all these reasons, selection of new therapeutic approaches that specifically target CSCs is a particularly challenging task. To achieve this goal, it is important to define optimal therapeutic targets in CSC sub-populations as well as to implement the improved drug screening systems.

In our opinion a modern and more effective antitumor therapy should include both CSC and non-CSC drugs, ideally targeting both cell populations with high efficacy. Therapeutic eradication of CSCs by their selective targeting with antitumor drugs may be a very dangerous therapeutic approach for several reasons. First, paradoxically many available literature data suggest that very selective antitumor drugs frequently are not efficacious in the clinical practice. Second, we still do not know how many cell generations are required for a tumor to degenerate, as a result of CSC depletion. It is possible that by targeting only CSCs the remaining non-CSCs may well kill the patient before a tumor disappears. In addition to that, although formally non-CSC tumor cells are more sensitive to anticancer agents, so they should not survive drug treatment, there is still a possibility that drugs can initiate cellular processes leading to trans-differentiation of non-CSC to CSC phenotype (de-polyploidization, EMT etc.).

Together, more detailed fundamental knowledge is still required about molecular mechanisms responsible for CSC formation, both inherent and therapy-induced, and CSC phenotype in general. Only after understanding these mechanisms will it be possible to find new anticancer treatment modalities which will be able to kill or arrest CSC growth by inhibiting critical intracellular pathways associated with stemness or CSC differentiation or both.

6. Disclosure statement

The authors are not aware of any biases that might affect the objectivity of this review.

7. References

Angelastro, J.M.; Lamé MW. (2010). Overexpression of CD133 promotes drug resistance in C6 glioma cells. *Molecular Cancer Research*, 8, 8, 1105-1115.

Adhikari, A.S.; Agarwal, N.; Wood, B.M.; Porretta, C.; Ruiz, B.; Pochampally, R.R.; Iwakuma, T. (2010). CD117 and Stro-1 identify osteosarcoma tumor-initiating cells associated with metastasis and drug resistance. *Cancer Research*, 70, 11, 4602-4612.

Baker, M. (2008). Melanoma in mice casts doubt on scarcity of cancer stem cells. *Nature*, 456, 7222, 553.

Banito, A.; Rashid, S.T.; Acosta, J.C.; Li, S.; Pereira, C.F.; Geti, I.; Pinho, S.; Silva, J.C.; Azuara, V.; Walsh, M.; Vallier, L.; Gil, J. (2009). Senescence impairs successful reprogramming to pluripotent stem cells. *Genes & Development*, 23, 18, 2134-2139.

Bao, S.; Wu, Q.; McLendon, R.E.; Hao, Y.; Shi, Q.; Hjelmeland, A.B.; Dewhirst, M.W.; Bigner, D.D.; Rich, J.N. (2006). Glioma stem cells promote radioresistance by preferential activation of the DNA damage response. *Nature*, 444, 7120, 756-760.

Beier, D.; Hau, P.; Proescholdt, M.; Lohmeier, A.; Wischhusen, J.; Oefner, P.J.; Aigner, L.; Brawanski, A.; Bogdahn, U.; Beier, C.P. (2007). CD133(+) and CD133(-) glioblastoma-derived cancer stem cells show differential growth characteristics and molecular profiles. *Cancer Research*, 67, 9, 4010-4015.

Beier, D.; Röhrl, S.; Pillai, D.R.; Schwarz, S.; Kunz-Schughart, L.A.; Leukel, P.; Proescholdt, M.; Brawanski, A.; Bogdahn, U.; Trampe-Kieslich, A.; Giebel, B.; Wischhusen, J.; Reifenberger, G.; Hau, P.; Beier, C.P. (2008). Temozolomide preferentially depletes cancer stem cells in glioblastoma. *Cancer Research*, 68, 14, 5706 -5715.

Bertolini, G.; Roz, L.; Perego, P.; Tortoreto, M.; Fontanella, E.; Gatti, L.; Pratesi, G.; Fabbri, A.; Andriani, F.; Tinelli, S.; Roz, E.; Caserini, R.; Lo Vullo, S.; Camerini, T.; Mariani, L.; Delia, D.; Calabrò, E.; Pastorino, U.; Sozzi, G. (2009). Highly tumorigenic lung cancer CD133+ cells display stem-like features and are spared by cisplatin treatment. *Proceedings of the National Academy of Sciences USA*, 106, 38, 16281-16286.

Bourguignon, L.Y.; Peyrollier, K.; Xia, W.; Gilad, E. (2008). Hyaluronan-CD44 interaction activates stem cell marker Nanog, Stat-3-mediated MDR1 gene expression, and ankyrin-regulated multidrug efflux in breast and ovarian tumor cells. *The Journal of Biological Chemistry*, 283, 25, 17635-17651.

Blagosklonny, M.V. (2005). Why therapeutic response may not prolong the life of a cancer patient: selection for oncogenic resistance. *Cell Cycle*, 4, 12, 1693–1698.

Breitman, T.R.; He, R.Y. (1990). Combinations of retinoic acid with either sodium butyrate, dimethyl sulfoxide, or hexamethylene bisacetamide synergistically induce differentiation of the human myeloid leukemia cell line HL60. *Cancer Research*, 50, 19, 6268-6273.

Bruce, W.R.; Van Der Gaag, H. (1963). A quantitative assay for the number of murine lymphoma cells capable of proliferation in vivo. *Nature*, 199, 4888, 79–80.

Chakrabarty, S. (1992). Regulation of human colon-carcinoma cell adhesion to extracellular matrix by transforming growth factor beta 1. *International Journal of Cancer*, 50, 6, 968–973.

Chen, R.; Nishimura, M.C.; Bumbaca, S.M.; Kharbanda, S.; Forrest, W.F.; Kasman, I.M.; Greve, J.M.; Soriano, R.H.; Gilmour, L.L.; Rivers, C.S.; Modrusan, Z.; Nacu, S.; Guerrero, S.; Edgar, K.A.; Wallin, J.J.; Lamszus, K.; Westphal, M.; Heim, S.; James, C.D.; VandenBerg, S.R.; Costello, J.F.; Moorefield, S.; Cowdrey, C.J.; Prados, M.; Phillips, H.S. (2010). A hierarchy of self-renewing tumor-initiating cell types in glioblastoma. *Cancer Cell*, 17, 4, 362-375.

Choi, S.R.; Cho, M.; Kim, H.R.; Ahn, D.H.; Sleisenger, M.H.; Kim, Y.S. (2000). Biological properties and expression of mucins in 5-fluorouracil resistant HT29 human colon cancer cells. *International Journal of Oncology*, 17, 1, 141–147.

Das, B.; Tsuchida, R.; Malkin, D.; Koren, G.; Baruchel, S.; Yeger, H. (2008). Hypoxia enhances tumor stemness by increasing the invasive and tumorigenic side population fraction. *Stem Cells*, 26, 7, 1818-1830.

Demers MJ, Thibodeau S, Noël D, Fujita N, Tsuruo T, Gauthier R, Arguin M, Vachon PH. (2009). Intestinal epithelial cancer cell anoikis resistance: EGFR-mediated sustained activation of Src overrides Fak-dependent signaling to MEK/Erk and/or PI3-K/Akt-1. *Journal of Cellular Biochemistry*, 107, 4, 639–654.

Dittfeld, C.; Dietrich, A.; Peickert, S.; Hering, S.; Baumann, M.; Grade, M.; Ried, T.; Kunz-Schughart, L.A. (2009). CD133 expression is not selective for tumor-initiating or radioresistant cell populations in the CRC cell lines HCT-116. *Radiotherapy & Oncology*, 92, 3, 353-361.

Dittmar, T.; Nagler, C.; Schwitalla, S.; Reith, G.; Niggemann, B.; Zänker, K.S. (2009). Recurrence cancer stem cells--made by cell fusion? *Medical Hypotheses*, 73, 4, 542-57.

Erenpreisa, J.; Cragg, M.S. (2010). MOS, aneuploidy and the ploidy cycle of cancer cells. *Oncogene*, [Epub ahead of print]

Essers, M.A.; Trumpp, A. (2010). Targeting leukemic stem cells by breaking their dormancy. *Molecular Oncology*, [Epub ahead of print]

Evers, P.; Lee, P.P.; DeMarco, J.; Agazaryan, N.; Sayre, J.W.; Selch, M.; Pajonk, F. (2010). Irradiation of the potential cancer stem cell niches in the adult brain improves progression-free survival of patients with malignant glioma. *BMC Cancer*, 21, 10, 384.

Facchino, S.; Abdouh, M.; Chatoo, W.; Bernier, G. (2010). BMI1 confers radioresistance to normal and cancerous neural stem cells through recruitment of the DNA damage response machinery. *Journal of Neuroscience*, 30, 30, 10096-10111.

Gasparini, P.; Bertolini, G.; Binda, M.; Magnifico, A.; Albano, L.; Tortoreto, M.; Pratesi, G.; Facchinetti, F.; Abolafio, G.; Roz, L.; Tagliabue, E.; Daidone, M.G.; Sozzi, G. (2010). Molecular cytogenetic characterization of stem-like cancer cells isolated from established cell lines. *Cancer Letters*, 296, 2, 206-215.

Golding, S.E.; Rosenberg, E.; Valerie, N.; Hussaini, I.; Frigerio, M.; Cockcroft, X.F.; Chong, W.Y.; Hummersone, M.; Rigoreau, L.; Menear, K.A.; O'Connor, M.J.; Povirk, L.F.; van Meter, T.; Valerie, K. (2009). Improved ATM kinase inhibitor KU-60019 radiosensitizes glioma cells, compromises insulin, AKT and ERK prosurvival signaling, and inhibits migration and invasion. *Molecular Cancer Therapeutics*, 8, 10, 2894-2902.

Guilbaud, N.F.; Gas, N.; Dupont, M.A.; Valette, A. (1990). Effects of differentiation-inducing agents on maturation of human MCF-7 breast cancer cells. *Journal of Cell Physiology*, 145, 1, 162-172.

Gupta, P.B.; Onder, T.T.; Jiang, G.; Tao, K.; Kuperwasser, C.; Weinberg, R.A.; Lander, E.S. (2009). Identification of selective inhibitors of cancer stem cells by high-throughput screening. *Cell*, 138, 4, 645-659.

Hamburger, A.W.; Salmon, S.E. (1977). Primary bioassay of human tumor stem cells. *Science* 197, 4302, 461–463.

Harper, L.J.; Costea, D.E.; Gammon, L.; Fazil, B.; Biddle, A.; Mackenzie, I.C. (2010). Normal and malignant epithelial cells with stem-like properties have an extended G2 cell cycle phase that is associated with apoptotic resistance. *BMC Cancer*, 28, 10, 166.

Hirschmann-Jax, C.; Foster, A.E.; Wulf, G.G.; Nuchtern, J.G.; Jax, T.W.; Gobel, U.; Goodell, M.A.; Brenner, M.K. (2004). A distinct "side population" of cells with high drug efflux capacity in human tumor cells. *Proceedings of the National Academy of Sciences USA*, 101, 39, 14228-14233.

Hochedlinger, K.; Blelloch, R.; Brennan, C.; Yamada, Y.; Kim, M.; Chin, L.; Jaenisch, R. (2004). Reprogramming of a melanoma genome by nuclear transplantation. *Genes & Development*, 18, 15, 1875-1885.

Hong, D.; Gupta, R.; Ancliff, P.; Atzberger, A.; Brown, J.; Soneji, S.; Green, J.; Colman, S.; Piacibello, W.; Buckle, V.; Tsuzuki, S.; Greaves, M.; Enver, T. (2008). Initiating and cancer-propagating cells in TEL-AML1-associated childhood leukemia. *Science*, 319, 5861, 336–339.

Ishimoto, T.; Oshima, H.; Oshima, M.; Kai, K.; Torii, R.; Masuko, T.; Baba, H.; Saya, H.; Nagano, O. (2010). CD44+ slow-cycling tumor cell expansion is triggered by cooperative actions of Wnt and prostaglandin E2 in gastric tumorigenesis. *Cancer Science*, 101, 3, 673-678.

Jin, F.; Zhao, L.; Guo, Y.J.; Zhao, W.J.; Zhang, H.; Wang, H.T.; Shao, T.; Zhang, S.L.; Wei, Y.J.; Feng, J.; Jiang, X.B.; Zhao, H.Y. (2010). Influence of etoposide on anti-apoptotic and multidrug resistance-associated protein genes in CD133 positive U251 glioblastoma stem-like cells. *Brain Research*, 1336, 103-111.

Kai, K.; Nagano, O.; Sugihara, E.; Arima, Y.; Sampetrean, O.; Ishimoto, T.; Nakanishi, M.; Ueno, N.T.; Iwase, H.; Saya, H. (2009). Maintenance of HCT116 colon cancer cell line conforms to a stochastic model but not a cancer stem cell model. *Cancer Science*, 100, 12, 2275-2282.

Kelly, P.N.; Dakic, A.; Adams, J.M.; Nutt, S.L.; Strasser, A. (2007). Tumor growth need not be driven by rare cancer stem cells. *Science*, 317, 5836, 337.

Kobayashi, H.; Man, S.; Graham, C.H.; Kapitain, S.J.; Teicher, B.A.; Kerbel, R.S. (1993). Acquired multicellular-mediated resistance to alkylating agents in cancer. *Proceedings of the National Academy of Sciences USA*, 90, 8, 3294-3298.

Kulesa, P.M.; Kasemeier, J.C.; Teddy, J.M.; Margaryan, N.V.; Seftor, E.A.; Seftor, R.E.; Hendrix, M.J. (2006). Reprogramming metastatic melanoma cells to assume a neural crest-like phenotype in an embryonic microenvironment. *Proceedings of the National Academy of Sciences USA*, 103, 10, 3752–3757.

Lee, J.; Kotliarova, S.; Kotliarov, Y.; Li, A.; Su, Q.; Donin, N.M.; Pastorino, S.; Purow, B.W.; Christopher, N.; Zhang, W.; Park, J.K.; Fine, H.A. (2006). Tumor stem cells derived from glioblastomas cultured in bFGF and EGF more closely mirror the phenotype and genotype of primary tumors than do serum-cultured cell lines. *Cancer Cell*, 9, 5, 391-403.

Levina, V.; Marrangoni, A.M.; DeMarco, R.; Gorelik, E.; Lokshin, A.E. (2008). Drug-selected human lung cancer stem cells: cytokine network, tumorigenic and metastatic properties. *PLoS One*, 3, 8, e3077.

Levina, V.; Marrangoni, A.; Wang, T.; Parikh, S.; Su, Y.; Herberman, R.; Lokshin, A.; Gorelik, E. (2010). Elimination of human lung cancer stem cells through targeting of the stem cell factor-c-kit autocrine signaling loop. *Cancer Research*, 70, 1, 338-346.

Li, H.; Chen, X.; Calhoun-Davis, T.; Claypool, K.; Tang, D.G. (2008). PC3 human prostate carcinoma cell holoclones contain self-renewing tumor-initiating cells. *Cancer Research*, 68, 6, 1820-1825.

Li, H.; Collado, M.; Villasante, A.; Strati, K.; Ortega, S.; Cañamero, M.; Blasco, M.A.; Serrano, M. (2009). The Ink4/Arf locus is a barrier for iPS cell reprogramming. *Nature*, 460, 7259, 1136-1139.

Lin, S.Y.; Elledge, S.J. (2003). Multiple tumor suppressor pathways negatively regulate telomerase. *Cell*, 113, 7, 881-889.

Locke, M.; Heywood, M.; Fawell, S.; Mackenzie, I.C. (2005) Retention of intrinsic stem cell hierarchies in carcinoma-derived cell lines. *Cancer Research*, 65, 19, 8944 -8950.

Mani, S.A.; Guo, W.; Liao, M.J.; Eaton, E.N.; Ayyanan, A.; Zhou, A.Y.; Brooks, M.; Reinhard, F.; Zhang, C.C.; Shipitsin, M.; Campbell, L.L.; Polyak, K.; Brisken, C.; Yang, J.; Weinberg, R.A. (2008). The epithelial-mesenchymal transition generates cells with properties of stem cells. *Cell*, 133, 4, 704-715.

Marian, C.O.; Cho, S.K.; Hatanpaa, K.J.; Wright, W.E.; Maher, E.; Madden, C.; Mickey, B.; Yang, X.-L.; Shay, J.W.; Bachoo, R. (2010). The telomerase antagonist, imetelstat, efficiently targets glioblastoma tumor-initiating cells leading to decreased proliferation and tumor growth. *Clinical Cancer Research*, 16, 1, 154–163.

Marian, C.O.; Wright, W.E.; Shay, J.W. (2010). The effect of telomerase inhibition on prostate tumor-initiating cells. *International Journal of Cancer*, 127, 2, 321–331.

Marsh, W.; Sicheri, D.; Center, M.S. (1986). Isolation and characterization of adriamycin-resistant HL-60 cells which are not defective in the initial intracellular accumulation of drug. *Cancer Research*, 46, 8, 4053-4057.

Meng, X.; Li, M.; Wang, X.; Wang, Y.; Ma, D. (2009). Both CD133+ and CD133- subpopulations of A549 and H446 cells contain cancer-initiating cells. *Cancer Science*, 100, 6, 1040-1046.

Meng, X.; Wang, X.; Wang, Y. (2009). More than 45% of A549 and H446 cells are cancer initiating cells: evidence from cloning and tumorigenic analyses. *Oncology Reports*, 21, 4, 995-1000.

McCord, A.M.; Jamal, M.; Williams, E.S.; Camphausen, K.; Tofilon, P.J. (2009). CD133+ glioblastoma stem-like cells are radiosensitive with a defective DNA damage response compared with established cell lines. *Clinical Cancer Research*, 15, 16, 5145-5153

McCord, A.M.; Jamal, M.; Shankavaram, U.T.; Lang, F.F.; Camphausen, K.; Tofilon, P.J. (2009). Physiologic oxygen concentration enhances the stem-like properties of CD133+ human glioblastoma cells in vitro. *Molecular Cancer Research*, 7, 4, 489-497.

Molina, J.R.; Hayashi, Y.; Stephens, C.; Georgescu, M.M. (2010). Invasive glioblastoma cells acquire stemness and increased Akt activation. *Neoplasia*, 12, 6, 453-463.

Morel, A.P.; Lièvre, M.; Thomas, C.; Hinkal, G.; Ansieau, S.; Puisieux, A. (2008). Generation of breast cancer stem cells through epithelial-mesenchymal transition. *PLoS One*, 3, 8, e2888.

Mueller, M.T.; Hermann, P.C.; Witthauer, J.; Rubio-Viqueira, B.; Leicht, S.F.; Huber, S.; Ellwart, J.W.; Mustafa, M.; Bartenstein, P.; D'Haese, J.G.; Schoenberg, M.H.; Berger, F.; Jauch, K.W.; Hidalgo, M.; Heeschen, C. (2009). Combined targeted treatment to eliminate tumorigenic cancer stem cells in human pancreatic cancer. *Gastroenterology*, 137, 3, 1102-1113.

Mumcuoglu, M.; Bagislar, S.; Yuzugullu, H.; Alotaibi, H.; Senturk, S.; Telkoparan, P.; Gur-Dedeoglu, B.; Cingoz, B.; Bozkurt, B.; Tazebay, U.H.; Yulug, I.G.; Akcali, K.C.; Ozturk, M. (2010). The ability to generate senescent progeny as a mechanism underlying breast cancer cell heterogeneity. *PLoS One*, 5, 6, e11288.

Nakai, E.; Park, K.; Yawata, T.; Chihara, T.; Kumazawa, A.; Nakabayashi, H.; Shimizu, K. (2009). Enhanced MDR1 expression and chemoresistance of cancer stem cells derived from glioblastoma. *Cancer Investigations,* 27, 9, 901-908.

Ozturk, N.; Erdal, E.; Mumcuoglu, M.; Akcali, K.C.; Yalcin, O.; Senturk, S.; Arslan-Ergul, A.; Gur, B.; Yulug, I.; Cetin-Atalay, R.; Yakicier, C.; Yagci, T.; Tez, M.; Ozturk, M. (2006). Reprogramming of replicative senescence in hepatocellular carcinoma-derived cells. *Proceedings of the National Academy of Sciences USA,* 103, 7, 2178-2183.

Quintana, E.; Shackleton, M.; Sabel, M.S.; Fullen, D.R.; Johnson, T.M.; Morrison, S.J. (2008). Efficient tumour formation by single human melanoma cells. *Nature,* 456, 7222, 593-598.

Pardal, R.; Clarke, M.F.; Morrison, S.J. (2003). Applying the principles of stem-cell biology to cancer. *Nature Reviews on Cancer,* 3, 12, 895-902.

Patrawala, L.; Calhoun, T.; Schneider-Broussard, R.; Zhou, J.; Claypool, K.; Tang, D.G. (2005). Side population is enriched in tumorigenic, stem-like cancer cells, whereas ABCG2+ and ABCG2- cancer cells are similarly tumorigenic. *Cancer Research,* 65, 14, 6207-6219.

Pralong, D.; Trounson, A.O.; Verma, P.J. (2006). Cell fusion for reprogramming pluripotency: toward elimination of the pluripotent genome. *Stem Cell Reviews,* 2, 4, 331-340.

Raaijmakers, M.H.; Mukherjee, S.; Guo, S.; Zhang, S.; Kobayashi, T.; Schoonmaker, J.A.; Ebert, B.L.; Al-Shahrour, F.; Hasserjian, R.P.; Scadden, E.O.; Aung, Z.; Matza, M.; Merkenschlager, M.; Lin, C.; Rommens, J.M.; Scadden, D.T. (2010). Bone progenitor dysfunction induces myelodysplasia and secondary leukaemia. *Nature,* 464, 7290, 852-857.

Reya, T.; Morrison, S.J.; Clarke, M.F.; Weissman, I.L. (2001). Stem cells, cancer, and cancer stem cells. *Nature,* 414, 6859, 105-111.

Riccioni, R.; Dupuis, M.L.; Bernabei, M.; Petrucci, E.; Pasquini, L.; Mariani, G.; Cianfriglia, M.; Testa, U. (2010). The cancer stem cell selective inhibitor salinomycin is a p-glycoprotein inhibitor. *Blood Cells, Molecules and Diseases,* 45, 1, 86-92.

Rizvi, A.Z.; Swain, J.R.; Davies, P.S.; Bailey, A.S.; Decker, A.D.; Willenbring, H.; Grompe, M.; Fleming, W.H.; Wong, M.H. (2006). Bone marrow-derived cells fuse with normal and transformed intestinal stem cells. *Proceedings of the National Academy of Sciences USA,* 103, 16, 6321-6315.

Ron-Bigger, S.; Bar-Nur, O.; Isaac, S.; Bocker, M.; Lyko, F.; Eden, A. (2010). Aberrant epigenetic silencing of tumor suppressor genes is reversed by direct reprogramming. *Stem Cells,* [Epub ahead of print]

Roninson, I.B. (2003). Tumor cell senescence in cancer treatment. *Cancer Research,* 63, 11, 2705-2715.

Ropolo, M.; Daga, A.; Griffero, F.; Foresta, M.; Casartelli, G.; Zunino, A.; Poggi, A.; Cappelli, E.; Zona, G.; Spaziante, R.; Corte, G.; Frosina G. (2009). Comparative analysis of DNA repair in stem and nonstem glioma cell cultures. *Molecular Cancer Research,* 7, 3, 383-392.

Sabisz, M.; Skladanowski, A. (2009). Cancer stem cells and escape from drug-induced premature senescence in human lung tumor cells: implications for drug resistance and in vitro drug screening models. *Cell Cycle,* 8, 19, 3208-3217.

Saito, Y.; Kitamura, H.; Hijikata, A.; Tomizawa-Murasawa, M.; Tanaka, S.; Takagi, S.; Uchida, N.; Suzuki, N.; Sone, A.; Najima, Y.; Ozawa, H.; Wake, A.; Taniguchi, S.; Shultz, L.D.; Ohara, O.; Ishikawa, F. (2010). Identification of therapeutic targets for quiescent, chemotherapy-resistant human leukemia stem cells. *Science Translational Medicine,* 2, 17, 17ra9.

Salmina, K.; Jankevics, E.; Huna, A.; Perminov, D.; Radovica, I.; Klymenko, T.; Ivanov, A.; Jascenko, E.; Scherthan, H.; Cragg, M.; Erenpreisa, J. (2010). Up-regulation of the embryonic self-renewal network through reversible polyploidy in irradiated p53-mutant tumour cells. *Experimental Cell Research,* 316, 13, 2099-2112.

Santisteban, M.; Reiman, J.M.; Asiedu, M,K,.; Behrens, M.D.; Nassar, A.; Kalli, K.R.; Haluska, P.; Ingle, J.N.; Hartmann, L.C.; Manjili, M.H.; Radisky, D.C.; Ferrone, S.; Knutson, K.L. (2009). Immune-induced epithelial to mesenchymal transition in vivo generates breast cancer stem cells. *Cancer Research*, 69, 7, 2887-2895.

Setoguchi, T.; Taga, T.; Kondo, T. (2004). Cancer stem cells persist in many cancer cell lines. *Cell Cycle*, 3, 4, 414-15.

Shen, G.; Shen, F.; Shi, Z.; Liu, W.; Hu, W.; Zheng, X.; Wen, L.; Yang, X. (2008). Identification of cancer stem-like cells in the C6 glioma cell line and the limitation of current identification methods. *In Vitro Cellular and Developmental Biology - Animal*, 44, 7, 280-9.

Souza, G.R.; Molina, J.R.; Raphael, R.M.; Ozawa, M.G.; Stark, D.J.; Levin, C.S.; Bronk, L.F.; Ananta, J.S.; Mandelin, J.; Georgescu, M.M.; Bankson, J.A.; Gelovani, J.G.; Killian, T.C.; Arap, W.; Pasqualini, R. (2010). Three-dimensional tissue culture based on magnetic cell levitation. *Nature Nanotechnology*, 5, 4, 291-296.

Skladanowski, A.; Bozko, P.; Sabisz, M. (2009). DNA structure and integrity checkpoints during the cell cycle and their role in drug targeting and sensitivity of tumor cells to anticancer treatment. *Chemical Reviews*, 109, 7, 2951-2973.

Soddu, S.; Blandino, G.; Citro, G.; Scardigli, R.; Piaggio, G.; Ferber, A.; Calabretta, B.; Sacchi, A. (1994). Wild-type p53 gene expression induces granulocytic differentiation of HL-60 cells. *Blood*, 83, 8, 2230-2237.

Sussman, R.T.; Ricci, M.S.; Hart, L.S.; Sun, S.Y.; El-Deiry, W.S. (2007) Chemotherapy-resistant side-population of colon cancer cells has a higher sensitivity to TRAIL than the non-SP, a higher expression of c-Myc and TRAIL-receptor DR4. *Cancer Biology & Therapy*, 6, 9, 1490-1495.

Tilkorn, D.J.; Lokmic, Z.; Chaffer, C.L.; Mitchell, G.M.; Morrison, W.A.; Thompson, E.W. (2010). Disparate companions: tissue engineering meets cancer research. *Cells Tissues & Organs*, 192, 3, 141-157.

Thomas, X.; Cannas, G. (2010). Leukemia stem cells and new strategies to overcome resistance to therapy. *Current Stem Cell Research and Therapy*, 5, 3, 277-286.

Vakifahmetoglu, H.; Olsson, M.; Zhivotovsky, B. (2008). Death through a tragedy: mitotic catastrophe. *Cell Death & Differentiation*, 15, 7, 1153-1162.

Vermeulen, L.; De Sousa, E.; Melo, F.; van der Heijden, M.; Cameron, K.; de Jong, J.H.; Borovski, T.; Tuynman, J.B.; Todaro, M.; Merz, C.; Rodermond, H.; Sprick, M.R.; Kemper, K.; Richel, D.J.; Stassi, G.; Medema, J.P. (2010). Wnt activity defines colon cancer stem cells and is regulated by the microenvironment. *Nature Cell Biology*, 12, 5, 468-476.

Verschueren, K.; Remacle, J.E.; Collart, C.; Kraft, H.; Baker, B.S.; Tylzanowski, P.; Nelles, L.; Wuytens, G.; Su, M.T.; Bodmer, R.; Smith, J.C.; Huylebroeck, D. (1999). SIP1, a novel zinc finger/homeodomain repressor, interacts with Smad proteins and binds to 5'-CACCT sequences in candidate target genes. *The Journal of Biological Chemistry,* 274, 29, 20489-2098.

Wang, F.; Weaver, V.M.; Petersen, O.W.; Larabell, C.A.; Dedhar, S.; Briand, P.; Lupu, R.; Bissell, M.J. (1998). Reciprocal interactions between beta1-integrin and epidermal growth factor receptor in three-dimensional basement membrane breast cultures: a different perspective in epithelial biology. *Proceedings of the National Academy of Sciences USA,* 95, 25, 14821-14826.

Wang, J.; Xie, L.Y.; Allan, S.; Beach, D.; Hannon, G.J. (1998). Myc activates telomerase. *Genes & Development,* 12, 12, 1769-1774.

Wang, X.Q.; Ongkeko, W.M.; Chen, L.; Yang, Z.F.; Lu, P.; Chen, K.K.; Lopez, J.P.; Poon, R.T.; Fan, S.T. (2010). Octamer 4 (Oct4) mediates chemotherapeutic drug resistance in liver cancer cells through a potential Oct4-AKT-ATP-binding cassette G2 pathway. *Hepatology,* 52, 2, 528-539.

Wang, Y.K.l; Zhu, Y.L.; Qiu, F.M.; Zhang, T.; Chen, Z.G.; Zheng, S.; Huang, J. (2010) Activation of Akt and MAPK pathways enhances the tumorigenicity of CD133+ primary colon cancer cells. *Carcinogenesis,* 31, 8, 1376-1380.

Wasserman, L.; Nordenberg, J.; Beery, E.; Deutsch, A.A.; Novogrodsky, A. (1987). Differential effects of sodium butyrate and dimethylsulfoxide on gamma-glutamyl transpeptidase and alkaline phosphatase activities in MCF-7 breast cancer cells. *Experimental Cell Biology,* 55, 4, 188-193.

Wicha, M.S.; Liu, S.; Dontu, G. (2006). Cancer stem cells: an old idea--a paradigm shift. *Cancer Research,* 66, 4, 1883-1890.

Yamamoto, A.; Shofuda, T.; Islam, M.O.; Nakamura, Y.; Yamasaki, M.; Okano, H.; Kanemura, Y. (2009). ABCB1 is predominantly expressed in human fetal neural stem/progenitor cells at an early development stage. *J Neuroscience Research, 87,* 12, 2615-2623.

Yamanaka, S.; Blau, H.M. (2010). Nuclear reprogramming to a pluripotent state by three approaches. *Nature,* 465, 7299, 704-712.

Yeung, T.M.; Gandhi, S.C.; Wilding, J.L.; Muschel, R.; Bodmer, W.F. (2010). Cancer stem cells from colorectal cancer-derived cell lines. *Proceedings of the National Academy of Sciences USA,* 107, 8, 3722-3727.

Ying, Q-L.;Wray, J.; Nichols, J.; Batlle-Morera, L.; Doble, B, Woodgett J, Cohen P, Smith A. (2008). The ground state of embryonic stem cell self-renewal. *Nature,* 453, 7194, 519–523

Qian, Y.; Drewe, J.A.; Shi, J.; McClurg, M.; Li, W.; Campbell, T.N. Tumorase™: *In vivo* efficacy data for novel localized proteinase treatment applicable to solid tumors of varied tissue origins, *Proceedings of the American Association for Cancer Research,* Washington DC, April, 2010, Cadmus Publishing, Richmond VA.

Zhang, M.; Atkinson, R.L.; Rosen, J.M. (2010). Selective targeting of radiation-resistant tumor-initiating cells. *Proceedings of the National Academy of Sciences USA,* 107, 8, 3522-3527.

Zheng, X.; Shen, G.; Yang, X.; Liu, W. (2007). Most C6 cells are cancer stem cells: evidence from clonal and population analyses. *Cancer Research,* 67, 8, 3691-3697.

Acronyms and Abbreviations

5-FU: 5-fluorocytosine
5α-R: 5α-reductase;
AAs: anaplastic astrocytomas
ABC transporters: Adenosine triphosphate-binding cassette
ACTH: adrenocorticotropic hormone;
ADC: adenocarcinoma
AKT: subfamily of the serine/threonine protein kinases
ALDH: aldehyde dehydrogenase
ALL: acute lymphoblastic leukemia
AML: acute myelogenous leukemia
Ang1: angiopoietin-1
antagomiR: anti-miRNA oligonucleotide
APC: antigen presenting cell
APC: adenomatous poliposys coli
AR: androgen receptor
ASC: adult stem cells (see OSC)
ASCL1: achaete-scute complex homolog 1
ATM/ATR: ataxia telangiectasia mutated/AT Rad3-related
BAA: BODIPY-aminoacetate (fluorescent substrate)
BCR: B cell receptor
bFGF: basic fibroblast growth factor
BLI: bioluminescence imaging
BM: bone marrow
BMP: bone morphogenetic protein
BMSC: bone marrow-derived stem cells
BrdU: 5′- bromo-2′-deoxyuridine
CDK: cyclin-dependent kinase
CII: Mitochondrial complex II
CAF: cancer (carcinoma)-associated fibroblasts
cAMP: cyclic adenosine monophosphate
CCC: cancer cache cell
CCL5: chemokine (C-C motif) ligand 5
CD: co-diffusing (surface markers)
CD::UPRT: cytosine deaminase::uracil phosphoribosyltransferase (a suicide gene)
Cdc: cyclin dependent kinase
CD_y-AT-MSC: cytosine deaminase expressing AT-MSCs
CGH: comparative genomic hybridization
CGNP: cerebellar granule neuron precursors
CIC: cancer initiating cell (aka TIC, CSC)
CK: cytokeratin

CK1: casein kinase 1
CLP: common lymphoid progenitor
CML: chronic myeloid leukemia
CMP: common myeloid progenitor
CNS: central nervous system
CoA: nuclear co-activator proteins
CoR: nuclear co-repressor proteins
CRT: chemoradiotherapy
CSC: cancer stem cell (aka cancer-maintaining cell, CIC, TIC)
CTAC: cancer transit amplifying cell
CTL: cytotoxic T lymphocyte
DDR: DNA damage response
DHT: 5a- dihydrotestosterone
DKK: Dikkopf (a secreted Wnt antagonist)
DNA: deoxyribonucleic acid
DSH or DVL (also DSH/DVL): Dishevelled phosphoprotein
ECM: extracellular matrix
EGF: epidermal growth factor
EGFR: epidermal growth factor receptor
ELP: early lymphocyte progenitor
EMT: epithelial to mesenchymal transformation
EPC: endothelial progenitor cells
ER: estrogen receptor
ESC: embryonic stem cell
ESCC: embryonic stem cells cell cycle
ET: endothelium
ETS factor: epithelium-specific transcription factor
FACS: fluorescence-activated cell sorting
FFPE: formalin-fixed paraffin embedded (specimen)
FGF: fibroblast growth factor
FLT: fetal liver tyrosine kinase
FLT3: FMS-like tyrosine kinase 3 (
FRP (also sFRP): Frizzled related proteins (a secreted Wnt antagonist)
G_0: post-mitotic dormancy
G_1: post-mitotic gap
G_2: pre-mitotic gap
GBM: glioblastoma multiforme
GC: germinal centre
GFAP: glial fibrillary acidic protein
GFP: green fluorescent protein
GIN: genomic instability
GPCR: G-protein coupled receptor
GRNs: gene regulatory networks
GSC: germ-line stem cell (aka gonocyte)
GSEA: gene set enrichment analysis
GSIs: gamma secretase inhibitors

GSK3: glycogen syntase kinase 3
HDAC: histone deacetylase
HER2-targeting agent: Herceptin (trastuzumab)
Hh: Hedgehog
HHM humoral hypocalcaemia of malignancy
HHMI: Howard Hughes Medical Institute
HIF: hypoxia-inducible factor
HMEC: human mammary epithelial cell
HNSCC: Head and neck squamous cell carcinoma
HPC: hematopoietic progenitor cell
HPPC: hematopoietic proliferative precursor cell
HSC: hematopoietic stem cell
ICP: immortal cell progenitor
IDO: indoleamine-2,3-dioxygenase
IFN: interferon
IGF: insulin-like growth factor
IGFBP: insulin-like growth factor binding protein
IGS: invasiveness gene signature
IL: interleukin
iPSC: induced-pluripotency stem cell
JNK: Wnt/ jun N-terminal kinase or Wnt/calcium pathway
KLK: kallikerin-related peptidase
LCC: large cell carcinoma
LCM: laser capture microdissection
LH: luteinizing hormone
LH-RH: luteinizing hormone releasing hormone;
LMPP: lymphoid-primed multipotent progenitor
LRC: label-retaining cell
LRP: lung resistance-related protein
LRP: low density lipoprotein receptor related protein
LSC: leukemic stem cell
M: mitosis (ordinarily referring to chromosomal events accompanying cell division)
Mac: macrophage antigen
malESC: malignant embryonic stem cell
malHSC: malignant hematopoietic stem cell
MAPC: multipotent adult progenitor cell
MELK: maternal embryonic leucine zipper kinase
MGMT: O^6-methylguanine-DNAmethyltransferase
MIM: mitochondrial inner membrane
miRNA: micro-ribonucleic acid
MitoVES: mitochondrially targeted vitamin E succinate
MM: multiple myeloma
MMP: matrix metalloproteinase
MP: main population (as opposed to side population [SP])
MPP: multipotent progenitor
mRNA: messenger RNA

MRP: multiple resistance-associated proteins
MSC: marrow stromal cell or mesenchymal stem cell
MSC: multipotent stromal stem cell
MV: mosaic vessels
NF-κB: Nuclear factor of kB
NICD: Notch intracellular domain
NK: natural killer cell
NKT: natural killer T-cell
NLS: nuclear localization sequence
NMSC: normal mammary stem cells
NOD/SCID: non-obese diabetic/severe combined immunodeficiency
NSCLC: non-small cell lung cancer (carcinoma)
oncomiR: oncogenic miRNA
OSC: organ stem cell (aka somatic/adult stem cell)
PAP: prostate acid phosphotase
PDEF: prostate-derived epithelium-specific transcription factor
PDGF: platelet-derived growth factor
PI: propidium iodide
PI3K: phosphoinositide 3-kinase
PIG: placental growth factor
PINS: Partner of Inscuteable (a cortical cell polarity determinant)
PLK: fetal liver tyrosine kinase
PMA: phorbol 12-myristate 13-acetate
primiRNA: primary-miRNA
PSA: prostate specific antigen
PSC: prostate stem cell
PTEN: Phosphatase and tensin homolog
PTH: parathyroid hormone
PTHrP: parathyroid hormone-related protein
PTL: parthenolide
RARE: retinoic acid response element
RDGN: retinal determination gene network
RNA: ribonucleic acid
RNAi: RNA interference
ROS: reactive oxygen species
RTK: receptor tyrosine kinase
RT-PCR: real-time reverse transcription- polymerase chain reaction
S: period of DNA synthesis or replication in the cell cycle
SAA: serum amyloid A
SC: stem cell
SCF: stem cell factor
SCID: severe combined immunodeficiency
SCLC: small cell lung carcinoma
SCP: senescent cell progenitor
SDF: stromal derived factor
SHh (also Shh): Sonic Hedgehog

siRNA: small interfering RNA
SP: side population (as opposed to main population [MP])
SQC: squamous cell carcinoma
SSEA: Stage Specific Embryonic Antigen
T: testosterone
TAC: transition amplifying cell
TCF/LEF: T cell factor/ lymphoid enhancer factor
TF: transferrin protein
TFR: transferrin protein receptor
TGF-β: transforming growth factor beta
TIC: tumor initiator cell (aka CIC, CSC)
TNF-α: tumor necrosis factor alpha
α-TOS: α-tocopheryl succinate
TPP+: positively charged triphenylphosphonium
TRBP: transactivating response RNA binding protein
TSA: trichostatin
TSmiR: tumor suppressor miRNA
TSC: tumor stem cell (aka CSC)
TTF: Thyroid transcription factor
TVPC: Tumor vasculogenic stem/progenitor cell
UCLA: University of California, Los Angeles
UTR: untraslated region (of mRNA)
VEGF: vascular endothelial growth factor
VEGFR: vascular endothelial growth factor receptor
VSEL-SC: very small embryonic-like stem cell
VM: vasculogenic mimicry